SPIRAL CT

Principles, Techniques,
and
Clinical Applications

Second Edition

SPIRAL CT

Principles, Techniques, and Clinical Applications

Second Edition

Editors

Elliot K. Fishman, M.D.
Professor
Departments of Radiology and Oncology
The Johns Hopkins University School of Medicine
Baltimore, Maryland

R. Brooke Jeffrey, Jr., M.D.
Professor
Department of Radiology
Stanford University School of Medicine
Stanford, California

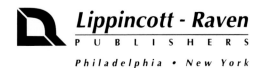

Lippincott - Raven PUBLISHERS

Philadelphia • New York

Acquisitions Editor: James Ryan
Developmental Editor: Brian Brown
Manufacturing Manager: Dennis Teston
Production Manager: Jodi Borgenicht
Production Editor: Karen Edmonson
Cover Designer: Diana Andrews
Indexer: Gerry Lynn Messner
Compositor: Maryland Composition, Inc.
Printer: Courier Westford

Printed in the United States of America

9 8 7 6 5 4 3 2 1

Library of Congress Cataloging-in-Publication Data

Spiral CT : principles, techniques, and clinical applications /
    editors, Elliot K. Fishman, R. Brooke Jeffrey, Jr. — 2nd ed.
        p.   cm.
    Includes bibliographical references and index.
    ISBN 0-7817-1251-3
    1. Spiral computed tomography.   I. Fishman, Elliot K.
II. Jeffrey, R. Brooke.
    [DNLM: 1. Tomography, X-Ray Computed—methods.   2. Tomography
Scanners, X-Ray Computed. WN 206 S759 1998]
RC78.7.T6S65 1998
616.07′572--dc21
DNLM/DLC
for Library of Congress

Care has been taken to confirm the accuracy of the information presented and to describe generally accepted practices. However, the authors, editors, and publishers are not responsible for errors or omissions or for any consequences from application of the information in this book and make no warranty, express or implied, with respect to the contents of the publication.

The authors, editors, and publisher have exerted every effort to ensure that drug selection and dosage set forth in this text are in accordance with current recommendations and practice at the time of publication. However, in view of ongoing research, changes in government regulations, and the constant flow of information relating to drug therapy and drug reactions, the reader is urged to check the package insert for each drug for any change in indications and dosage and for added warnings and precautions. This is particularly important when the recommended agent is a new or infrequently employed drug.

Some drugs and medical devices presented in this publication have Food and Drug Administration (FDA) clearance for limited use in restricted research settings. It is the responsibility of the health care provider to ascertain the FDA status of each drug or device planned for use in their clinical practice.

To Whitney, Torrey, and Lori.

E.K.F.

To Stefanie, Catherine, Luke, and Elizabeth.

R.B.J.

Contents

Contributing Authors

Christopher F. Beaulieu, M.D., Ph.D. *Department of Radiology, Stanford University School of Medicine, 300 Pasteur Drive, Room S056, Stanford, California 94305-5105*

David A. Bluemke, M.D., Ph.D. *Assistant Professor of Radiology, Department of Radiology, The Johns Hopkins University School of Medicine, 600 North Wolfe Street, Baltimore, Maryland 21287*

Elliot K. Fishman, M.D., F.A.C.R. *Professor, Departments of Radiology and Oncology, The Johns Hopkins University School of Medicine, 600 North Wolfe Street, Baltimore, Maryland 21287*

Karen M. Horton, M.D. *Instructor, Department of Radiology, The Johns Hopkins University School of Medicine, 600 North Wolfe Street, Baltimore, Maryland 21287*

R. Brooke Jeffrey, Jr., M.D. *Professor, Department of Radiology, Stanford University School of Medicine, 300 Pasteur Drive, Room H-1307, Stanford, California 94305-5105*

Janet E. Kuhlman, M.D. *Professor of Radiology and Chief of Thoracic Imaging, Department of Radiology, University of Wisconsin Hospital and Clinics, D41346 Clinical Science Center, 600 Highland Avenue, Madison, Wisconsin 53792-3252*

Michael P. Marks, M.D. *Assistant Professor, Departments of Radiology and Neurosurgery, Director of Neuroradiology, Stanford Stroke Center, Stanford University Medical Center, 300 Pasteur Drive, Stanford, California 94305-5105*

Sandy A. Napel, B.S.E.E., M.S.E.E., Ph.D. *Associate Professor of Radiology, Associate Professor of Electrical Engineering and Medicine (Medical Informatics) by courtesy, Stanford University School of Medicine, 1201 Welch Road, Room P-268, Stanford, California 94305-5488*

Anwar R. Padhani, M.R.C.P., F.R.C.R. *Senior Lecturer in Radiology, Department of Diagnostic Radiology, The Royal Marsden NHS Trust, Downs Road, Sutton, Surrey, SM1 5PT, United Kingdom*

Geoffrey D. Rubin, M.D. *Assistant Professor of Radiology, Department of Radiology, S-027B, Stanford University School of Medicine, 300 Pasteur Drive, Stanford, California 94305-5105*

Paul M. Silverman, M.D. *Professor of Radiology and Medical Oncology, Department of Radiology, Division of Abdominal Imaging, Georgetown University Medical Center, 3800 Reservoir Road, N.W., Washington, DC 20007*

George A. Taylor, M.D. *Professor of Radiology (Pediatrics), Department of Radiology, Harvard Medical School, Children's Hospital, 300 Longwood Avenue, Boston, Massachusetts 02115*

Bruce A. Urban, M.D. *Assistant Professor of Radiology, Department of Radiology, The Johns Hopkins University School of Medicine, 600 North Wolfe Street, Baltimore, Maryland 21287*

Foreword

Ring Out the Old, Ring in the New

Spiral CT, described in our foreword to the First Edition as a seminal development, has rapidly matured to become a standard technology. In 1998 we are presented with engineering advances and x-ray tubes of greater heat capacity to yield shorter examination times with comparable image quality. Spiral CT has emerged as the current state-of-the art for the routine CT examination.

Although only three years have elapsed, a Second Edition of this text was mandated and expanded to deal with the wealth of additional clinical experience. The book has been totally updated, revised, to 21 chapters. There are new chapters on subsecond scanning, perspective rendering, examination of the esophagus and stomach, and dual phase spiral CT of the liver.

With the exception of a single chapter from Dr. Silverman, all of the authors are either current faculty from the Stanford University School of Medicine, and current or former faculty from the Johns Hopkins University Medical Center. The authors have distilled the essentials of the very extensive clinical experience with spiral CT at these facilities.

Spiral CT: Principles, Techniques, and Clinical Applications is a primer for physicians making the transition from standard to spiral CT studies. The differences in the proper administration of contrast media, the usual patterns of enhancement of the vasculature and viscera, and the sequencing of images make this book required reading. There is no doubt that spiral CT is here to stay for a number of years. Those who master the contents of this book will be well prepared to practice first rate CT imaging at the beginning of the next century.

Stanley S. Siegelman, M.D.
The Johns Hopkins University School of Medicine
Baltimore, Maryland

Preface to First Edition

Computed tomography (CT) evolved from a study requiring 1 to 2 minute scan times per slice, 1 to 5 minute reconstruction times per slice, and limited resolution in the late 1970s to 1 second scan times, instantaneous reconstruction, and .35 mm resolution in the late 1980s. However, despite the advances, CT was still limited by the speed of data acquisition that typically ranged from 8 to 12 scans per minute on the best of systems. Acquiring sets of data in a manner needed to optimize lesion detection was difficult, as best exemplified by the countless articles describing a new strategy for evaluating the liver to optimize lesion detection. Similarly, data acquisition was done at a fixed phase of respiration (typically suspended inspiration) and assumed identical respiratory efforts for anywhere between 30 and 60 breathholds. Inability by patients to perform this ''Herculean'' task often resulted in the missing of lesions (false negative study) in the lung and/or liver due to gaps in the scanning volume.

In 1990, many of the long-standing problems with standard dynamic CT were overcome with the introduction of spiral CT scanning as a commercial product. To generate true volume datasets with CT, spiral CT combined the goal of a volume acquisition in a single breathhold. Although the initial spiral CT scan parameters included only 12 second volumes, 110 mAs, and poor slice profiles, there has been a rapid evolution of the technology to the current state-of-the art, which includes 30 to 40 second spiral acquisitions, 250 to 300 mAs, and slice profiles nearly identical to standard CT scan slices. In fact, it is nearly as hard to write an article describing the technical state of spiral CT as it is to draw a picture of a moving object because spiral CT is constantly changing. The recent introduction of back-to-back spirals acquisitions, higher mAs values, and a range of three-dimensional protocols with an emphasis on vascular imaging are a few of the changes we are continuing to see in this exciting and rapidly changing field.

Writing a textbook on such a rapidly changing field is daunting. Techniques used became obsolete as a chapter was being written. Despite this difficulty, we present a book by many of the experts who are driving spiral CT into the future. The book can be used as a companion text to optimize scanning protocols as well as to understand the specific advantages of spiral CT compared with standard CT in the head and body. Exciting new applications of spiral CT including vascular 3D imaging are all discussed in detail. Commonplace clinical applications, such as evaluation of the liver, pancreas, and kidneys, are all addressed with the specific advantages of spiral CT defined.

Elliot K. Fishman, M.D.
R. Brooke Jeffrey, Jr., M.D.

Preface

After reading the preface to the First Edition of this book we were struck by how much change had occurred in a span of only three years. Many of our predictions for the evolution of spiral CT have not only been met, but exceeded. We anxiously await the future advances in spiral CT scanning, including multi-detector scanners and scan times less than .5 seconds. Once again, technical advances will drive the clinical advances in areas including vascular imaging, virtual reality, and oncology. We hope that the information provided in this book will help the reader in his/her daily practice, as well as stimulate the search for new opportunities for this exciting technology.

Elliot K. Fishman, M.D.
R. Brooke Jeffrey, Jr., M.D.

Acknowledgments

We thank everyone who so generously contributed their time and material to this book, especially the staff, fellows, residents, and technologists at The Johns Hopkins Hospital and Stanford University Medical Center. A special thanks to Adeline Alonso, who coordinated the manuscript flow and expedited the completion of this book. This book is truly a cross-country endeavor and would not have been possible without the encouragement of our families, who are always our first priorities. Finally, we would be remiss if we did not thank Mary Rogers and the staff at Lippincott-Raven Publishers for their effort in bringing this book to print in a prompt and quality manner. We would especially like to thank James Ryan and Brian Brown at Lippincott-Raven Publishers for their help in making this book a reality.

PART 1

Basic Principles

CHAPTER 1

Basic Principles of Spiral CT

Sandy Napel

Computed tomography (CT) has evolved continuously since its introduction to medical imaging in the early 1970s. Over the years, all major aspects (e.g., spatial resolution, low-contrast detectability, and acquisition speed) have improved, through changes both to hardware and to software. The latest stage in the development of CT has come with the introduction of CT scanners where patient translation and data acquisition occur simultaneously through the use of a continuously rotating gantry and a high-heat-capacity x-ray tube. Two terms arose to describe this technology: *spiral* and *helical* CT. Initially, there was some controversy as to which was the more correct and/or precise term, and individual vendors took different stands on the issue. In 1994, Kalender's eloquent letter to the editor of *Radiology,* and the editor's reply, ended the controversy; thereafter both terms were equally acceptable (1). For the sake of consistency, we shall refer to this methodology for CT scanning as *spiral CT.*

This chapter describes several important technical aspects and implications of spiral CT. To set the stage, the chapter begins with an overview of the evolution of CT, from its beginnings up to the advent of spiral CT. (The reader is referred to ref. 2 for an in-depth treatment.) Next, the basic principles of spiral CT are covered, including scanner designs and techniques for reconstruction of spirally acquired image data. The chapter concludes with a discussion of spiral CT image quality issues such as longitudinal spatial resolution, noise, and artifacts.

THE EVOLUTION OF COMPUTED TOMOGRAPHY

The impact of CT on the practice of diagnostic imaging was so profound that CT's inventors, Godsfrey Hounsfield and Alan Cormack, were awarded the Nobel Prize in 1979. Computed tomography derives its superb contrast resolution by dividing up the measurement of the x-ray attenuation due to a thin (1–10 mm) section along hundreds of thousands of precisely defined directions and using these measurements to reconstruct a cross-sectional image. The sequential acquisition and reconstruction of multiple parallel sections comprised the first truly three-dimensional (3D) medical imaging modality.

Since its introduction in the early 1970s, CT has progressed through several generations of scanner design (2). First-generation scanners employed a single x-ray detector. The x-ray source and detector simultaneously translated along parallel lines on opposite sides of the patient as measurements were gathered along lines that passed through the patient perpendicular to the direction of translation. After a given projection was acquired in this manner, the entire apparatus was rotated by a fraction of a degree and the measurements were repeated until 180 degrees of projection data were acquired. These scanners were characterized by an acquisition time that lasted several minutes and thus initial applications were limited to parts of the body whose motion could be restrained, the major applications being in the head. Second-generation scanners added multiple detectors so that several projections could be acquired simultaneously, thereby reducing acquisition time. However, third-generation scanners, with a continuously rotating fan beam consisting of an x-ray tube and an opposing arc of several hundred detectors, made CT truly practical by reducing scanning time to several seconds per section. After this development, thousands of CT scanners were installed in hospitals around the world, with applications ranging from the lower extremities through the pelvis, abdomen, chest, neck, and head. A fourth-generation design, in which the detectors remained fixed in space and the only moving part was the x-ray source, was also introduced, but no advantages were ever proven in practice and its installed customer base remained small.

Exposures on the order of seconds are still long compared with some physiological motions, and so fifth-generation scanners, which have no moving parts, were developed and introduced (3,4). Electron beam scanners (4), the only fifth-generation technology in production, create a moving focus of x-rays by sweeping an electron beam along a tungsten target arranged in a ring surrounding the patient. Fixed detectors opposite the target ring record the transmitted radiation, and a single section can be acquired in 50–100 ms. Thus cardiac pulsations can be time-resolved within a single section, with artifact and blurring from respiratory and peristaltic motion nearly (if not completely) eliminated.

Even though electron beam scanners have temporal resolution on the order of fractions of a second per section, the time required to reposition to an adjacent section is no better than that required with conventional CT. That is, volume acquisitions are limited in speed not by the number of projections acquired per second, but by the time wasted between section acquisitions. This "dead time" is caused in part by the need to accelerate, translate, and decelerate the patient and in part by the need to cool the x-ray tube. For example, a very popular conventional scanner in the late 1980s had a "quick" mode in which a 16-s interscan delay occurred between 2-s section acquisitions. If we define the duty factor D as

$$D = \frac{\text{section acquisition time}}{(\text{section acquisition time} + \text{interscan delay})},$$

(1)

this scanner, though quick for its time, had a duty factor of only 11%.

In an effort to improve this, most scanners of this era permitted a "dynamic mode" of scanning, wherein a "group" of consecutive scans (e.g., three) with minimal interscan delay between them (e.g., 3 s) was performed during a breath-holding interval. Following this, the patient was allowed to breathe for 6–8 s before another group was acquired. Using this dynamic paradigm, an average interscan delay of 6–8 s could be achieved, resulting in a duty factor improvement to $D = 20\%$ to 25%.

Spiral CT scanners employ slip-ring technology to acquire data continuously as the patient is translated through the gantry (5–7). With the patient translating inside the rotating gantry, the path of the x-ray source describes a spiral, or helix, with its focus along a line passing through the rotational isocenter perpendicular to the plane of rotation. Because there are no interscan delays, $D = 100\%$, and the rate of coverage along this line is equal to the table speed. Thus in the same amount of time, spiral scanners can acquire a volume of CT data four to nine times larger than the conventional scanner of the 1980s described earlier. For example, a 30-s spiral scan with the patient table moving at 5 cm/s allows for the coverage of a 15-cm volume of patient anatomy. In contrast, the 1.67–3.75 cm that could be acquired during the same amount of time by the 1980s scanner can hardly be called a volume at all. (It should also be noted that electron beam scanners achieve similar gains by translating the patient table during scanning. This "continuous volume" mode of scanning has recently been demonstrated, but few clinical results are available at this time.)

The increased rate of coverage along the long axis of the patient has led to a virtual renaissance of CT, improving its capabilities in existing applications and creating new ones. As an example of an existing application that has been improved by spiral CT, consider CT in the chest. An increase in the number of sections that may be acquired per breath-hold greatly reduces the incidence of missed or doubly scanned anatomy due to respiratory misregistration (8–10) and reduces the volume of iodinated contrast required for lesion detection (11). A new application that has rapidly gained acceptance is CT angiography (see Chapters 19–21), in which the first pass of a bolus of iodinated contrast is captured in transit through a volume of target vasculature (12–23). More recently, advances in computer graphics, combined with spiral CT's high resolution and rapid data acquisition, have resulted in "virtual endoscopy" (24–29) applications (see Chapter 3), such as virtual colonoscopy (30,31), virtual bronchoscopy (32,33), and virtual cystoscopy (34), appearing in the literature. The new applications and improvements to existing ones have been made possible by conceptually simple extensions to scanner design. However, it is important to understand the principles of spiral CT both to appreciate the new capabilities it affords and to be aware of its limitations.

TECHNICAL ASPECTS

This section begins with a description of a typical spiral CT scanner design. This leads to a discussion of the implications of this design, including acquired volume size, image reconstruction techniques, artifacts, and temporal and spatial resolution.

Spiral CT Hardware

At first glance, spiral CT scanners look quite similar to conventional scanners. However, several of the major components have been completely redesigned for spiral CT. Figure 1-1 shows a basic block diagram of a spiral CT scanner. A discussion of the portions of the design that are unique or especially important for the case of spiral CT acquisitions follows.

Rotating Gantry

Third-generation scanners have both the x-ray tube and the detectors mounted on a rotating gantry. Fourth-generation designs are simpler in that only the x-ray tube rotates; the detectors are fixed. In each case, however, no more than two complete rotations are possible before the gantry is required to reverse its direction. This constraint is due to the fact that electrical cables are used to supply power to the x-ray tube, collect data from the detectors, and power other moving parts such as filters and collimators. (A major part of the mechanical design of these scanners is the cable wind/unwind mechanism.) However, spiral CT requires a continuously rotating gantry, and so mechanisms that do not require

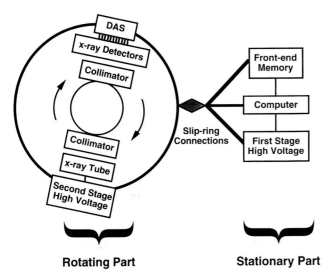

Rotating Part   **Stationary Part**

FIG. 1-1. Spiral CT system block diagram. The continuously rotating gantry communicates with the stationary components via multiple parallel slip-rings (i.e., brushes and contactors). Current implementations limit the minimum gantry rotational period to 0.75 s, though not all vendors yet offer this capability and limit the speed to one rotation per second. In the design illustrated, the high-voltage generator is split into two parts, with the second and final stage on the rotating gantry. The data acquisition system (DAS) digitizes detector signals and transmits these data across the slip rings to the front-end memory. Signals that originate at the computer also cross the slip-ring connections to direct the collimator adjustment motors.

the use of cables must be in place to get the appropriate power and signals on to and off of it. Spiral CT scanners accomplish this by means of a "slip-ring" design. Typically, multiple electrically conductive brushes on the stationary part contact a set of parallel conductive rings on the rotating part (or vice versa).

High-Voltage Power Supply

The most straightforward approach to delivering high voltage to the rotating x-ray tube is to pass it directly across one of the slip-rings. However, because CT x-ray tubes operate in the 80–140-kV range, there is a high probability of arcing between the brushes and the rings of the continuously rotating gantry. Thus a special high-voltage insulator must surround the slip-ring in order to guard against arcing. Other designs split the power supply into two parts. The first stage, which steps up the voltage to an intermediate alternating current (AC) value, is stationary, and the final stage, which further steps up and rectifies the voltage to its final direct current (DC) potential, is mounted on the rotating gantry. In other designs, low-voltage DC is passed across the slip-ring and converted to high-voltage DC by a high-frequency generator mounted on the gantry. In both cases, only a low to intermediate voltage has to cross the brush/slip-ring contact, thus reducing the chances of arcing. However, positioning

part or all of an x-ray generator on the gantry adds considerable weight and imposes a requirement for increased cooling in the room that houses the gantry.

X-ray Tube

Conventional CT scanners use the interscan delays for tube cooling. A spiral CT scan, however, may require that the tube be turned on for up to 60 s without a pause for cooling. (Technique factors for a typical spiral scan sequence with a 1-s gantry rotation might be 120 kV at 300 mA for 60 s, or more than 2 million J.) Initial implementations of spiral CT accommodated this by requiring that the beam current be reduced considerably for a spiral scanning sequence (e.g., 165 mA for a 40-s scan) and that very long cooling periods followed all spiral sequences. However, the increased noise in these low-milliampere scans was limiting, particularly in obese patients. The maximum current allowed for a particular scan is a function not only of the desired scan time, but also of the current tube temperature; thus greater tube current is available for the first scan of the day than after several spiral examinations. Improved designs have resulted in higher available dose, but the tube current available at any given time is still less than would be used for a nonspiral scanning sequence, and up to 20% of all spiral scans may still suffer from higher noise than desirable. Therefore x-ray tubes with high-energy dissipation ratings and detectors with high capture and geometric efficiency are especially important for spiral CT. Further improvements in tube design are expected to close the gap completely and reduce the requirement for long interspiral cooling delays.

Front-End Memory

Heat is not the only thing that must be removed between acquisitions. Given that approximately 1,000 x-ray detectors must be sampled approximately 1,000 times per rotation and that each sample requires 16 bits of computer storage, projection data may accumulate at a rate of 2 MB/s. For a 60-s scan, 120 MB of computer memory must be written at this high rate. Thus the development of fast and inexpensive solid-state and magnetic disk computer memory was an important factor that helped make spiral CT possible.

Spiral Scanning

Implementation of the preceding improvements permits a 100% duty factor over a long period of time. Combining this capability with simultaneous patient translation results in spiral CT. Figure 1-2 shows the three-dimensional geometry of spiral CT data acquisition. Patient translation in the cranial direction may be thought of as gantry translation in the caudal direction. By imagining gantry translation during scanning, it is easy to see that the x-ray source describes a spiral path that surrounds the patient.

Two parameters control the details of the spiral scanning

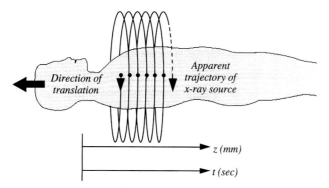

FIG. 1-2. Spiral CT data acquisition geometry. Translation of the patient in the direction shown is equivalent to translation of the scanning apparatus in the opposite direction. The apparent trajectory of the x-ray source is a spiral or helix surrounding the patient. The projection of the source as a function of time onto the scanner axis (*z-axis*) is a line segment that begins at the position from which the patient begins to move and whose end point travels at the same speed as the patient, but in the opposite direction.

geometry. The first of these is the collimator width w (mm). For conventional CT, w is the principal determinant of the width of the section sensitivity profile (SSP), and thus we would expect it to have major influence over spatial resolution in the z direction for spiral CT as well. As in conventional CT, larger w's permit greater photon flux (and therefore reduced noise and greater contrast sensitivity) for a given set of technique factors, but this occurs at the expense of loss of information regarding density distribution in the z direction. Indeed, it is well known that relatively large section thicknesses can result in partial volume errors and artifacts (35,36).

The second parameter is the patient translation speed s (mm/s). The length of coverage in the z direction is the product of the speed and the time during which the x-ray tube is energized. Faster speeds result in greater coverage. Although w and s may be chosen independently, it is convenient to define the dimensionless quantity called pitch (P) as follows:

$$P = \frac{s \text{ (mm/s)}}{w \text{ (mm)}} \times \text{gantry rotational period (s).} \quad (2)$$

(See Fig. 1-3.) Pitch can also be thought of as the number of collimator widths covered in one gantry rotation. Note that conventional CT is the trivial case of spiral CT with a pitch of zero; the exposed section through the patient is identical for all projection angles. For cranial-to-caudal scanning with $P = 0.5$, two complete rotations occur before the cranial edge of the collimator aligns with the initial location of the caudal edge of the collimator. If $P = 1.0$, this alignment occurs after a single rotation. And if $P = 2.0$, this situation is repeated after only one-half of a gantry rotation. The motion of the patient under the collimator (which can be thought of as the motion of the collimator across the patient in the

opposite direction) during scanning has two major consequences: SSP broadening and the potential for motion-related artifacts. Because the manifestations of these effects are also influenced by image reconstruction algorithms, we defer the discussion until the section entitled ''Longitudinal Spatial Resolution'' later in this chapter.

Image Reconstruction

In addition to hardware upgrades, spiral CT requires enhancements to image reconstruction software. The mathematics of image reconstruction from projections dates back to a paper published by Radon in 1917 (37). More recent treatments of the subject, particularly with respect to medical imaging applications, can be found in several textbooks (e.g., see refs. 38 and 39). A basic assumption of CT reconstruction is that the imaged object is completely stationary during the course of the scan. Motion during scanning not only creates blurring, but also may create severe artifacts that obscure even stationary parts of the image (36). In practice, the no-motion assumption is almost always violated due to voluntary (e.g., discomfort) and involuntary (e.g., cardiac, respiratory, peristaltic) patient movements, and an incredible amount of effort has been expended to reduce motion at the source (e.g., mechanical or pharmaceutical patient restraints,

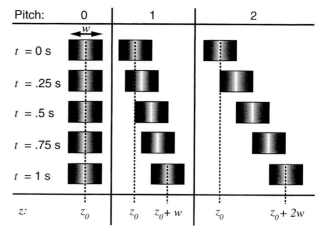

FIG. 1-3. The position of the collimator along the patient axis as a function of time for three different choices of pitch. The gantry rotational period is assumed to be 1 s and w is the collimator width; z is the position of the section center as a function of time, with z_0 its position at $t = 0$. Note that spiral CT with a pitch of zero reduces to conventional CT. A pitch of 1 implies translation of one collimator width per gantry rotation; a pitch of 2 implies translation of two collimator widths per rotation. The most consistent projection data are acquired when the pitch is zero and inconsistency (and, therefore, possibility of artifacts) increases with increasing pitch. Assuming a full 360 degrees of projection data will be used to reconstruct an image, note that the section width (and, in general, the SSP) is broadened by increased pitch. Note also the increased distance covered along the z-axis per unit time, which, in many cases, justifies the broadened SSP and possible increase in artifacts.

breath-holding), to reduce the probability of motion in each scan (e.g., faster scanners) and to develop artifact-suppressing computer algorithms that reduce the detrimental effects of motion during scanning.

Spiral CT is, then, an interesting development in that it *requires* motion during scanning. In fact, spiral CT trades some deleterious effects of motion during scanning for a large increase in coverage rate. However, the motion that spiral CT entails is relatively well behaved compared with the usual sources, because patient velocity is smooth and well known. (In fact, all current implementations of spiral CT employ constant table velocity, though Crawford [6] describes other possibilities that we will not consider here.) This fact can be used to derive reconstruction methods that minimize resulting artifacts, as described next. However, it must be noted that other motion artifacts—such as those caused by cardiac pulsations, patient breathing, and peristalsis—are not reduced by corrections for table motion during gantry rotation. The following paragraphs discuss the basic approaches that have been described in the literature. The conceptually simplest approach, mid-plane synthesis using linear interpolation and 720 degrees of projection data, is described in detail. Other approaches are described in relation to the first, with appropriate references to the literature. All these methods produce a set of projec-

tion data that can be input to a standard CT reconstruction algorithm.

The simplest approach can be best understood as a technique that attempts to synthesize from the spirally acquired projection data a set of projections that would have been obtained with the table stationary (8,40,41). It requires the generation of a complete rotation's worth (i.e., 360 degrees) of projection data and begins with the assumption that an estimate of a projection p, at table location $z = z_0$ and angle θ, can be estimated from other projections obtained at different table positions but at identical projection angles. In theory any number of projections acquired at the desired projection angle can be used for interpolation. However, in practice only the two projections that are closest to z_0 (along the z axis) are used and are combined linearly to estimate the projection at z_0 and angle θ:

$$p(z_0, \theta) = (1 - f)\, p\, (z', \theta) + fp(z + d, \theta). \quad (3)$$

Here z' refers to the table position that is closest to and less than z_0 at which a projection was acquired at the desired angle θ. Equation (3) also assumes that the table speed s equals d mm per period of the gantry rotation; thus $p(z' + d, \theta)$ is also acquired and is linearly combined with $p(z', \theta)$. Figure 1-4 illustrates this procedure graphically. The weighing fraction f is computed as follows:

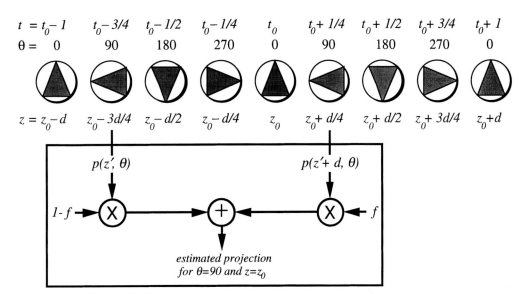

FIG. 1-4. Sequence of projection angles θ and table positions z as a function of time t for a spiral scan with a rotational period of 1 s and a table speed d mm/s. Triangular symbols indicate angular position of the rotating gantry every 1/4 s for 2 s starting at $t = t_0 - 1$. Note that the scanner acquires a unique projection angle at each table position. The linear interpolation mid-plane synthesis approach estimates projections that would have been acquired with the table stationary by interpolating between available projections using equations (3) and (4). Suppose we wish to estimate planar projection data at $z = z_0$. Only the projection $\theta = 0$ was actually acquired at this position, and so we must interpolate projection data for all the other required angles. For example, to compute the projection for $\theta = 90$, we use the nearest (along z) projections that occurred at $\theta = 90$: $z' = z_0 - 3d/4$ and $z' + d = z_0 + d/4$. Because $z_0 + d/4$ is closer (along z) to the desired table position than $z_0 - 3d/4$, equations (3) and (4) will weight the former more heavily than the latter. Interpolation of other projection angles can be envisioned by sliding the box, above, to the left or right, and adjusting the weighting fraction f according to equation (4).

$$f = \frac{(z_0 - z')}{d}; \qquad (4)$$

Thus, for example, if $z_0 = z'$ or if $z_0 = z' + d$ (i.e., the desired projection was actually acquired), then only the corresponding acquired projection is used. In between (i.e., $z' < z_0 < z' < d$), the two nearest projections at angle θ are weighted linearly and inversely proportional to their distance from z_0. (Note that for simplicity this discussion assumed that all samples of the projection [i.e., all detector readings] were acquired simultaneously. In practice, this may not be true. However, the rotation angle at which each detector is sampled is known, and so the preceding argument would hold if we were to define p as a single detector reading.)

The preceding approach, called *360-degree linear interpolation*, requires data from two complete gantry rotations (i.e., 720 degrees). This requirement has both positive and negative implications. The good news is that, independent of table speed, the increased exposure time used per reconstructed section reduces noise compared with a conventional fan-beam reconstruction using 360 degrees of projection data. However, there are three negative implications: First, it is impossible to reconstruct sections centered at table positions that are scanned during the first or last rotation. Second, because two rotation's worth of projection data are used, the temporal resolution of each reconstructed section is reduced by a factor of 2 compared with a conventional single-rotation reconstruction. Finally, and perhaps the most regrettable effect, broadening of the SSP results from the increased range of projection data used along the z-axis (81% and 325% full width at tenth maximum [FWTM]* increase for pitch 1 and pitch 2 scanning, respectively [41]).

Several techniques were quickly developed in an effort to recover some of the reduced temporal and spatial resolution. Two of these, utilization of a higher-order interpolation function and reduction of the total amount of projection data required for mid-plane synthesis, have been detailed by both Polacin (41) and Crawford (6). Polacin showed that higher-order interpolation functions for mid-plane synthesis result in minimal improvement of the SSP with a large cost in image reconstruction time. However, he proposed a method that exploited the notion that images may be reconstructed on conventional scanners using projection data acquired over only 180 degrees plus the angle subtended by the arc of x-ray detectors (the ''fan angle'') (42). The resulting 180-degree linear interpolation algorithm thereby reduced the total amount of projection data from 720 to 2 × (180 + fan angle) degrees. This in turn resulted in a considerable improvement of the SSP, at the expense of a small increase in noise, and has since replaced the two-rotation algorithm in scanners employing it.

Crawford (6) describes and compares seven reconstruction methods for spiral data acquired at constant table speed. One mid-plane synthesis approach, called *half-scan with extrapolation*, uses data from only one complete rotation to synthesize a set of projection data covering 180 degrees plus the fan angle. Thus it is similar to Polacin's approach (41) but requires less projection data per reconstructed section by twice the fan angle, and therefore would be expected to produce a narrower SSP with possibly increased noise. In addition to several other mid-plane synthesis approaches, Crawford (6) presents several methods that do not attempt to synthesize the mid-plane. Instead, these ideas arise from the realization that motion causes certain portions of the data, which should be nearly identical, to be inconsistent. One of these approaches, called *underscan*, focuses on the fact that the table motion causes a large discontinuity in the projection data at projection angles of 0 and 360 degrees. To reduce the discontinuity, data acquired near zero and 360 degrees are underweighted compared with the more centrally located projections. Crawford concludes that of all the methods he compared, half-scan with extrapolation and underscan produce the best results in terms of SSP, noise, and structured artifacts.

Longitudinal Spatial Resolution

SSP Broadening

Spatial resolution in the longitudinal direction (i.e., along the z-axis) is completely described by the SSP. Complete description of a spiral SSP requires knowledge of the collimation, table speed, and image reconstruction algorithm. In general, the spiral SSP can be described as a convolution of a *table motion function* with the zero-velocity SSP. For both 360- and 180-degree linear interpolation (see the preceding section), the table motion functions are triangle functions (5,43,44).

Given a fixed collimator setting, the SSP broadens with increasing pitch because each reconstructed image uses projection data from a region along the z-axis whose length is proportional to the table speed (44,45). Because different spiral reconstruction algorithms use different ranges of projection data along the z-axis and each weights the projection data differently, the magnitude of SSP broadening at any pitch is a function of the algorithm used. For example, using Polacin's 180-degree linear interpolation algorithm, scanning with pitch = 1.0 increases the FWTM of the SSP by 31% relative to zero pitch (i.e., conventional CT); scanning with pitch = 2.0 broadens the FWTM of the SSP by 85% relative to zero pitch (41).

The incremental impact of going from pitch 1.0 to pitch 2.0 has interesting implications. Suppose that the desired coverage and maximum desirable scan time dictate a 5-mm/s table speed, and consider the following two options: (a) 5-mm collimation, pitch 1.0, or (b) 3-mm collimation, pitch 1.7. Both achieve the same coverage rate. However, for op-

---

*Polacin (41) describes and compares several ways to parameterize the width of a SSP (e.g., full width at half maximum [FWHM], full width at tenth maximum [FWTM], and full width at tenth area [FWTA]). We use FWTM here because it emphasizes contributions from the ''tails'' of the SSP.

tion a the FWTM of the SSP is 6.6 mm and for option (b) the FWTM of the SSP is equal to 5.0 mm (assuming 65% broadening at pitch = 1.7). Thus the second option results in less partial volume and therefore higher longitudinal resolution. The narrower collimator, of course, results in increased image noise and therefore reduced low-contrast detectability for option b. This tradeoff tends to be beneficial in cases where the inherent contrast is high, such as CT angiography or thoracic CT (46–48) but might not be the proper choice in larger patients and/or when exploring for low-contrast lesions (49).

The following are some final notes about the SSP for spiral CT: The measurement of SSPs in spiral CT requires more care than for conventional CT. The use of the usual ramp phantom results in an erroneous slice profile that varies with longitudinal position; accurate SSPs are, however, obtainable with a precisely aligned thin-sheet phantom, which simulates an impulse function in the longitudinal direction (50). Further, just as with conventional CT, the SSP may not be uniform across the transaxial section because of the finite dimension of the source and detector, and any nonidealities of collimation (51). In spiral CT, even ideal conditions can result in variation of the SSP as a function of in-plane position (52,53). The magnitude and spatial distribution of this variation are functions of the interpolation algorithm used. Recent work has focused on more general reconstruction methods that attempt to reduce spatial variations in SSP and noise (53) (see the following section entitled "Image Noise"), but implementations in clinical scanners are not yet available.

Arbitrary Choice of Section Location and Spacing

A major advantage of spiral over conventional CT is that the center of the reconstructed section can be retrospectively and arbitrarily placed along the z-axis. In addition, reconstructed sections may have a very high degree of overlap. These capabilities may be used to reduce through-plane partial volume effects, thereby improving small lesion conspicuity, and to create off-axis and/or 3D reconstructions with reduced "stair-step" artifact. These two implications are described next.

Consider a lesion whose extent along the z-axis is on the order of the width of the SSP. Because conventional CT reconstructions occur at fixed intervals from the location of the first acquired section, it is quite possible that the lesion will be only partially covered by the reconstruction of a given section. (See Fig. 1-5.) For example, one-half of the lesion may be covered by section k and the other half by section k + 1. Thus the total attenuation experienced by rays that pass through a voxel that includes the lesion will, owing to the partial volume effect, be somewhere in between the attenuation caused by the lesion and that caused by the surrounding tissue (35). Now suppose it is possible to position the section at position k′ as shown by the dotted lines. In this case, the attenuation of rays passing through the voxel

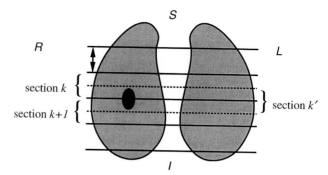

FIG. 1-5. Illustration of intensity loss due to through-plane partial volume effect. Consider a relatively high-density lesion (*black ellipse*) surrounded by low-density soft tissue. The full width at half maximum of the SSP is given by the separation between solid lines. The lesion is only partly imaged by sections k and k + 1; thus its intensity will be decreased due to volume averaging with the surrounding soft tissue. However, section k′, which can be positioned and reconstructed from the acquired spiral projection data, images the lesion with less volume averaging from above and below and, therefore, with greater intensity.

will be caused only by the lesion itself. Therefore if the lesion is a high-density one surrounded by lower-density soft tissue, section k′ will depict it with greater contrast compared with section k or k + 1. Thus improved lesion detectability results from the capability of spiral CT to center the position of the reconstructed section at an arbitrary location. This can be accomplished by retrospectively adjusting the section center or by reconstructing overlapping sections to increase the likelihood of optimal lesion centering in one or more sections.

The capability for production of overlapping sections (absent from conventional CT without overlapping exposures and therefore increased patient dose) also results in smoother 3D renderings and/or off-axis (i.e., sagittal, coronal, or oblique) reformatted images. For example, consider Fig. 1-6, which illustrates two maximum-intensity projections (MIP; see Chapter 19) of a rod lying in the coronal plane passing through a spirally acquired volume at a 45-degree angle with respect to the z-axis. Figure 1-6A shows a coronal MIP of images reconstructed with section spacing equal to the collimation. Thus the sequence of reconstructed sections depicts elliptical cross-sections of the rod with a 10-pixel shift of its center from section to section. In this case, the ratio of section spacing to in-plane pixel spacing was b/a = 10. Thus for every line in the MIP image that passes through the center of an acquired section, there are nine lines that must be interpolated between sections. This interpolation stage generates the familiar stair-step artifact. Alternatively, reconstruction of the spiral CT data every 1 mm along the z-axis generates a sequence of elliptical cross-sections with centers shifted from section to section by only two pixels. Since in this case b/a = 2, only interpolation of alternate lines is required. This results in an image that is much more representative of the continuous object (see Fig. 1-6B). This

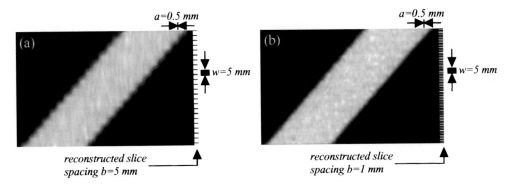

FIG. 1-6. Maximum-intensity projections of spiral CT images of a rod in the coronal plane at 45 degrees to the longitudinal axis. The in-plane pixel size *a* was 0.5 mm, the collimator width *w* was 5 mm, and the table speed *s* was 5 mm/s. **(A)** Reconstructed slice spacing, *b*, was 5 mm (one image per gantry rotation). **(B)** Reconstructed slice spacing *b* was 1 mm (five images per gantry rotation). Note: residual stair-step artifacts are due to spiral interpolation algorithms; see the section on artifacts and Fig. 1-9.

improvement is similarly enjoyed by other 3D renderings, such as shaded-surface displays, as well as coronal, sagittal, and oblique reformations. Of course, reconstruction of five sections for each gantry rotation increases image reconstruction time fivefold. However, the resulting image quality is a function of the ratio *b/a*, and therefore intermediate improvements may be expected for intermediate ratios. The improvement in image quality is also a function of the object being imaged. For example, a coronal MIP of a rod parallel to the *z*-axis would be unchanged by the reconstruction of overlapping sections. However, patient scans are never so uncomplicated; there are always structures passing through the acquired sections at oblique angles whose depiction benefits from overlapping reconstructions. Note that although this technique minimizes the major cause of stair-step artifacts, some spiral reconstruction algorithms can cause a similar artifact; we defer this discussion until the section entitled "Artifacts."

Maximizing Longitudinal Spatial Resolution

We have seen earlier that the possibility afforded by spiral CT for increased spatial sampling along the *z*-axis without increasing patient dose reduces the partial volume effect and permits improved low-contrast detectability. But without a priori knowledge of where the lesions are located, how are we to choose section locations to maximize their contrast? One possibility is to prospectively reconstruct many images with a high degree of overlap between pairs. Indeed, two theoretical studies by Wang (43,44) and one experimental study by Kalender (54) conclude that longitudinal spatial resolution improves as the number of slices reconstructed per gantry rotation increases. For the 180-degree linear interpolation reconstruction algorithm and pitch = 1, the theoretical maximum is approached when one reconstructs three to five slices per collimation width; at pitch = 2, the maximum is approached when one reconstructs two or three scans per collimation width. Perhaps a more surprising conclusion

is that if this recommendation is followed, spiral CT provides better longitudinal resolution than conventional CT with equivalent collimation and equal patient dose. Note that to achieve this requires multiplying the number of reconstructed sections per exam by 4 or 5 which, in turn, greatly increases reconstruction time and the number of images to be interpreted and stored.

In-plane Spatial Resolution

Spatial resolution in CT is related to several design parameters, including focal spot size, detector aperture, and collimator width (51). In-plane resolution is defined as a function of the first two of these, and through-plane resolution is primarily a function of the third. Initial descriptions of spiral CT asserted that the in-plane spatial resolution of spiral CT was identical to that of conventional CT on the same scanner. Although this is of course true, measurements of spatial resolution are done using phantoms whose geometry is constant along the *z*-axis. Structures that do change size or position along the *z*-axis suffer increased blurring as a function of increasing section width (Fig. 1-7). Thus spiral CT may cause a decrease in perceived in-plane spatial resolution for structures that do change size or position along the *z*-axis of the scanner dependent on the imaged anatomy and the degree of SSP broadening. SSP broadening may also result in certain structures appearing elongated in the cranial-to-caudal direction (5).

In the previous sections, we have seen that the ability to center sections arbitrarily and/or reconstruct overlapping sections can result in improved small-lesion visibility, 3D renderings, and off-axis reformatted images. Most vendors, however, delete the raw projection data sometime after the scans are acquired. Thus today it is important to view the reconstructed images as soon as possible in order to retain this flexibility afforded by spiral CT. In the future, the whole concept of what constitutes an examination archive will need to be rethought; perhaps when image reconstruction is fast

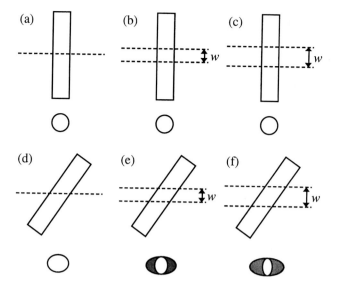

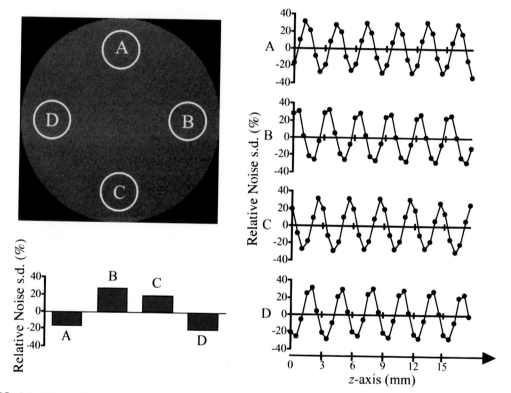

FIG. 1-7. Illustration of perceived loss of in-plane spatial resolution with increasing section thickness. Each subfigure shows a coronal view of a cylinder (*solid line*) and a measure of the section thickness *w* for the axial view below (*ellipse*). **(A)** Cylinder is perfectly aligned perpendicular to an infinitely thin-section plane. Axial image is a sharply defined circle. **(B,C)** Axial image is unchanged when scanned with thicker sections. **(D)** Cylinder is inclined with respect to the section plane. For the infinitely thin-section plane, the axial image is a sharply defined ellipse. **(E,F)** As the section becomes thicker, the edges of the ellipse are less sharply resolved due to partial volume. The result is that the ellipse appears less sharp with increasing section thickness. Note: The transition from **(E)** to **(F)** occurs when for any reason the SSP broadens (e.g., increase in collimator width [conventional or spiral CT] or same collimator width with increase in table speed [spiral CT]). Thus **(E)** could be taken to be conventional CT (pitch = 0.0) and **(F)** spiral CT with pitch = 1.0 and the same collimation as **(E)**.

FIG. 1-8. Nonuniform noise in spiral CT. The image (top left) shows a reconstructed cross-section from a spiral CT scan of a 480 mm diameter uniform calibration phantom. Scan parameters were 1 s gantry rotation, 3-mm collimation, 3-mm/s table speed (pitch = 1), 100 kV, 350 mA, standard reconstruction kernel, and reconstructed section spacing of 0.5 mm. Column plot below image shows the percentage of variation of the noise s.d. from the mean noise s.d. in the four regions of interest (ROIs) labeled A–D. Plots on the right show the percentage variation of the s.d. of the noise from the mean s.d. as a function of section location along the *z*-axis (tick marks correspond to the distance covered in one gantry rotation) for each of the four ROIs. Note that noise variation with this particular spiral reconstruction algorithm may be as high as ±32% about the average noise level and is periodic in the distance moved per gantry rotation. This periodic spatial variation in the noise level may cause problems when looking for low-contrast lesions (58) and is the major cause of "zebra" stripe artifact in maximum-intensity projection images (52,59).

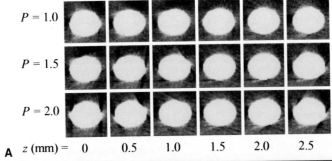

$P = 1.0$

$P = 1.5$

$P = 2.0$

A z (mm) =   0   0.5   1.0   1.5   2.0   2.5

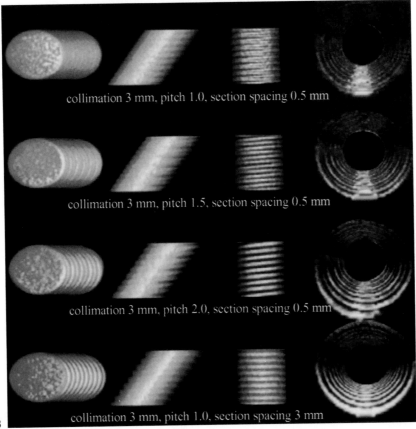

collimation 3 mm, pitch 1.0, section spacing 0.5 mm

collimation 3 mm, pitch 1.5, section spacing 0.5 mm

collimation 3 mm, pitch 2.0, section spacing 0.5 mm

collimation 3 mm, pitch 1.0, section spacing 3 mm

B

FIG. 1-9. Spiral artifacts in 3D reconstructions. All images were made from spiral CT scans of a plastic rod in air oriented in the coronal plane, making an angle with the sagittal plane of 45 degrees. Other relevant scan parameters were the following: gantry rotation interval 1 s, display field of view 256 mm, section interval 0.5 mm. Three scans were made at pitches (P) of 1.0, 1.5, and 2.0, respectively. **(A)** Overlapping cross-sections positioned as shown along the z-axis displayed with a 25-HU window show rotating artifact that worsens with increasing pitch. **(B)** Volume renderings with lighting adjusted to exaggerate the appearance of this artifact in 3D images. First three columns, from left to right, show views perpendicular to axial, coronal, and sagittal directions, respectively. Rightmost column shows perspective volume-rendered internal view of the outer edge of the rod, simulating virtual angioscopy (27). Top three rows show increase of magnitude and pitch of corkscrew pattern with increasing scan pitch when sections are reconstructed with relatively large percentage overlap. Smaller pitches result in smoother renderings but do not completely eliminate the artifact. Bottom row shows $P = 1$ scans (same as top row) but with nominally contiguous section reconstruction. Note artifact in this case appears as concentric rings, not a corkscrew pattern. (Volume renderings done with VoxelView 2.5.3, Vital Images, Inc., Fairfield, IA.)

enough, raw projection data will be archived instead of reconstructed images, thereby allowing the full fidelity of the spiral CT exam to be available at any time (55).

Image Noise

Image noise in spiral CT is dominated by the same factors that influence its magnitude in conventional CT: photon noise, collimation, tube output, scanning time per image, geometric and detector efficiencies (56). In addition, however, unique contributions to image noise are made by the spiral geometry and image reconstruction algorithms. There are two effects to consider: noise level, generally measured in the center of the image, and uniformity of noise as a function of transaxial position.

Several authors have compared the noise in the center of a spiral CT image with that of conventional CT. At identical collimator width and dose, noise is determined by the number of projections used, and the projection weighting employed by the individual image-reconstruction algorithms. Originally, 360-degree linear interpolation was touted with respect to its lower noise (83% of conventional CT at identical collimation and dose). However, as mentioned earlier, this advantage is far outweighed by the disadvantageous SSP broadening described earlier in the section on image reconstruction. In general, the ratio of the noise (s.d.) in the center a spiral CT image to the noise in the center of a nonspiral scan made by the same scanner at equivalent collimation and dose is between 1.1 and 1.4 (5,6,41,57).

Perhaps more interesting is that noise is not generally independent of in-plane spatial position (58–60). Figure 1-8 demonstrates this effect for one particular CT scanner. This effect varies in magnitude among the various interpolation algorithms, and in one case the spatial variation of the noise s.d. was determined to be as high as 40% (58). Again we mention Hsieh's work (53,60) as a precursor for potential future improvements in this area.

Artifacts

The theory of CT reconstruction assumes consistency of the projection data for the duration of the data collection. Patient motion, of course, violates this assumption, and spiral CT requires patient motion. With reference to Fig. 1-3, one can see that the further the patient moves between the collection of the first and last projections used to reconstruct a cross-section, the less consistent are the projection data. That is, projection data consistency decreases with increasing pitch. And as projection data consistency decreases, artifactual content increases. Many reconstruction algorithms weight each projection according to its distance (along the z-axis) from the nominal center of the cross-section being reconstructed; the closer each projection is to the center, the larger the multiplicative weight. Although this weighting reduces the artifactual energy, the algorithms may introduce asymmetries that distort the reconstructed images (6,61–63).

(See Fig. 1-9.) Note, however, that in many cases these spiral artifacts are minimal and are justified by the increased coverage per unit time afforded by higher pitch (47).

SUMMARY

Spiral CT represents a major step forward in the evolution of CT scanning. As will be shown in the following chapters, the advent of spiral CT has resulted in improved efficiency of existing applications of CT and the creation of new applications. Where appropriate, spiral CT examinations permit coverage rates in the cranial-to-caudal direction to be increased by almost an order of magnitude compared with conventional CT studies. This improved scanning rate may translate into improved iodinated contrast utilization, reduced respiratory misregistration, reduction in partial volume effects, and an increase in the number of patients that can be scanned in a given amount of time.

ACKNOWLEDGMENTS

I gratefully acknowledge support from Siemens Medical Systems, the Lucas Foundation, the National Institutes of Health, the Whitaker Foundation, and General Electric Medical Systems. I offer sincere thanks to my physician collaborators, including Michael D. Dake, Dieter R. Enzmann, Robert J. Herfkens, R. Brooke Jeffrey, Jr., David A. Katz, Michael P. Marks, and Geoffrey D. Rubin. Thanks also to Shin Yi Yen, M.S., whose careful reading of this chapter led to a scientifically correct and coherent discussion. Further thanks go to Dr. Stanley Fox and Dr. Rolf Hupke, for thoughtful criticism and historical perspective. Finally, thanks to my wife Lyn Furness, my son Walt, and my daughter Madeline, who offer continued support and encouragement and put up with my frequent absences to get things like this done.

REFERENCES

1. Kalender WA. Spiral or helical CT: right or wrong? [letter]. *Radiology* 1994;193:583.
2. Zatz LM. General overview of computed tomography instrumentation. In: Newton TH and Potts DG, eds. *Radiology of the skull and brain: technical aspects of computed tomography.* St Louis: CV Mosby; 1981: 4025–4057.
3. Robb RA, Ritman EL, Gilbert BK, Kinsey JH, Harris LD, Wood EH. The DSR: a high speed three-dimensional x-ray computed tomography system for dynamic spatial reconstruction of the heart and circulation. *IEEE Trans Nucl Sci* 1979;NS-26:2713–2717.
4. Peschmann KR, Napel SA, Couch JL, et al. High speed computed tomography, system and performance. *Appl Optics* 1985;24:4052.
5. Kalender WA, Polacin A. Physical performance characteristics of spiral CT scanning. *Med Phys* 1991;18:910–915.
6. Crawford CR, King KF. Computed tomography scanning with simultaneous patient translation. *Med Phys* 1990;17:967–982.
7. Yamada T, Harada J, Tada S. Complex congenital cardiovascular anomalies evaluated by continuous-rotation computed tomography in children. *Pediatr Cardiol* 1989;10:65–74.
8. Kalender WA, Seissler W, Klotz E, Vock P. Spiral volumetric CT with single-breath-hold technique, continuous transport, and continuous scanner rotation. *Radiology* 1990;176:181–183.
9. Vock P, Soucek M, Daepp M, Kalender WA. Lung: spiral volumetric CT with single-breath-hold technique. *Radiology* 1990;176:864–867.

10. Remy-Jardin M, Remy J, Giraud F, Marquette CH. Pulmonary nodules: detection with thick-section spiral CT versus conventional CT. *Radiology* 1993;187:513–520.

11. Costello P, Dupuy DE, Ecker CP, Tello R. Spiral CT of the thorax with reduced volume of contrast material: a comparative study. *Radiology* 1992;183:663–666.

12. Hupke R, Ezrielev J, Fisler R. Three-dimensional imaging in CT. In: Felix R and Langer M, eds. *Advances in CT II,* 2nd European Scientific User Conference Somatom Plus. Berlin: Springer-Verlag; 1992: 147–154.

13. Schaefer C, Prokop M, Nischelsky J, Riemer P, Bonk K, Galanski M. Vascular imaging with spiral CT. In: Felix R and Langer M, eds. *Advances in CT II,* vol. 1, 2nd European Scientific User Conference Somatom Plus. Berlin: Springer-Verlag; 1992:109–116.

14. Napel S, Marks MP, Rubin GD, et al. CT angiography with spiral CT and maximum intensity projection. *Radiology* 1992;185:607–610.

15. Aoki S, Sasaki Y, Machida T, Ohkubo T, Minami M, Sasaki Y. Cerebral aneurysms: detection and delineation using 3D-CT angiography. *AJNR* 1992;13:1115–1120.

16. Schwartz RB, Jones KM, Chernoff DM, et al. Common carotid artery bifurcation: evaluation with spiral CT. Work in progress. *Radiology* 1992;185:513–519.

17. Marks MP, Napel S, Jordan JE, Enzmann DR. Diagnosis of carotid artery disease: preliminary experience with maximum-intensity-projection spiral CT angiography. *AJR* 1993;160:1267–1271.

18. Rubin GD, Dake MD, Napel S, McDonnell CH, Jeffrey RB Jr. Three-dimensional spiral CT angiography of the abdomen: initial clinical experience. *Radiology* 1993;186:147–152.

19. Rubin GD, Walker PJ, Dake MD, et al. 3D spiral CT angiography: an alternative imaging modality for the abdominal aorta and its branches. *J Vasc Surg* 1993;18:656–665.

20. Rubin GD, Dake MD, Napel S, et al. Spiral CT of renal artery stenosis: comparison of three-dimensional rendering techniques. *Radiology* 1994;190:181–189.

21. Helmberger H, Bautz W, Vogel U, Lenz M. [CT arterioportography in the spiral technique for the demonstration of liver metastases]. *Rofo Fortschr Geb Roentgenstr Neuen Bildgeb Verfahr* 1993;158:410–415.

22. Lenz M, Wunderlich AP, Helmberger H, Gross M. [Spiral CT in aortic aneurysms. 2D and 3D reconstructions and CT angiography]. *Rofo Fortschr Geb Roentgenstr Neuen Bildgeb Verfahr* 1993;158:393–404.

23. Remy-Jardin M, Remy J, Wattinne L, Giraud F. Central pulmonary thromboembolism: diagnosis with spiral volumetric CT with the single-breath-hold technique: comparison with pulmonary angiography. *Radiology* 1992;185:381–387.

24. Gieger B, Kikinis R. Simulation of endoscopy. AAAI Spring Symposium Series: Applications of Computer Vision in Medical Image Processing, Stanford, CA, 1994:138–140.

25. Higgins WE, Ramaswamy K. Toward dynamic visualization for endoscopy simulation. In: Sheppard NF, Jr, Eden M, and Kantor G, eds. *Proceedings of the 16th Annual International Conference of the IEEE Engineering in Medicine and Biology Society.* Engineering Advances: New Opportunities for Biomedical Engineers (Cat. No. 94CH3474-4). New York: IEEE Press; 1994;700–701.

26. Lorensen WE, Jolesz FA, Kikinis R. The exploration of cross-sectional data with a virtual endoscope. In: Satava RM, Morgan K, Sieburg HB, Mattheus R, Christensen JP, eds. Interactive technology and the new Paradigm for health care. Amsterdam, Netherlands: IOS Press; 1995: 221–230.

27. Rubin GD, Beaulieu CF, Argiro V, et al. Perspective volume rendering of CT and MR images: applications for endoscopic viewing. *Radiology* 1996;199:321–330.

28. Vining DJ. Virtual endoscopy: is it reality? [editorial; comment]. *Radiology* 1996;200:30–31.

29. Sommer FG, Olcott E, Ch'en I, Beaulieu CF. Volume rendering of CT data: applications to the genitourinary tract. *AJR Am J Roentgenol* 1997; 168:1223–1226.

30. Hara AK, Johnson CD, Reed JE, Ehman RL, Ilstrup DM. Colorectal polyp detection with CT colography: two-versus three-dimensional techniques. Work in progress. *Radiology* 1996;200:49–54.

31. Hara AK, Johnson CD, Reed JE, et al. Detection of colorectal polyps by computed tomographic colography: feasibility of a novel technique. *Gastroenterology* 1996;110:284–290.

32. Vining DJ, Liu K, Choplin RH, Haponik EF. Virtual bronchoscopy: relationships of virtual reality endobronchial simulations to actual bronchoscopic findings. *Chest* 1996;109:549–553.

33. Ferretti GR, Vining DJ, Knoplioch J, Coulomb M. Tracheobronchial tree: three-dimensional spiral CT with bronchoscopic perspective. *J Comput Assist Tomogr* 1996;20:777–781.

34. Vining DJ, Zagoria RJ, Liu K, Stelts D. CT cystoscopy: an innovation in bladder imaging. *AJR* 1996;166:409–410.

35. Glover GH, Pelc NJ. Nonlinear partial volume artifacts in x-ray computed tomography. *Med Phys* 1980;7:238–248.

36. Joseph P. Artifacts in computed tomography. In: Newton TH and Potts DG, eds. *Radiology of the skull and brain: technical aspects of computed tomography.* St Louis: CV Mosby; 1981:3956–3992.

37. Radon J. Uber die bestimmung von funktionen durch ihre Integralwerte langs gewisser Mannigfaltigkeiten. *Saechsische Akademie der Wissenschaften.* Liepzig: Berichte uber die Verhandlungen; 1917;69: 262–277.

38. Herman GT. *Image reconstruction from projections: the fundamentals of computerized tomography.* New York: Academic Press; 1980.

39. Kak AC, Slaney M. *Principles of computerized tomographic imaging.* New York: IEEE Press; 1988.

40. Kalender WA, Vock P, Polacin A, Soucek M. Spiral-CT: a new technique for volumetric scans. I. Basic principles and methodology. *Roentgenpraxis* 1990;43:323–330.

41. Polacin A, Kalender WA, Marchal G. Evaluation of section sensitivity profiles and image noise in spiral CT. *Radiology* 1992;185:29–35.

42. Parker DL. Optimal short scan convolution reconstruction for fan beam CT. *Med Phys* 1982;9:254–257.

43. Wang G, Vannier MW. Longitudinal resolution in volumetric x-ray computerized tomography: analytical comparison between conventional and helical computerized tomography. *Med Phys* 1994;21: 429–433.

44. Wang G, Brink JA, Vannier MW. Theoretical FWTM values in helical CT. *Med Phys* 1994;21:753–754.

45. Brink JA, Heiken JP, Balfe DM, Sagel SS, DiCroce J, Vannier MW. Spiral CT: decreased spatial resolution *in vivo* due to broadening of section-sensitivity profile. *Radiology* 1992;185:469–474.

46. Brink JA, Lim JT, Wang G, Heiken JP, Deyoe LA, Vannier MW. Technical optimization of spiral CT for depiction of renal artery stenosis: in vitro analysis. *Radiology* 1995;194:157–163.

47. Rubin GD, Napel S. Increased scan pitch for vascular and thoracic spiral CT [letter to editor]. *Radiology* 1995;197:316.

48. Kallmes DF, Evans AJ, Woodcock RJ, et al. Optimization of parameters for the detection of cerebral aneurysms: CT angiography of a model. *Radiology* 1996;200:403–405.

49. Wright AR, Collie DA, Williams JR, Hashemi-Malayeri B, Stevenson AJ, Turnbull CM. Pulmonary nodules: effect on detection of spiral CT pitch. *Radiology* 1996;199:837–841.

50. Polacin A, Kalender WA, Brink J, Vannier MA. Measurement of slice sensitivity profiles in spiral CT. *Med Phys* 1994;21:133–140.

51. Blumenfeld SM, Glover GH. Spatial resolution in computed tomography. In: Newton TH and Potts DG, eds. *Radiology of the skull and brain: technical aspects of computed tomography.* St Louis: CV Mosby; 1981:3918–3940.

52. Wang G, Vannier MW. Spatial variation of section sensitivity profile in spiral computed tomography. *Med Phys* 1994;21:1491–1497.

53. Hsieh J. A general approach to the reconstruction of x-ray helical computed tomography. *Med Phys* 1996;23:221–229.

54. Kalender WA, Polacin A, Suss C. A comparison of conventional and spiral CT: an experimental study on the detection of spherical lesions. *J Comput Assist Tomogr* 1994;18:167–176.

55. Rubin GD, Napel S, Leung AN. Volumetric analysis of volumetric data: achieving a paradigm shift. *Radiology* 1996;200:312–317.

56. Hanson KM. Noise and contrast discrimination in computed tomography. In: Newton TH and Potts DG, eds. *Radiology of the skull and brain: technical aspects of computed tomography.* St Louis: CV Mosby; 1981:3941–3955.

57. Wang G, Vannier MW. Helical CT image noise: analytical results. *Med Phys* 1993;20:1635–1640.

58. Polacin A, Kalender WA. Evaluation of spatial resolution and noise in spiral CT. 80th RSNA. *Abstract in Radiology* 1994;193(P):171.

59. Crawford CR, King CF, Hu H. Helical CT noise reduction with optimum starting angles. 80th RSNA. *Abstract in Radiology* 1994;193(P):171.

60. Hsieh J. Nonstationary helical CT noise characteristics and their effect on MIP images. 82nd RSNA. *Abstract in Radiology* 1996;201(P):325.

61. Wang G, Vannier MW. Stair-step artifacts in three-dimensional helical CT: an experimental study. *Radiology* 1994;191:79–83.

62. Brink JA, Heiken JP, Wang G, McEnery KW, Schlueter FJ, Vannier MW. Helical CT: principles and technical considerations. *Radiographics* 1994;14:887–893.

63. Wilting JE, Timmer J. Artifacts on spiral CT images and their relation to pitch and the imaged structure. 82nd RSNA. *Abstract in Radiology* 1996;201(P):189.

CHAPTER 2

Pharmacokinetics of Contrast Enhancement in Body CT: Implications for Helical (Spiral) Scanning

Paul M. Silverman

The use of contrast agents for body computed tomography (CT) is now almost two decades old. During this time there has been considerable evolution and controversy in CT protocols as noted in a recent commentary by Dodd et al. (1) with regard to the detection of hepatic and abdominal abnormalities by CT. They stated, ''Despite nearly fifteen years of research it is hard to find more than a handful of radiologists who can agree on what constitutes the optimal method of contrast administration'' (1). However, the following basic concepts are generally accepted: (a) Rapid power injection of contrast material is preferable to a drip infusion; (b) scanning of the liver should be completed prior to equilibrium phase; and (c) the degree of parenchymal enhancement is directly related to the amount of contrast material administered (2–5).

With the development of rapid dynamic CT scanning attention to specific protocols for contrast administration is increasingly important even with conventional CT scanning. Now helical (spiral) CT with slip-ring technology has cut scan times in half, to 1 s, and, more importantly, has eliminated the 6–7-s interscan delay. The combination of these improvements provides scan times six to seven times faster than could be achieved by the best conventional ''step and shoot CT.'' Thus a complete reassessment of our methods of using iodinated contrast material and the timing of scans is required. Although this is a challenge, the potential rewards are extensive and include the use of less contrast (decreased expense), decreased motion artifact, improved definition of vascular structures, lack of misregistration artifacts, routine use of thinner sections, rapid imaging of multiple body parts, and ability to perform three-dimensional (3D) reconstructions.

To begin to develop protocols for helical CT, one must thoroughly appreciate the pharmacokinetics of contrast and particularly an understanding of the concept of time–density curves related to scanning. The scanning protocols must be adapted to these curves to take maximal advantage of the contrast used and to determine the optimal injection rates, delays between injection and scan initiation, and subtle effects of variations in contrast concentration.

CONTRAST AGENTS FOR CT

Over the years various novel contrast agents have been tried, including ethiodized oil emulsion 13 (EOE-13), liposomes, and perfluorocarbons, but because of unacceptable toxic side effects, none has become commercially accepted for widespread clinical use (6–9). The standard agents for clinical use in CT are the iodinated urographic contrast materials. These agents are water-soluble, have a high safety index, and are easily administered intravenously. They differentially enhance normal and abnormal tissues and thus improve discrimination and tumor or inflammatory processes from normal tissues (9).

The most widely utilized agents, ionic contrast materials, have a wide margin of safety in the range of the common antibiotic penicillin. Although they typically range from 30% to 76% iodine, the most effective concentration for routine body CT is 60% iodine. Ionic agents tend to have a very high osmolality compared with blood. The osmolality for 60% contrast agents is on the order of 1,500 mOsm.

The introduction of nonionic, low-osmolality contrast has significantly impacted radiology practice. With an osmolarity of 520–675 mOsm they are associated with a lower frequency and severity of allergic reactions. Newer, nonionic agents are now available that are iso-osmolar with blood but are not generally used in computed tomography (10). Despite the much wider utilization of nonionic contrast agents recently, no studies have definitively demonstrated a significant decrease in mortality to offset their greater expense compared with standard ionic contrast agents (11–16). They are, however, less cardiotoxic and neurotoxic, and are better tolerated by patients (17–20). This makes nonionic contrast especially advantageous in high-risk patients or in patients receiving large volumes of contrast. There is not a clinically significant difference in relative enhancement of the liver when ionic and nonionic contrast materials are compared when controlled for total iodine dose. Since the iodinated water-soluble contrast agents commonly used are hyperosmolar compared with blood, their physiological behavior is similar to different degrees. These agents expand the blood pool, causing intravascular dilution. Over time, they diffuse into the extravascular space that can cause lesions to become isodense and indistinguishable from normal tissues.

A recent study has shown that nonionic contrast use has increased in response to patient safety concerns (20). The resulting dramatic increase in expense to the health care system has caused additional controversy. An article by Levin et al. found that the upwardly spiraling use of nonionic contrast material can be controlled while adhering to the American College of Radiology (ACR) guidelines with appropriate monitoring and controls (21).

Helical technology can benefit from the use of nonionic contrast for a number of reasons. These agents have decreased minor side effects, including nausea and vomiting. Not only is minimizing these effects important with conventional CT, but it is critical in helical CT especially when high rates of administration are used. Since helical CT involves a continuous acquisition, potential motion during the scan can ruin the helical scan sequence. Since helical examinations are often performed with the plan of performing 3D reconstructions, it is important that when 3D reconstructions are considered, the scans be generated without misregistration or motion artifact that can render the 3D images useless. Thus many departments have committed to using nonionic contrast for helical scanning to avoid motion that may occur from the minor adverse reactions of nausea or motion artifact from the uncomfortable feelings that are more commonly associated with ionic contrast.

CONTRAST INJECTION TECHNIQUES: POWER INJECTOR TECHNOLOGY

One practical consideration related to CT scanning is the common use of power injector technology for administration of contrast material compared with other radiographic procedures such as intravenous urography in which injections are made using a standard hand-generated bolus or, rarely, drip technique with direct patient monitoring during the administration of contrast. The use of power injectors creates a significant difference in the approach of radiologists to their selection of contrast material. Although the initial portion of the power injection is monitored by the physician or designated professional, the person monitoring the injection is

removed from the patient while contrast is being administered. This allows for the potential of contrast extravasation into the soft tissues as an adverse reaction. This is one area where nonionic contrast material have previously been shown to be safer than ionic contrast material in terms of adverse reactions, including tissue necrosis (22). This has driven many radiologists to the use of nonionic contrast material despite its higher expense and the issues of cost containment now being firmly exerted by hospitals and third-party insurers. This will undoubtedly be a continuing source of controversy until the cost differential between ionic and nonionic contrast agents is diminished or the overall cost of the nonionic contrast agent per examination can be reduced, such as by dose reduction. Further study is needed in this area.

HISTORICAL PERSPECTIVE

The use of contrast in helical CT scanning is best appreciated in a historical context. Even during the early days of body scanning, the need for faster scanners to optimally utilize contrast kinetics was recognized. Studies performed between 1976 and 1979 by Dean et al. demonstrated that between 0 and 2 min of contrast enhancement was specific for individual tissues, but by 5 min there was equilibration of contrast into the extracellular tissues (3,23–25). Further delayed scanning thus reflected recirculation of contrast and renal excretion. The greatest contrast enhancement occurred at the conclusion of the infusion of contrast material. Enhancement was found to be proportional to the dose and the rapidity of administration.

A major problem in assessing current literature is the variation in the definition of phases of contrast. In 1981, Burgener and Hamlin defined three phases of enhancement that are still in use (26). The bolus phase occurs when the arteriovenous iodine difference (AVID) (i.e., aorta versus inferior vena cava) enhancement difference is greater than 30 Hounsfield units (HU), which coincides with the end of the bolus. The second phase, the nonequilibrium phase, is present when the AVID drops to 10–30 HU, occurring 1 min after the bolus or any time during contrast infusion. Finally, the equilibrium phase corresponds to a less than 10-HU difference and occurs 2 min after the bolus phase or following drip infusion. Since a 10-HU difference is difficult to discriminate visually, this work suggests hepatic scanning should *not* be performed during the equilibrium phase to attempt to detect lesions. A second, and very different definition of the nonequilibrium and equilibrium phase has been proposed by Foley and his colleagues (27,28). Their definition of the equilibrium phase is much earlier and is defined at the point in which the aortic and hepatic enhancement curves become parallel. The aortic enhancement increases rapidly during the bolus phase, which may last 1 min or longer. Vascular enhancement increases progressively until the end of the injection. Aortic enhancement then decreases rapidly during the nonequilibrium phase. During this phase there is redistribution of the contrast from the intravascular to the extravascular space. The resulting effect is an increase in attenuation or Hounsfield units within the hepatic parenchyma, creating the intense liver enhancement. Peak hepatic enhancement occurs late in the nonequilibrium phase toward the end of the portal venous enhancement. Finally, when the intravascular and extravascular contrast material equilibrate, the *equilibrium phase,* contrast enhancement declines at a rate determined by renal excretion. This is initiated at the point at which the aortic and hepatic curves begin to become parallel. They assume equilibrium occurs at approximately 2 min after initiation of constant injection of contrast material. They believe a standard single injection rate (monophasic technique) does not leave enough time to scan the liver (assuming approximately 2 min of scanning time).

PRACTICAL IMPLICATIONS OF CONTRAST ON IMAGING

Young et al. studied the bolus versus drip infusion technique for the detection of liver neoplasms (29). They found that the best diagnostic images were obtained soon after the bolus, prior to diffusion of contrast into the tumor. In fact, scans performed during the equilibrium phase were less effective at detecting hepatic lesions than noncontrast scans.

Dean et al. studied the relationship of iodine dose to contrast enhancement. Their results showed that doubling the iodine dose resulted in a similar increase in enhancement and that tripling the dose increased enhancement approximately threefold (23–25). Prolonged infusion times increased the length of time enhancement remains at acceptable levels and thus allowed a longer scanning time. Their conclusions resulted in the concept that increasing the iodine dose per kilogram produces the greatest relative increase in parenchymal organ attenuation. This translates clinically into the concept that high levels of contrast enhancement improve detectability of hepatic lesions. In contrast to brain CT, where enhancement is moderated by the blood-brain barrier in body CT, it is necessary to maximize contrast enhancement of parenchymal organs in the body for optimal lesion detectability, but below contrast levels associated with renal toxicity. Dean et al. recommended that bolus or very rapid infusion techniques were optimal to obtain the greatest possible enhancement.

Moss et al., because of conflicting reports concerning the clinical need of intravenous contrast material as an aid to enhancing the detection of liver lesions, evaluated 61 patients with proven liver metastases (30). At the time of the study there were some centers that still felt that "intravenous contrast enhancement is generally not necessary to detect space-occupying lesions." Their results concluded that 84% of focal liver lesions were seen as well or better after enhancement. These results have been supported by subsequent studies. In most cases, the preferred method for CT evaluation of patients with suspected liver lesions has become dependent on postcontrast CT scans (31).

PRACTICAL ASPECTS OF CONTRAST ADMINISTRATION

Uniphasic vs. Biphasic Injection Protocols

The two different definitions of the onset of equilibrium have resulted in two distinctly different approaches to administering contrast for body CT, specifically when the liver is the target organ. Those who accept the definition proposed by Burgener and Hamlin assume that equilibrium occurs much later, many minutes after the onset of a constant or *uniphasic* injection of contrast (26). Thus they feel comfortable using the technique even with conventional scans because they feel that scanning of the upper abdomen can be easily completed before equilibrium. In contrast, *biphasic* proponents such as Foley and his colleagues accept the definition of equilibrium as occurring within 2–2.5 min after the onset of a uniphasic injection. Therefore they recommend that to avoid scanning during equilibrium, the method of contrast administration be changed to a biphasic approach with a rapid initial and slower secondary injection rate. This significantly delays the onset of equilibrium and provides a longer period (termed the *optimal temporal window*) in which to scan. The details of these two approaches and their major advocates are outlined.

Using conventional CT, most investigators have employed a dose equivalent of 150 mL of 60% contrast material administered as a uniphasic or a biphasic injection technique. Proponents of a *uniphasic injection technique* claim certain advantages (32):

1. Seventy percent of peak hepatic enhancement occurs after the termination of 150 mL of 60% contrast material at the widely used rates of 2–3 mL/s. Thus a 50–75-s delay from the onset of injection to initiation of conventional scanning (assuming a 2-s scan time and 6-s interscan delay [ISD]) would achieve optimal enhancement. This is a slightly longer injection delay than previously advocated by multiple other investigators (45 s) (33).
2. Since time–density curves of hepatic enhancement have shown that the upward slope of the hepatic enhancement is steeper than the downward slope, scanning too early yields suboptimal hepatic enhancement. When scanning occurs prior to portal venous enhancement, small unopacified venous structures may mimic small hepatic metastases.
3. Enhancement curves have shown that higher peak enhancement is achieved with monophasic injections despite a lower initial rate of enhancement. Enhancement of the liver is superior at all points in time for rapid monophasic injection techniques compared with biphasic methodology (Fig. 2-1).
4. Unfortunately, advocates of monophasic techniques accept a much different definition of the equilibrium phase, making it difficult to compare monophasic and biphasic approaches objectively (32).

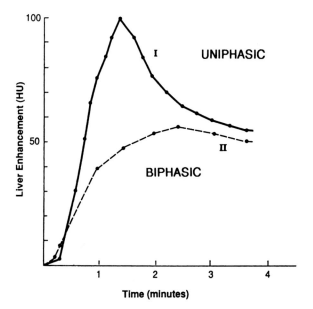

FIG. 2-1. Hepatic enhancement curves demonstrate that there is better enhancement of the liver with a monophasic injection than with a biphasic injection. **(I)** Monophasic injection at 2.5 mL/s. **(II)** Biphasic injection of 50 mL at 5 mL/s followed by 130 mL at 1 mL/s. (From Walkey MM. *Radiology* 1991;181:21.)

Biphasic proponents recommend a very different set of parameters as accepted by Foley and his colleagues:

1. They suggest an earlier scanning delay, 45 s (27,28).
2. Their approach to contrast administration and scanning techniques is built upon the premise of prolonging contrast administration as an adaptation to the time necessary to scan the upper abdomen prior to the onset of the equilibrium phase using conventional CT, which they define as occurring approximately a couple of minutes after onset of injection. The biphasic injection, which prolongs the bolus and nonequilibrium phases, delays

the onset of equilibrium. This allows scanning to be completed prior to their definition of equilibrium, in contrast to the uniphasic approach (Fig. 2-2). They have recommended high initial rates of 5 mL/s for 50 mL followed by 1 mL/s for 130 mL. This much higher rate is set to achieve adequate peak enhancement. These authors employ a shorter 45-s delay from initiation of contrast injection to scan initiation to increase the so-called optimal temporal window for liver CT. Others have experimented with lower initial rates ranging from 2.0 to 4.5 mL/s (34). An optimized imaging protocol would initiate the first scan at as high a point on the upward slope of the hepatic enhancement curve as possible while completing the examination prior to equilibrium.

Since neither of these definitions of equilibrium has been experimentally confirmed, the debate is expected to continue, although most researchers accept the more stringent criteria applied by biphasic proponents. Unfortunately, complex factors are involved in patients, creating a great degree of individual variation in the effect of enhancement on anatomic structures despite similar injection and scanning techniques. Factors such as patients' size (weight), cardiac status, degree of hydration, age, and sex have considerable effect on the actual enhancement of critical structures such as the liver.

In terms of practical acceptability, the monophasic technique has been more widely utilized in the radiologic community because of its simplicity. Additionally, many radiologists are not comfortable with the higher rates recommended by many biphasic proponents for fear of an increase of complications from contrast extravasation. This can be minimized by the radiologist monitoring the patient closely within the CT suite until the rapid initial phase is completed. Biphasic proponents feel that such injection protocols are easy to implement with current day power injectors and should not deter the practicing radiologist from using this technique. Subtle refinements in injection rates and

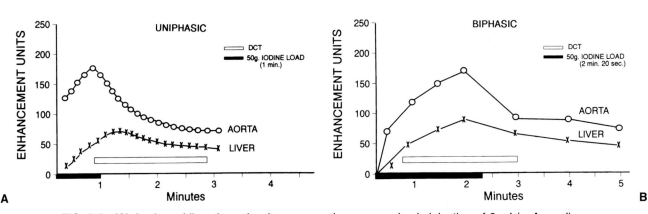

FIG. 2-2. (A) Aortic and liver time–density curves using a monophasic injection of 3 mL/s. According to the criteria of Foley and colleagues, the time requirement for conventional scanning extends well into the equilibrium phase. (From Walkey MM. *Radiology* 1991;181:19.) **(B)** Time–density curves using a biphasic injection of 50 mL at 5 mL/s, 130 at 1 mL/s. Using dynamic scanning with a 45-s delay, a 2-min and 15-s temporal window was provided prior to the onset of equilibrium.

volumes may allow the technique to be adopted to different practices.

CLINICAL IMPACT OF CONTRAST INJECTION METHODOLOGY

In 1993, Heiken et al. investigated biphasic and uniphasic injections at high and low flow rates to determine their effects on parenchymal liver enhancement (35). They assessed (a) the optimal scanning interval (i.e., the duration between the onset of a desired hepatic enhancement threshold and the decline of enhancement below that threshold or onset of equilibrium) and (b) the contrast enhancement index (CEI). (The CEI is the area under the hepatic enhancement curve above a desired threshold during the nonequilibrium phase, which was considered an appropriate measure for determining the relative merits of the different injection techniques [Fig. 2-3].) The low flow rates consisted of 2.5 mL/s and the high flow rates consisted of 5 mL/s. They found that for most thresholds of hepatic enhancement, the optimal scanning intervals were longer and the CEIs were significantly higher for the biphasic protocols. The biphasic protocol with the high initial flow rate produced the highest peak enhancement and the greatest delay to the onset of equilibrium providing the widest temporal window. As suspected, the most rapid contrast medium injection protocol, the uniphasic high-flow-rate protocol (5 mL/s) resulted not only in the earliest peak hepatic enhancement, but also in the shortest optimal scanning interval. This is a consequence of the fact that short, rapid injections of contrast material, although having higher initial parenchymal enhancement, also demonstrate a precipitous fall of parenchymal enhancement compared with other techniques. If one takes a threshold of 40 HU of enhancement, then the biphasic techniques allowed approximately 1.5 min of scanning time prior to equilibrium, whereas the uniphasic low flow rate allowed only 30 s and the uniphasic high flow rate permitted only 12 s. The optimal scanning interval was defined as the length of time between the onset of the desired level of hepatic enhancement to begin scanning and the onset of equilibrium. For conventional scanners one can see that the biphasic protocols would be preferable because they provide a long enough time during which there is high contrast enhancement for optimal hepatic imaging.

The introduction of helical CT has again challenged the approach of injecting contrast material. Nowhere is the impact of the brief scan time for helical CT as critical as in the liver. Birnbaum et al. evaluated patients using either a uniphasic injection at 2 or 3 mL/s or a biphasic injection (3 mL/s for 50 mL, followed by 1 mL/s for 100-mL) technique. Peak enhancement occurred at 73 s (64 HU) for the fast uniphasic injection, 96 s (62 HU) for slow uniphasic injection, and 141 s (52 HU) for the biphasic technique (36). The two uniphasic approaches resulted in time–density enhancement curves that showed a more rapid and greater peak enhancement than with the biphasic approach. When helical CT windows are centered near peak hepatic enhancement,

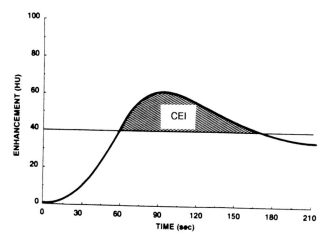

FIG. 2-3. Example of contrast enhancement index (CEI) or a means of evaluating the value of theoretically different methods of contrast enhancement. The greater the CEI, the better the protocol should be to detect hepatic metastases (From Heiken et al. *Radiology* 1993;87:327–331.)

biphasic injections provide less hepatic enhancement while also requiring a prohibitively longer delay times that compromise patient throughput. The differences between Heiken et al. and this study relate to the fact that these data were specifically modeled for helical CT.

Thus when current helical CT of the liver is considered, scan times on the order of only 15–30 s will require an adaptation of protocols of either a moderate uniphasic injection or biphasic injectors with much closer initial and secondary rates.

Garcia et al. evaluated the rate of contrast administration on hepatic enhancement (37). They found that the time to peak enhancement was shorter for faster rates of injection, as expected. However, they did not find a significant effect on maximum liver enhancement within the rates tested, including a comparison of 3 mL/s versus 6 mL/s. The difference in times to peak enhancement only reached statistical significance in comparison with 2 mL/s versus 4.5 mL/s, and 3 mL/s versus 6 mL/s groups. Previous studies have confirmed that the time to peak liver enhancement depends mainly on the duration of injection, with the shorter injection times resulting in shorter times to peak enhancement. Chambers et al. did demonstrate that in the same patient, peak liver enhancement increased by 10 HU and that mean time to peak enhancement was shorter by 15 s when using a rate of injection of 3 mL/s as opposed to 2 mL/s (38). In this study, the mean liver enhancement increased by a statistically significant amount only with the faster rate of injection during the earliest time interval (55–79 s). This reflects not an overall increase in liver enhancement, but rather a shift toward the left of the time-enhancing curve when a faster rate of injection is used. It is unclear why the rate of injection does not modify peak liver enhancement. It is possible that regardless of the rate of injection, the bolus of contrast medium is dissipated in either the systemic or splanchnic circu-

MONOPHASIC-CONVENTIONAL VS HELICAL CT
(150 ml, 2 ml/s)

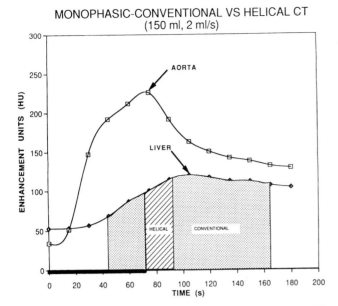

FIG. 2-4. Graph demonstrating the superiority of helical CT compared with conventional CT. Because helical CT takes such a relatively short time, we can afford to begin scanning higher on the peak liver enhancement curve yet still avoid equilibrium. Additionally, a longer delay should be used before scan initiation prior to helical CT.

lation. Caution should be exercised because these results related to enhancement of normal liver should not be interpreted as suggesting that higher rates are always beneficial for detecting liver lesions such as metastases in which the rate of seepage of contrast into the lesion, decreasing its conspicuity, is important. The complex dynamics between normal tissue and tumor are critical in determining lesion detectability.

Using helical technology, Silverman et al. determined that a significantly longer delay than that used for conventional scans was appropriate for helical CT (39). Most importantly, the much briefer scanning time of helical compared with conventional CT allows one to scan closer to the peak of liver enhancement yet avoid the equilibrium phase (Fig. 2-4). This illustrates an important benefit of helical CT, with contrast enhancement providing improved efficiency and exam quality. Specifics regarding clinical protocols for liver CT are elaborated upon in the following section dedicated to clinical applications.

CLINICAL APPLICATIONS OF CONTRAST

Head and Neck

High-quality scans of the head and neck can be performed in one or two scan helices. This is especially important in minimizing artifacts from swallowing and respiratory motion.

Excellent vascular enhancement of medical structures is achieved using helical CT with 45–85 mL (13–26 g of io-

dine) compared with 36 g of iodine usually required with conventional studies (40–42). Slightly greater doses can be advantageous to demonstrate tumor enhancement and for staging malignancies. Using routine doses of contrast, helical CT can allow rapid imaging of the circle of Willis with quality similar to that of magnetic resonance imaging (MRI). Helical CT of the extracranial carotid arteries is an area of great interest (40–43). The preliminary results of such studies have demonstrated good visualization of the carotid arteries and carotid bifurcation, producing 3D angiograms that will presumably be competitive with MRI. Advantages of of helical CT over MRI include multiple methods of display and the lack of flow-related artifacts that are prevalent with MRI (Fig. 2-5). Techniques are variable but scans initiated 20 s after the injection of approximately 75 mL of the equivalent of 60% contrast at 2–3 mL/s with 2–4-mm slice thickness provide excellent 3D imaging. In one study, the degree of carotid stenosis determined with helical CT correlated with that determined from conventional angiography in 92% of all cases (40). The major disadvantage to the technique was the need to postprocess the data, time, and expertise required in removing veins, bony structures, and overlying structures. Also, significant intersubject variability in opacification of the carotid bifurcation opacification occurred. This relates primarily to variations in cardiac output. Other factors that may affect the examination are the location of the carotid bifurcation and any delay in flow when significant stenoses are present. Ideally, the carotid arteries should be well opacified, but scanning should occur before significant contrast reaches the jugular veins.

Thorax

Noncontrast scans were routinely performed when CT was first used to evaluate the chest. Contrast enhancement was specifically reserved for distinguishing vascular from nonvascular structures. Contrast enhancement was only routinely utilized to evaluate aortic aneurysms, exclude aortic dissection, identify vascular anomalies, or assess the vascularity of specific lesions usually identified on plain films of the chest. In the past decade, contrast enhancement of the chest has generally become routine with conventional CT. In part, this is because improved scanner technology has allowed better evaluation of mediastinum and hilar structures. This allows a much clearer definition of normal and abnormal structures and provides the ability to detect hila lymphadenopathy that often would not be appreciated on noncontrast scans.

Specific applications in the thorax depend on optimal contrast enhancement. These include the staging of primary lung carcinoma, evaluation of venous clot in the mediastinum, detection of pulmonary emboli, and assessment of aortic aneurysms and dissections. With conventional CT, scans were routinely performed at 1-cm collimation thickness through the chest and required minutes to complete the entire thorax. To achieve adequate enhancement of the chest, significant amounts of contrast material (125–150 mL) were

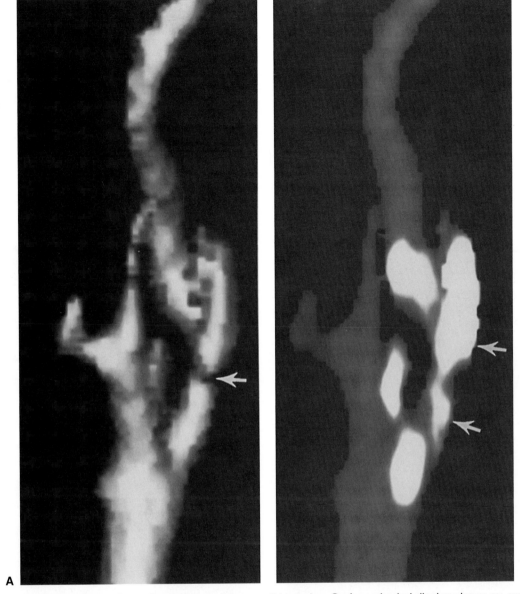

FIG. 2-5. (A) Three-dimensional image of the carotid arteries. Surface-shaded display shows an area of stenosis in the interval carotid artery (*arrow*). **(B)** A maximum-intensity projection (MIP) image of the same data shows additional information by demonstrating the extensive calcification (*arrows*) associated with the carotid artery.

routinely used to provide adequate opacification of mediastinum and hila structures.

Specific protocols for evaluating aortic dissections evolved with single-level dynamic scanning at the site of the mid-ascending aorta, to exclude ascending aortic dissections, and subsequent scanning of the entire thorax. These techniques are time-consuming and cumbersome, often employing multiple boluses of contrast. To scan the entire mediastinum and upper abdomen to determine the extent of dissections, up to 200 mL might be used. Patients with low clinical suspicion for ascending aortic dissections would undergo CT, whereas those with high clinical suspicion would often be sent for angiography. Subsequently, the evolution of MR technology has made this a valuable technique for assessing the aorta, with its multiplanar capabilities. However, sick patients requiring constant monitoring, particularly those in greatest need for diagnostic imaging, are excluded from study.

With helical CT, the entire thorax can be examined in a single breath-hold. Thus scans can be made from the lung apex to the diaphragms in a single breath-hold, thereby greatly simplifying the protocol. For routine surveys of the mediastinum, less than 100 mL of contrast can effectively be used. Costello et al. have demonstrated the effectiveness of helical CT with as little as 60 mL of 60% contrast material compared with the standard approach of 120 mL in patients undergoing conventional CT (44,45). They found that vascular opacification and image quality were better with helical than with conventional CT despite the increased amount of contrast used for conventional study.

The introduction of helical technology has completely changed the approach to evaluating patients with aortic dissections. Routine helical protocol for aortic dissection uses less contrast and usually requires only one set of scans performed in a single breath-hold to adequately evaluate the thoracic aorta. This makes a rapid and highly effective tech-

nique in noninvasively evaluating for thoracic aorta dissections. Helical technology impacts other aspects of chest imaging. Although helical CT cannot replace pulmonary angiography in detection of small peripheral emboli, this technique has been used to successfully demonstrate central emboli and even emboli within second- to fourth-order pulmonary arteries with high sensitivity. This has been achieved with doses of as little as 90–120 mL of 30% contrast material (46). Importantly, current practices often require scanning of the chest and multiple other body parts. With helical CT, this can be possible, with conservative doses of contrast, yielding images far superior to conventional CT (Fig. 2-6).

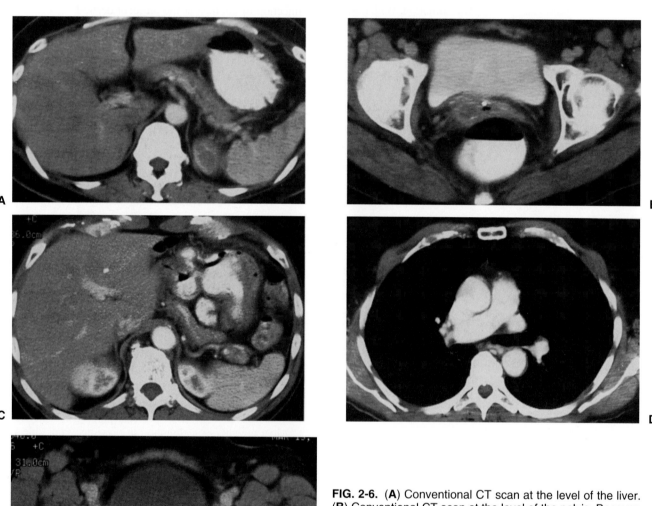

FIG. 2-6. (A) Conventional CT scan at the level of the liver. (B) Conventional CT scan at the level of the pelvis. Because of the long time it takes for scanning, contrast opacification of the pelvic vasculature is already poor. (C) Helical CT scan at the level of the liver of high quality. (D) Helical CT scans were performed through the entire chest with the same amount of contrast, yielding beautiful vascular opacification. (E) Study in the same patient at the level of the pelvis after completion of the abdomen and chest. There is better opacification of the external iliacs on the helical study despite scanning of the chest, abdomen, and pelvis than with just the abdomen and pelvis with conventional CT and the same amount of contrast.

Liver

As previously discussed, most work related to the pharmacokinetics of contrast material has targeted the liver because it is the major intra-abdominal focus for metastatic disease. The dynamics of contrast enhancement vary predictably within the liver; therefore precise timing to detect metastases is critical. Dynamic scanning of the liver during the nonequilibrium phase is the preferred method for examining the liver. Our experience has been that a longer delay allows scanning during the peak of hepatic enhancement, thereby avoiding the pitfalls of insufficiently enhanced hepatic parenchyma and unopacified hepatic venous structures that mimic lesions. With conventional scanners, 10-mm collimation was routinely used. Helical scanners promote the routine use of thinner sections, 7- or 8-mm collimation. With thinner collimations, more lesions are detected and the entire liver can be adequately covered with single or multiple helices. With hyperventilation prior to the examination and adequate coaching, patients usually can tolerate a 30-s breath-hold. An alternative in patients unable to hold their breath for 24–30 s is to perform multiple helices (two 15-s helices or three 10-s helices to cover the same volume). No consensus has yet been achieved as to the optimal technique for scanning the liver with helical CT; there are a number of practical approaches. The simplest means would be to determine the optimal temporal window and scan with a single pass during this period of time (e.g., a scan delay 60–80 s). Using 1-cm collimation the recommended delay is approximately 80 s to achieve the optimal temporal window for helical liver CT using a monophasic technique. Rapid scanning on helical CT allows a more flexible temporal window for enhancement compared with the actual scan time. By decreasing the scan delay slightly, thinner sections can be used in an attempt to identify smaller hepatic lesions without significantly sacrificing enhancement. Using 8-mm sections, we suggest approximately a 75-s delay. Using 7-mm sections, a 70-s delay is possible (see Fig. 2-4). By comparing helical CT scans done on the same patients with liver metastases, Silverman et al. have demonstrated that a 75-s delay between injection and scan initiation is preferable to a 50-s scan delay (47). In their study radiologists found 94% of lesions more conspicuous with the longer delay time. Depending on the technique and scanner, imaging the liver during different contrast phases may sometimes improve detection hepatic lesions.

Despite improvements attributed to helical technology, the continued use of fixed delays between contrast injection and scan initiation results in varied degrees of hepatic enhancement. The variability is partly the result of controllable factors, such as the rate of injection and the volume and concentration of contrast material. Other factors are attributed to individual patient variability and cannot be completely compensated. Problems caused by differences in patients' weights can be partially controlled by stratifying patients into groups, with smaller patients receiving a relatively lower iodine load (48,49). However, accurately predicting the impact of factors such as metabolic and clincal status, cardiac output, and splanchnic blood supply remains difficult. We have recently introduced the concept of an individualized scan delay technology as a means of compensating for such individual patient variability. This computer-automated scan technology (CAST) does not require a test dose of contrast. The operator first performs a baseline low-radiation-dose single CT scan at the level of the target organ, in this case the liver, and subsequently performs a series of low-dose monitoring scans in rapid succession. Region-of-interest (ROI) cursors are placed on various structures that one wishes to monitor. In addition, the operator sets a desired threshold of enhancement over baseline for the target structure, in this case the liver. A 50-HU enhancement over baseline liver values is a reasonable level. Following the routine injection of contrast at the protocol desired, software plots the relative enhancement over baseline of the liver over time. When the operator notices that the enhancement has reached the desired threshold (50 HU), independent of the duration of the injection, the technologist manually initiates a transition from this monitoring to a diagnostic helical scan series. Despite the fact that there is a brief lag time for this transition, we have found that there is a significant improvement in the level of enhancement of the liver, as well as decreased variability when compared with the standard approach of a fixed time delay (50) (Fig. 2-7).

A more recent study compared a volume of 150 mL using a standard fixed delay against a lower-volume group (125 mL) using the individualized scan delay technology. The mean hepatic enhancement achieved was similar, indicating that this technology could provide the same degree of enhancement with a savings of contrast material. If one wished to utilize the full dose of 150 mL of contrast, a significantly greater degree of enhancement could be achieved (51).

When a more flexible approach is desired, additional passes can be made through the liver, both early and late within the nonequilibrium phase, to improve lesion detection (Fig. 2-8). This would allow detection of lesions with different degrees of vascularity that might be better visualized during one phase of contrast enhancement than during another (4). Another advantage is the ability to distinguish unopacified vessels from lesions (Fig. 2-9).

Most recently, a technique not previously possible with conventional CT scanning has been advocated for improved hypervascular lesions. This technique has been termed *dual-phase* or *double-pass CT* (52–54). A noncontrast scan can often be used as a triple-phase study. The dual phase study consists of a series of CT scans through the liver during the hepatic arterial phase (HAP), approximately 15–30 s after the injection of contrast material, followed by rescanning the liver during the portal venous phase (PVP), approximately 60–80 s after contrast injection. This approach is only used in selective cases of hypervascular tumor, such as hepatocellular carcinoma and metastases from renal cell carcinoma, pancreatic islet cell tumors, and breast carcinoma. Other tumors include sarcomas, thyroid carcinoma, melanoma, and benign tumors, such as focal nodular hyperplasia (FNH) and

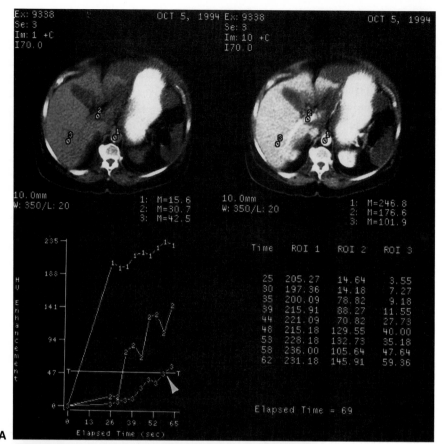

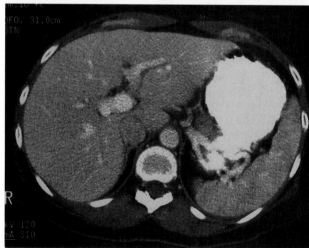

FIG. 2-7. (**A**) Computer-automated scan technology (CAST) for providing an individualized scan delay technology approach. The top left represents the baseline image. The top right is the most recently reconstructed image. The bottom left is a graphic display of aortic (1) portal venous (2), and liver (3) enhancement. When the liver enhancement reaches threshold (T), the diagnostic scan series is instituted (*arrow*). (**B**) CT scan of the liver using 150 mL, 2.5 mL/s, showing poor enhancement of the liver parenchyma secondary to individual patient variability. *(continued)*

hepatic adenoma. The approach takes advantage of the dual blood supply of the liver, which receives 75% to 80% of its blood flow from the portal vein, and the remainder from the hepatic artery. Because hypervascular tumors receive virtually all their functional blood supply from the hepatic artery, early scanning can take advantage of this by demonstrating a blush of contrast enhancement compared with a much lower background liver attenuation. Experience has suggested that when the helical CT examination using moderate injection rates (2.5–3.0 mL/s) is compared with that

using higher (4.0–6.0 mL/s) injection rates, the higher injection rates increase tumor conspicuity and improve tumor detection. This technique can be employed with the previously discussed CAST approach by placing an ROI cursor over the abdominal aorta at the level corresponding to the most cephalad extent of the liver and using a threshold of 100-HU enhancement over baseline. When this threshold is reached, the technologist can begin scanning the liver. This may provide more consistency for examinations, especially in patients with underlying circulatory disturbances. Alterna-

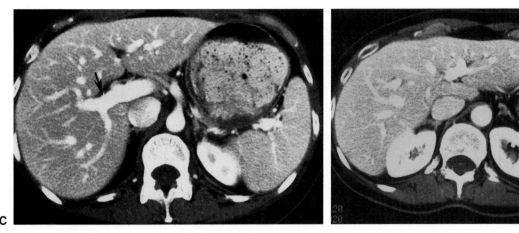

FIG. 2-7. *Continued.* (**C**) CT scan of the liver in another patient using exactly the same technique. There is much-improved liver enhancement and portal vein enhancement (*arrow*) related to individual patient differences. (**D**) CT scan of the liver in another patient using the same injection protocol but employing (CAST) technology (SmartPrep, General Electric Medical Systems, Milwaukee, WI). Note superb liver parenchymal and vascular enhancement. Consistent results can be obtained employing this technology with a savings of contrast material.

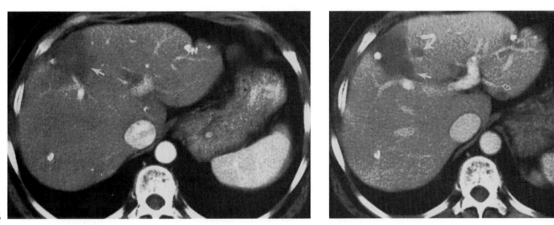

FIG. 2-8. (**A**) CT scan of the liver at 50 s following initiation of contrast administration (3 mL/s). A lesion is noted in the right lobe with peripheral calcification (*arrow*). (**B**) CT scan at 70 s. Much better background enhancement is noted of the liver. The original lesion is more easily seen (*arrow*). Small, satellite lesions (*curved arrow*) are now detected as well as a small lesion in the left lobe (*open arrowhead*).

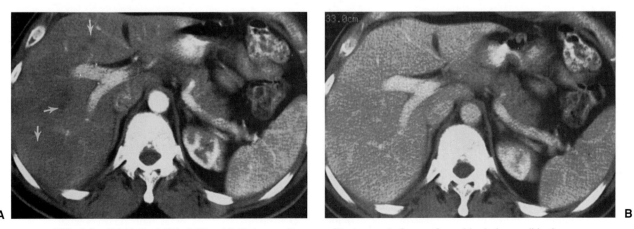

FIG. 2-9. (**A**) Helical CT at 50 s. Multiple small unopacified vessels (*arrows*) could mimic small lesions. (**B**) Scan at 74 s. All the low-attenuation areas "fill in," indicating they simply represented vessels.

tively, a small test bolus of 10–20 mL of contrast could be used. In general, a 20-s scanning delay at a rate of 4.0 mL/s and a 28-s scanning delay at injection rates of less than 4.0 mL/s generally are reliable for the HAP. A 7-mm collimation and 1.5:1 pitch generally provides excellent images. However, with patients who have difficulty suspending respiration, increased pitches of up to 2:1 may be used. One should be aware of various pitfalls that are present on the HAP phase of the examination, similar to that seen with CT arterial portography (CTAP). The most prominent artifacts are those of transient hepatic attenuation differences (THAD). These are most often areas of focal increased hepatic enhancement or physiological enhancement differences that can mimic hypervascular lesions. Hyperenhancing foci may appear as lobar, segmental, or small subsegmental lesions. These may result from the lack of unenhanced portal venous flow to these regions to dilute the contrast material supplied by the hepatic artery. Such lesions are almost always wedge shaped and peripheral, often with straight-line margins and the presence of normal vessels coursing through them, allowing them to be distinguished from pathology.

Pancreas

Helical CT is better able to image pancreatic carcinoma. After localizing the pancreas with precontrast slices, contrast is generally injected at a rate of 2–3 mL/s, for a total of 125–150 mL with approximately a 70-s delay. Five-mm collimation is selected for the pancreas and subsequently the remainder of the liver at 5- or 7-mm intervals. Alternatively, the pancreas can be evaluated with a lower dose (90 mL) with a biphasic injection, and images with superior vascular opacification and reduced respiratory artifact can be achieved (55). The additional use of retrospective imaging can be especially helpful in the pancreas. Often by saving raw data and performing overlapping slices of up to 50% of the initial slice thickness, lesions are visible that were not evident on the initial examinations. There seems to be more value in this approach to the pancreas than in using it with the liver because most lesions in the pancreas tend to be of pathological significance, whereas those in the liver are often benign. Scanning the pancreas during multiple phases can be helpful in accurately assessing lesion size (Fig. 2-10). Specific pitfalls can arise from the flow phenomenon in vascular structures. This includes the false appearance of clot within even small venous structures (Fig. 2-11).

Most recently, Lu et al. have evaluated two-phase helical CT for pancreatic tumors (56). These examiners have taken advantage of the speed of the helical CT by performing the first acquisition during the pancreatic phase (40–70 s after contrast administration), and subsequently rescanning the pancreas during the optimal hepatic phase (70–100 s after contrast administration). These authors found that the tumor–pancreas enhancement was significantly greater during the early pancreatic phase. This was the result of both greater enhancement of the normal pancreas and lesser enhancement of the tumor. In addition, better opacification of vascular structures, including the portal vein, was achieved during this phase. Previous studies assessing the sensitivity for detecting vascular invasion have shown a sensitivity of only as low as 50%. Thus optimization of technique is critical to improving this result. Fortunately, this requires optimizing number of factors, including tumor–pancreas contrast, visualization of parapancreatic vessels, and detection of liver metastases. This is challenging to perform with a single diagnostic study, because structures and organs have different optimal enhancement times relative to contrast administration. For this reason such a two-phase sequence has been recommended. High-quality CT with thin sections for detection of pancreatic carcinoma shows sensitivities of up to 97% and an accuracy of 93%. Nevertheless, other studies have demonstrated that the sensitivity for detection of unre-

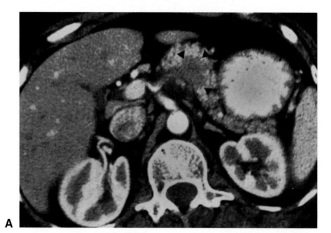
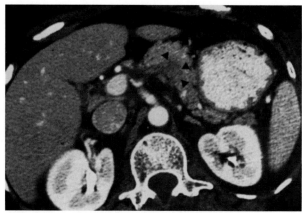

FIG. 2-10. (**A**) CT scan at the level of the pancreas after a 50-s delay. A low-attenuation mass is seen in the body of the pancreas, representing a primary adenocarcinoma (*arrowheads*). (**B**) A scan at 75 s demonstrates that there is significant filling in of the mass (*arrowheads*). Thus, what might be an optimal time for one organ may not be the optimal time for scanning another organ, and different tumors may behave differently.

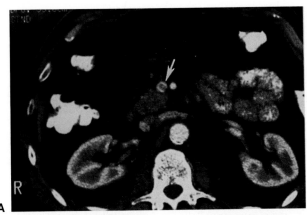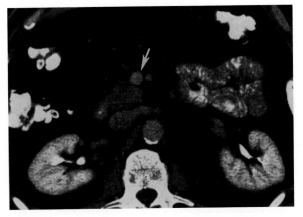

FIG. 2-11. **(A)** CT scans at the level of the superior mesenteric artery and vein. On a scan early in the bolus phase low attenuation is present within the SMV (*arrow*), which could easily mimic clot. **(B)** A scan approximately 30 s later demonstrates filling in of the SMV, indicating that this simply represented flow artifact (*arrow*).

sectable disease is about 50%, which is reflected in a substantial number of unnecessary laparotomies with unresectable disease. Although excellent arterial and portal venous opacification were achieved during the early phase, true arterial visualization probably would have been improved if scanning were to occur even earlier, but the critical question of portal vein involvement would not be answered.

In terms of producing 3D models of the portal venous system, arterial system, and parapancreatic vessels, even relatively conservative doses of contrast yield high-quality studies. Although 3D studies often are somewhat time-consuming in terms of constructing models, they can be extremely helpful in identifying vascular encasement, which aids the surgeon in determining potential resectability. Current helical CT has been able to demonstrate splenic–portal venous anatomic detail with great clarity out to second- to fourth-order branches.

Kidneys

In contrast to the intra-abdominal organs, renal imaging is often more problematic with helical CT. Following a standard injection of 125–150 mL at 2 mL/s with a 50–70-s delay, initially excellent differentiation is achieved between the densely enhanced renal cortex and the lower attenuation renal medulla (i.e., the corticomedullary phase [CMP]). Delayed scanning during the nephrogram phase (NP) is necessary to opacify the medullary portion of the kidney, and even later scans may be needed if one wishes to identify opacified renal collecting system and ureter. Users of helical CT routinely note that small low-attenuation lesions in the medulla may be missed if only the early bolus phase prior to medullary enhancement is evaluated (Fig. 2-12). They become apparent only later, when the medullary portion of the kidney enhances. Fortunately, most of these lesions are clinically insignificant cysts, but small neoplasms could be missed as well. Also in bolus phase, particularly on sections through

the upper and lower poles of the kidney, unenhanced medulla surrounded by densely enhanced cortex can stimulate low-density lesions. The value of scanning during the NP compared with the CMP has been described (57). In one study, the difference in lesion detection rate was greatest for small (less than 11 mm) medullary lesions, with approximately seven times more of these detected in the NP than in the CMP. These authors recommended a modification of renal CT protocols to include thin-section helical-mode unenhanced scans followed by thin-section scans in the CMP beginning 40 s after initiation of contrast material and a second set of scans in the NP obtained beginning 100 s after initiation of contrast. Such NP images also have been found to be more valuable in demonstrating many of the key features of small renal masses that help to distinguish benign from malignant lesions (58). Caution should be exercised regarding the ROI attenuation measurements from helical images, because these may be less accurate than those from standard axial images. A subsequent study compared scanning early (60–70 s) after initiation of contrast injection with delayed scans (2–4 min after contrast injection) (59). The sensitivity for lesion detection was 77% to 89% for early scans, and 97% for delayed scans. It was found that observers were more likely to miss a neoplastic lesion than a non-neoplastic lesion on early scans. The earlier study by Cohan evaluated predominantly cystic or complicated renal cysts, whereas this study included a wide range of cysts, complex cysts, and tumors. Evaluation of early scans alone resulted in a significantly greater likelihood of missing neoplastic lesions than of missing nonneoplastic ones. Less experienced observers tended to have greater difficulty in characterizing lesions on early scans. When the integrity of the collecting system must be assessed, as in cases of trauma, even more delayed images are required.

Although no clear data are available for the accuracy of helical CT compared with conventional CT in the staging of renal carcinoma, we have found excellent opacification of

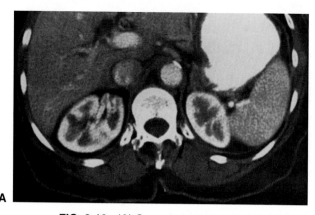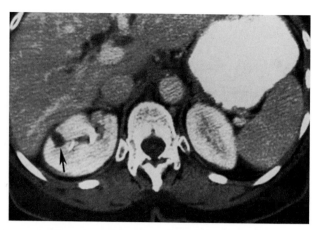

A   B

FIG. 2-12. (A) Scan during the early bolus phase demonstrating excellent corticomedullary differentiation in the kidneys. **(B)** A low-attenuation cystic lesion (*arrow*) is demonstrated in the right kidney that was not as obvious on the early scan that lacked medullary enhancement.

the renal veins with helical CT. However, characteristically inhomogeneous opacification of the inferior vena cava (IVC) because of mixing unopacified blood from lower extremities can make it more difficult to exclude caval thrombosis than with conventional CT because they are more accentuated on helical CT than on conventional CT (Fig. 2-13). These flow artifacts can be much more difficult to distinguish from clot (60). In practical situations if the renal vein is not involved, then the findings within the inferior vena cava can be presumed to represent flow-related artifacts from unopacified blood returning from the lower extremities. When there is any question of clot, a second set of helical scans or repeat single-slice images can be used.

Most recently, 3D imaging of the renal vasculature has become an exciting area of investigation for the noninvasive evaluation of renal artery stenosis (61,62). One study evaluated patients with suspected renovascular hypertension with helical CT compared with digital subtraction angiography (61). These authors found that helical CT was successful in

detecting stenoses and occlusions in the renal vasculature they studied. The grading of stenoses with helical CT was identical to that with angiography in most cases. The authors noted that precise timing was important to ensure adequate contrast within the aorta and renal arteries and to minimize interference from the overlying renal veins.

There is generally a narrow time period for optimal scanning. Usually, viewing of the axial images and reformatted images proved most helpful. In specific cases, the 3D reconstructions were useful, but mainly effective because of their ability to demonstrate pathology on one image. The maximum-intensity projection (MIP) reconstructions have developed as the technique of choice for image presentation because they produce angiography-like images, allowing discrimination between the vessel lumen and wall calcifications. The 3D surface shaded display (SSD) of reconstructions, although able to depict the stenosis within a single image, was least informative because demonstration of stenosis depends on the specific threshold selected for viewing.

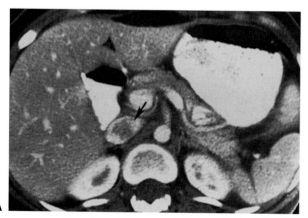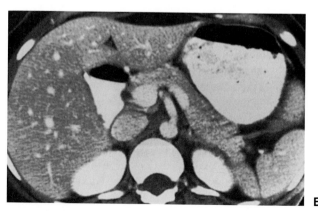

A   B

FIG. 2-13. (A) Helical CT scan during the corticomedullary phase of renal enhancement demonstrates a rounded low-attenuation area within the inferior vena cava (*arrow*) that could easily mimic thrombosis. **(B)** A delayed scan demonstrates that the inferior vena cava fills homogeneously; thus this was simply flow artifact accentuated by the rapidity of helical scanning.

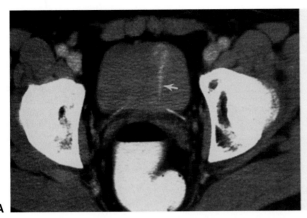 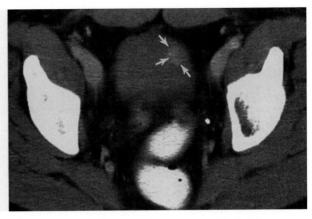

A
B

FIG. 2-14. (A) Helical CT at the level of the bladder, showing ureteral jets. The one on the left is prominently noted (*arrow*). **(B)** Rounded density along anterior bladder represents mixed contrast simulating a bladder lesion (*arrows*).

A definite measurement of the actual vessel diameter to grade the stenosis was impossible. Wall calcifications and the vessel lumen also could not be differentiated with this SSD technique. Areas generally limited in their ability to be evaluated by helical CT include segmental vessels with peripheral stenosis (because of their small size). Moreover, high-grade stenosis could actually appear as occlusions. It has been concluded that helical CT angiography represents a promising screening technique for renal artery stenosis.

Rubin et al. have also evaluated helical CT in renal artery stenosis with 3D techniques (62). They similarly found that MIP angiography was highly sensitive (92%) and very specific (83%) for the detection of stenosis greater than 70%. SSDs were much less sensitive (59%) and 82% specific for similar stenosis. The accuracy of stenosis grading was 80% with MIP and 55% with SSD. Thus the actual type of 3D study performed reflects on the accuracy of the diagnosis. Contrast administered with a power injector at rates ranging from 3 mL/s for 90 mL to 5 mL/s for 150 mL produces excellent 3D studies. To provide optimal timing these authors took a more vigorous approach by injecting a preliminary 10–20-mL volume of contrast material injected at the same rate as that anticipated to be used at CT angiography as a test dose. Scans were used to develop a time–density curve. From this curve an appropriate time delay was calculated. The results demonstrated delay times ranging from 12 to 25 s, with a mean of 18 s.

Abdominal Aorta

We have found that helical CT provides excellent delineation of the presence and extent of abdominal aortic aneurysms. The ability to cover a large extent of the abdomen in a short period of time is extremely advantageous using conservative rates and volumes of contrast. In addition, the relationship of the aneurysms can be established related to the renal arteries, and 3D imaging has been found to assist the surgeon in planning operative therapy.

Spleen

Bolus artifacts in the spleen are a well-recognized phenomenon in conventional CT. They generally appear as inhomogeneous areas of enhancement. This phenomenon is greatly exaggerated in helical CT. Inhomogeneous enhancement may actually mimic focal lesions. Delayed routine or cluster scanning or a subsequent helical scan can be helpful to further evaluate for splenic pathology.

Bladder

Ureteral jets are a common finding on helical CT. Even when the abdomen and pelvis are scanned, images at the level of the pelvis still show contrast emanating from the ureter because of the rapid scan time. We have noted that when the jet extends to the anterior bladder wall, it can create the false impression of a bladder lesion (Fig. 2-14) (60).

SUMMARY

In summary, helical CT requires an appreciation of the pharmacokinetics of contrast administration and the impact made by very rapid scanning. The present discussion focused on some of the more pertinent issues in what will surely be an ongoing evolution in the literature as to the most effective scanning procedures for helical CT.

REFERENCES

1. Dodd, GE, Baron RL. Investigation of contrast enhancement in CT of the liver: the need for improved methods. *AJR* 1993;160:643–646.
2. Dean PB, Violante MR, Mahoney JA. Hepatic CT contrast enhancement: effect of dose, duration of infusion, and time elapsed following infusion. *Invest Radiol* 1980;15:158–161.
3. Kormano M, Dean PB. Extravascular contrast material major component of contrast enhancement. *Radiology* 1976;121:379–382.
4. Burgener FA, Hamlin DJ. Contrast enhancement in abdominal CT: bolus vs. infusion. *AJR* 1981;137:351–358.
5. Claussen CD, Bander D. Pfretzschner C, Kalender WA, Schorner W. Bolus geometry and dynamics after intravenous contrast medium injection. *Radiology* 1984;153:365–368.

6. Miller DL, Vermess M, Doppman JL, et al. CT of the liver and spleen with EOE-13 review of 225 examinations. *AJR* 1984;143:235–243.

7. Lamarque JL, Burel JM, Dondelinger R, et al. The use of iodolipids in hepatosplenic computed tomograph. *J Comput Assist Tomogr* 1979;3:21–24.

8. Long DM, Multer FK, Greenburg AG, et al. Tumor imaging with x-rays using macrophage uptake of radiopaque fluorocarbon emulsions. *Surgery* 1978;84:104–112.

9. Wegener OH, Mutzel W, Soudron R. Contrast medical for computed tomograph of the liver. *Acta Radiol [Diagn]* 1980;21:239–247.

10. Lee JT, Caroline DF, Thornburg JR. A randomized comparison of iodixanol and iohexol in adult computed tomography scanning. *Acad Radiol* 1996;3:5500–5506.

11. Morris TW, Fisher HW. The pharmacology of intravascular radiocontrast media. *Ann Rev Pharmacol Toxicol* 1986;26:143–160.

12. Katayama H, Kozuka T, Takashima T, Matsuura K, Yamaguchi K. Adverse reactions to contrast media: high-osmolality versus low-osmolality media. Presented as a Scientific Exhibit at the 74th Assembly and Annual Meeting of the Radiological Society of North America, Chicago, November 1988.

13. Amin MM, Cohan RH, Dunnick MR. Ionic and nonionic contrast media: current status and controversies. *Appl Radiol* 1993;(Nov.):41–54.

14. McClennan BL. Low-osmolality contrast media: premises and promises. *Radiology* 1987;162:1–9.

15. Katayama J, Yamaguchi K, Kozukat, et al. Adverse reaction to ionic and nonionic contrast media. Report from the Japanese Committee on the Safety of Contrast Media. *Radiology* 1990;175:621–628.

16. Almen T. Contrast media: the relation of chemical structure, animal toxicity, and adverse clinical effects. *Am J Cardiol* 1990;66:2F–8F

17. Spring DB, Quesenberry CP. Cost of low-osmolar contrast media. *JAMA* 1991;266:1081–1082.

18. McClennan BL, Stolberg HO. Intravascular contrast media, ionic versus nonionic, current status. *Radiol Clin North Am* 1991;29:437–454.

19. Palmer TO. The RACR survey of intravenous media reactions: final report. *Australas Radiol* 1988;32:426–428.

20. Debatin J, Cohan RH, Leder RA, Zakrzewski CB, Dunnick NR. Selective use of low-osmolar contrast media. *Invest Radiol* 1991;26:17–21.

21. Levin DC, Gardiner GA, Karasick S, et al. Cost containment in the use of low-osmolar contrast agents: effect of guidelines, monitoring, and feedback mechanisms. *Radiology* 1993;189:753–757.

22. Cohan RH, Dunnick NR, Leder RA, et al. Extravasation of nonionic contrast media: efficacy of conservative treatment. *Radiology* 1990;176:65–67.

23. Dean PB, Kivisaari L, Kormano M. The diagnostic potential of contrast enhancement pharmacokinetics. *Invest Radiol* 1978;13:533–540.

24. Dean PB, Kormano M. Intravenous bolus of ^{125}I labelled meglumine diatrizoate: early extravascular distribution. *Acta Radiol* (Diagn) 1977;18:293–304.

25. Dean PB, Violante MR, Mahoney BS. Hepatic CT contrast enhancement: effect of dose, duration of infusion, and time elapsed following infusion. *Invest Radiol* 1980;15:158–161.

26. Burgener FA, Hamlin DJ. Contrast-enhancement of hepatic tumors in CT: comparison between bolus and infusion techniques. *AJR* 1983;140:291–295.

27. Foley WD. Dynamic hepatic CT. *Radiology* 1989;170:617–622.

28. Foley WD, Berland LL, Lawson TL, Smith DF, Thorsen MK. Contrast enhancement technique for dynamic hepatic computed tomographic scanning. *Radiology* 1983;147:797–803.

29. Young SW, Turner RJ, Castellino RA. A strategy for the contrast enhancement of malignant tumors using dynamic computed tomograph and intravascular pharmacokinetics. *Radiology* 1980;137:137–147.

30. Moss AA, Schrumpf J, Schnyder P, Korobkin M, Shimshak RR. Computed tomography of focal hepatic lesions: a blind clinical evaluation of the effect of contrast enhancement. *Radiology* 1979;131:427–430.

31. Berland LL, Lawson TL, Foley D, Melrose L, Chintapalli KN, Taylor AJ. Comparison of pre- and post-contrast CT in hepatic masses. *AJR* 1992;138:853–858.

32. Walkey MM. Dynamic hepatic CT: how many years will it take 'til we learn? *Radiology* 1991;181:17–24.

33. Zeman RK, Clements LA, Silverman PM, et al. CT of the liver: a survey of prevailing methods for administration of contrast material. *AJR* 1988;150:107–109.

34. Berland L. Additional comment: dynamic hepatic CT. *Radiology* 1991;22–23.

35. Heiken JP, Brink JA, McClennan BL, Sagel SS, Forman HP, DiGroce J. Dynamic contrast-enhanced CT of the liver: comparison of contrast medium injections rates and uniphasic and biphasic injection protocols. *Radiology* 1993;187:327–333.

36. Birnbaum BA, Jacobs JE, Dongping Y. Hepatic enhancement during helical CT: a comparison of moderate rate uniphasic and biphasic contrast injection protocols. *AJR* 1995;165:853–858.

37. Garcia PA, Bonaldi VM, Bret PM, Liang L, Reinhold C, Atri M. Effect of rate of contrast medium injection on hepatic enhancement. *Radiology* 1996;199:185–189.

38. Chambers TP, Baron RL, Lush RM. Hepatic CT enhancement, part II: alterations in contrast material volume and rate of injection within the same patients. *Radiology* 1994;193:518–522.

39. Silverman PM, Cooper C, Mahmud S, et al. Establishing the optimal temporal window for liver CT using a time density analysis: implications for helical CT. *J Comput Assist Tomogr* 1995;19(1):73–79.

40. Suojanen JN, Mukherji SK, Dupuy DE, Takahashi JH, Costello P. Spiral CT in evaluation of head and neck lesions: work in progress. *Radiology* 1992;183:281–283.

41. Napel S, Marks MP, Rubin GD, et al. Angiography with spiral CT and maximum intensity projection. *Radiology* 1992;185:607–610.

42. Schwartz, Jones KM, Chernoff DM. Common carotid artery bifurcation: evaluation with spiral CT. *Radiology* 1992;185:513–519.

43. Moran CJ, Vaniier MW, Erickson KK, et al. Diagnosing extra-cranial atherosclerotic disease with spiral CT. *Radiology* 1991;181(P):162.

44. Costello P, Dupuy DE, Ecker CP, Tello R. Spiral CT of the thorax with reduced volume of contrast material: a comparative study. *Radiology* 1992;183:663–666.

45. Costello P, Ecker, Tello R, Hartnell GG. Assessment of the thoracic by spiral CT. *AJR* 1992;158:1127–1130.

46. Remy-Jardin M, Remy J, Wattinne L, Giraud F. Central pulmonary thromboembolism: diagnosis with spiral volumetric CT with the single-breath-hold technique: comparison with pulmonary angiography. *Radiology* 1992;185:381–387.

47. Silverman PM, O'Malley J, Tefft MC, Cooper C, Zeman RK. Conspicuity of hepatic metastases on helical CT: effect of different time delays between contrast administration and scanning. *AJR* 1995;164:619–623.

48. Heiken JP, Brink JA, McClennan BL, Sagel SS, Crow TM, Gaines MMV. Dynamic incremental CT: effect of volume and concentration of contrast material and patient weight on hepatic enhancement. *Radiology* 1995;195:353–357.

49. Brink, JA, Heiken JP, Forman HP, Sagel SS, Molina PL, Brown PC. Reduction of intravenous contrast material required for hepatic spiral CT. *Radiology* 1995;197:83–88.

50. Silverman PM, Roberts SC, Tefft MC, et al. Helical CT of the liver: clinical application of an automated computer technique, smart prep for obtaining images with optimal contrast enhancement. *AJR* 1995;165:73–78.

51. Silverman PM, Roberts SC, Ducic I, et al. Assessment of a technology that permits individualized scan delays on helical hepatic CT: a Technique to improve efficiency and use of contrast material. *AJR* 1996;167;79–84.

52. Oliver JH, Baron RL. Helical biphasic contrast-enhanced CT of the liver: technique, indications, interpretation, and pitfalls. *Radiology* 1996;201:1–14.

53. Baron RL, Oliver JH, Dodd GD, Nalesnik M, Holbert BL, Carr, BI. Hepatocellular carcinoma: evaluate for biphasic contrast-enhanced, helical CT. *Radiology* 1996;199:505–511.

54. Baron RL. Understanding and optimizing use of contrast material for CT of the liver. *AJR* 1994;163:323–331.

55. Dupuy DE, Costello P, Ecker CP. Spiral CT of the pancreas. *Radiology* 1992;183:815–818.

56. Lu DSK, Vedantham S, Krasny RM, Kadell B, Berger WL, Reber HA. Two-phase helical CT for pancreatic tumors: pancreatic versus hepatic phase enhancement of tumor, pancreas, and vascular structures. *Radiology* 1996;97–701.

57. Cohan RH, Sherman LS, Korobkin M, Bass JC, Francis IR. Renal masses: assessment of corticomedullary-phase and nephrographic-phase CT scans. *Radiology* 1995;196:445–451.

58. Silverman SG, Lee BY, Seltzer SE, Bloom DA, Corless CL, Adams DF. Small (<3 cm) renal masses: correlation of spiral CT features and pathologic findings. *AJR* 1994;163:597–605.

59. Zeman RK, Zeiberg A, Hayes WS, Silverman PM, Cooper C, Garra BS. Helical CT of renal masses: the value of delayed scans. *AJR* 1996; 167;771–776.

60. Silverman PM, Cooper C, Weltman DI, Zeman RL. Helical (spiral) CT: practical considerations and potential pitfalls. *Radiographics* 1995; 15:25–36.

61. Galanski M, Prokop M, Chavan A, Schaefer CM, Jandeleit, Nischelsky JE. Renal arterial stenoses: spiral CT angiography. *Radiology* 1993; 189:185–192.

62. Rubin GD, Dake MD, Napel S, Jeffrey RB Jr, et al. Spiral CT of renal artery stenosis: comparison of three-dimensional rendering techniques. *Radiology* 1994;190:181–189.

CHAPTER 3

Perspective Rendering of Spiral CT Data: Flying Through and Around Normal and Pathologic Anatomy

Christopher F. Beaulieu and Geoffrey D. Rubin

Shortly after the introduction of spiral computed tomography (CT) in 1990 (1–3), new clinical applications of CT began to emerge. Some of the most notable developments have been CT angiography (4,5) and multiphasic and thin-section imaging of solid organs such as the liver and pancreas (6–8). These new CT techniques stimulated interest in nonconventional means of data visualization (4,9) that could take advantage of the excellent spatial registration of successive sections obtained during a breath-holding interval and of the improvement in longitudinal resolution that is achieved with narrower collimators and reconstruction of overlapping sections (10).

Developing in parallel with improvements in CT acquisition technology have been computer graphics hardware and software tools that enable sophisticated image processing and display at a progressively more acceptable performance-for-price ratio. By combining high-quality, volumetric CT data with powerful graphics computers and innovative ideas, a new era in cross-sectional imaging has begun. Roadblocks of the past such as inadequate source image data (thick, nonoverlapping sections with slice-to-slice misregistration) and slow rendering times for three-dimensional (3D) displays, even on prohibitively expensive workstations, have all but vanished. As a result, we can now realistically consider that improved diagnostic information might be obtained by exploring CT volumes with tools other than the conventional review of a stack of static sections. This is a very exciting and fast-moving new era, as well as one that is in its infancy. Although at this time there exists only scant literature to support the concept that the new tools improve diagnosis and patient outcome, the early clinical experience is quite compelling, so that a bright future for the visualization of spiral CT data with sophisticated computer graphics tools seems likely.

A significant recent innovation of the spiral CT–computer graphics era began with the recognition that the spatial position of the observer for 3D visualization need not be confined to locations outside the volume. In other words, unlike the live patient, there are no risks or barriers to penetrating inside the virtual body represented by imaging data. Graphics tools that permit viewing of the data from inside, or so-called perspective techniques, have been rapidly embraced and have stimulated new data interpretation methods that are loosely called virtual reality applications, such as virtual colonoscopy and virtual bronchoscopy. Initial applications of these new techniques appear promising and have generated widespread interest (11,12).

This chapter provides an overview of perspective-rendering methods applied to spiral CT data. Although the fundamental principles of 3D rendering will be covered in Chapter 19, key concepts of perspective are discussed here. Current applications are illustrated for various organ systems, and potential future developments are discussed.

PRINCIPLES OF PERSPECTIVE VISUALIZATION

Volumetric Data

The primary image data (in this context the group of reconstructed cross-sections) are the most basic representation of the patient's anatomy and have a fundamental impact on the quality of 3D renderings. Fortunately, in cooperative patients, carefully performed spiral CT acquisition and reconstruction can result in superb input data in terms of spatial resolution, image contrast, and signal-to-noise ratio (SNR). The physical principles underlying these important parameters have been discussed in Chapter 1. Another key attribute of the input data relates to anisotropy in spatial resolution between the in-plane (*x-y* plane) and through-plane (*x-z* or *y-z* plane) dimensions. Ideally, CT data input to the graphics computer would be isotropic (i.e., contain the same voxel dimensions and spatial resolution in *x-y* as in *x-z*). The practical situation is that even at the narrowest collimator settings (typically 1 mm), the *x-y* plane voxel dimensions are usually smaller by a factor of 1–2 than the *x-z* voxel dimension. This amounts to slightly inferior spatial resolution in the *x-z* direction compared with *x-y*. Wider collimator settings for a fixed *x-y* pixel size result in even further anisotropy in

voxel dimensions and spatial resolution. This issue must be kept in mind when planning a volumetric scan for 3D reconstruction, as it influences the relative amount of in-plane versus through-plane partial volume averaging, which in turn influences the shape and apparent size of objects in the rendering. As with other forms of visualization such as multiplanar reformations, maximum-intensity projections (MIPs), and external 3D renderings, use of the narrowest collimator possible for a given longitudinal coverage and reconstruction of overlapping sections is highly desirable in

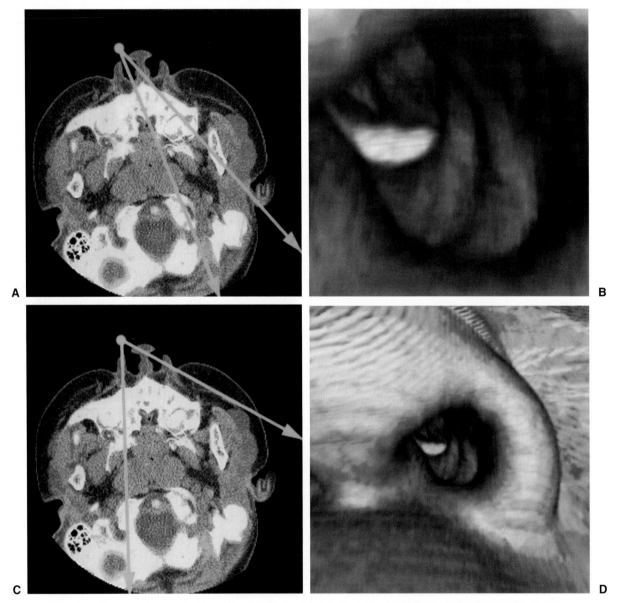

FIG. 3-1. Perspective rendering: effective visual field of view (FOV). Pairs of images representing the axial CT section and a corresponding 3D volume-rendered view are given for three different visual fields of view: 20, 60, and 120 degrees. Images are from a facial bone study with 1-mm collimation, pitch 1.5, reconstruction interval 1 mm, bone reconstruction kernel, reconstruction field of view (DFOV) 18 cm. **(A)** Axial CT section with arrows indicating 20-degree FOV. **(B)** Perspective-volume-rendered (PVR) view showing the nasal passage. Without prior knowledge, it might be difficult to identify the anatomy being displayed. **(C)** Axial CT section with arrows indicating 60-degree FOV. **(D)** Corresponding 60-degree PVR image. Even though the viewpoint is unchanged from that in **(A)**, more of the surrounding anatomy is visible, allowing recognition of anatomic features that represent the nose. *(continued)*

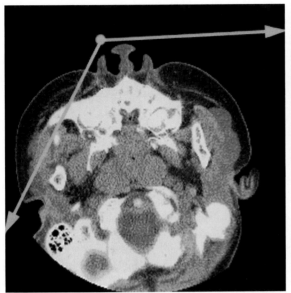

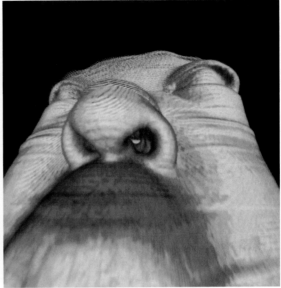

E   F

FIG. 3-1. *Continued.* **(E)** Axial CT section with arrows indicating 120-degree FOV. **(F)** Corresponding 120-degree PVR image. At this wide camera angle, nearly the entire face becomes visible. Image distortion in the form of an elongated upper lip is evident. Similar concepts apply to perspective rendering inside the body, such that a wider FOV allows visualization of more surrounding anatomy and structures close to the observer appear further away than they actually are.

the creation of perspective renderings, as long as SNR is sufficient. Further discussion on these issues is given in Chapters 1, 19, and 20 and in publications by Kalender (13) and Wang et al. (14). Although no optimal acquisition and reconstruction parameters have been established for many of the applications illustrated, those currently in use and used to create the images shown are indicated.

Perspective

Because we have binocular vision, humans perceive the world in three dimensions. Our visual field or cone of vision is approximately 37 degrees horizontal and 28 degrees vertical (15) and is determined by the physiological optics of the eye for reception of light rays converging on the retina. Traditional methods of 3D visualization have relied on the creation of models of the data in which the computed rays forming the rendering are parallel and viewing is as if one were using magnification from an infinite distance. Although this creates renderings that have 3D cues owing to occlusion of far objects by near ones and shading–lighting effects, the observer's effective cone of vision amounts to tunnel vision, a situation in which further magnification gives the impression of moving closer to the object, but spatial context is quickly lost as only a small fraction of the object becomes visible. Such close-up views are difficult to interpret and are in large part the reason that internal exploration of data sets has not been useful in the past. In addition to the difficulties in exploring surfaces and objects from close range, visualization of parallel ray renderings is limited because unimportant anatomic structures may obscure visualization of the anat-

omy of interest. Removal of unwanted structures requires editing in the form of thresholding, segmentation, or manual editing. These processes not only are time-consuming, but may inadvertently result in the loss of important information about the patient or create artifacts that result in misinterpretation.

In art, *perspective* is defined as the means by which an impression of three dimensions is produced upon a two-dimensional plane (15). Similarly, in computer graphics, perspective rendering lends objects in the scene the impression of relative positions, shapes, and distance. Their appearance depends on the position of the eye or virtual camera (the viewpoint) as well as on the observer's *effective* cone, or field of vision (FOV). Perspective effects are created by graphics software that utilizes divergent, rather than parallel, rays to generate the image. By adjusting the amount of divergence of the rendering rays, one can expand the FOV analogous to wide-angle camera lens and capture more of the surrounding scene from a given viewpoint. Furthermore, a wider FOV results in the impression that objects appear further away than they actually are; this is the fundamental attribute of perspective rendering that enables exploration from within the volume and close to surfaces without loss of visual context. Figure 3-1 illustrates the effect of different degrees of rendering ray divergence on 3D renderings of a facial CT study. From the same viewpoint, at a distance of approximately 1 cm from the tip of the nose, rays with wider divergence (a larger effective FOV) show more of the surrounding anatomy and make the nose and face appear farther away.

When perspective effects are combined with other display

features such as color and lighting models, varying a voxel's opacity in volume rendering, or simulating motion along a flight path, one can create images that mimic naturally occurring anatomic scenes, with the possibility for striking visualization of nearly any surface or anatomic feature that has sufficient image contrast compared with neighboring structures. Another useful feature of perspective rendering lies in the ability to change the observer's viewpoint to get around structures that would otherwise obscure the line of sight; this can obviate the need for spatial editing and reduce the risk of information loss and artifact generation inherent to editing techniques in conventional 3D.

Rendering Techniques

Perspective-rendering techniques can be implemented with either shaded surface display (SSD) or volume rendering (VR) graphics systems. Many laboratories have developed their own software for perspective rendering (16–19), and systems for perspective surface rendering (PSR) and perspective volume rendering (PVR) are commercially available (PSR, Navigator, GE Medical Systems, Milwaukee, WI; PVR, VoxelView 2.5/Vitrea 1.0, Vital Images, Fairfield, IA). Although a full discussion of rendering techniques is beyond the scope of this chapter, it is worth emphasizing that the same advantages and disadvantages of SSD and VR that apply to conventional external renderings also apply to perspective rendering with these algorithms (20,21) and that at present no consensus exists on a single most

effective or efficient technique. Shaded-surface displays rely on thresholding of the data to create a model in which a binary classification is made in which voxels are either kept or deleted from the data (9,22). Because the size of the data set is greatly reduced when a surface model is created, SSDs can be rapidly computed. However, such displays cannot simultaneously represent voxels with a range of attenuation values, and artifacts such as surface discontinuities and floating pixels are common. Volume rendering has advantages in that simultaneous visualization of structures with a range of attenuation values is possible (11,20,23), and the effective display of interfaces between structures with different attenuation values can be achieved with few inherent artifacts. Computationally, however, volume-rendering techniques are much more intensive, as potentially all the voxels in the data set are being rendered to create the image. With recent advances in computer graphics technology, volume-rendering techniques have become interactive, with some laboratories having achieved real-time volume rendering of large spiral CT data sets (24). An example of the display differences between PSR and PVR is shown in Fig. 3-2. Endoluminal perspective renderings of the colon effectively display a 5-mm polyp with both PSR and PVR, but the PSR image (at the selected threshold) exhibits surface artifacts that might be misleading for diagnostic interpretation.

Our own experience with perspective rendering is heavily weighted toward PVR. In our early work (11,25) we believed that the superior display qualities of PVR outweighed the disadvantages of needing higher-priced workstations with

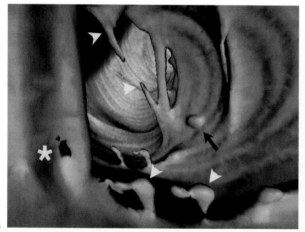
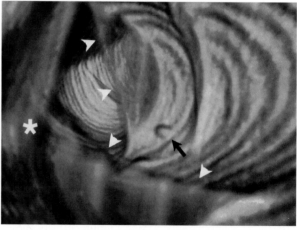

A

B

FIG. 3-2. Rendering techniques: perspective surface rendering (PSR) versus perspective volume rendering (PVR). (**A**) Simulated endoscopic view of the ascending colon created with PSR, threshold −960 HU. At this threshold, haustral folds that are thin and subject to partial volume averaging with adjacent air are rendered as incomplete structures that can take on a polypoid appearance (*arrowheads*). A 5-mm adenomatous polyp is depicted by the *black arrow*. Because of the thresholding inherent in PSR, haustra may also develop surface discontinuities (*asterisk*). (**B**) Same view of the colon created with PVR, with an opacity table that renders the thin haustra as semitransparent (*arrowheads*). Although it depicts the 5-mm polyp as well as PSR, carefully performed PVR is less susceptible to creating artifactual polypoid structures and holes (*asterisk*). In addition, PSR techniques typically compute the surface for a fixed threshold value and require complete recomputation to change the threshold. With PVR, the user can interactively adjust the opacity table to optimize the rendering and see the results in a few seconds.

relatively slow rendering times compared with PSR. The images shown are representative of our work with PVR using VoxelView 2.5 (Vital Images, Fairfield, IA) running on Silicon Graphics workstations (Onyx with Reality Engine or Infinite Reality Graphics; Indigo Impact, or O2 with minimums of 256 MB RAM; Mountain View, CA).

Animations and Virtual Reality

With perspective rendering, body cavities and hollow viscera can be viewed from a unique internal perspective that simulates fiberoptic endoscopy. Indeed, as long as sufficient image contrast is present for visualization, the virtual endoscope has no limitations on what spaces can be explored, unlike the mechanical device. When a series of images is strung together, the series representing a logical progression through the data set—whether through spatial movement, changes in viewing direction, or systematic variation of other rendering parameters—one obtains an animated sequence or movie that simulates flying through the data. To consider that this represents virtual reality has a certain high-tech appeal and may be useful as a familiar term for communication. However, true virtual reality displays assume that interaction with the data is a real-time computation/display experience, with scenes updating many times each second. (What constitutes real time is a matter of debate. The concept is that the scene updates with a rate sufficient to allow user input to be displayed essentially instantaneously, so that a truly interactive environment is simulated. Computer graphics engineers often assume that the benchmark for real time is the standard frame rate for video playback, or 30 frames per second [fps].) Perspective-rendering systems currently in use encompass a wide range of rendering rates. PSR systems are generally the fastest, with update rates of several fps in some laboratories (17,19). In practice, scenes that update at rates as slow as 1–2 fps appear to be useful for simulating motion. With such fast rendering rates, the observer can use input devices such as the mouse, a joystick, or the keyboard to explore a data set interactively. One is limited, however, to the precomputed surface determined by the thresholding operation, and selection of a different threshold requires building a new model. Because of slower rendering rates, varying from about 0.1 to 0.5 fps (image display every 2–10 s, or longer), initial work with PVR required precomputation of animations. To create such animations, the observer selects a series of key-frames that form a logical spatial progression through the data set. Each key-frame encodes a viewpoint, viewing direction and FOV, and may systematically vary other parameters, such as opacity or lighting properties. A scripted animation is created by stringing together a series of key-frames, and the graphics computer then interpolates scenes between key-frames to create an animation that is played back interactively. The disadvantage of this method is that the observer is limited to precomputed views and can only interact with the animation in the form of selecting a playback rate and running the loop in a forward or reverse direction.

In the early work with perspective rendering, it often took many hours of interacting with the computer to simply generate key frames for animation. New tools were quickly developed that allowed a user to point and click on axial sections or reformatted sagittal or coronal sections with a mouse to determine the viewpoint and view direction (VoxelView 2.5, Vital Images, Fairfield, IA; Navigator, GE Advantage Windows, Milwaukee, WI). This markedly simplified the flight planning but left the often tedious job of determining the flight path up to the observer. More recently, a number of semi-automated path-planning tools have been developed that use segmentation of the data and central axis determination to generate automatically the key frames that are used for scripted animations (16,26). Such semi-automated paths may also be useful as guidepaths for real-time interactive navigation, in which the operator could fly along a prescribed flight path, but stop and look around by changing the camera angle or FOV at a selected point.

Since many current implementations of perspective visualization in spiral CT require precomputation of animations, they do not constitute virtual reality in the pure sense. For this reason, we have adopted the terms *fly-through* and *fly-around* as more broadly applicable, encompassing techniques that actually render in real time as well as precomputed animations. In this scheme, a fly-through is usually visualization of a specific organ when confined within the organ's boundaries, and the term *fly-around* describes visualization of an organ from outside its boundaries but from a viewpoint that remains within the boundaries of the volume (27).

Virtual Endoscopy

Some of the earliest and most promising techniques enabled by perspective visualization are those that create renderings that simulate the views traditionally obtained by inserting a fiberoptic endoscope into a body cavity. The virtual endoscope, on the other hand, is not limited by the anatomic boundaries of the body, but relies on natural (or generated, with iodinated contrast enhancement) image contrast for visualization. The chief requirement to create an adequate endoscopic view is a sufficient attenuation difference (image contrast) between the voxels to be viewed and those comprising the viewpoint. The higher the image contrast, the less overlap there is between voxels of interest and voxels one wishes to make transparent. This is true whether the transparent voxels are assigned by thresholding, effectively eliminating them from the data, as in SSD, or by assignment of minimal or zero opacity to a range of attenuation in continuous VR. Several natural situations exist in which the image contrast is excellent for creation of endoscopic renderings from CT data. The roughly 1,000 Hounsfield units (HU) of attenuation difference between air ($-1,000$ HU) and tissues (~ -100–100 HU) provide high contrast and are taken advantage of in such applications as virtual colonoscopy and virtual bronchoscopy. For orthopedic applications, the high attenuation of bone relative to neighboring structures serves as a high-contrast tissue relative to its surroundings. Finally, just as it increases conspicuity in axial CT imaging, the administration of intravenous iodine generates high contrast between enhancing structures and their neighbors.

The Overall Process

Computation of perspective renderings is only one step in the overall process of advanced visualization. For each type of study, there are four essential elements: patient preparation, data acquisition, rendering, and interpretation. Patient preparation may involve cleansing the colon of stool and fluid and air-insufflation for polyp detection, or ensuring adequate hydration when intravenous iodinated contrast is administered for evaluation of vascular structures or solid organs. Data acquisition is a critical phase in which the projection data are acquired and reconstructed into a series of cross-sections. Rendering involves the transfer of data to a graphics workstation and creation of images, whether snapshots, computed animations, or models for real-time interactivity. Finally, interpretation of the newly generated information is necessary, whether the study is for scientific validation or clinical use. At present, there is no consensus on the optimal means of presentation of 3D data to provide the highest diagnostic accuracy. Issues such as the use of color, lighting, and motion cues are relatively foreign to diagnostic radiology, and the individual or collective value of these advance visual cues in depicting normality or pathology is unknown. As work progresses, developing insight into these visual psychophysical properties of these new applications will become increasingly important.

APPLICATIONS OF PERSPECTIVE VISUALIZATION

Colon: Virtual Colonoscopy

The clinical rationale for examining the colon with spiral CT and computer graphics, known as virtual colonoscopy or 3D computed tomography colonography (3DCTC), is that the technique might be able to serve as a tool for detection of colonic polyps and masses that are malignant or premalignant (12). Lesions ≥1.0 cm in diameter are the target size for detection, because the risk of malignancy in lesions <1.0 cm is only 1%, but the risk of malignancy increases to 37% for a 2-cm polyp (28). A technique that could serve as a minimally invasive tool for detection of early cancers could be well accepted by patients and potentially eliminate fatal cases of colon carcinoma.

Initial applications of 3DCTC have relied on patient preparation in the form of an osmotic bowel preparation regimen to cleanse the colon of stool and fluid (17,29,30). Subsequently, the colon is inflated with room air or carbon dioxide through a small rectal catheter. A spiral CT acquisition is then performed during suspended respiration. Most investigators have utilized 5-mm collimation and pitch values of 1.4 (31,32) to 2.0 (29). Studies with 3-mm collimation, pitch 2.0, have also been undertaken (33). Slice reconstruction intervals of 1–3 mm have been used. The general rule of thumb of creating two or three reconstructions per collimator thickness to optimize longitudinal resolution and reformation quality applies to 3D perspective rendering just as it does to multiplanar reformation and conventional 3D displays (13).

Figure 3-3A illustrates the process of selecting a viewpoint within the distended colon lumen and pointing the camera toward a structure of interest, such as a constricting adenocarcinoma in this patient. Figure 3-3B (see color plate 1 following page 48) shows the resulting PVR image, which demonstrates a nodular mass with a constricted residual lumen. By systematically moving the viewpoint along the lumen of the colon and capturing successive PVR frames as a movie, a colon fly-through is created.

Initial reports of the efficacy of 3DCTC are encouraging and suggest that the technique can compete favorably with such existing modalities as the barium enema (31). There is also the potential for the technique to exceed fiberoptic colonoscopy in visualizing the entire colon, because in some series up to 36% of colonoscopic exams fail to reach the cecum (34). In addition, support for the concept that 3D renderings improve the detection of colonic lesions over viewing of 2D cross-sections alone has been reported (35). It is important to recognize, however, that viewing 3D images alone is often insufficient for characterization of a colonic lesion. This is because 3D images are usually optimized to display the colonic mucosa as a continuous, opaque structure, whether created with PSR or PVR, such that the attenuation of the underlying tissue is not apparent on the 3D image. In Fig. 3-4A (see color plate 2 following p. 48), a polypoid colonic lesion displayed with PVR shows the same color and lighting reflectance characteristics as the normal surrounding colon. On axial CT, however (Fig. 3-4B), the lesion is seen to have the attenuation of fat, and the diagnosis of benign lipoma can be made with confidence. In a similar way, evaluating the attenuation characteristics of polypoid foci of retained fecal matter may reveal internal foci of gas, which helps differentiate such a pseudopolyp from a true lesion (32).

With advanced visualization tools and high-quality image data, images with a very broad range of appearances can be created. Figure 3-5 shows an example of how fly-around concepts can be used to visualize a constricting colon carcinoma. The PVR view in Fig. 3-5B (see color plate 3 following p. 48) simulates an applecore lesion, as may be depicted on a barium enema.

For 3DCTC to become widely accepted, all phases of the process—from patient preparation through CT acquisition methods to rendering techniques and interpretation—need to be studied systematically (36). Based on initial experience, we believe that further validation will allow 3DCTC to become an accurate, minimally invasive, and cost-effective colon-imaging method.

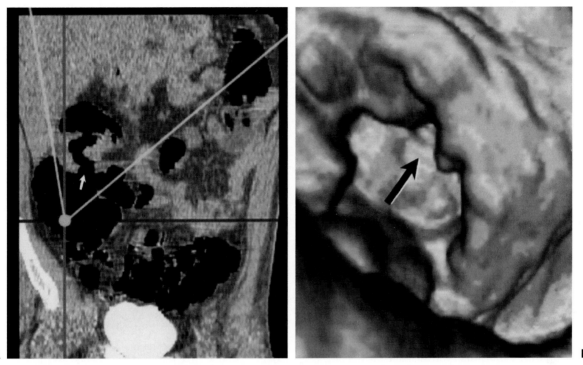

A　　　　　　　　　　　　　　　　　　　　　　　　　　B

FIG. 3-3. Conceptual basis of virtual colonoscopy (3DCTC). Spiral CT data were obtained at 3-mm collimation, pitch 2; they were reconstructed at 1-mm intervals at a 36-cm DFOV. The patient had undergone colonic cleansing for fiberoptic colonoscopy and had air insufflated into the colon with a Foley catheter. (**A**) Coronal reformation through the abdomen and pelvis indicating the viewpoint as a circle and a 60-degree FOV for the virtual camera as delimited by the lines. *Arrow:* Lumen of constricting adenocarcinoma of the ascending colon. (Contrast in the urinary bladder is a result of a preceding hepatic CT acquisition.) (**B**) PVR view of the carcinoma with 60-degree FOV. Note the nodularity of the inner colonic surface. *Arrow:* Residual lumen through the lesion. Rendering a series of images obtained at viewpoints coursing through the lumen, one can create an animation simulating fiberoptic colonoscopy. In this patient, the virtual camera captured the proximal aspect of the lesion and permitted endoscopic views of the cecum; the fiberoptic scope could not be passed through the constricted lumen.

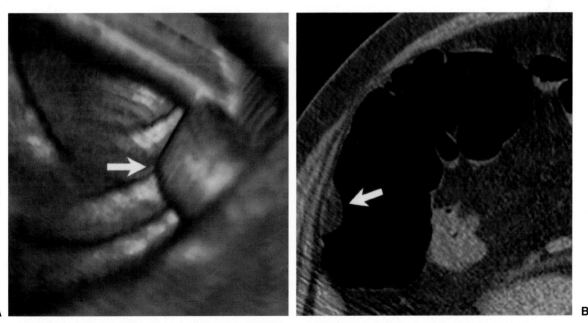

A　　　　　　　　　　　　　　　　　　　　　　　　　　B

FIG. 3-4. Virtual colonoscopy (3DCTC) of a hepatic flexure mass. (**A**) PVR view at a 60-degree FOV demonstrates a sessile, 2-cm-diameter lesion (*arrow*). Since the air–wall interface has been rendered relatively opaque, the interior of the lesion cannot be characterized on the PVR view alone. (**B**) Corresponding axial CT image (3-mm collimation) shows that the lesion has fat attenuation and represents a lipoma. Both surface feature anatomy as displayed by (**A**) and attenuation information in the axial CT section (**B**) are important in characterization of colonic lesions with virtual colonoscopy.

41

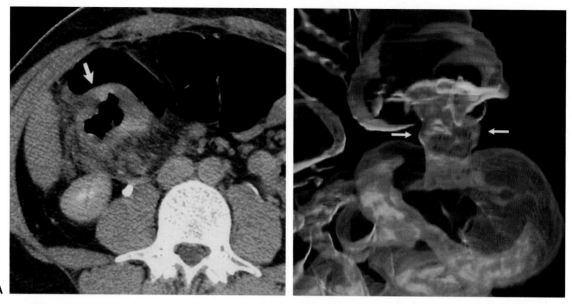

FIG. 3-5. Annular adenocarcinoma of the ascending colon. (**A**) Axial CT section shows annular mass (*arrow*) with surrounding infiltration of abdominal fat. Colon has been cleansed and insufflated with air, and imaged with 3-mm collimation, pitch 2. (**B**) Perspective volume rendering in which only voxels contributing to the air–wall interface are rendered (semi)opaque, resulting in a view that simulates a barium enema of an apple core lesion (*arrows*). A series of such images from different viewpoints could constitute a fly-around visualization of the colon.

Liver

Three-dimensional rendering of hepatic masses is performed in some centers to help guide surgical therapy and assess response of malignancies to medical therapy (20,24). To the best of our knowledge, perspective visualization of the liver has only been applied to anecdotal cases; systematic studies on any incremental value of the technique are lacking. An example of PVR of the liver in a patient with multiple masses due to focal nodular hyperplasia is shown in Fig. 3-6 (see color plates 4A, B and C following p. 48). In this example, high CT contrast was achieved by acquisition of a spiral volume during the arterial phase of intravenous contrast injection. This permitted creation of high-quality PVR images because the voxels representing tumor and those representing normal liver had approximately 150 HU difference in attenuation, allowing assignment of high opacity to tumor voxels and low opacity to normal liver voxels. In general, as the lesion-to-background contrast decreases, it becomes increasingly difficult to classify voxels as either tumor or normal liver, in turn making it difficult (or impossible) to create meaningful renderings without the use of manual tracing of individual lesions. In Fig. 3-6C, a different opacity table has been applied to the same data as those shown in Figs. 3-6A and 3-6B, and a 50-mm-thick volume-rendered slab of the data is rendered as viewed in the conventional CT orientation. This type of visualization combines features of advanced visualization with conventional CT viewing and is somewhat analogous to sliding-thin-slab maximum intensity projection (STS-MIP) imaging (37). With sliding-slab VR, however, an individual image encodes depth information that is unavailable in MIP.

Airways: Virtual Bronchoscopy

For spiral CT of the tracheobronchial tree, no specific patient preparation is necessary, as the natural image contrast between the lumen and walls of airways is on the order of 1,000 HU. The clinical rationale for evaluating the airways lies in the potential for providing information beyond that provided by evaluation of routine cross-sections and reformatted images, and ultimately, in the potential of the technique to replace fiberoptic bronchoscopy in some patients (38). We have experience with approximately 20 patients performing virtual bronchoscopy for a number of indications. Examples of the types of images that can be created using PVR techniques are shown in Fig. 3-7 (see color plate 5 following p. 48).

In a preliminary study by Vining and colleagues, spiral acquisitions with 3-mm collimation, pitch 2, and 1-mm reconstruction intervals were used to compare virtual bronchoscopy with fiberoptic bronchoscopy in 20 patients (19). Although virtual bronchoscopy accurately identified endobronchial tumor in five patients, airway distortion and/or ectasia in four, and an accessory bronchus in the remaining case, suboptimal examinations limited evaluation in half the cases. Summers and colleagues used virtual bronchoscopy with 3-mm collimation, pitch 2, and 1-mm reconstruction intervals to evaluate 14 patients with a variety of airway abnormalities (39). These authors found that third-order bronchi were depicted in up to 90% of cases. However, only 76% of segmental airways were identified. Axial CT and the virtual endoscopic images were of equal accuracy in estimating the maximal luminal diameter and cross-sectional area of the central airways (when the airways could be identi-

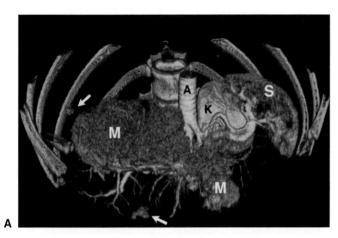

A

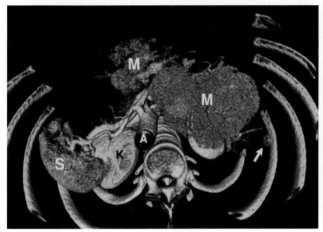

B

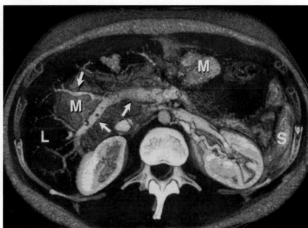

C

FIG. 3-6. Fly-around of focal hepatic masses: focal nodular hyperplasia (FNH). (**A,B**) Two different perspective volume renderings of hyperenhancing hepatic lesions imaged with 5-mm collimation, pitch 1.5, in the arterial phase of bolus intravenous contrast enhancement. Images were created with VoxelView 2.5 with a 60-degree FOV and the opacity table adjusted to emphasize contrast enhancement and osseous structures. Normal liver parenchyma is transparent. The relationship of the multiple masses (M) to the portal venous system can be visualized on static images or when a series of images is viewed as an animation. *Arrows* = small foci of FNH; A = abdominal aorta; K = left kidney; S = spleen. (**C**) Volume-rendered view of a slab of data 50 mm thick from the same patient. In this view, normal liver parenchyma is semitransparent and the relationship of the FNH foci to the portal venous system (*arrows*) is illustrated. Note that the hepatic masses (M) are assigned the same color as the spleen owing to similar attenuation values achieved with contrast enhancement.

fied). Although many investigators rely on 3-mm collimation imaging, we prefer 1-mm collimation with pitch 2. Using this protocol, we can routinely visualize sixth- and seventh-order bronchial branches, as seen in Fig. 3-7H.

There is potential for the virtual examination to replace fiberoptic bronchoscopy in some patients requiring frequent screening for bronchial anastomotic strictures, such as the pulmonary transplant population or patients with endobronchial stents. For initial diagnosis of airway abnormalities that are not detected on axial sections or routine reformatted tomograms, it remains to be proved that perspective imaging of the airways provides an incremental benefit (38). Preliminary studies have suggested that virtual bronchoscopy may aid in planning of fiberoptic bronchoscopy by displaying simultaneously the airway walls and surrounding anatomy (40). By obtaining a 3D mental image of a particular patient's anatomy and disease, transbronchial biopsy of technically difficult or risky areas may become possible. Ultimately, image fusion of virtual endoscopy data with the actual invasive procedure may be possible, and could be helpful for anatomically complex instrumentations.

The nasal cavity and paranasal sinuses are also attractive anatomic structures for perspective visualization, because of high image contrast inherent in the air-containing cavities.

Figure 3-8 illustrates some of the detailed anatomy that can be rendered with high-quality spiral CT data. Such renderings may be useful for planning or follow-up of endoscopic sinus surgery and for teaching the principles of sinus endoscopy to trainees (41). When affordable real-time display of perspective rendering becomes a reality, we should expect further innovations in the form of head-mounted displays, systems to detect collisions with walls or organ boundaries, and methods for realistic surgical simulation.

As with the colon, initial results on perspective rendering of the airways are encouraging. To what extent the techniques will replace invasive procedure is not currently clear, however, nor is the extent to which the 3D endoluminal perspective influences the accuracy of interpretation of the CT study relative to more conventional means of CT interpretation. Ongoing trials at a number of centers are likely to provide some answers to these questions in the near future.

Blood Vessels: Virtual Angioscopy

Whereas virtual colonoscopy and bronchoscopy have their fiberoptic correlates, there is no means of directly visualizing the inner walls of blood vessels with an optical technique, because of the opaqueness of blood. With administra-

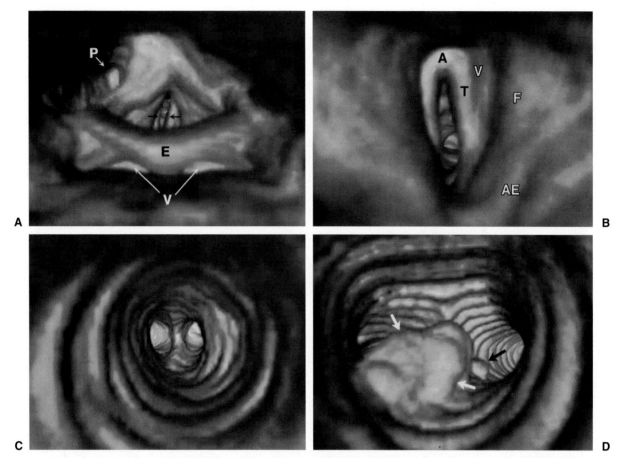

FIG. 3-7. Perspective rendering of the airways. Spiral CT volumes were acquired with 1-mm collimation, pitch 2, and were reconstructed at 0.5–1.0-mm intervals, unless indicated otherwise, and rendered with a 60-degree FOV. (**A**) Orohypopharynx. Supero-inferior view from a viewpoint at the base of the tongue shows the epiglottis (E), lingual valleculae (V), and the right pyriform sinus (P). Further inferiorly, the true vocal cords are seen (*black arrows*). (**B**) Larynx viewed from above. Aryepiglottic folds (AE), false (F) and true (T) vocal cords are seen along with the anterior commissure (A) and the laryngeal ventricle (V). (**C**) Normal trachea. PVR of a scan with 3-mm collimation, pitch 2, shows carina and mainstem bronchi. Corrugations in the tracheal wall may represent normal cartilaginous rings; however, spatial variations in spiral CT noise can also cause a ribbed or corrugated appearance, especially with extended-pitch scanning, requiring that the viewer appreciate spiral CT artifacts and the influence of scan parameters (38). (**D**) Endobronchial coccidiomycosis. Inferior viewing PVR image of a patient with a large tracheal lesion (*white arrows*) and several smaller endobronchial lesions, one of which is shown by the *black arrow*. (**E**) Bronchogenic carcinoma. Supero-inferior view of the left mainstem bronchus shows marked narrowing of the lumen (*arrows*) due to tumor (T). *(continued)*

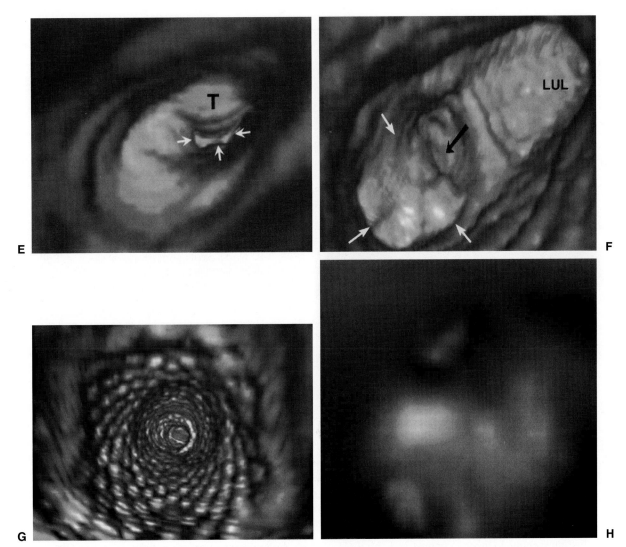

FIG. 3-7. *Continued.* **(F)** Bronchial carcinoid. Lobular endobronchial mass lesion (*white arrows*) is seen in the proximal bronchus intermedius. *Black arrow* = residual lumen; LUL = takeoff of normal left upper lobe bronchus. **(G)** Tracheal stent. Follow-up PVR view (80-degree FOV) of spiral CT in a patient with tracheal stenosis shows wide patency of the trachea after placement of expandable metallic stents. The stent could be assigned a different color from that of the tracheal wall because of the higher attenuation values in the metal, which aids in visualization. **(H)** Small airways. Seventh-order bronchial branching is demonstrated within a subsegment of the anterior segment of the right upper lobe. This level of detail is only possible with thin (1 mm) collimation. ([**A**], [**C**], and [**E**] reprinted with permission from Rubin et al., *Radiology* 1996;199:321–330; [**D**] reprinted with permission from Rubin et al., *Radiology* 1996;200:312–317.)

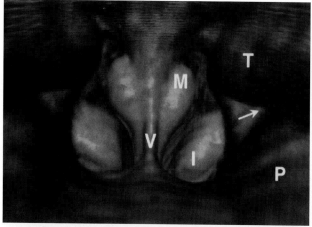

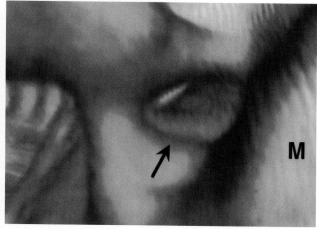

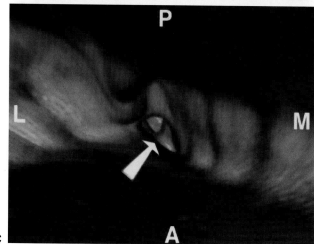

FIG. 3-8. Nasal cavity and paranasal sinuses. Spiral CT volume was acquired with 1-mm collimation, pitch 2, and reconstructed at 1-mm intervals. (**A**) Nasal cavity viewed postero-anteriorly from the upper surface of the soft palate. The midline vomer (V), middle (M), and inferior (I) turbinates, torus tubarii (T), eustachian tube hiatus (*arrow*), and the mucosal covering of the levator veli palatini muscles (P) are well depicted. (**B**) Antero-posterior view of the ostium to the right maxillary sinus (*arrow*) as viewed from within the maxillary sinus. The ability to choose a perspective that looks into or outward from a sinus cavity may be valuable to plan endoscopic sinus surgery or re-evaluate previously operated patients. (**C**) Supero-inferior view from within the right frontal sinus demonstrates the ostium of the sinus (*arrow*). The anterior margin (A) that underlies the calvarial outer table, the posterior margin (P) that underlies the inner calvarial table, and the lateral (L) and medial (M) aspects of the sinus are labeled for orientation. Rendering was performed by Helmut Ringl. (Reprinted with permission from Rubin et al., *Radiology* 1996;199:321–330.)

tion of bolus intravenous iodinated contrast and spiral CT, sufficient image contrast is generated to enable simulated angioscopy (27,42). This technique affords a unique perspective of intraluminal relationships of branch origins and various lesions, such as intimal flaps and atherosclerotic plaques, and, potentially, an improved means of interrogation of stents and stent grafts to determine their relationship to normal structures, adequacy of deployment, and complications. A key feature of perspective rendering as applied to the cardiovascular system is that the time-intensive steps of manual editing of the source CT images to remove unwanted structures can be avoided; if the ribs or other structures obscure the line of sight, one can simply move inside or around them to obtain the desired view. Figures 3-9 and 3-10 (see color plates 6 and 7 following p. 48) illustrate PVR techniques applied to the thoracic aorta and the abdominal aorta, respectively. Figure 3-11 (see color plate 8 following p. 48) illustrates the concept of flying around for viewing spiral CT data from outside the structure of interest, but within the boundaries of the volume. Figure 3-12 shows PVR applied to the intracranial arteries. Such images may be helpful in determining the optimal surgical or endoluminal approach to aneurysms.

Although perspective rendering of spiral CT angiography data provides unique displays, systematic studies need to be performed to show that the additional expense and effort provide either incremental diagnostic accuracy or uniquely valuable means of communication with treating physicians. In addition, competitive technology exists in the form of volumetric Fourier-transform magnetic resonance imaging (MRI) with dynamic intravenous gadolinium infusion, which can also be used to create perspective renderings (43). As computer hardware and software technology continue to advance, we expect that semi-automated rendering and path-planning methods will become available that will allow the efficient creation of renderings from an endoluminal or extraluminal perspective. These renderings can then be compared directly with traditional CT review, with other studies (such as MRI and endovascular ultrasound), and with surgical findings to determine their relative value.

Kidneys and Urinary Collecting System

Pilot studies on perspective visualization applied to the genitourinary (GU) system have been reported. In the uri-

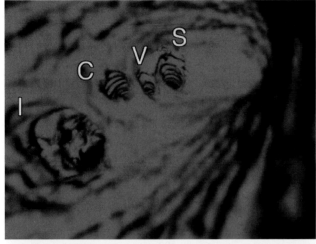

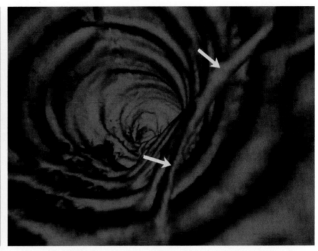

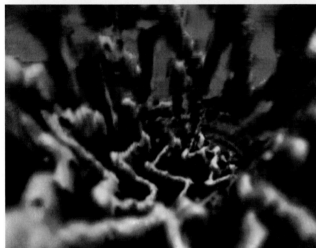

FIG. 3-9. Endoscopic imaging of the thoracic aorta. Images were acquired with 3-mm collimation, pitch 1.5–2.0 during bolus intravenous injection of iodinated contrast at 4–5 mL/s and rendered with perspective volume rendering. (**A**) PVR view showing the innominate (I), left common carotid (C), left vertebral (V), and left subclavian (S) arteries arising from the aortic arch as viewed from the ascending aorta. (**B**) Type B aortic dissection. Infero-superior view from the descending thoracic aorta shows a dissection flap (*arrows*) demarcating the true and false lumina. Prominent corrugations in the aortic wall predominantly reflect pulsatility of the thoracic aorta during the CT acquisition. (**C**) Aortic stent-graft. Metallic struts of a covered thoracic aortic stent-graft can be depicted along the aortic wall to visualize adequacy of stent deployment and the configuration of the aortic lumen.

nary bladder, distention with air, and potentially with iodinated contrast, can be used to generate surface-rendered displays (44) and volume-rendered displays (45) that depict the inner contour of the bladder. Figure 3-13 (see color plate 9 following p. 48) shows a volume-rendered display of a large bladder neoplasm obtained by imaging the bladder at 3-mm collimation, pitch 1.5, after distention of the bladder with air. Systematic clinical studies will be necessary to evaluate if the CT examination could replace conventional cystoscopic evaluation in some patients. One issue that has not been carefully addressed is the efficacy with which CT virtual examinations can depict relatively flat mucosal lesions, which can be nonetheless malignant and need to be detected (44). The ability of perspective rendering, particularly with volume-rendering graphics, to depict relationships of masses to normal structures has been applied anecdotally to the kidneys (45). Figure 3-14 shows several images demonstrating the relationship of a renal cell carcinoma to the kidney and the renal collecting system in a patient with a horseshoe kidney. Figure 3-14C–F (see color plate 10 following p. 48) demonstrates the use of perspective to create images that simulate the view of an endoscope in the renal

pelvis, although mechanical endoscopy from this perspective would not be easily accomplished. In this example, the high image contrast afforded by dense iodine in the collecting system allows creation of effective renderings of the interface between the renal pelvis and surrounding structures, including the renal mass. Where complex surgical planning is necessary, exploration of the patient's anatomy and pathology with multiplanar reformations, 3D, and perspective techniques may improve the outcome. A significant problem, however, is that it is difficult to quantify how such displays change the operating surgeon's mental image or level of confidence when treating a given patient, so that it is not easy to design studies to help validate whether or not the additional effort and expense involved in creating advanced renderings are justified.

Joints: Virtual Arthroscopy

Initial applications of perspective rendering to articular disorders, particularly with MRI (46), have been encouraging. Because the majority of clinical imaging of joints is done with MRI, capitalizing on the ability to supplement

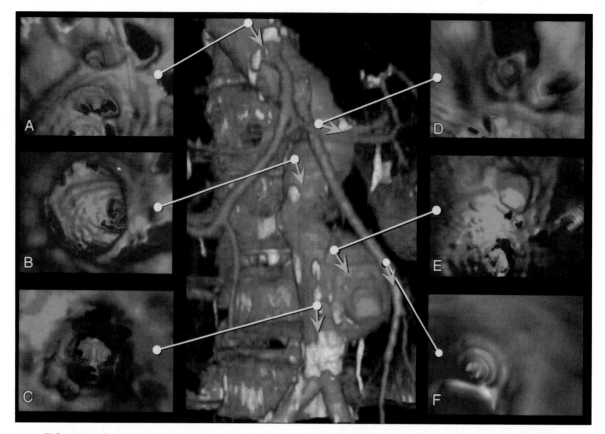

FIG. 3-10. Endoscopic imaging of the abdominal aorta. Multiple frames were captured from an endoscopic fly-through of a patient with an infrarenal abdominal aortic aneurysm performed with perspective volume rendering on spiral CT data obtained with 3-mm collimation, pitch 2, during injection of intravenous iodinated contrast at 5 mL/s. Center image depicts the general morphology of the abdominal aorta. Calcific plaque has been assigned a white color and can be depicted as distinct from contrast column because of its attenuation, which is higher than that of the aortic lumen. Lines with arrows show viewpoint and viewing directions for multiple endoluminal views shown in (A–F). **(A)** Celiac and superior mesenteric artery (SMA) origins. Note foci of atherosclerotic plaque at the ostium of the SMA. **(B)** Mid-aortic view showing plaque and proximal neck of aneurysm. **(C)** Caudal aorta showing aortic bifurcation and heavy calcific plaque. **(D)** Left renal artery origin with ostial plaque but no significant stenosis. **(E)** Endoluminal view of focal ulcer in the anterior/left aspect of the aneurysm. The aortic bifurcation is visible in the lower portion of image but better shown in (C). **(F)** SMA fly-through. Second- through fourth-order branch vessels can be routinely be viewed from an endoscopic perspective provided adequate vascular enhancement. Focal calcific plaque in the distal SMA is seen in the lower portion of the image, and branching is seen in the distance. Renderings performed by Yasayuki Kobayashi.

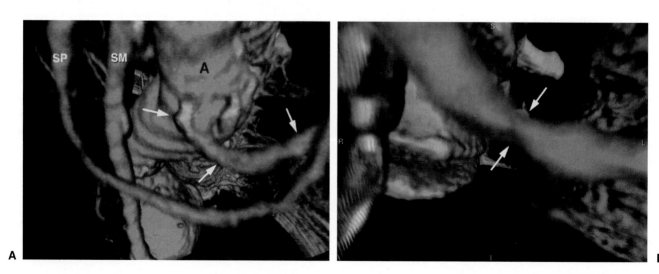

A

B

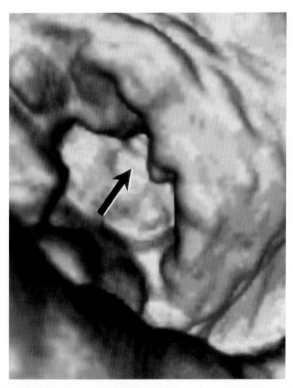

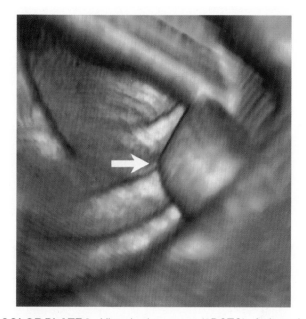

COLOR PLATE 2. Virtual colonoscopy (3DCTC) of a hepatic flexure mass. PVR view at a 60-degree FOV demonstrates a sessile, 2-cm-diameter lesion (*arrow*). Since the air–wall interface has been rendered relatively opaque, the interior of the lesion cannot be characterized on the PVR view alone.

COLOR PLATE 1. PVR view of the carcinoma with 60-degree FOV. Note the nodularity of the inner colonic surface. *Arrow:* Residual lumen through the lesion. Rendering a series of images obtained at viewpoints coursing through the lumen, one can create an animation simulating fiberoptic colonoscopy. In this patient, the virtual camera captured the proximal aspect of the lesion and permitted endoscopic views of the cecum; the fiberoptic scope could not be passed through the constricted lumen.

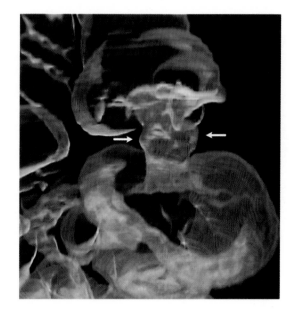

COLOR PLATE 3. Perspective volume rendering in which only voxels contributing to the air–wall interface are rendered (semi)opaque, resulting in a view that simulates a barium enema of an apple core lesion (*arrows*). A series of such images from different viewpoints could constitute a fly-around visualization of the colon.

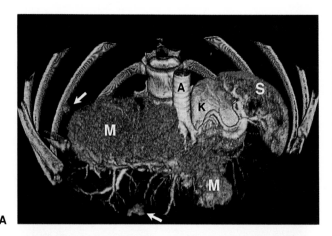

A

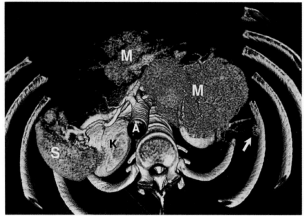

B

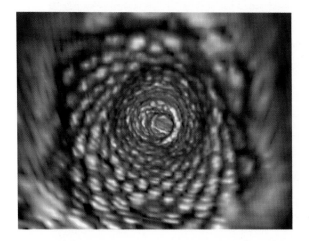

C

COLOR PLATES 4A, B, and C. Fly-around of focal hepatic masses: focal nodular hyperplasia (FNH). (**A,B**) Two different perspective volume renderings of hyperenhancing hepatic lesions imaged with 5-mm collimation, pitch 1.5, in the arterial phase of bolus intravenous contrast enhancement. Images were created with VoxelView 2.5 with a 60-degree FOV and the opacity table adjusted to emphasize contrast enhancement and osseous structures. Normal liver parenchyma is transparent. The relationship of the multiple masses (M) to the portal venous system can be visualized on static images or when a series of images is viewed as an animation. *Arrows* = small foci of FNH; A = abdominal aorta; K = left kidney; S = spleen. (**C**) Volume-rendered view of a slab of data 50 mm thick from the same patient. In this view, normal liver parenchyma is semi-transparent and the relationship of the FNH foci to the portal venous system (*arrows*) is illustrated. Note that the hepatic masses (M) are assigned the same color as the spleen owing to similar attenuation values achieved with contrast enhancement.

COLOR PLATE 5. Tracheal stent. Follow-up PVR view (80-degree FOV) of spiral CT in a patient with tracheal stenosis shows wide patency of the trachea after placement of expandable metallic stents. The stent could be assigned a different color from that of the tracheal wall because of the higher attenuation values in the metal, which aids in visualization.

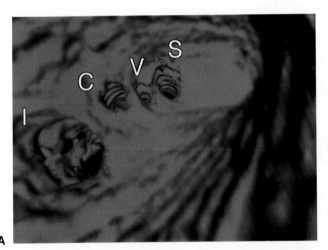

A

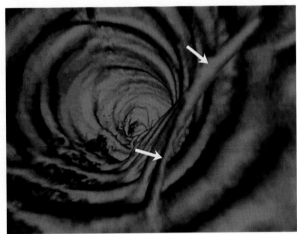

B

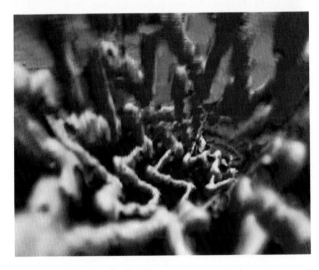

C

COLOR PLATES 6A, B, and C. PVR view showing the innominate (I), left common carotid (C), left vertebral (V), and left subclavian (S) arteries arising from the aortic arch as viewed from the ascending aorta. Type B aortic dissection. Infero-superior view from the descending thoracic aorta shows a dissection flap (*arrows*) demarcating the true and false lumina. Prominent corrugations in the aortic wall predominantly reflect pulsatility of the thoracic aorta during the CT acquisition. Aortic stent-graft. Metallic struts of a covered thoracic aortic stent-graft can be depicted along the aortic wall to visualize adequacy of stent deployment and the configuration of the aortic lumen.

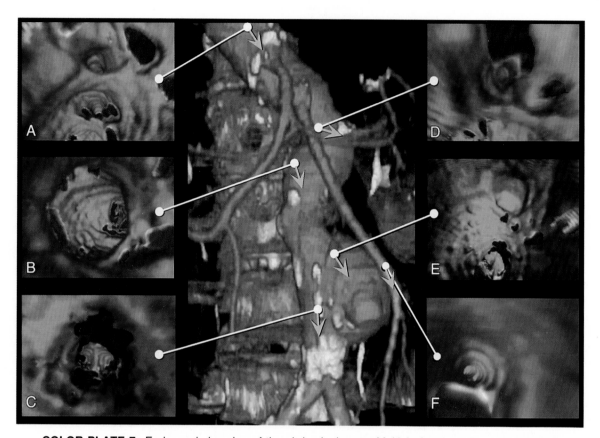

COLOR PLATE 7. Endoscopic imaging of the abdominal aorta. Multiple frames were captured from an endoscopic fly-through of a patient with an infrarenal abdominal aortic aneurysm performed with perspective volume rendering on spiral CT data obtained with 3-mm collimation, pitch 2, during injection of intravenous iodinated contrast at 5 mL/s. Center image depicts the general morphology of the abdominal aorta. Calcific plaque has been assigned a white color and can be depicted as distinct from contrast column because of its attenuation, which is higher than that of the aortic lumen. Lines with arrows show viewpoint and viewing directions for multiple endoluminal views shown in (A–F). (**A**) Celiac and superior mesenteric artery (SMA) origins. Note foci of atherosclerotic plaque at the ostium of the SMA. (**B**) Mid-aortic view showing plaque and proximal neck of aneurysm. (**C**) Caudal aorta showing aortic bifurcation and heavy calcific plaque. (**D**) Left renal artery origin with ostial plaque but no significant stenosis. (**E**) Endoluminal view of focal ulcer in the anterior/left aspect of the aneurysm. The aortic bifurcation is visible in the lower portion of image but better shown in (C). (**F**) SMA fly-through. Second- through fourth-order branch vessels can be routinely be viewed from an endoscopic perspective provided adequate vascular enhancement. Focal calcific plaque in the distal SMA is seen in the lower portion of the image, and branching is seen in the distance. Renderings performed by Yasayuki Kobayashi.

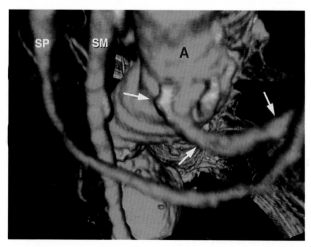

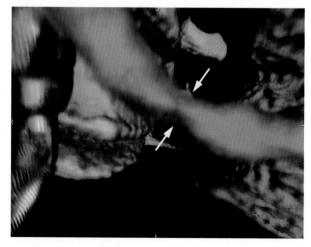

A

B

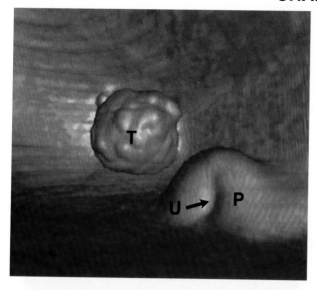

COLOR PLATE 9. Virtual cystoscopy. Endoluminal view (80-degree FOV) of a large, lobulated transitional cell carcinoma (T) obtained with PVR of the air-distended bladder. Spiral CT volume was acquired with 3-mm collimation, pitch 1.5, and images were reconstructed at 1-mm intervals. Prostatic impression (P) is clearly visible, and the urethral orifice (U) is seen. Whether or not such techniques will be sensitive or specific enough to enable screening for bladder malignancies is unknown. (Data courtesy of F. Graham Sommer and Eric W. Olcott.)

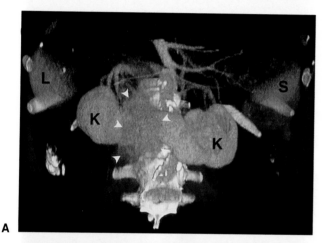

A

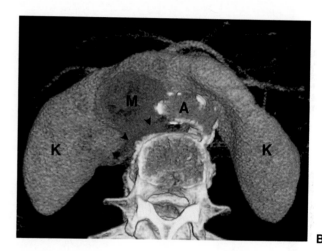

B

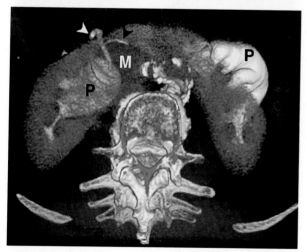

C

COLOR PLATES 10A, B, and C. Oblique, antero-posterior view of nephrographic phase showing morphology of horseshoe kidney with mass (*arrowheads*) in the right moiety and isthmus. L = liver; S = spleen. Infero-superior view showing kidney (K) and mass (M) adjacent to the abdominal aorta and effacing the inferior vena cava (*arrowheads*). Infero-superior view similar to (**B**), but for the excretion phase. Attenuation in the renal parenchyma now exceeds that of the mass (M), which is seen as a defect in the parenchyma. Renal pelves (P) are well delineated and mass effect on right-sided calyces is evident (*black arrowhead*). The right ureter is seen coursing anterior to the kidney (*white arrowhead*).

COLOR PLATES 8A and B. Oblique supero-inferior view (60 degrees) of the left renal artery (*arrows*) in a patient with an infrarenal abdominal aortic aneurysm. Calcific plaque at the ostium is evident. The splenic (SP) and superior mesenteric (SM) arteries are also visible. A = aorta. Antero-posterior view of the left renal artery (80-degree FOV) in a patient with moderate renal artery stenosis (*arrows*). In this case, early enhancement of the left renal vein obscured visualization of the renal artery, so the viewpoint was positioned between the renal artery and the vein, obviating the need to perform spatial editing of the data.

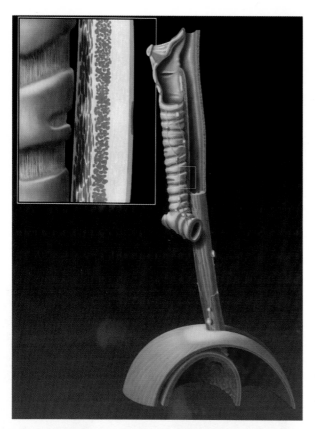

A

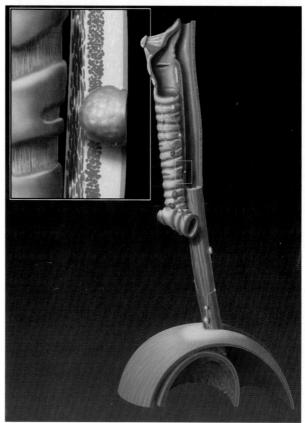

B

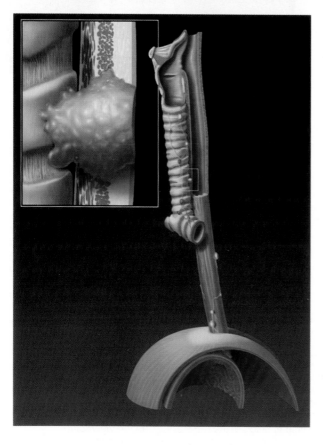

C

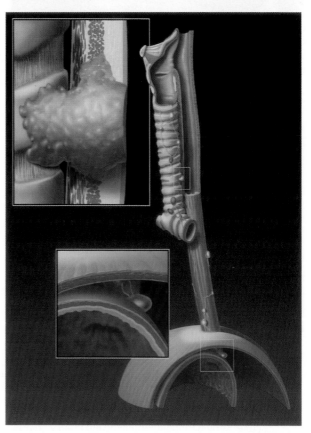

D

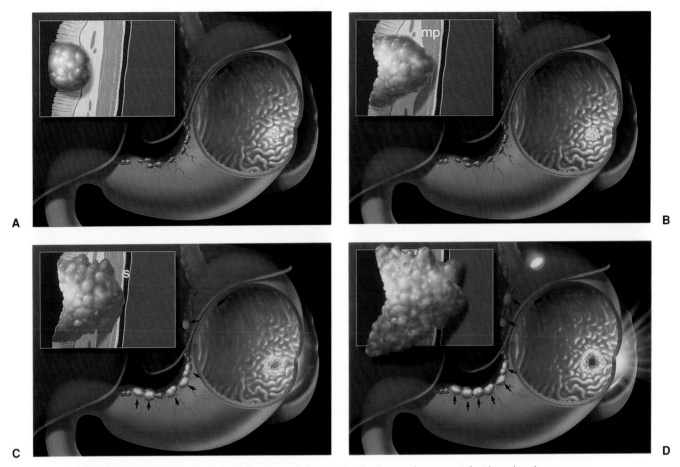

COLOR PLATES 12A, B, C, and D. Stage I. An intraluminal mass is present that invades the mucosa without deeper tumor spread. Stage II. There is greater than 1-cm wall thickness that invades through the submucosa into the muscularis propria (mp). There is no evidence of extragastric spread. Stage III. The tumor invades through the muscularis propria and serosa (s). Enlarged nodes are seen (*arrows*). Stage IV. Tumor has extended through the serosa into the peritoneal cavity. Enlarged nodes and liver metastases are also present.

COLOR PLATES 11A, B, C, and D. Stage O. Carcinoma in situ. Stage II (T2, N1, M0). Tumor invasion into muscularis propria with regional nodal involvement. Note that the nodes in red are malignant while those in white are normal. Stage III (T4, N1, MO). Tumor extension through the esophageal wall with involvement of the trachea. Regional lymph nodes are also involved. Stage IV (T4, N1, M1). Extraesophageal spread of tumor with involvement of regional nodes, trachea, and distant metastases.

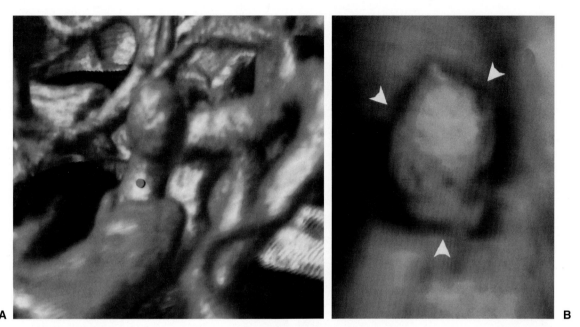

FIG. 3-12. Intracranial arteries. Spiral CT volume was acquired during intravenous contrast administration with 1-mm collimation, pitch 2, and images were reconstructed at 0.5-mm intervals. (**A**) Oblique PVR view of a supraclinoid carotid aneurysm. (**B**) Endoluminal view of the broad aneurysm neck (*arrowheads*) viewing from the point in (**A**) indicated by the circle. Evaluation of the cerebrovascular system with spiral CT and perspective rendering may aid detection of aneurysms and in planning the surgical approach for optimal clipping of aneurysms. (Data courtesy of Michael Marks, Alexander Norbash, and Ramin Shahidi, Stanford Medical Center.)

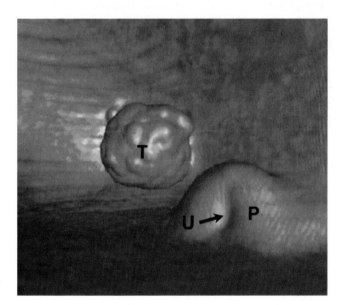

FIG. 3-13. Virtual cystoscopy. Endoluminal view (80-degree FOV) of a large, lobulated transitional cell carcinoma (T) obtained with PVR of the air-distended bladder. Spiral CT volume was acquired with 3-mm collimation, pitch 1.5, and images were reconstructed at 1-mm intervals. Prostatic impression (P) is clearly visible, and the urethral orifice (U) is seen. Whether or not such techniques will be sensitive or specific enough to enable screening for bladder malignancies is unknown. (Data courtesy of F. Graham Sommer and Eric W. Olcott.)

FIG. 3-11. Fly-around of the abdominal aorta. By assuming a viewpoint inside the volume, a unique perspective can be obtained that allows the viewer to move around and between structures to optimize visualization of the anatomy of interest. (**A**) Oblique supero-inferior view (60 degrees) of the left renal artery (*arrows*) in a patient with an infrarenal abdominal aortic aneurysm. Calcific plaque at the ostium is evident. The splenic (SP) and superior mesenteric (SM) arteries are also visible. A = aorta. (**B**) Antero-posterior view of the left renal artery (80-degree FOV) in a patient with moderate renal artery stenosis (*arrows*). In this case, early enhancement of the left renal vein obscured visualization of the renal artery, so the viewpoint was positioned between the renal artery and the vein, obviating the need to perform spatial editing of the data.

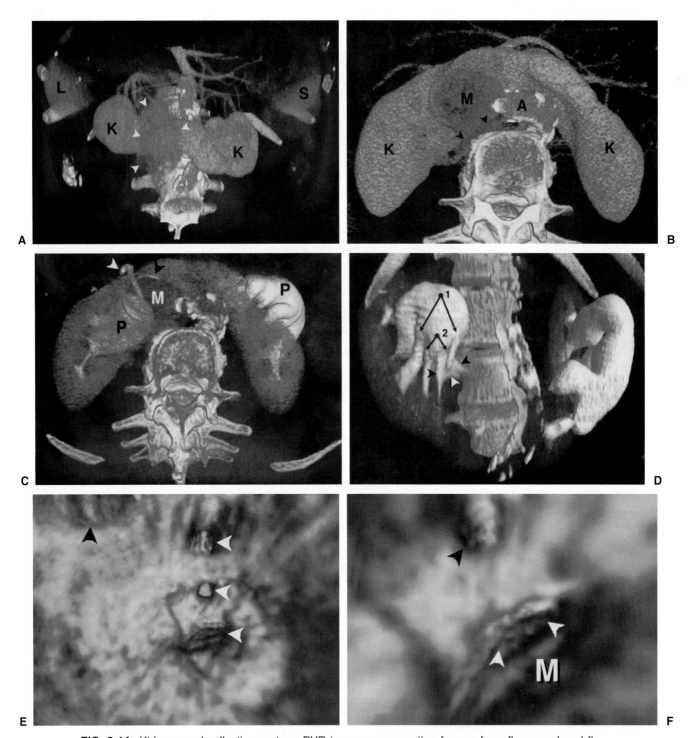

FIG. 3-14. Kidneys and collecting system. PVR images representing frames from fly-around and fly-through animations of a patient with renal cell carcinoma arising in a horseshoe kidney. Sequential spiral CT volumes were acquired with 5-mm collimation, pitch 1.5. at 70 s (nephrographic phase) and 180 s (excretion phase) after intravenous injection of iodinated contrast medium. Images were reconstructed at 2.5-mm intervals. (**A**) Oblique, antero-posterior view of nephrographic phase showing morphology of horseshoe kidney with mass (*arrowheads*) in the right moiety and isthmus. L = liver; S = spleen. (**B**) Infero-superior view showing kidney (K) and mass (M) adjacent to the abdominal aorta and effacing the inferior vena cava (*arrowheads*). (**C**) Infero-superior view similar to (**B**), but for the excretion phase. Attenuation in the renal parenchyma now exceeds that of the mass (M), which is seen as a defect in the parenchyma. Renal pelves (P) are well delineated and mass effect on right-sided calyces is evident (*black arrowhead*). The right ureter is seen coursing anterior to the kidney (*white arrowhead*). (**D**) Oblique antero-posterior view in the excretion phase shows splayed calyces (*arrowheads*) due to the mass. (**E**) Endoluminal view corresponding to viewpoint (1) in (**D**) shows several infundibulae (*white arrowheads*) and part of the ureteropelvic junction (*black arrowhead*). (**F**) Close-up view of infundibulae allows comparison of normal infundibulum (*black arrowhead*) with effaced infundibulum (*white arrowheads*) due to mass (M). (Data courtesy of F. Graham Sommer and Eric W. Olcott.)

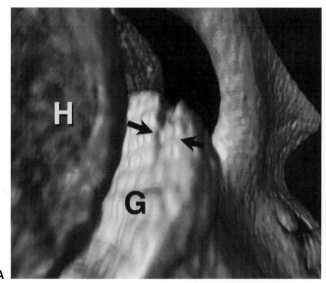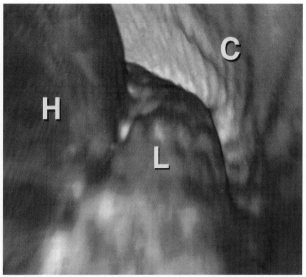

A   B

FIG. 3-15. Virtual arthroscopy. In a patient with subacute posterior dislocation of the glenohumeral joint, a spiral CT volume was acquired with 3-mm collimation, pitch 1, after injection of air into the shoulder joint under fluoroscopy. Images were reconstructed at 0.5-mm intervals with the standard reconstruction kernel. (**A**) PVR image of osseous structures. Opacity table adjusted to render only bone opaque, so that glenoid fossa (G) and humeral head (H) are depicted. *Arrows* denote posterior glenoid fracture. (**B**) PVR image of soft tissues. Opacity table adjusted to render the glenoid labrum (L) and air-distended capsule (C) from the same viewpoint as that in (**A**). By creating an animation that slowly alternates between osseous and soft-tissue visualization, one obtains a unique understanding of how soft-tissue anatomy relates to the underlying bones. Since the normal joint capsule is closely applied to the bones, adequate visualization requires distention of the joint with air or positive contrast.

routine MR examinations with acquisition of 3D Fourier volume data sets is appealing. In spiral CT, there is the potential for virtual arthroscopic examination if iodinated contrast material or air is injected into the joint. Injection of the joint of interest is necessary both to provide sufficient image contrast and to distend the joint capsule for visualization of its surface anatomy. Figure 3-15 shows a perspective image of the posterior glenohumeral joint obtained after injection of the joint with air. In Fig. 3-15A, the opacity has been adjusted so that only bone-attenuation voxels are opaque; a posterior glenoid fracture is evident. By applying a new opacity table that makes the soft tissues of the glenoid labrum relatively more opaque, one can visualize how the posterior labrum is applied to the glenoid and ascertain that there is no significant labral injury (Fig. 3-15B). In the future, virtual arthroscopy with spiral CT may be helpful in communicating results of studies to orthopedic surgeons and in surgical planning, but stiff competition from volumetric MR arthrography can be expected.

CONCLUSIONS

Improvements in scanner technology, coupled with affordable and powerful computer graphics systems, have resulted in superb image generation and visualization tools for the radiologist and clinician. Perspective rendering of spiral CT data may be the best current example, but the concepts may be equally applicable to any imaging system providing

a volumetric data set, such as MRI and ultrasound. Although the advanced visualization techniques do not actually create new anatomic *data* above and beyond the source cross-sections, using these tools to display the data in new ways that more closely simulate natural, 3D scenes may create additional new visual *information* about the patient. This new information can now be created efficiently and affordably, and the current challenge is to prove that the additional effort and expense are justified by improving patient care through more accurate diagnosis, improved patient outcome, or measurably improved communication with referring physicians. When considering the more distant future of computer graphics and spiral CT, we should be limited only by our imaginations in terms of how imaging data will be manipulated and visualized. At the same time, we need to remain ever conscious of the fact that advanced visualization tools can never increase the quality of the source image data.

ACKNOWLEDGMENTS

We offer thanks to our scientific and physician collaborators, including Sandy Napel, R. Brooke Jeffrey, Jr., Vincent Argiro, David Paik, Harvey Young, Ted Slosberg, Scott Mitchell, Christopher Zarins, Craig Miller, James Mark, Norman Rizk, and Gary Fanton. A high level of enthusiasm for our work from the late John Flynn of the Silicon Graphics Corporation is gratefully acknowledged. Support from the Lucas Foundation, the Society for Gastrointestinal Radiology, and NIH grant

RO1 CA72023 is also appreciated. Finally, thanks to our wives Patti and Rhesa, and to our children Marielle and Elena, and Rainier, Magellan, Giulianna, and Elka, who help us keep things in perspective.

REFERENCES

1. Kalender WA, Vock P, Polacin A, Soucek M. Spiral CT: a new technique for volumetric scans. I. Basic principles and methodology. *Roentgenpraxis* 1990;43:323–330.
2. Kalender WA, Seissler W, Klotz E, Vock P. Spiral volumetric CT with single-breath-hold technique, continuous transport, and continuous scanner rotation. *Radiology* 1990;176:181–183.
3. Crawford CR, King KF. Computed tomography scanning with simultaneous patient translation. *Med Phys* 1990;17:967–982.
4. Napel S, Marks MP, Rubin GD. CT angiography with spiral CT and maximum intensity projection. *Radiology* 1992;185:607–610.
5. Rubin GD, Dake MD, Napel SA, Mcdonnell Jr. CH, Jeffrey RB. Abdominal spiral CT angiography: initial clinical experience. *Radiology* 1993;186:147–152.
6. Honda H, Matsuura Y, Onitsuka H, et al. Differential diagnosis of hepatic tumors (hepatoma, hemangioma, and metastasis) with CT: value of two-phase incremental imaging. *Am J Roentgenol* 1992;159:735–740.
7. Bluemke DA, Soyer P, Fishman EK. Helical (spiral) CT of the liver. *Radiol Clin North Am* 1995;33:863.
8. Bluemke DA, Cameran JL, Hruban RH, et al. Potentially resectable pancreatic adenocarcinoma: spiral CT assessment with surgical and pathologic correlation. *Radiology* 1995;197:381.
9. Magnusson M, Lenz R, Danielsson PE. Evaluation of methods for shaded surface display of CT volumes. *Comput Med Imaging Graph* 1991;15:247–256.
10. Kalender WA, Polacin A, Suss C. A comparison of conventional and spiral CT: an experimental study on the detection of spherical lesions. *J Comput Assist Tomogr* 1994;18:167–176.
11. Rubin GD, Beaulieu CF, Argiro V, et al. Perspective volume rendering of CT and MR images: applications for endoscopic imaging. *Radiology* 1996;199:321–330.
12. Vining DJ. Virtual endoscopy: is it reality? *Radiology* 200;1996:30–31.
13. Kalender WA. Thin-section three-dimensional spiral CT: is isotropic imaging possible? *Radiology* 1995;197:578–580.
14. Wang G, Vannier MW. Longitudinal resolution in volumetric x-ray computerized tomography: analytical comparison between conventional and helical computerized tomography. *Med Phys* 1994;21:429–433.
15. West K. *Basic perspective for artists.* New York: Watson-Guptill; 1995:10.
16. Summers RM. Navigational aids for virtual endoscopy. *Radiology* 1996;201(P):248(abst).
17. Lorensen WE, Jolesz FA, Kikinis R. The exploration of cross-sectional data with a virtual endoscope—interactive technology and the new paradigm for health care: medicine meets virtual reality III. *Proceedings.* Amsterdam, Holland: IOS Press; 1995.
18. Jolesz FA, Lorensen WE, Shinmoto H, Atsumi H, et al. Interactive virtual endoscopy. *Am J. Roentgenol* 1997;*169*:1229–35.
19. Vining DJ, Liu K, Choplin RH, Haponik EF. Virtual bronchoscopy: relationships of virtual reality endobronchial simulations to actual bronchoscopic findings. *Chest* 1996;109:549–553.
20. Fishman EK, Magid D, Ney DR, et al. Three-dimensional imaging. *Radiology* 1991;181:321–337.
21. Heath DG, Soyer PA, Kuszyk BS, et al. Three-dimensional spiral CT during arterial portography: comparison of three rendering techniques. *Radiographics* 1995;15:1001–1011.
22. Rubin GD, Dake MD, Napel S, et al. Spiral CT of renal artery stenosis: comparison of three-dimensional rendering techniques. *Radiology* 1994;190:181–189.
23. Drebin RA, Carpenter L, Hanrahan P. Volume rendering. *Comput Graph* 1988;22:65–74.
24. Johnson PT, Heath HG, Bliss DF, Cabral B, Fishman EK. Three-dimensional CT: real-time interactive volume rendering. *Radiology* 1996;200:581–583.
25. Beaulieu CF, Baker ME, Chotas HG, McCann R, Kurylo WC, Johnson GA. Volume rendering for 3D helical CT of the abdominal aorta. *Radiology* 1993;189(P):173(abst).
26. Paik D, Beaulieu CF, Rubin GD, Jeffrey RB, Napel S. Automated path planning for virtual endoscopy. *Med Phys* May, 1998.
27. Kobayashi Y, Rubin GD, Napel S, et al. Intraluminal and extraluminal images of the vasculature: perspective volume rendering of CT angiograms without editing or thresholding. *Radiology* 1996;201(P):316(abst).
28. Hermanek P. Dysplasia-carcinoma sequence, types of adenomas and early colorectal carcinoma. *Eur J Surg Oncol* 1987;13:141–143.
29. Vining DJ, Shifrin RY, Grishaw EK, Liu K, Gelfand DW. Virtual colonoscopy. 80th RSNA. *Radiology* 1994;193(P):446.
30. Vining DJ, Gelfand DW, Bechtold RE, Scharling ES, Grishaw EK, Shifrin RY. Technical feasibility of colon imaging with helical CT and virtual reality. *Am J Roentgenol* 1994;162[Suppl]:104(abst).
31. Hara AK, Johnson CD, Reed JE, et al. Colorectal polyp detection with CT colography: initial assessment of sensitivity and specificity. *Radiology* 1997;205:59–65.
32. Hara AK, Johnson CD, Reed JE, et al. Detection of colorectal polyps by computed tomographic colography: feasibility of a novel technique. *Gastroenterology* 1996;110:284–290.
33. Beaulieu CF, Napel S, Ch'en IY, Daniel BD, Rubin Jr GD, Jeffrey RB. Optimization of CT parameters for virtual colonoscopy. Society of Computed Body Tomography and Magnetic Resonance, Phoenix, AZ, 1996.
34. MacCarthy RL. Colorectal cancer: the case for the barium enema. *Mayo Clin Proc* 1992;67:253–257.
35. Hara AK, Johnson CD, Reed JE, Ehman RL, Ilstrup DM. Colorectal polyp detection with CT colography: two versus three-dimensional techniques. *Radiology* 1996;200:49–54.
36. Dachman AH, Lieberman J, Osnis RB, et al. Small simulated polyps in pig colon: sensitivity of CT virtual colography. *Radiology* 1997;203:427–430.
37. Napel S, Rubin Jr GD, Jeffrey RB. STS-MIP: a new reconstruction technique for CT of the chest. *J Comput Tomogr* 1993;17:832–838.
38. Naidich DP, Gruden JF, McGuinness G, McCauley DI, Bhalla M. Volumetric (helical/spiral) CT (VCT) of the airways. *J Thorac Imaging* 1997;12:11–28.
39. Summers RM, Feng DH, Holland SM, Sneller MC, Shelhamer JH. Virtual bronchoscopy: segmentation method for real-time display. *Radiology* 1996;1996:857–862.
40. McAdams HP, Erasmus JJ, Shahidi R, Argiro V, Tapson V, Kussin P. Virtual bronchoscopy: principles, pitfalls and clinical applications. *Radiology* 1996;201(P):480(abst).
41. Gilani S, Norbash AM, Ringl H, Rubin GD, Napel S, Terris DJ. Virtual endoscopy of the paranasal sinuses using perspective volume rendered helical sinus computed tomography. *Laryngoscope* 1997;107:25–29.
42. Rubin GD, Napel S, Beaulieu CF, et al. Virtual angioscopy using volume rendered CT angiograms. Three-dimensional rendering without editing or thresholding. *Radiology* 1995;197(P):144(abst).
43. Davis CP, Ladd ME, Romanowski BJ, Wildermuth S, Knoplioch JF, Debatin JF. Human aorta: preliminary results with virtual endoscopy based on three-dimensional MR imaging data sets. *Radiology* 1996;199:37–40.
44. Vining DJ, Zagoria RJ, Liu K, Stelts D. CT cystoscopy: an innovation in bladder imaging. *Am J Roentgenol* 1996;166:409–410.
45. Sommer FG, Olcott EW, Ch'en IY, Beaulieu CF. Volume rendering of CT data: applications to the genitourinary tract. *Am J Roentgenol* 1997;168:1223–1226.
46. Feller JF, Rubin GD, Tirman PF, Fanton GS, et al. MR virtual arthroscopy. *Radiology* 1995;197(P):227(abst).

CHAPTER 4

Subsecond Spiral CT Scanning: Clinical Applications with Emphasis on 3D Imaging

Elliot K. Fishman

Spiral computed tomography (CT) continues to evolve with each new scanner introduced, providing specific and unique features designed to either optimize classic scanning protocols or to develop newer study protocols or even completely new applications. Total length of single spiral CT acquisitions has increased from the 20–24-s range in 1993 to the 40–50-s range in 1998. Similarly, initial scan parameters included values in the 140–210-mA range, where current systems provide values in the 280–320-mA range, making spiral protocols similar to standard dynamic CT protocol parameters.

The most recent advance has been the introduction of subsecond spiral CT scanning. Classically, spiral CT scanners complete a single 360-degree scanner rotation in 1 s, which means that the gantry rotates at a rate of 60 revolutions per minute (rpm). Introduction of advanced scanner technology permits the gantry to rotate at 80 rpm, so that 360 degrees are transversed in 0.75 s. This means that 1.33 rotations/s are achieved, with the rotation speed 33% faster. Thus when using subsecond spiral CT we are able to acquire a 33% larger volume with identical resolution and pitch. For example, a pitch of 1 and 10-mm collimation set for a 1-s spiral CT scan will travel 10 mm/s, whereas at 0.75 s the same pitch and collimation settings will travel 13.33 mm/s. With 0.75-s scanners we can cover a larger distance with similar collimation, or we can use narrower collimation and still acquire a large volume of data. For example, by maintaining a 3-mm collimation and a pitch of 2 (resulting in 6-mm/s table speed), we have improved *z*-axis resolution, which yields sharper images and better data sets for three-dimensional (3D) rendering while retaining the capability for large-volume scanning (Fig. 4-1). Similarly, we can do a 40-s spiral scan and maintain a 5-mm collimation and a pitch of 1 and scan 26.6 cm with a 0.75-s scan rather than only 20 cm with classic 1-s spiral CT (1).

Although the concept of subsecond scanning is an exciting

one at first glance, one would be concerned that the CT images might be of lower overall quality or that the images might have increased noise. Herts et al. (2) compared the abdominal and pelvic CT scans in patients with 0.75- and 1-s spiral CT scans. The authors looked at organ sharpness, vessel visibility and enhancement, and possible breathing-related motion. The authors found there was little difference between the two studies and none that was clinically relevant in most applications. Image quality appeared to be nearly equal for both data sets. The typical parameters that were looked at were such variables as liver and splenic edge sharpness, renal edge sharpness, and definition of vessels such as the portal vein, celiac axis, superior mesenteric artery (SMA), and renal arteries.

The key advantage, then, with subsecond scanning revolves around the ability either to complete a scan faster using parameters similar to a 1-s scan or to create protocols that take advantage of the increased length of the spiral study with different parameters, usually by using narrower scan collimation. We can look at both of these opportunities in terms of clinical day-to-day CT operations.

We currently use the 0.75-s scan as our standard protocol for scanning the chest, abdomen, or pelvis. As implemented on a Somatom Siemens Plus-4 Scanner (Siemens Medical Systems; Iselin, NJ), we routinely scan the chest using 0.75-s scans, 280 mA, 120-kilovolt peak (kVp), 5-mm collimation, and 8-mm/s table speed (pitch 1.6). Images are reconstructed at 5-mm intervals. Standard abdominal imaging uses these same protocols. Both studies are done as single-breath-hold examinations. Scanning typically begins approximately 40–50 s after initiation of iodinated contrast injection.

For vascular imaging, such as evaluation of suspected aortic aneurysm or dissection (see Fig. 4-1) or for vascular mapping of the liver, 3-mm collimation, with 3–6-mm/s table speed or 1–2 pitch (depending on the volume to be covered)

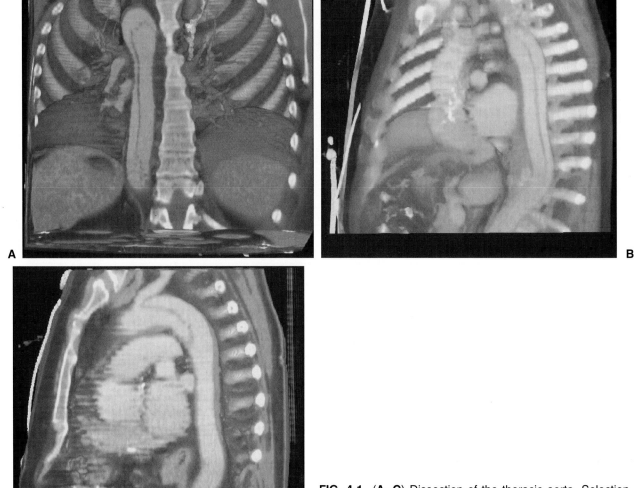

FIG. 4-1. (A–C) Dissection of the thoracic aorta. Selection of infinite numbers of views or projections allows clear definition of the dissection including the extent of the dissection to the origin of the subclavian artery.

is used. With this protocol a subsecond scanner is especially valuable. With the 0.75-s study a total maximum distance of 32 cm is possible (3-mm collimation, 6-mm/s table speed, 40-s study). This is usually acceptable to study the entire thoracic or abdominal aorta in a single breath-hold. This protocol is used for studies of the liver or liver and pancreas, but because the area to scan is less, a table speed of 4–5 mm/s is usually sufficient.

The advantages of subsecond protocols are especially evident with 3D imaging, regardless of whether volume rendering or maximum-intensity projection (MIP) techniques are used. Several recent articles have focused on the importance of scan protocols in generating satisfactory data sets for 3D imaging (3–5). Some of the key factors discussed in these articles includes narrow collimation at the expense of pitch. Thick-scan sections (5–8 mm) are simply not satisfactory for generating high-quality 3D data sets. Therefore we routinely use 0.75-s scans coupled with 3-mm collimation and a pitch of 1–2, depending on the anatomic zone to be scanned. We typically use a pitch of 2 if we couple dual-

phase imaging (i.e., arterial and portal-venous phase) with a 3D acquisition. This is done to limit tube-heat loading and minimize the time delay between the two spiral acquisitions to 5 s. Similar decisions and compromises are made on all scanners, so it is essential that radiologists understand the capabilities of their own systems to optimize the study protocols.

A number of unique applications that take advantage of subsecond scanning are being developed. Space does not permit a review of them all but we will review a representative sampling.

PREOPERATIVE LIVER TRANSPLANT EVALUATION

Liver transplants are used for a wide range of conditions that have caused destruction of the native hepatic tissue (6–8). This can range anywhere from children with primary biliary cirrhosis or biliary atresia to adults with end-stage liver disease resulting from toxins, hepatitis C, or tumor. In

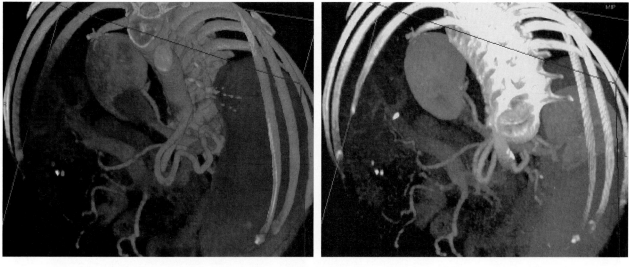

A   B

FIG. 4-2. (A,B) Vascular map of the celiac and hepatic artery. The study of these cutaway views is done with volume rendering and MIP techniques, respectively. Note that with MIP additional rendering is needed to define the aorta and proximal vessels in this perspective.

the classic radiologic preoperative evaluation of these patients, imaging studies--including angiography, Doppler ultrasound, CT, and magnetic resonance (MR)—are done to define several important parameters or features. The first feature is vascular anatomy, specifically the origin of the hepatic artery, be it a classic pattern arising off the celiac axis or variations, including the SMA or directly from the aorta (Figs. 4-2, 4-3). The status of the portal vein and its patency must also be evaluated. Another important component of the preoperative evaluation is to exclude the possibility of underlying tumor, such as hepatoma, in patients who have processes such as hepatitis C or cirrhosis. In many centers transplantation will not be done if underlying tumor is present. Finally, the studies should exclude extrahepatic tumor, because this will make the patient ineligible for a transplant.

We are now performing a dual-phase CT angiographic study of the liver with 3D rendering for vascular reconstruction (9). The study consists of the injection of 150 mL of Omnipaque-350 (Nycomed, Inc.; Princeton, NJ) at a rate of 3 mL/s via a 20-gauge angiocatheter placed in an antecubital vein. Arterial phase imaging begins at 30 s after initiation of contrast injection with scan parameters of 3-mm collimation, 5–6-mm/s table speed, 280 mA, and 120 kVp. This is followed by a second spiral study that begins within 5–8 s of the arterial-phase images and typically is around 60–70 s after initiation of contrast injection. The arterial data sets are reconstructed at 1-mm intervals, whereas the venous-phase images are reconstructed at 3-mm intervals. My personal experience to date has been that reconstruction at 1-mm intervals does give better vessel detail, especially for small branching vessels, which are critical for 3D imaging

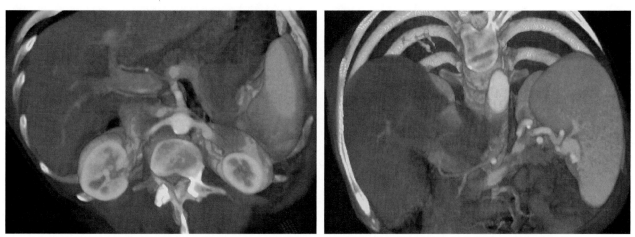

A   B

FIG. 4-3. (A,B) Vascular mapping of a liver transplant candidate. Arterial-phase mapping of hepatic arteries and their branching. Note the texture display of the liver and spleen in the patient with biopsy-proven cirrhosis.

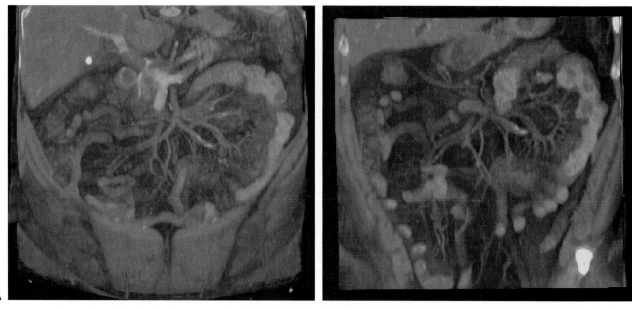

FIG. 4-4. (A,B) Vascular map of the mesenteric vessels. 3D renderings define in detail the branching of the SMA and SMV with colic vessels to the colon defined.

(Fig. 4-4). All data are then sent via the fiberoptic network to a workstation (Infinite Reality; Silicon Graphics, Inc.; Mountain View, CA) for further analysis and 3D rendering. We have examined more than 50 patients and have been successful in all cases in performing the examination. The initial review of our first 50 patients has shown that 20%, or 10 cases, had aberrant origin of the hepatic artery. In all cases, the origin and branching patterns of the hepatic artery was clearly defined. The presence of tumors was noted in five cases, including one case of hepatoma, two cases of hepatic adenoma, and one case of focal nodular hyperplasia. In only one of the 50 cases was an additional study (MRI) requested, and this was the patient with hepatoma, who required further evaluation of this suspected mass. Patient compliance with the protocol is excellent because the entire process, from needle stick to data acquisition to exam completion takes 5–10 min.

A subgroup of liver transplant patients is composed of children who will be getting liver transplants from living donors (10). In these cases, two spiral CT scans are performed. The first is done on the child to obtain a shape and volume of the native liver. The second typically is done on a parent who will be donating part of his or her liver. The lateral segment of the left lobe or the portion of the left lobe lateral to the falciform ligament is typically used. Spiral CT is done for two reasons: (a) for defining vascular anatomy and (b) for determining the volume of the left lobe (Fig. 4-5). By calculating the volumes of liver, the surgeon can determine how much liver should be removed. It would be problematic if the left lobe were removed from the donor and then found to be larger than the fossa from the native liver during transplantation. Simulation of liver shapes for placement into the patient is also possible on computer workstations.

The advantages of these techniques are obvious. Unlike angiography, spiral CT with angiography is noninvasive. Other techniques, including Doppler ultrasound and MRI, have been used for evaluating transplant patients but are more expensive and do not usually provide all the information necessary. Although further detailed work on exam accuracy and cost models will need to be done in this area to determine if spiral CT can replace all other studies, initial results are very promising.

RENAL TRANSPLANT DONORS

Several articles have documented the role of spiral CT with CT angiography in the evaluation of the renal arteries in patients who are potential renal donors (11–12). Spiral CT has been shown both to determine accurately the number and location of renal arteries and to detect the presence of any pathology, including stenosis (Fig. 4-6). An additional advantage of spiral CT with 3D angiography when compared with standard angiography or MRI is the ability to detect incidental renal tumors, which can occur particularly when donors are older.

The role of CT angiography in renal transplant evaluation will increase with the introduction of newer surgical techniques, including laparoscopic removal of donor kidneys. With these minimally invasive procedures the left kidney is usually harvested (13). In addition to the information regarding the renal artery, the surgeon needs information on renal venous anatomy and on the presence of any unusual vessels, such as the lumbar vessels, or any aberrant vessel that may be in the course of the laparoscopic field. Using dual-phase spiral CT with CT angiography we are able to define arterial as well as venous variations (Figs. 4-7–4-9). This is helpful

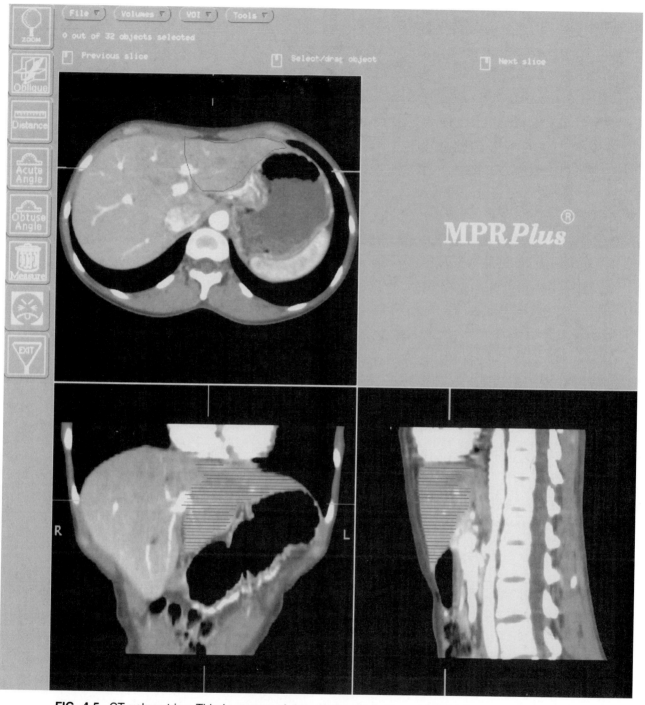

FIG. 4-5. CT volumetrics. This is a copy of the volume study for a potential liver related transplant donor. The volume of the lateral portion of the left lobe was 180 cc.

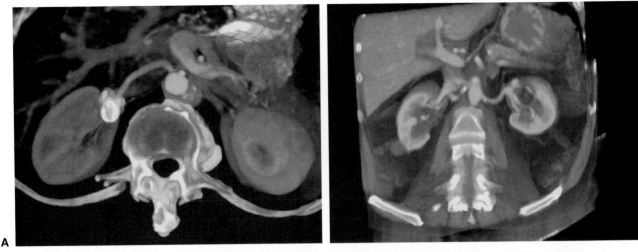

FIG. 4-6. (A,B) Renal artery disease. Two examples of renal artery pathology defined with CT angiography. **(A)** Demonstrates an aneurysm of the right renal artery and **(B)** calcifications near the origins of both the right and left renal artery.

in preoperative planning, including determining whether or not the left kidney can be used as the donor organ. We are currently using this technique and have found it to be successful in essentially all cases; it has become the standard of care at our institution. Our standard protocol is to obtain arterial-phase images beginning approximately 30 s after initiation of contrast injection, which is quickly followed by venous-phase imaging, usually at around 50–60 s after contrast injection began. Scan protocols include 3-mm collimation, a table speed of 5–6 mm/s with arterial-phase data reconstruction at 1-mm intervals, and venous-phase reconstruction at 3-mm intervals. It is important to remember that in the arterial phase of the study one needs to scan from the

level of the celiac axis through the aortic bifurcation to detect all accessory renal arteries.

In these studies all images are analyzed in detail with volumetric interactive 3D reconstructions (14–15). This technique is ideal because interactive editing allows careful definition of renal vasculature regardless of the plane of the vessels. We also find that virtual angioscopy, which allows us to look inside such vessels as the aorta, proves very useful for locating small accessory renal arteries. Similarly, we can study the surface of the aorta, which also will help optimize vessel detection. Our experience has been that looking only at transaxial images may make it difficult to detect all accessory renal arteries. A combination of reviewing the transaxial im-

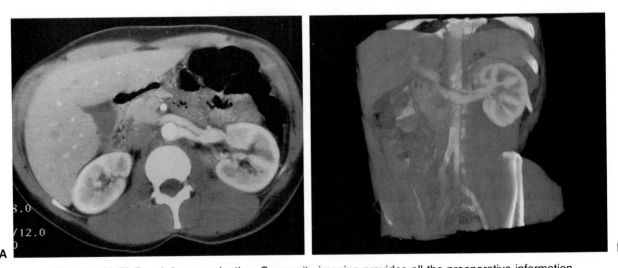

FIG. 4-7. (A,B) Renal donor evaluation. Composite imaging provides all the preoperative information needed by the surgeon. **(A)** Defines a transaxial slice at the level of the renal hilum. **(B,C)** provide a 3D map of the single left renal artery and vein and their normal course. The cutaway angled view shows the left renal vein (*curved arrow*) and the orifice for the single left renal artery (*straight arrow*). **(D)** is a delayed topogram for defining the ureters. *(continued)*

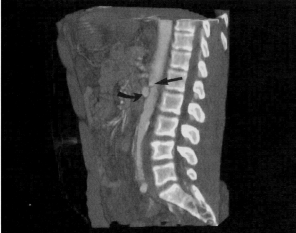

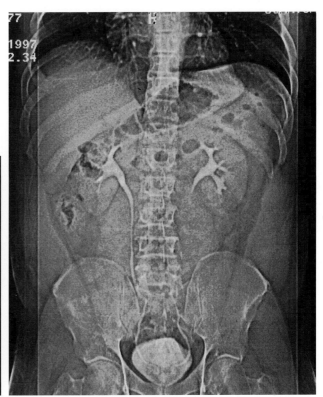

C   D

FIG. 4-7. *Continued.*

ages and the 3D maps has proven most successful. To date, we have studied more than 50 patients with this technique.

PANCREATIC CANCER STAGING

The role of CT in the evaluation of pancreatic cancer is discussed in Chapter 10. The value of spiral CT when compared with dynamic CT is carefully addressed in that chapter,

which details the advantages in detecting primary tumors and in determining the local spread of the tumor as well as distant metastasis to such areas as the liver (16–18). An important role of subsecond scanning is to create data sets that allow the creation of vascular maps of patients who are potential surgical candidates (Figs. 4-10–4-11). In these cases vascular maps generated and defined the appearance and status of the celiac and SMA axis. The presence of steno-

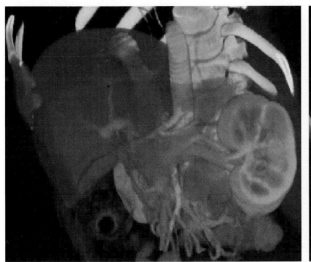

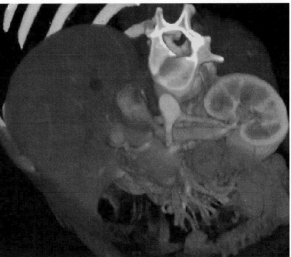

A   B

FIG. 4-8. (**A,B**) Vascular mapping of a renal transplant donor. Vascular map defines single left renal artery and vein with no vascular variants.

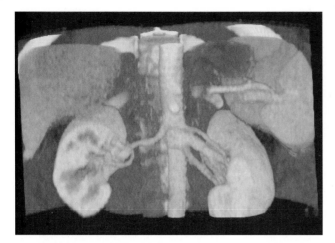

FIG. 4-9. Renal donor evaluation. This study demonstrates two left renal arteries and veins.

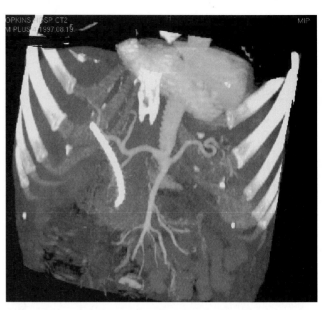

FIG. 4-10. Normal mesenteric arterial anatomy. Three-dimensional with MIP technique defines the celiac axis with the hepatic and splenic arteries. The SMA and its branching are also seen.

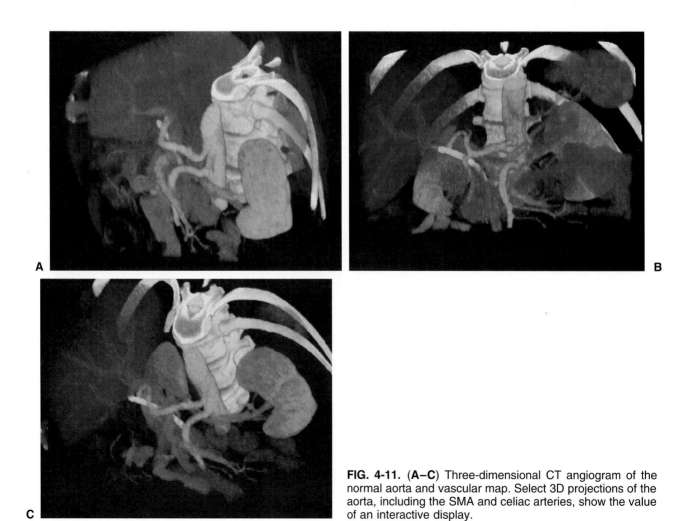

FIG. 4-11. (**A–C**) Three-dimensional CT angiogram of the normal aorta and vascular map. Select 3D projections of the aorta, including the SMA and celiac arteries, show the value of an interactive display.

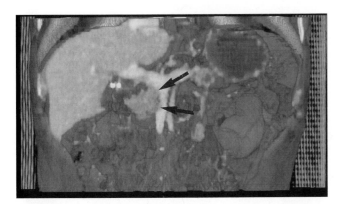

FIG. 4-12. Carcinoma of the pancreas invading the SMV/ portal vein confluence. The patient looked potentially resectable on the transaxial images, although this image clearly defines the tumor invasion of these vessels (*arrows*).

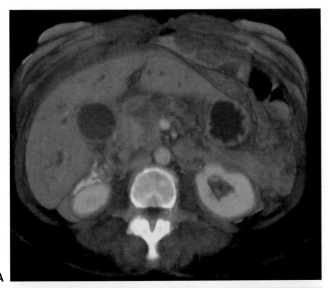

A

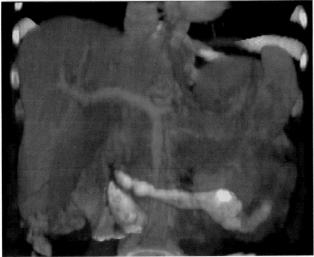

B

FIG. 4-13. **(A,B)** Carcinoma of the pancreas with early portal vein encasement. Three-dimensional rendering defines a mass in the head of the pancreas without vascular encasement. On the coronal plane 3D view the early encasement of the junction of the SMV and portal vein was noted.

sis or encasement of these vessels is better defined on 3D reconstructions than on the standard transaxial images. We believe that with subsecond scanning a single comprehensive examination that both accurately stages patients and helps plan surgery can be performed in less than 5 min.

At many institutions, catheter angiography is still performed prior to Whipple's procedure to define vascular anatomy and look at vessel patency. Classic articles from Freeny et al. (19) have documented that a carefully tailored CT study can determine SMA/superior-mesenteric-vein (SMV) patency or tumor encasement with an accuracy equal to that of angiography. With spiral CT and 3D angiography we can even improve on these results. The 3D CT angiogram provides additional information in equivocal cases that occur when a tumor abuts a vessel and the decision is between tumor encasement and simple tumor/vessel adjacency. Using 3D reconstructions through multiple planes, we have found that this decision can be more accurately made (Figs. 4-12–4-16). We are able to show whether there is or is not vessel encasement. In these cases narrow collimation (3 mm) and close interscan spacing (1 mm) become critical. We believe this technology will become part of the standard protocol for imaging the pancreas in the near future.

PULMONARY EMBOLISM EVALUATION

One of the most exciting and newest applications for spiral CT is the evaluation of suspected pulmonary embolism. The classic use of ventilation–perfusion studies (VQ scans) has always been less than satisfactory because of a high percentage of indeterminate cases, and classic angiography is often felt to be too invasive or complicated.

The potential role of spiral CT for the evaluation of suspected pulmonary thromboembolism has been the subject of controversy since the earliest days of spiral CT. Remy-Jardin et al. (20) initially reviewed a series of 42 patients with suspected pulmonary embolism who had both spiral CT and selective pulmonary arteriography and found that spiral CT could reliably depict thromboemboli in second- to fourth-division pulmonary vessels. Blum et al. (21) performed a similar study and were equally successful.

Other groups, including Goodman et al. (22), were less optimistic, and in their series spiral CT was only 63% sensitive, with subsegmental emboli difficult to diagnose. Their conclusion was that CT had a limited role in the evaluation of suspected pulmonary embolism. Oser et al. (23) helped bring the problem with CT into sharper focus by studying a group of 88 consecutive pulmonary angiograms and looking at the distribution of the pulmonary emboli. They concluded that if CT could only image emboli in segmental or larger arterial branches, then emboli in 30% of patients would have been missed.

With continued improvements in technique there still was continuing optimism. Gefter et al. (24) and Van Erkel et al. (25) felt that the technique had potential especially from the standpoint of cost effectiveness. Van Erkel et al. found that "the use of spiral CT angiography is likely to reduce the

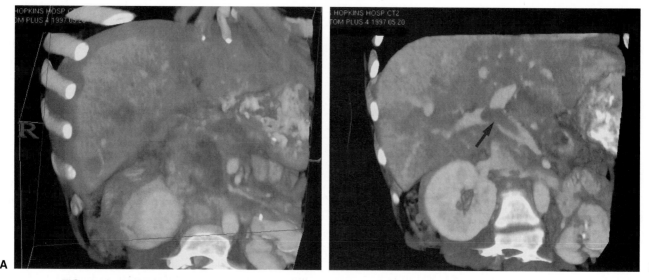

FIG. 4-14. (A,B) Carcinoma of the pancreas with portal vein thrombosis. Three-dimensional display defines the pancreatic head tumor as well as the multiple liver metastases. Portal venous thrombosis (*arrow*) is also well defined.

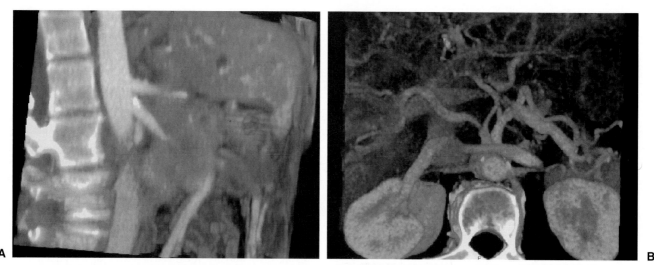

FIG. 4-15. (A,B) Carcinoma of the pancreas with vascular invasion. Vascular maps demonstrate encasement of the celiac and SMA by tumor. Three-dimensional CT angiography provides unique views that can best define vascular involvement.

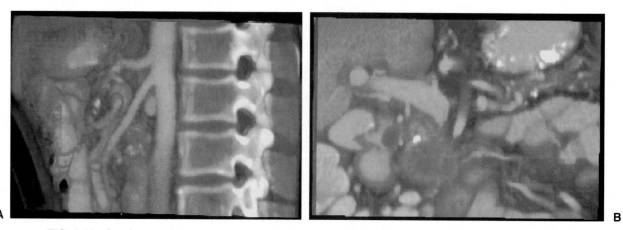

FIG. 4-16. Carcinoma of the pancreas with venous involvement. The 3D map from a lateral perspective (**A**) demonstrates patency of the celiac and SMA. However, on other views (**B**) encasement of the confluence of the portal vein and SMV is seen (*arrow*).

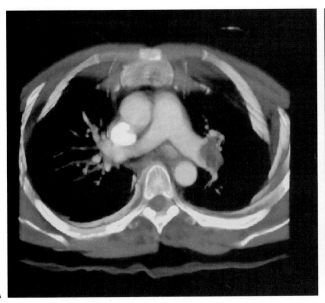

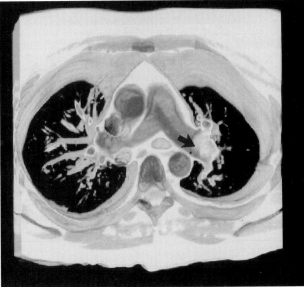

FIG. 4-17. Pulmonary embolism. **(A)** Spiral CT demonstrates a thrombus in the left main pulmonary artery. **(B)** Angioscopic view nicely defines the full extent of thrombus (*arrow*).

mortality and improve cost-effectiveness in the diagnostic work-up of suspected pulmonary embolism.''

Further work by Remy-Jardin and colleagues (26) focused on optimizing the technique for detecting pulmonary embolism by using multiplanar reconstruction. They found that this proved helpful in indeterminate cases, especially for central emboli, by helping distinguish between clot and small nodes. Most recently, they investigated the use of thin-section subsecond spiral CT (27) and found that a technique of 0.75-s, 2-mm collimation and pitch of 2 enabled marked improvement in the analysis of segmental and subsegmental pulmonary arteries. This is the technique we are currently using in our clinical practice (Figs. 4-17–4-18).

Whether or not spiral CT can totally replace classic angi-

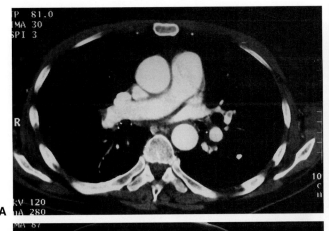

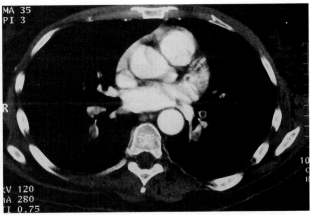

FIG. 4-18. Multiple pulmonary emboli and infarcted spleen. **(A,B)** Spiral CT demonstrates multiple bilateral pulmonary emboli in this patient being evaluated for left upper quadrant pain. **(C)** Global infarction of the spleen is also seen and was the cause of the patients symptoms. A pulmonary embolus was never considered prior to the CT.

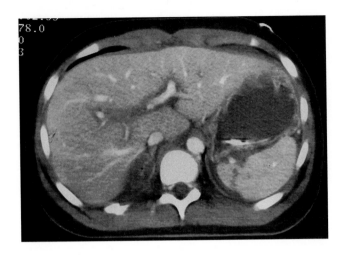

FIG. 4-19. Multiorgan abdominal trauma. Spiral CT defines the presence of right adrenal hemorrhage, a splenic laceration and blood in the periportal region due to a liver laceration (not seen).

ography is still a subject of debate. However, it is a little less controversial to state that spiral CT can probably replace classic ventilation perfusion scanning as the initial exam for the detection of suspected pulmonary emboli. The high interobserver variability rate of interpretation of VQ scans as well as the high rate of indeterminate scans has always made the technique suspect in the eyes of the referring physician.

TRAUMA IMAGING

Details about the advantages of evaluating the trauma patient (28) with spiral CT are discussed in Chapter 18. How-

ever, we can reemphasize that subsecond scanning has special value in the unstable or uncooperative emergency room patient. With a 5-mm collimation and a pitch of 2, essentially the entire chest and abdomen can be imaged in a single breath-hold or acquisition in under 50 s. Even if the patients cannot hold their breaths for the entire scan, the minimal respiration present does not routinely interfere with scan acquisition or interpretation (Fig. 4-19). Interestingly, with subsecond spiral CT and long scan times, the longest part of the study is often the logistics of moving the patient on and off the scanning table and injecting the IV contrast. The actual scanning is an ever smaller portion of examination

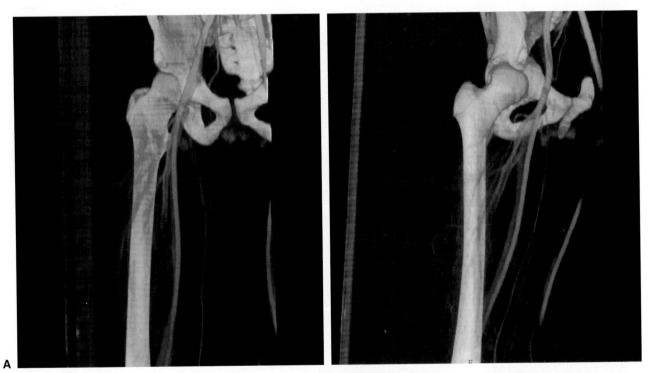

A

B

FIG. 4-20. CT Angiogram of the pelvis and thigh. The study was done to rule out vascular injury in this patient with a gunshot wound to the thigh. Using volume rendering (**A,B**) and MIP (**C**) excellent vascular maps can be generated. The need for diagnostic angiography may be eliminated in these cases. *(continued)*

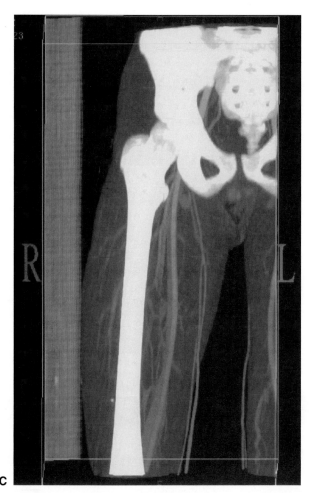

FIG. 4-20. *Continued.*

time. Subsecond data sets even with 5-mm collimation can be used for basic 3D reconstruction, although a narrower collimation would be preferred, as discussed earlier.

An important aspect of trauma imaging is the role of subsecond scanning for 3D CT angiography (Fig. 4-20). Whether it be for suspected thoracic aortic injury caused by a steering wheel injury or vascular injury to the carotid artery or pelvic vessels due to a gunshot wound, 3D CT angiography can often replace classic angiography. The capability of spiral CT for these and other applications is undoubtedly one of the forces pushing for the physical placement of scanners in the emergency room.

CONCLUSION

Subsecond spiral scanning has several significant advantages for the acquisition of high-quality volume data sets, which are of value especially for studies requiring 3D reconstruction or other vascular imaging. At present there are no definite disadvantages using subsecond scanning. The ability to complete the study faster or obtain extended coverage is tremendously advantageous in the angiographic arena (Figs. 4-21–4-22). We believe that subsecond scanning will continue to evolve, with the potential for spiral CT to be accomplished in about 0.5 s. It is important to recognize that true subsecond scanning in the range of 100 ms is possible with electron-beam scanners such as the Evolution Scanner (Siemens Medical Systems, Iselin, NJ) or Imatron (Imatron, Oyster Bay, CA). However, this technology is far more expensive and to date has been less reliable than standard spiral CT scanning. However, with faster subsecond scanning we can expand potential applications, including evaluation of coronary artery stenosis (29) and possible increased accuracy in the evaluation of suspected pulmonary embolism (Fig. 4-23).

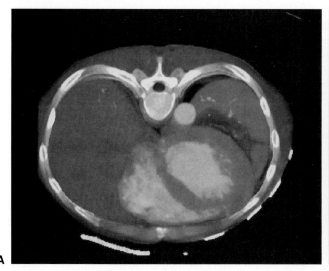
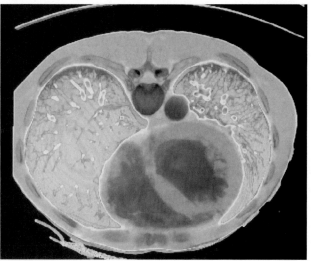

FIG. 4-21. **(A,B)** Three-dimensional imaging of the heart. **(A)** Defines the heart and especially the left ventricle. With varying rendering parameters the internal details of the cardiac chambers are well defined. (Image orientation is as if viewed from above the head, looking caudally.)

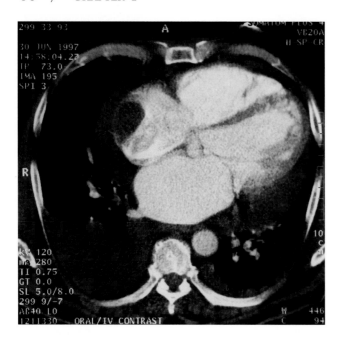

FIG. 4-22. Thrombus in right atrium. Spiral CT demonstrates a filling defect in the right atrium, which was a surgically confirmed thrombus.

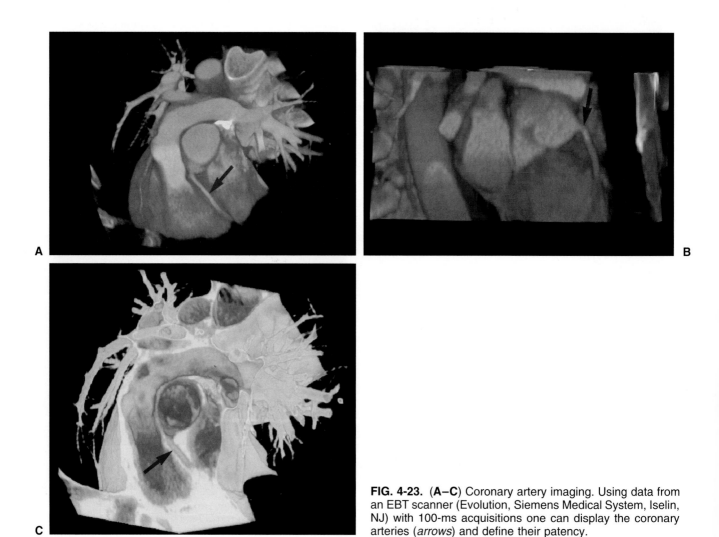

FIG. 4-23. (A–C) Coronary artery imaging. Using data from an EBT scanner (Evolution, Siemens Medical System, Iselin, NJ) with 100-ms acquisitions one can display the coronary arteries (*arrows*) and define their patency.

Nevertheless, we believe spiral CT will continue to advance and, coupled with advances in image processing and computer simulations, will provide exciting and innovative solutions to many of the common problems that we evaluate radiologically in a more comprehensive and substantive fashion.

REFERENCES

1. Fishman EK. High-resolution three-dimensional imaging from subsecond helical CT data sets: applications in vascular imaging. *AJR* 1997; 169:441–443.
2. Herts B, Baker ME, Davros WJ, et al. Helical CT of the abdomen: comparison of image quality between scan times of 0.75 and 1 sec per revolution. *AJR* 1996;167:58–60.
3. Zeiberg AS, Silverman PM, Sessions RB, et al. Helical (spiral) CT of the upper airway with three-dimensional imaging: technique and clinical assessment. *AJR* 1996;166:293–299.
4. Brink JA. Technical aspects of helical (spiral) CT. *Radiol Clin North Am* 1995;33:825–841.
5. Rubin GD, Dake MD, Semba CP. Current status of three-dimensional spiral CT scanning for imaging the vasculature. *Radiol Clin North Am* 1995;33:51–70.
6. Ferris J, Marsh J, Little A. Presurgical evaluation of the liver transplantation candidate. *Radiol Clin North Am* 1995;33(3):497–520.
7. Redvanly R, Nelson R, Stieber A, Dodd G. Imaging in the preoperative evaluation of adult liver-transplant candidates: goals, merits of various procedures, and recommendations. *AJR* 1995;164:611–617.
8. Van Thiel D, Wright H, Fagiuoli S, Caraceni P, Rodriguez-Rilo H. Preoperative evaluation of a patient for hepatic surgery. *J Surg Oncol* 1993;3:49–51.
9. Smith PA, Klein AS, Heath DG, Chavin KD, Fishman EK. Dual-phase spiral CT angiography with volumetric 3-D rendering for preoperative liver transplant evaluation: preliminary observations. *AJR* 1997 (*in press*).
10. Broelsch CE, Lloyd DM. Living related donors for liver transplants. In: Cameron JL, ed. *Advances in surgery*. St Louis: Mosby Year Book, 1993;26:209–231.
11. Alfrey EJ, Rubin GD, Kuo PC, et al. The use of spiral computed tomography in the evaluation of living donors for kidney transplantation. *Transplantation* 1995;59(4):643–645.
12. Rubin GD, Alfrey EJ, Dake MD, et al. Assessment of living renal donors with spiral CT. *Urol Radiol* 1995;195(2):457–462.
13. Ratner LE, Kavoussi LR, Schulam PG, et al. Comparison of laparoscopic live donor nephrectomy versus the standard open approach. *Transplantation* 1997;29:138–139.
14. Smith PA, Marshall FF, Fishman EK. Spiral CT evaluation of the kidneys: state of the art. *Urology* 1998;51(1):3–11.
15. Smith PA, Urban BA, Marshall FF, Heath DG, Fishman EK. Three-dimensional CT stereoscopic visualization of renal masses: impact on diagnosis and patient management. *AJR* 1997;169:1331–1334.
16. Novick SL, Fishman EK. Three-dimensional CT angiography of pancreatic carcinoma: role in staging extent of disease. *AJR* 1998;170: 139–143.
17. Fishman EK, Wyatt SH, Ney DR, Kuhlman JE, Siegelman SS. Spiral CT of the pancreas with multiplanar display. *AJR* 1992;159: 1209–1215.
18. Bluemke DA, Cameron JL, Hruban RH, et al. Potentially resectable pancreatic adenocarcinoma: spiral CT assessment with surgical and pathologic correlation. *Radiology* 1995;197:381–385.
19. Nghiem HV, Freeny PC. Radiologic staging of pancreatic adenocarcinoma. *Radiol Clin North Am* 1994;32:71–79.
20. Remy-Jardin M, Remy J, Wattinne L, Giraud F. Central pulmonary thromboembolism: diagnosis with spiral volumetric CT with the single-breath-hold technique: comparison with pulmonary angiography. *Radiology* 1992;185:381–387.
21. Blum AG, Delfau F, Grignon B, et al. Spiral-computed tomography versus pulmonary angiography in the diagnosis of acute massive pulmonary embolism. *Am J Cardiol* 1994;74:96–98.
22. Goodman LR, Curtin JJ, Mewissen MW, et al. Detection of pulmonary embolism in patients with unresolved clinical and scintigraphic diagnosis: helical CT versus angiography. *AJR* 1995;164:1369–1374.
23. Oser RF, Zuckerman DA, Gutierrez FR, Brink JA. Anatomic distribution of pulmonary emboli at pulmonary angiography: implications for cross-sectional imaging. *Radiology* 1996;199:31–35.
24. Gefter WB, Hatabu H, Holland GA, et al. Pulmonary thromboembolism: recent developments in diagnosis with CT and MR imaging. *Radiology* 1995;197:561–574.
25. Van Erkel AR, van Rossum AB, Bloem JL, Kievit J, Pattynama PMT. Spiral CT angiography for suspected pulmonary embolism: a cost-effectiveness analysis. *Radiology* 1996;201:29–36.
26. Remy-Jardin M, Remy J, Cauvain O, Petyt L, Wannebroucq J, Beregi JP. Diagnosis of central pulmonary embolism with helical CT: role of two-dimensional multiplanar reformations. *AJR* 1995;165:1131–1138.
27. Remy-Jardin M, Remy J, Artaud D, Deschildre F, Duhamel A. Peripheral pulmonary arteries: optimization of the spiral CT acquisition protocol. *Radiology* 1997;204:157–163.
28. Pretorius ES, Fishman EK. Spiral computed tomography of upper abdominal trauma. *Emer Radiol* 1995;2(5):285–289.
29. Achenbach S, Moshage W, Ropers D, et al. Noninvasive, three-dimensional visualization of coronary artery bypass grafts by electron beam tomography. *Am J Cardiol* 1997;79:856–861.

PART 2

Chest Applications

CHAPTER 5

Spiral CT: Thorax Applications

Janet E. Kuhlman

Spiral CT has revolutionized the way in which chest disorders are evaluated. With spiral CT, continuous table feed and synchronous data acquisition generate a volumetric acquisition that can be performed during a single breath-hold (1–3). By comparison, conventional CT is limited in the chest by variations in respiratory effort that can occur between each CT slice and create interscan gaps. This chapter reviews the advantages and disadvantages of using spiral CT for chest imaging. Operator-defined choices for section thickness, table speed, pitch, and reconstruction algorithms, as well as guidelines for contrast administration, are discussed in depth. Emphasis is placed on spiral CT approaches to specific chest problems, including: (a) evaluation of solitary and multiple pulmonary nodules, (b) assessment of the airways, (c) evaluation of peridiaphragmatic problems, (d) vascular assessment, (e) tumor staging, and (f) 2D/3D imaging of the lung and chest wall.

LIMITATIONS OF CONVENTIONAL CT FOR CHEST IMAGING

Conventional slice-by-slice CT has major limitations in the evaluation of chest disorders (3). The traditional stepwise technique with interscan delays of 3–10 s between axial slices often results in slice misregistration because of respiratory variations in depth of inspiration from one CT slice acquisition to the next. Slice misregistration, patient motion, and partial volume averaging with conventional CT increase the likelihood of missing significant pathology in the lung (3) (Fig. 5-1). Slice misregistration and motion artifacts also significantly degrade the quality of multiplanar and three-dimensional (3D) image reconstruction of the lung (3).

ADVANTAGES OF SPIRAL CT FOR CHEST IMAGING

Spiral CT is essentially a gapless scanning technique. Volume acquisition eliminates discontinuities between slices

(1,2). Spiral CT performed during a single breath-hold further limits respiratory motion (1,2). The resulting data set allows the generation of superior multiplanar and 3D images. An added benefit of spiral CT is that the faster scanning times eliminate delays during intravenous contrast injection, allowing for superior vascular enhancement with smaller amounts of intravenous contrast (2–5).

SPIRAL TECHNIQUE

Spiral CT Options for Chest Imaging

The optimal, single best spiral CT protocol for imaging the chest has yet to be determined. Indeed, one of the major advantages of spiral CT scanning is the increased flexibility that this mode of acquisition allows. When performing spiral CT examinations of the chest, the radiologist has a number of new parameters to manipulate compared with conventional CT scanning, including linear interpolation algorithms, reconstruction algorithms, slice acquisition thickness, slice reconstruction interval, table speed, duration of scan, and single versus variable mode of acquisition. By optimizing each of these parameters, the CT radiologist can customize a spiral CT examination by taking into account patient and equipment factors as well as the particulars of the chest problem to be investigated.

Linear Interpolation Algorithms

Image generation in spiral CT is accomplished through a process of linear interpolation that reconstructs planar images from the raw spiral data. The first generation of spiral CT scanners used a 360-degree linear interpolation algorithm. These older algorithms have now been replaced by newer, improved 180-degree linear interpolation algorithms that result in less broadening of the section sensitivity profile and less blurring of the images (6).

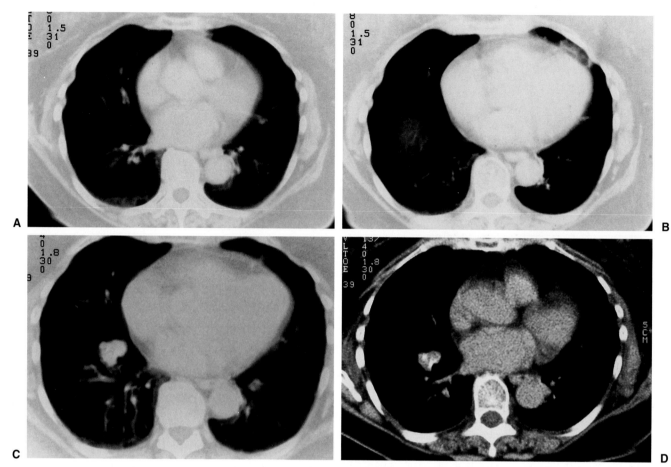

FIG. 5-1. **(A,B)** Conventional 8-mm × 8-mm CT scans obtained in a patient referred for evaluation of a right lower lobe nodule seen on plain films. These scans failed to identify the nodule **(C,D)**. A repeat spiral CT through the area of suspicion was performed using a 4-mm slice collimation, pitch of 1, with images reconstructed every 2 mm. The spiral CT demonstrates a relatively large nodule with scattered calcifications completely missed by the conventional CT because of respiratory variability between consecutive slices. Single-breath-hold techniques used with spiral CT eliminate this problem and facilitate pulmonary nodule evaluation.

Reconstruction Algorithms

Depending on the manufacturer, a number of image display reconstruction algorithms are also available. A standard or soft-tissue algorithm is usually chosen for display of soft-tissue structures of the mediastinum and chest wall, whereas a lung algorithm is preferable for displaying the lung parenchyma. Newer high-resolution lung algorithms available on some manufacturer's scanners, dramatically improve image quality for lung detail.

Reconstruction Interval

The interval at which each planar CT image is reconstructed (i.e., the degree of overlap between reconstructed axial images and the reconstruction incrementation) is a new spiral CT parameter that must be designated by the operator. For example, each 10-mm-thick slice may be reconstructed

every 10 mm with no overlap or every 5 mm, giving an overlap of 5 mm. As a general rule when performing chest studies, we have found reconstructing images at an interval that is one-half the slice thickness (two images per slice incrementation) increases the information gained from the spiral CT data set. Little additional information is gained by reconstructing at closer intervals, unless one is performing CT angiography or multidimensional imaging. Most authors agree that for most studies one or two images per slice incrementation are more than adequate for routine studies, whereas closer reconstruction intervals with three or four images may be preferred for multiplanar imaging (7–9). Reconstructing images at closer intervals increases the number of images that must be filmed and reviewed, increasing both the dollar and time cost of the examination (7). Some of the additional filming expense can be curtailed, however, by viewing the spiral study on an independent console rather than on hard-copy images.

KVP, mA, Duration of Spiral Scan, Scanning Mode

Specific spiral CT scanning parameters, such as kilovolt peak (kVp) and milliampere (mA) settings, vary by manufacturer and should be adjusted for patient characteristics. The maximum spiral imaging time for one spiral acquisition or the duration of scan depends on the manufacturer's available x-ray tube power and the patient's ability to hold his or her breath (7). The option to perform only a single spiral CT acquisition versus multiple spiral acquisitions in rapid succession—so-called variable-mode spiral CT—also varies among manufacturers. In variable-mode spiral CT, a series of shorter spiral CT acquisitions can be preprogrammed to be acquired sequentially with short breaks between the acquisitions to allow the patient to breathe (7,10–12). This mode of scanning is preferable for patients who cannot hold their breath for the extended 24–40 s required for a single-acquisition spiral scan. It is also ideal for combined chest and abdomen studies that use a single injection of intravenous contrast, as is often employed when screening cancer patients for lung and liver metastases. Variable-mode spiral CT allows both the pulmonary hila and the liver to be imaged during their optimal phases of the contrast enhancement (11,12).

Slice Acquisition Thickness and Table Speed

Slice acquisition thickness or beam collimation can be varied from 1 to 10 mm in thickness on most spiral CT scanners. Table speed can also be varied from 1 to 10 mm/s. Choice of slice thickness and table speed depends on the clinical question of concern and determines the pitch that is used.

Pitch

Pitch is defined as the "table feed distance per 360-degree tube rotation divided by the nominal section thickness." Because each 360-degree rotation occurs in 1 s,

$$\text{Pitch} = \text{Table speed/Slice thickness}$$

Using a pitch of 1 is generally a good compromise in the chest to achieve adequate area coverage with a minimum of z-axis blurring. A pitch of more than 1 is valuable if a larger volume needs to be covered in a single breath-hold acquisition (7).

Increasing pitch widens the section-sensitivity profile, which in turn causes increased partial volume averaging and z-axis blurring. The impact on image quality is lessened to a certain extent in the chest, where there is high inherent contrast between structures. Widening of the section sensitivity profile has also been markedly decreased by the newer 180-degree interpolation algorithms on modern spiral scanners (13). In the chest, pitches of 1.5–1.7 can be used with little apparent degradation of image quality caused by z-axis blurring.

By choosing a pitch of more than 1 and decreasing the slice collimation, the same volume of tissue can be scanned in the same time with higher spatial resolution (14). For example, by increasing the pitch to 1.7 and decreasing slice thickness from 10 mm to 6 mm, one can actually improve the spatial resolution within the axial plane but still cover the same territory in the chest in the same amount of time. However, decreasing slice collimation increases pixel noise (7,14,15).

There are, in addition, other disadvantages of increasing pitch beyond a certain point. Wright et al. studied the effect of increasing pitch on pulmonary nodule detection and found a tendency to undercount lung nodules as pitch increased above 1.5 (13). Spiral artifacts also become more noticeable at higher pitches. One such artifact consists of an area of image drop-out or low attenuation that occurs at branch points of vessels at pitches of more than 1.5 (13).

The trade-offs in the chest can be summarized as follows: increasing pitch allows the use of thinner-slice collimation with resultant higher spatial resolution and lower radiation dose, but at the expense of increased pixel noise and more noticeable spiral CT artifacts (7,13–15). Understanding these trade-offs allows one to choose the slice thickness and pitch that are most appropriate for the individual examination.

Choosing Spiral Options for Imaging the Chest

When choosing spiral CT parameters for thoracic imaging one should consider the

- Distance to be covered in the chest;
- Resolution required;
- Patient's respiratory status;
- Desirability of single-acquisition versus variable-mode scanning;
- Need for multiplanar reformation or 3D imaging.

Optimizing Spiral CT Technique for the Chest

At our institution, we have found two protocols practical for most chest imaging. For studies of the chest requiring fine detail and high resolution but a limited area of coverage, we choose the following parameters: 3–5-mm section acquisition thickness, table speed of 3–5 mm/s, pitch of 1, high-resolution algorithm (lung algorithm on GE system), and reconstruction of overlapping slices every 1–2 mm. The distance covered can be increased by increasing the pitch from 1 to 1.5–1.7. Evaluation of the pediatric airway provides an example of a study that might use this thin-section protocol with a higher pitch of 1.7. Thin collimation with overlapping slices is desirable in this type of study to achieve high-resolution images of this relatively small structure. At the same time, the entire airway needs to be imaged in a single breath-hold so that high-quality multiplanar and 3D reformatted images can be generated, which creates the need to increase pitch to cover more distance in the chest. By increasing the pitch, an additional benefit of lower radiation exposure to the child is also achieved.

Our second protocol is used when the entire chest must be covered in a routine fashion (e.g., as a screening or follow-up examination for pulmonary pathology). In this survey spiral scan we use 10-mm slice acquisition thickness, 10-mm/s table speed, pitch of 1, lung algorithm, and reconstruction of overlapping slices every 5 mm. We find using a 50% overlap of reconstructed images particularly useful when screening or following lung metastases. Using a variable-mode acquisition, a series of three or four back-to-back, 7–10-s helical scans is often chosen for patients who find it difficult to hold their breath for an extended period of time. If it is more desirable to scan the entire chest during a single breath-hold (e.g., to generate multiplanar or 3D images of the airways or vessels), a single 30–32-s spiral acquisition is chosen, pitch is increased from 1 to 1.5–1.7, and the narrowest slice collimation that will cover the distance required in the chest is chosen (usually 5–7 mm). The images can then be reconstructed at 2–3-mm intervals.

To further optimize the quality of the spiral CT images obtained, a few minutes should be spent on instructing the patient on breath-holding techniques. We find it helpful to hyperventilate the patient by having him take three deep breaths just before the spiral scan. After taking the three breaths in and out, we ask the patient to take in a deep breath and hold it. With this type of preparation, many patients can successfully hold their breath for 24–32 s.

EVALUATION OF PULMONARY NODULES

One of the first areas where spiral CT made an impact on clinical practice was in the detection and evaluation of pulmonary nodules (1–3,16–22) (see Fig. 5-1; Figs. 5-2–5-5). With conventional CT, variations in depth of inspiration result in interscan gaps. These gaps can cause one to miss significant pulmonary pathology, including moderate-sized pulmonary nodules (3) (see Fig. 5-1). Spiral CT's volume acquisition technique eliminates discontinuities between slices, lessening the chance of missing a lung nodule because of slice misregistration. Respiratory and other patient motion artifacts are also minimized (3).

Lesion Detection

A number of studies have now shown that spiral CT is more sensitive and accurate for detecting pulmonary nodules than conventional CT (17–19,22). Particularly when overlapping slice reconstruction is used, observer's true positive rates for detecting pulmonary nodules increase, their degree of confidence in reporting pulmonary nodules increases, and their rates of reporting false-positive nodules decrease (23) (see Fig. 5-2).

Lesion Characterization

In addition to lesion detection, spiral CT facilitates the process of lesion characterization (see Figs. 5-3–5-5). Spiral CT allows for more convincing densitometry assessment, because image reconstruction intervals can be chosen retrospectively by the operator. This more readily assures that at least one reconstructed slice will fall through the center of a pulmonary nodule, thus reducing partial volume averaging and generating better densitometry assessments of nodules (2,3). It is important to recognize, however, that the slice thickness does not change in this process (see Fig. 5-3). Slice thickness is determined by the beam collimation that is chosen at the time of data acquisition. Therefore even when performing a spiral CT examination for nodule densitometry, it is important to choose a slice collimation appropriate for the size of the nodule. For accurate measurements of CT density, slice thickness should be one-half the diameter of the lung lesion or less (3,24). So, in fact, if a small nodule in question cannot be identified on the scout topogram, an initial survey spiral CT exam through the chest

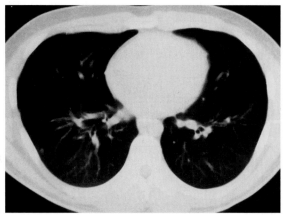
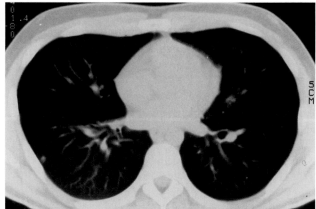

A   **B**

FIG. 5-2. (A,B) Conventional 8-mm × 8-mm CT barely catches the top of a small lung nodule in the right lower lobe. *(continued)*

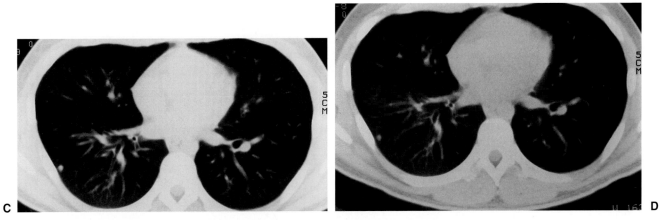

FIG. 5-2. *Continued.* **(C,D)** Spiral CT (4-mm slice thickness, pitch of 1, slice reconstruction every 2 mm) demonstrates the small lung nodule on multiple slices from its top to bottom, with at least one slice through the center of the lesion, allowing more confident detection and diagnosis.

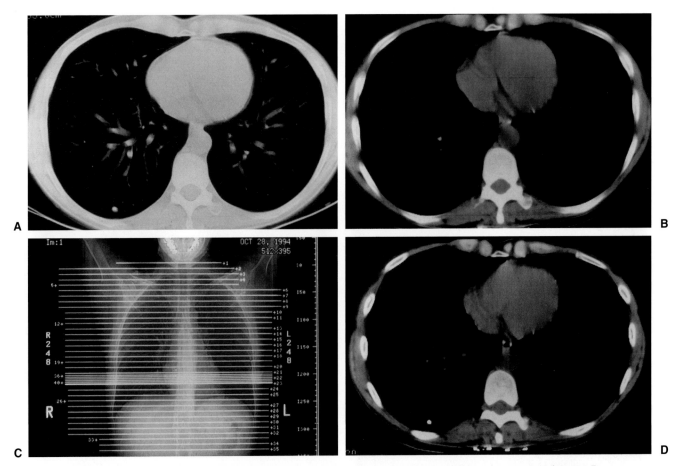

FIG. 5-3. **(A,B)** Survey spiral CT with 10-mm collimation, pitch of 1, and slices reconstructed every 5 mm. A small 6-mm nodule is identified in the right lower lobe on the lung window settings, but the nodule cannot be seen on the soft-tissue settings. To accurately assess the CT density of this lesion a thinner slice thickness is required to avoid partial volume averaging. Collimation should be one-half the diameter of the nodule or less. **(C,D)** A repeat, limited spiral CT using 3-mm collimation, pitch of 1, and slices reconstructed every 1 mm was performed. This is a rapid, efficient way to evaluate small nodules. With thin-section collimation we can ensure with spiral CT technique that the entire volume of tissue in the area of the nodule is covered without missing the nodule because of respiratory variation. And with overlapping reconstruction of the images, we can ensure that at least one image will be centered on the nodule. The repeat thin-section spiral CT shows the nodule to be densely calcified.

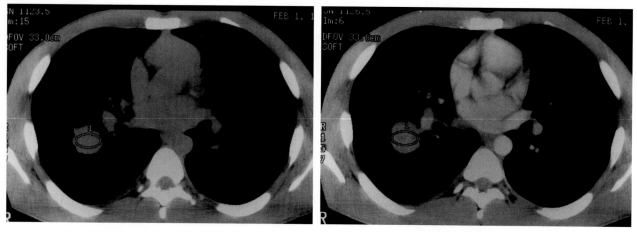

FIG. 5-4. (**A,B**) Assessing the degree of contrast enhancement of an indeterminate pulmonary nodule may indicate the likelihood of malignancy. Using variable-mode spiral CT, a series of sequential short spiral CT acquisitions can be obtained in rapid succession through the nodule following the administration of intravenous contrast.

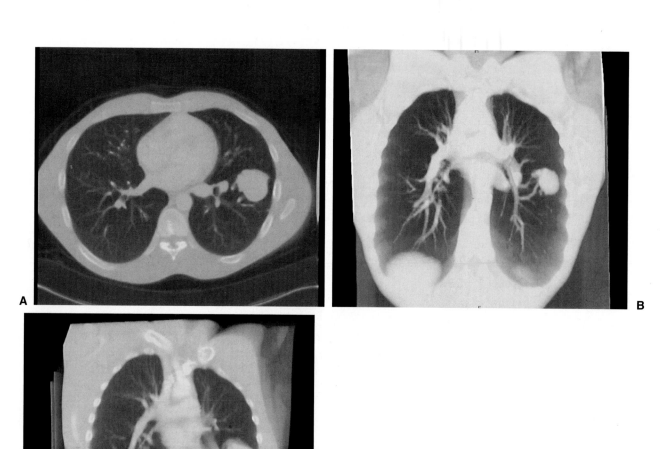

FIG. 5-5. (**A–C**) Spiral CT demonstration of pulmonary arteriovenous malformation. Characterization of pulmonary lesions with respect to vascular structures or airways is greatly facilitated with spiral CT techniques. Multiple spiral CT images through this nodule make use of a closely overlapping reconstruction interval to display the spiral CT data. Three-dimensional reconstructions may be especially helpful in allowing one to accurately follow the incoming artery and outgoing vein from this pulmonary arteriovenous malformation.

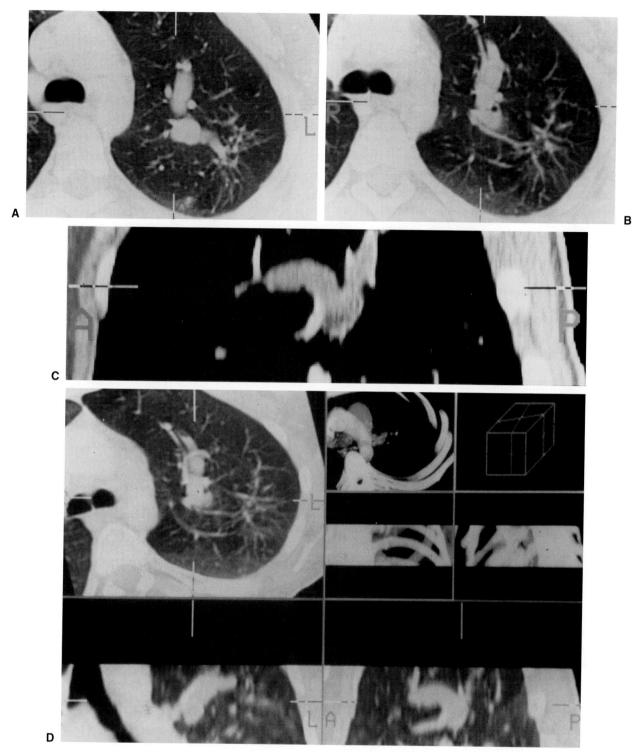

FIG. 5-6. Spiral CT demonstration of mucous plug in the (**A,B**) axial plane, (**C**) sagittal plane, and (**D**) multiformatted display. The relationship of the mucus-filled bronchus and its adjacent pulmonary artery branches is exquisitely detailed with spiral CT.

using wider collimation may be used to find the location of the nodule first. Then a second, limited spiral scan using thin collimation can be performed just through the nodule for the purposes of densitometry measurements. The combination of thin collimation, volume acquisition through the nodule during a single breath-hold, and ability to reconstruct those thin slices at 1–2-mm intervals allows one to determine density measurements of smaller pulmonary nodules with much greater ease and confidence. Similarly, the enhancement characteristics of indeterminate pulmonary nodules that are not calcified are more easily determined with spiral CT technique (see Fig. 5-4). Swenson and others have shown data to suggest that nodules that show significant contrast enhancement *during the first 3 min after intravenous contrast injection* are more likely to be neoplastic (25,26). By preprogramming a series of short helical scans sequentially through the nodule, one can accurately monitor nodule enhancement during a bolus injection of intravenous contrast.

Spiral CT also allows for more detailed analysis of the anatomic relationships between lung nodules and adjacent vascular and bronchial structures (see Fig. 5-5; Fig. 5-6). Thinly collimated, closely overlapping spiral CT slices that are free from respiratory gaps have proven clinically useful in the characterization of pulmonary arteriovenous malformations (27). They are also very useful in detecting segmental bronchi leading to lung masses for the purposes of bronchoscopy planning (3,28).

Another advantage of spiral CT data is that it can be used to generate accurate multiplanar and 3D images of the lung lesion (Fig. 5-7). Particularly with the increased use of thoracoscopy to remove small peripheral pulmonary nodules, it has become increasingly advantageous to be able to display lung pathology in multiple planes and in a 3D format.

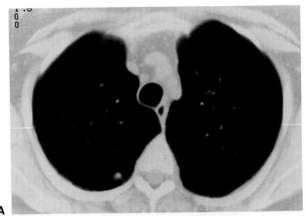

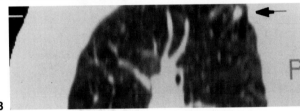

FIG. 5-7. (**A**) This patient had a history of surgery for lung cancer and was being followed for a small lung nodule in the right apex. After several frustrating attempts to follow this small lesion with conventional CT, serial spiral CTs were found to provide more consistent and reproducible follow-up. Spiral CT (4-mm collimation, pitch of 1, slice reconstruction interval of 2 mm) shows a small nodule with surrounding emphysema in the right upper lobe. (**B**) Another advantage of spiral CT is the ability to generate high-quality multiplanar reconstructions of lung pathology that are not degraded by respiratory motion. Sagittal multiplanar image showing the location of nodule. With the emergence of thoracoscopic surgery and the increasing use of wedge resections rather than formal lobectomies for removal of peripheral lung nodules, the ability to display lung pathology in three dimensions becomes increasingly important.

Peridiaphragmatic Pathology

Evaluation of peridiaphragmatic nodules and processes is particularly difficult with conventional CT because the degree of excursion of the lung bases and diaphragms from one breath to the next tends to be great (estimated to be up to 8 cm) and quite variable (3,15). Spiral CT acquired during a single breath-hold maneuver eliminates problems with respiratory excursions and facilitates examination of nodules and abnormalities near the diaphragm (3) (Figs. 5-8, 5-9). Additional information regarding the relationship of the lesion and the diaphragm can be gained from multiplanar images in the coronal and sagittal plane that are free of respiratory artifacts (3).

Multiple Nodules

Evaluation of multiple pulmonary nodules is also facilitated by spiral CT technique (Fig. 5-10). Reconstructing spi-

ral CT data at one-half the slice thickness increases the conspicuity of nodules, and in one study increased the observer's confidence in diagnosis, improving true-positive and lowering false-positive rates (23). How spiral images are viewed may also influence detection rate. One study has shown that simply viewing spiral images on an independent workstation using a cine mode to page through the images increased the observer's detection rate when compared with hard-copy review (29).

Reproducibility of Exam

Particularly in the oncological patient who may be undergoing serial examinations to determine response to treatment, accurate assessment of number and size of nodules on multiple serial CT examinations becomes critical for treatment planning decisions. Because spiral CT is much more reproducible from one examination to the next compared with conventional CT, making comparisons of tumor

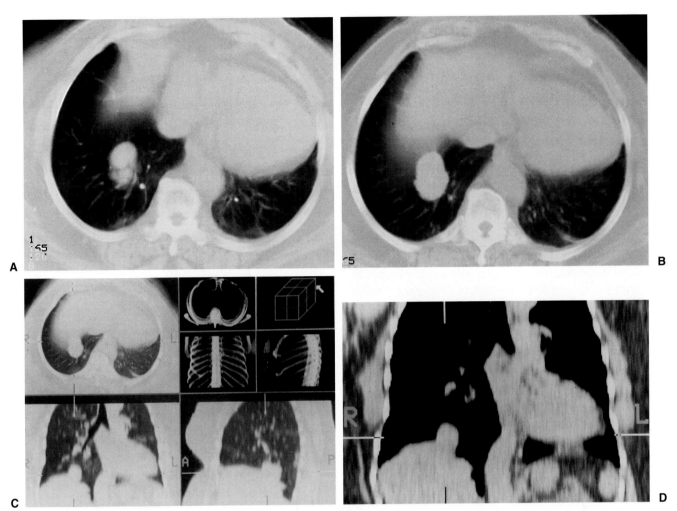

FIG. 5-8. (A–D) Metastatic thyroid cancer with involvement of the diaphragm proven at surgery. Peridiaphragmatic lesions are particularly difficult to evaluate with conventional CT because respiratory excursion of the lung tends to be greatest and most variable near the diaphragm. Spiral CT eliminates this problem and allows for confident evaluation of nodules near the diaphragm. As an added bonus, the data from the spiral CT acquisition can be used to generate high-quality multiplanar reconstructions, demonstrating the relationship of the lesion with respect to the diaphragm in multiple planes (**C,D**), thus providing additional information regarding diaphragmatic involvement.

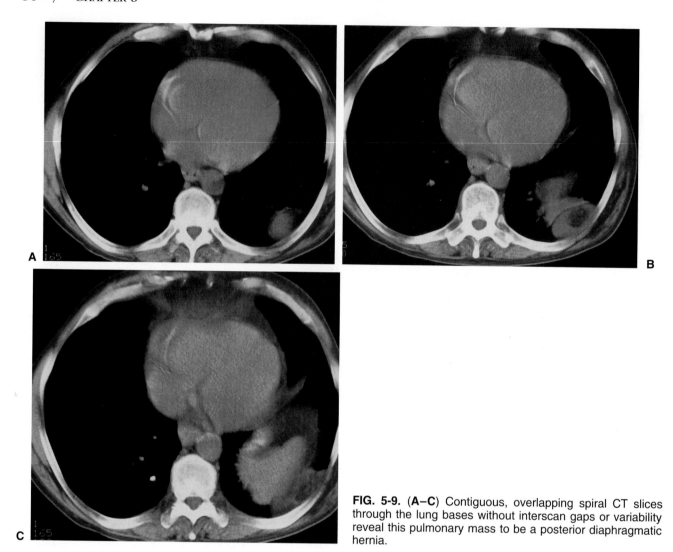

FIG. 5-9. (A–C) Contiguous, overlapping spiral CT slices through the lung bases without interscan gaps or variability reveal this pulmonary mass to be a posterior diaphragmatic hernia.

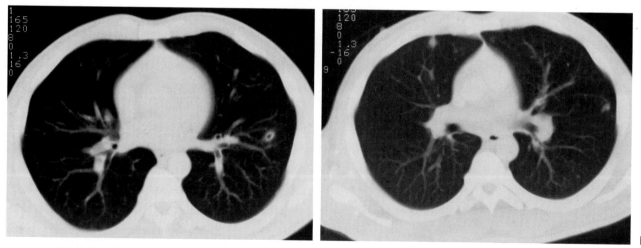

FIG. 5-10. (A,B) Spiral CT facilitates detection and characterization of multiple small pulmonary nodules in a 29-year-old HIV-positive intravenous drug user. A spiral CT using a survey protocol (8-mm beam collimation, pitch of 1, slice reconstruction interval 4 mm) shows one small cavitary nodule in the left lung and multiple other tiny peripheral nodules with feeding vessels compatible with septic emboli.

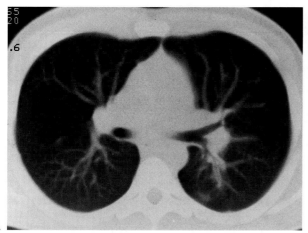
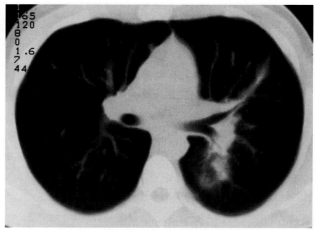

FIG. 5-11. **(A)** Spiral chest CT in HIV-positive male in March. **(B)** Follow-up spiral CT in July. The consistent, reproducible follow-up that spiral CT provides allowed confident comparison of one CT examination with the next, demonstrating unequivocal though subtle progression of the peribronchial lung disease. CT findings were compatible with Kaposi's sarcoma, confirmed at bronchoscopy.

size and extent is more reliable with spiral CT techniques (Fig. 5-11).

Disadvantages of Spiral CT

The increased conspicuity of small pulmonary nodules on spiral CT does create problems, however, since the likelihood of identifying intrapulmonary lymph nodes and other small benign densities increases (Fig. 5-12).

To summarize, the advantages of spiral CT for evaluating lung nodules are that spiral CT:

- Eliminates respiratory misregistration;
- Facilitates detection and characterization of small nodules;

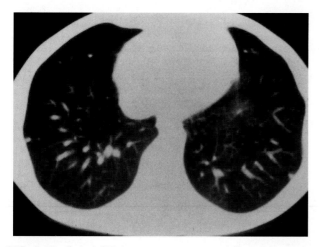

FIG. 5-12. Spiral CT demonstrates two small nodules in the lung bases that proved to be intrapulmonary lymph nodes. One disadvantage of spiral CT is the increased conspicuity of smaller lesions, a certain percentage of which will prove to be benign.

- Improves evaluation of peridiaphragmatic nodules;
- Allows for more reproducible follow-up.

EVALUATION OF THE AIRWAYS

Spiral CT has made it possible to examine the airways in a new and exciting way (3,30) (Figs. 5-13–5-16). By combining a single breath-hold acquisition with thin-section collimation and overlapping slice reconstruction, spiral CT provides a superior means of assessing the course and caliber of the trachea and proximal bronchi (31–35). It allows for generation of high-quality multiplanar and 3D images of the airways that are free from respiratory artifacts. Spiral CT's overlapping slice reconstruction decreases aliasing and partial-volume artifacts that typically degrade reformatted images from conventional CT scans (33–35). In fact, the quality of the spiral CT data set is such that sophisticated, virtual reality software can be applied to the data to generate bronchoscopic-like views of the airway, so-called virtual bronchoscopy (33–35).

Airways indications for spiral CT include detection of endobronchial lesions in patients with hemoptysis, evaluation of bronchial obstruction (see Figs. 5-14, 5-15), assessment of bronchial dehiscence or stenosis following lung transplantation (30), detection of tumor recurrence at bronchial stump sites (see Fig. 5-16), evaluation of endobronchial stents, and 2D/3D modeling of the trachea for planning reconstructive surgery (3) (Fig. 5-17). Functional imaging of the airway can also be performed by acquiring a spiral CT sequence of the airway in inspiration and expiration. This may be helpful in detecting or documenting an area of tracheomalacia (e.g., in the pediatric patient with a congenital tracheal anomaly or in the lung transplant patient with an anastomotic complication) (30).

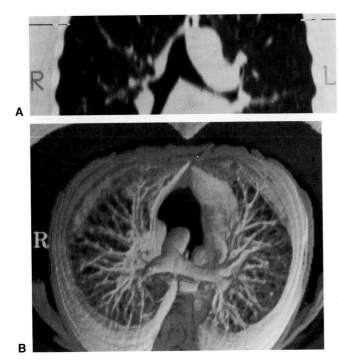

A

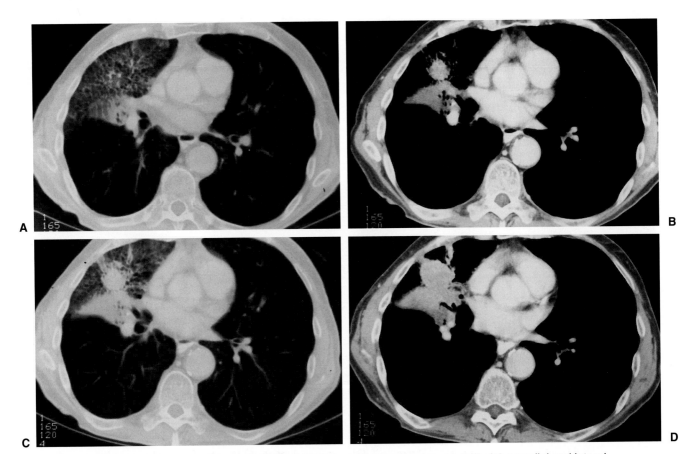

FIG. 5-13. Spiral CT of the airways. (**A**) Coronal reconstructions and (**B**) 3D images of the proximal airways using reformatted spiral CT data. Because it allows generation of multiplanar and 3D reconstructions free of respiratory artifacts, spiral CT provides a new way of displaying and evaluating the airways.

FIG. 5-14. (**A–D**) Spiral CT shows right middle lobe infiltrate with abrupt cutoff of the medial and lateral segment bronchi by a non–small-cell lung cancer. The ability to trace smaller bronchi from one CT slice to the next, at close intervals without interscan gaps, makes spiral CT the technique of choice for evaluating the cause of bronchial obstruction.

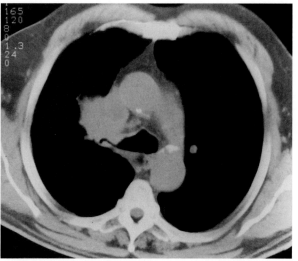
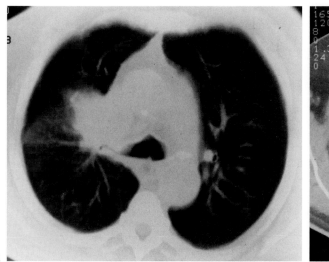

FIG. 5-15. (**A**) Spiral CT demonstrates a large lung cancer encasing and narrowing the right mainstem bronchus. On the soft-tissue windows (**B**) one can appreciate subtle thickening of the anterior wall of the right mainstem bronchus up to the carina due to tumor infiltration.

A typical protocol for examination of the trachea and central airways at our institution is a single-acquisition spiral CT scan using a 5-mm slice thickness, pitch of 1.5–1.7, and reconstruction interval every 2 mm. Images are transferred to an independent workstation where multiplanar coronal, sagittal, or curved reformats are performed. The same data may also be used to generate surface-rendered 3D images, as well as minimum-intensity projections (3). These are often very helpful in determining the location, length, and severity of the airway narrowing. Virtual bronchoscopy or rendering the spiral CT data set of the airway in a bronchoscopic-like projection provides additional information that can be helpful in planning bronchoscopic procedures and for selecting patients for endobronchial stents or laser or brachytherapy (33). Un-

like real bronchoscopy, virtual bronchoscopy allows the observer to view the airway beyond an obstruction as well to visualize the lung and soft tissues surrounding the airway on the other side of the bronchial wall (33).

VASCULAR ASSESSMENT

Spiral CT has become the CT scanning technique of choice for assessing vascular problems in the chest because excellent contrast enhancement is more consistently obtained with this technique than with conventional CT (4) (Fig. 5-18). To optimize spiral CT technique for vascular assessments the following become critical considerations: (a) the timing of the bolus injection of intravenous contrast

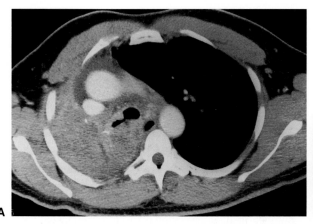
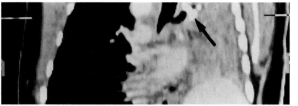

FIG. 5-16. Spiral CT can be used effectively to evaluate bronchial stump sites for recurrent tumor. (**A**) The spiral CT of this 56-year-old male with a history of right upper lobectomy for lung cancer shows a large tumor recurrence growing out from the stump site, encasing the right mainstem bronchus, and extensively infiltrating the mediastinum. (**B**) Multiplanar reconstructions show the surgical stump site (*arrow*) to better advantage using off-axis oblique views.

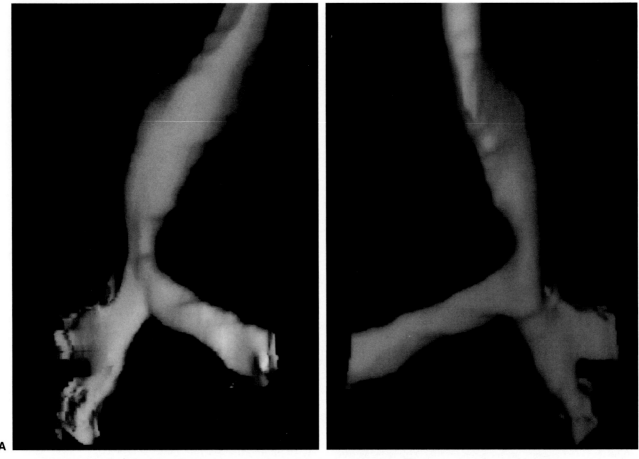

FIG. 5-17. (A,B) Spiral CT evaluation of pediatric airway. Single-breath-hold acquisition spiral CT using 5-mm collimation, pitch of 1.7, and slice reconstruction interval every 2 mm was obtained through the central airways of this child with a post-traumatic stricture of the lower trachea. Spiral CT data were used to generate 3D models of the central airways using a surface-rendering threshold program. The length and degree of narrowing of the trachea just above the carina are readily appreciated on the 3D model that can be rotated around the vertical axis.

with respect to the start of the spiral CT scan, (b) the volume of intravenous contrast administered, and (c) the rate of delivery of intravenous contrast.

For thoracic spiral CT examinations requiring contrast enhancement, a power injector should be used to deliver the intravenous contrast. Injection rates of 2–3 mL/s for a total of 100 mL of contrast are used for most routine chest cases. Faster injection rates (3–5 mL/s) are preferred for spiral CT angiography. We routinely use nonionic contrast material in all patients undergoing contrast enhanced spiral CT scanning of the chest, because in our experience, patients tolerate higher rates of contrast injection with the nonionic agents, experiencing fewer side effects such as nausea and vomiting that ordinarily would abort or interrupt the spiral CT examination (36).

Spiral CT data acquisition in the chest begins 20–40 s after the start of the intravenous contrast injection. The scan delay time will depend on whether venous anatomy (e.g., the SVC) or arterial structures (the aorta and great vessels) are of primary concern. A good rule of thumb for choosing

scan delay times is to remember that it takes approximately 15 s for intravenous contrast injected from a peripheral vein to reach the pulmonary arteries and about 20–25 s for the contrast to reach the aorta and great vessels. An optional upgrade available on some scanners (Smart Prep; General Electric Medical Systems; Milwaukee, WI) allows for visual on-line monitoring of the intravenous contrast enhancement by means of a series of very-low-mA scans and region-of-interest measurements (37) (Fig. 5-19). This allows one to customize contrast enhancement to the individual and to take into account such factors as cardiac output and circulation time. Enhancement of any selected structure in the chest can also be optimized by the operator with this software–hardware option (37).

When compared with conventional CT, spiral CT has a number of advantages with respect to contrast enhancement. Spiral CT is capable of scanning the entire area of interest within the chest in considerably less time than conventional CT. Because the duration of time required for vascular enhancement is decreased, reduced volumes of intravascular

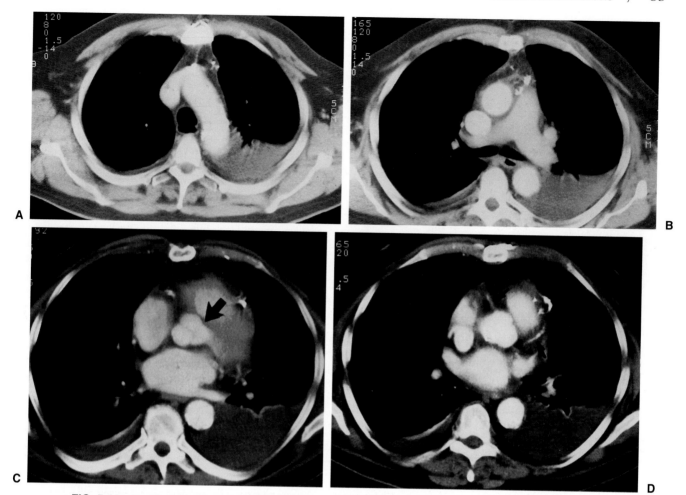

FIG. 5-18. (A–D) Optimal vascular enhancement is achieved routinely using spiral CT, because of the shorter scanning times. Timing of the bolus of intravenous contrast with respect to spiral CT data acquisition becomes more critical, however. In this case, opacification of the patient's coronary artery bypass grafts is demonstrated. Note also the detail of the aortic valve leaflets demonstrated by the spiral CT scan.

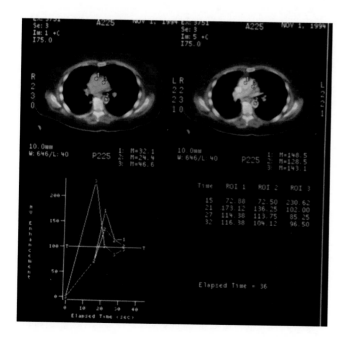

FIG. 5-19. Smart Prep (General Electric Medical Systems, Milwaukee, WI). Using a series of low-mA images and ROI measurements, the progress of contrast enhancement can be monitored on-line to determine the optimal time to start spiral CT scanning after the start of injection.

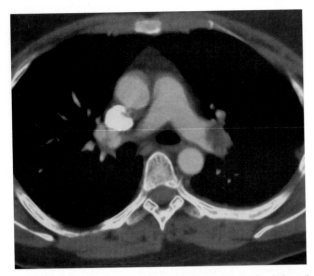

FIG. 5-20. Spiral CT demonstrating thrombus in the left main pulmonary artery. An increasing body of literature suggests that spiral CT is an accurate way to detect proximal pulmonary emboli.

contrast material can be used while still achieving optimal vascular phase enhancement throughout the spiral CT acquisition (4). The improved spiral CT data can also be used to generate excellent multiplanar and 3D images of vascular structures (see Fig. 5-19).

The number of vascular applications of spiral CT reported in the literature continues to grow (Figs. 5-20–5-23). Spiral CT has been shown to be valuable in the evaluation of the thoracic aorta (3,4,38,39) and to reliably identify central pulmonary thromboemboli (40) (see Figs. 5-20, 5-21). Spiral CT has been used to assess patency of coronary bypass grafts, and spiral CT angiographic techniques show promise as a potential alternative to conventional angiography in the evaluation of aortic vascular disease, vascular anomalies, and pulmonary arteriovenous malformations in the chest (5,27). Evaluation of venous obstruction within the thorax is also easily performed using spiral CT (see Fig. 5-23).

The role of spiral CT in the evaluation of suspected pulmonary emboli is evolving rapidly. Remy et al. showed spiral CT could, with a high degree of accuracy, identify central pulmonary emboli down to the second- to fourth-order pulmonary arteries (40,41) (see Figs. 5-20, 5-21). Data from several studies indicate that spiral CT has a sensitivity and specificity of approximately 89% and 93%, respectively, for the detection of central pulmonary emboli (5,38,40). All studies to date indicate lower sensitivity for detecting smaller peripheral emboli in subsegmental arteries, the importance of which remains controversial (5,38,42). One must also be very familiar with the appearance of normal-sized hilar and intersegmental lymph nodes that can be misinterpreted on spiral CT as emboli (40).

Our protocol for evaluating pulmonary emboli is as fol-

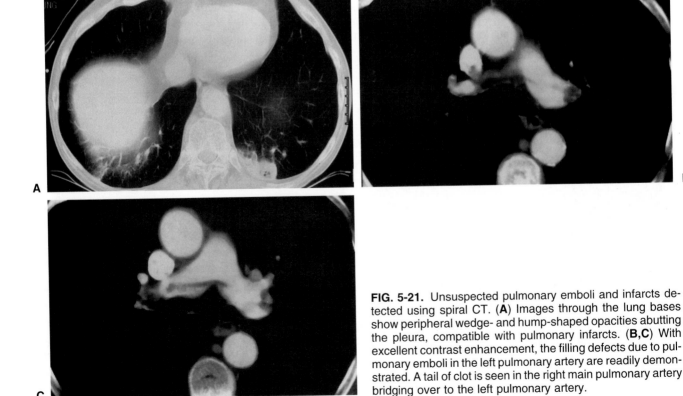

FIG. 5-21. Unsuspected pulmonary emboli and infarcts detected using spiral CT. (**A**) Images through the lung bases show peripheral wedge- and hump-shaped opacities abutting the pleura, compatible with pulmonary infarcts. (**B,C**) With excellent contrast enhancement, the filling defects due to pulmonary emboli in the left pulmonary artery are readily demonstrated. A tail of clot is seen in the right main pulmonary artery bridging over to the left pulmonary artery.

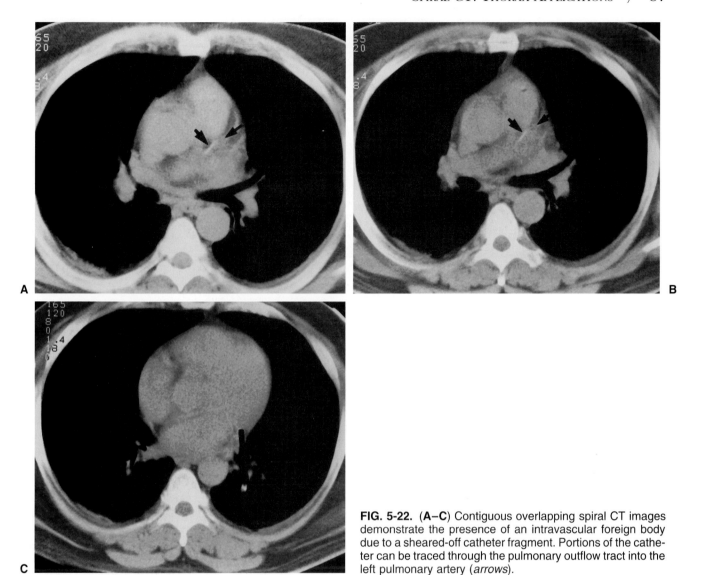

FIG. 5-22. (**A–C**) Contiguous overlapping spiral CT images demonstrate the presence of an intravascular foreign body due to a sheared-off catheter fragment. Portions of the catheter can be traced through the pulmonary outflow tract into the left pulmonary artery (*arrows*).

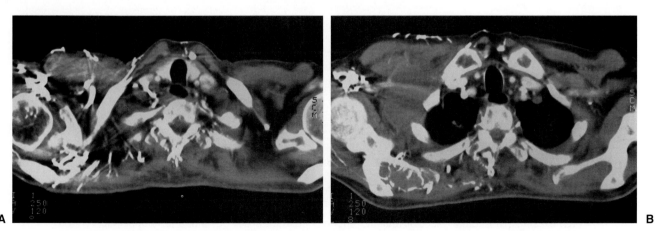

FIG. 5-23. (**A,B**) Spiral CT evaluation of venous obstruction caused by metastatic tumor. A large mass in the right axilla is causing obstruction of the axillary vessels. Extensive collaterals are identified in the chest wall anteriorly and posteriorly.

FIG. 5-24. (A,B) Vascular artifact commonly seen on spiral CT images obtained through the aortic root. The double curved line (*arrow*) is due to motion of the aortic root and *z*-axis blurring and should not be mistaken for a dissection flap.

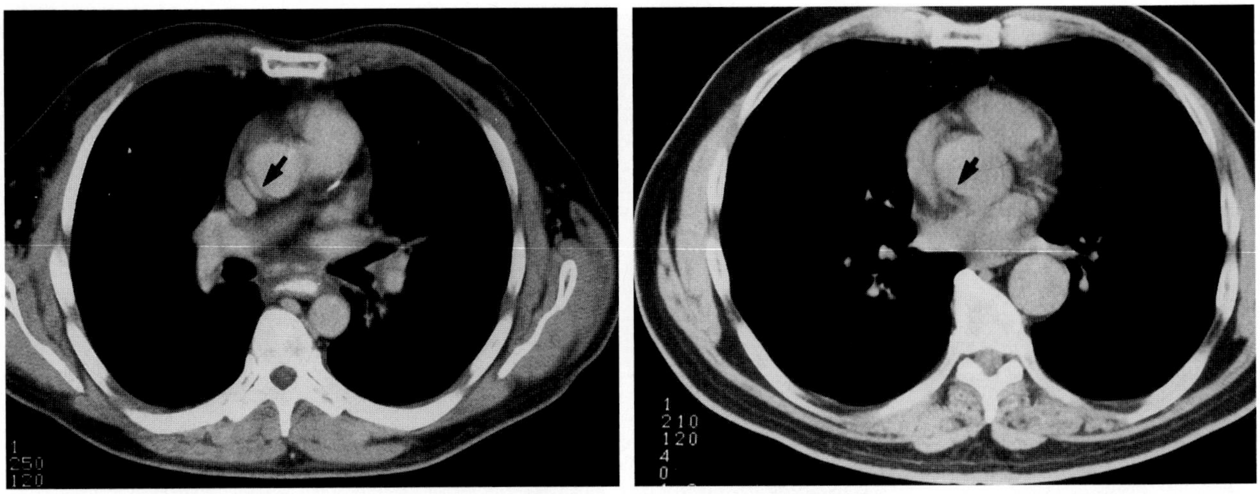

lows: 5-mm collimation, pitch 1.7 with a single breath-hold acquisition of 30–32 s. Scanning is performed from the diaphragm cephalad to above the main pulmonary artery using a contrast injection of 150 mL of 60% nonionic contrast at 4 mL/s after a 15-s delay. Images are reconstructed every 3 mm and transferred to an independent workstation where multiplanar and 3D reformats can be performed. Remy and others have shown that multiplanar images may provide complementary information to the axial images for detecting clot in vessels traveling obliquely through the imaging volume (41).

Findings of acute pulmonary emboli on spiral CT include filling defects that occlude or partially occlude the pulmonary arteries (see Figs. 5-20, 5-21). One may see a tail of clot within an opacified vessel (3,40). Chronic thrombi are also very apparent on spiral CT and appear as crescentic or laminar filling defects adherent to the walls of the pulmonary artery (3,40). Because chronic clots are more difficult to appreciate on conventional angiography, spiral CT may prove to be the best method for evaluating patients with pulmonary hypertension for the extent of chromic thrombo-embolism, particularly if surgical thrombectomy is contemplated (5).

What role should spiral CT play currently in the evaluation of patients with suspected acute pulmonary emboli? The answer will have to be determined by larger studies, including a multicenter comparative imaging trial (3). In the meantime, spiral CT should be considered in patients with suspected pulmonary emboli who have a contraindication for conventional angiography but require verification of a high

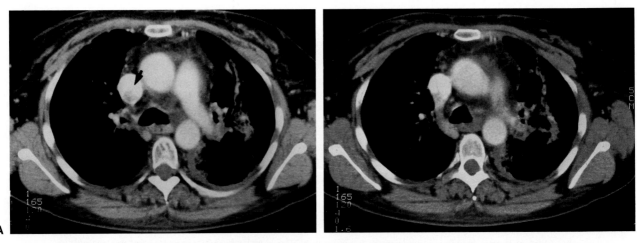

FIG. 5-25. (A,B) Another vascular artifact frequently seen on spiral CT is due to unopacified venous blood from the azygous system mimicking thrombus in the superior vena cava (*arrows*). Because spiral CT scanning occurs faster than conventional CT scanning, this region is often imaged during peak arterial opacification prior to enhancement of venous structures.

probability or indeterminate V/Q scan because of contraindications to anticoagulation or prior to filter placement (3). Spiral CT may also play a role in the follow-up of patients with proven pulmonary emboli, to follow clot lysis while undergoing anticoagulation or thrombolytic therapy (5).

When performing spiral CT for vascular disease, it is important to remember there are a few vascular artifacts that are particularly apparent on spiral CT images (43,44) (Figs. 5-24, 5-25). Pulsation artifacts near the aortic root can mimic a dissection flap and should not be mistaken for pathology (5,43,44) (see Fig. 5-24). Segmenting the CT data by using less than one 360-degree tube rotation's worth of data tends to diminish this artifact (5,43). Venous mixing artifacts due

to unopacified venous blood are also more prominent on spiral CT because of the faster scanning times through the chest (see Fig. 5-25).

TUMOR STAGING

Spiral CT is particularly advantageous for tumor staging of chest malignancies (see Fig. 5-15; Figs. 5-26–5-28). Assessment of airway encroachment (see Fig. 5-15), chest wall invasion, mediastinal infiltration (see Fig. 5-27), and vascular encasement (see Figs. 5-6, 5-28) is facilitated with spiral CT techniques. Spiral CT accurately evaluates hilar, perihilar, and aortopulmonary lymph nodes (45). Acquisition dur-

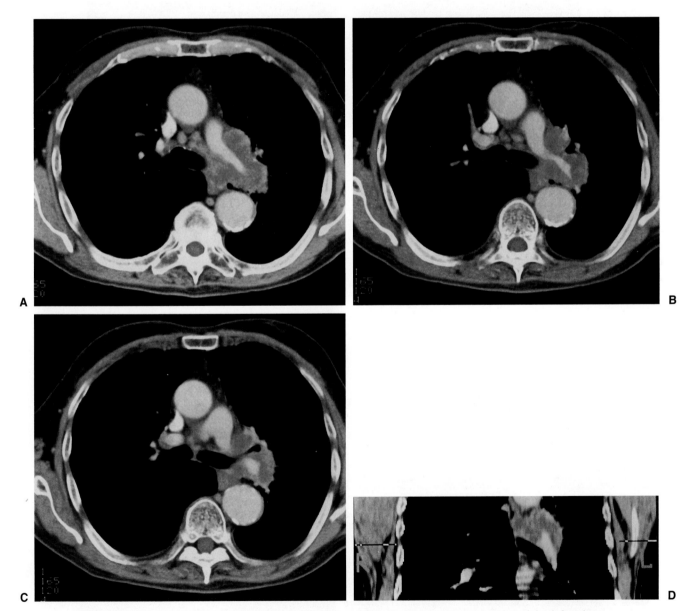

FIG. 5-26. Tumor staging of lung cancer using spiral CT to demonstrate encasement of the left pulmonary artery on (**A–C**) overlapping spiral axial views and (**D,E**) multiplanar reconstructions. (**D**) Coronal reconstruction demonstrating involvement of the aorto-pulmonary window. (**E**) Multiformatted views. *(continued)*

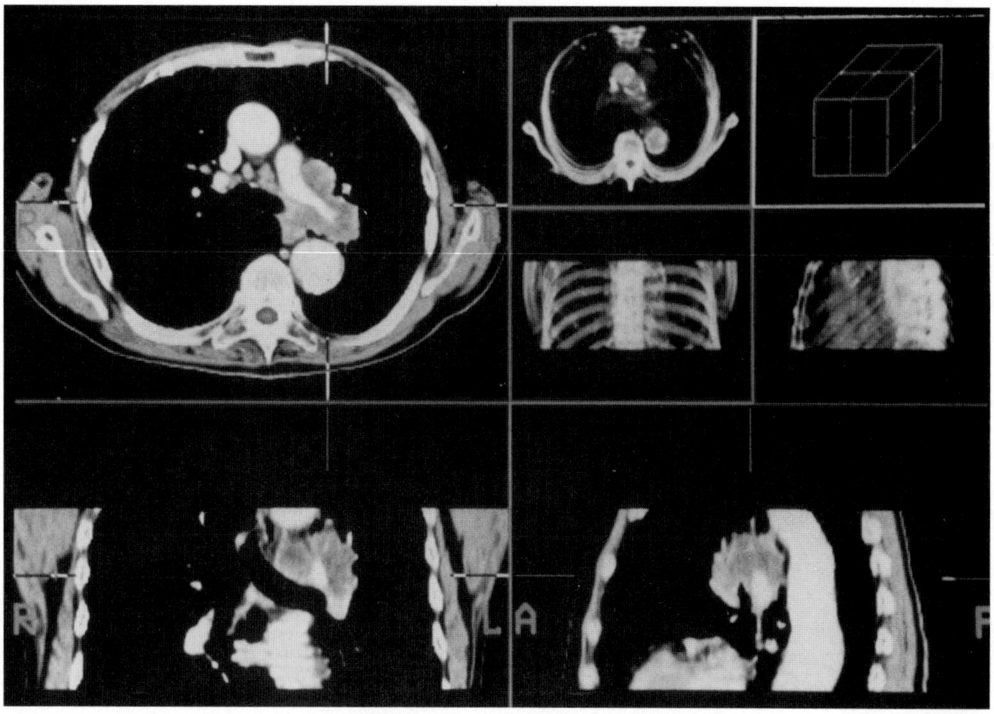

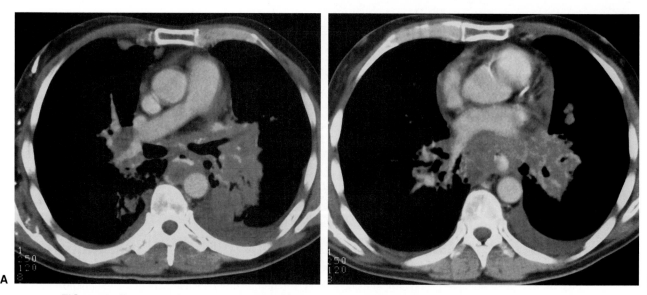

FIG. 5-26. *Continued.*

ing a single breath-hold, superior and more consistent vascular opacification, and the ability to obtain multiple thin sections through the hila without interslice gaps all contribute to improved image quality. These advantages of spiral CT are invaluable in identifying small lymph nodes and small tumor masses that would otherwise be missed by conventional CT. An added bonus of spiral CT is its ability to display hilar pathology in coronal, sagittal, and oblique planes, as well as in 3D images. Padhani et al. have recently described 3D imaging of the hilum using spiral CT (46). This is valuable not only in the diagnosis of hilar pathology, but also in tumor staging and for planning bronchoscopy, surgery, and radiation therapy. A future application of 2D/3D spiral CT may be in obtaining accurate 3D measurements

FIG. 5-27. Tumor staging of lung cancer. Spiral CT demonstrates the extent of tumor invasion of the mediastinum with involvement of the esophagus. (**A**) Extensive tumor involves the left hilum and right hilar lymph nodes. (**B**) The tumor surrounds, invades, and compresses the esophagus.

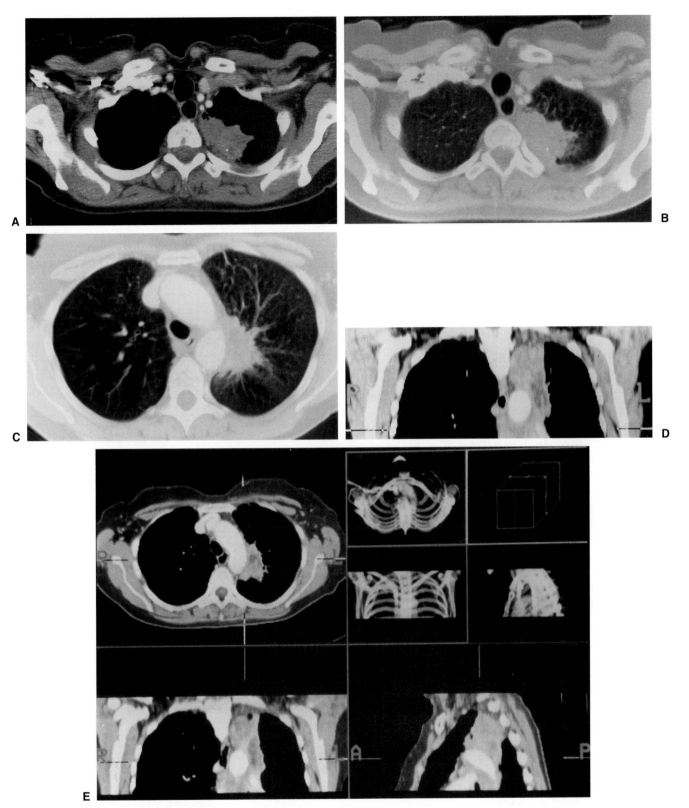

FIG. 5-28. Spiral CT staging of lung cancer—extent of disease. **(A–C)** Axial images show lung cancer in the posterior apical segment of the left upper lobe. **(D,E)** Multiplanar reconstructions of the spiral CT data set show that the tumor wraps around the aorta.

of tumor volumes and 2D/3D assessment of chest wall and pleural invasion by tumor (47).

2D/3D IMAGING OF THE THORAX

Since the introduction of conventional CT, a number of researchers have attempted multiplanar and 3D imaging of the lung with limited success. Early work by Ney et al. (34) using volumetric rendering techniques to image cadaveric lungs showed promising results; however, work on the *in vivo* lung resulted in 3D images of poorer quality because of widely spaced slices and respiratory motion between slices.

With the advent of spiral CT, high-quality multiplanar and 3D images of the *in vivo* lung are now possible. The improved quality of the reconstructed images is due to the fact that spiral CT is a volume acquisition obtained during a single breath-hold. This eliminates interslice variability and discontinuities between slices that degrade reformatted images.

A number of 3D techniques can be applied to spiral CT data sets, including thresholding and surface-rendering techniques, maximal- or minimal-intensity projections, and volumetric rendering (5).

The advantages of 2D and 3D imaging of spiral CT data are numerous. It allows for multiplanar and 3D display of the airways and pulmonary vasculature, enabling the bronchoscopist or surgeon to obtain a thorough understanding of the anatomy and pathology prior to procedures. In addition, the volume of a given region of interest can be measured in three dimensions. A future application of 2D/3D spiral CT may be in oncology, to generate sophisticated 3D tumor volumetrics for planning and assessing tumor response to chemotherapy and radiation therapy (47). Multiplanar and 3D spiral CT can also be used to display complex chest wall deformities and chest wall masses in a way that enables the surgeon to better understand the anatomy and plan complicated reconstructive surgery.

DISADVANTAGES AND LIMITATIONS

Spiral CT does have limitations and some disadvantages in thoracic imaging. Because of heat buildup in the x-ray tube, there are limits in the amount of milliamps that can be generated over an extended period of time during a spiral CT acquisition. Depending on the manufacturer, there are also some postprocessing delays that occur while the spiral CT images are being reconstructed. Computer and data storage capacities on many scanners do not allow for unreconstructed data to be stored indefinitely.

The nature of the spiral CT data acquisition process and reconstruction algorithm creates certain unique problems (8). When compared with conventional CT, spiral CT shows broadening of the section-sensitivity profile, demonstrating a greater full width at half maximum (FWHM = 1.8 for spiral CT using 360-degree LI) (2). Broadening of the slice thickness is due to table transport during the spiral CT scan. This results in z-axis blurring or blurring along the longitudinal table axis. Z-axis blur manifests itself on spiral CT images as lack of sharpness due to increased volume averaging. It is particularly noticeable for structures oriented obliquely to the z-axis or structures whose cross-sectional diameter changes rapidly along the table feed direction (6,20). Z-axis blur can be minimized by decreasing the speed of the table feed with respect to the beam collimation (i.e., decreasing pitch) and by narrowing the beam collimation with greater overlap of reconstructed images (8,16,48). Using a high-resolution or sharp algorithm also seems to help. Newer 180-degree interpolation algorithms also significantly decrease the amount of z-axis blur and demonstrate section-sensitivity profiles with FWHM as low as 1.1 (6,7).

Trade-offs for spiral CT are between (a) increasing speed, greater distance covered, and lower radiation dose, and (b) increasing z-axis blur and artifacts. For example, if a large area of interest needs to be scanned, one must choose a faster table speed and perhaps greater pitch, but at the cost of increased z-axis blurring. Another trade-off is between increasing spiral scan time and maximum milliamps allowed. For longer scan times of 32–40 s, only a lower maximum milliamperage is possible on many scanners. This will increase pixel noise and may be noticeable when examining larger patients.

Radiation dose to the patient from a spiral CT with a table speed of x cm/s is equivalent to a conventional CT with a slice thickness equal to x, given identical mA and kVp settings. In many instances, however, the milliamperage is set lower for spiral CT, so in fact the total radiation dose may actually be smaller. In addition, the need to rescan areas of interest is much less common with spiral CT than with conventional CT. This is particularly true for chest examinations when evaluating a small, solitary pulmonary nodule.

HIGH-RESOLUTION CT VERSUS SPIRAL CT

If spiral CT has so many advantages for chest imaging, should conventional CT ever be used in the chest? What about high-resolution CT (Fig. 5-29)? At our institution spiral CT has replaced conventional CT in the thorax, but it has not replaced high-resolution CT technique. If one compares a high-resolution CT with 1-mm-thick collimation to a spiral CT, the differences in resolution are clearly visible. Spatial resolution and linear edge detection are superior with high-resolution computed tomography (HRCT) techniques. Although linear structures are delineated better with HRCT, small nodules are better demonstrated with spiral CT (5). One approach that combines the advantages of both techniques is to start examination with a survey study of the chest using spiral CT technique and follow that with a few select high-resolution CT images as needed.

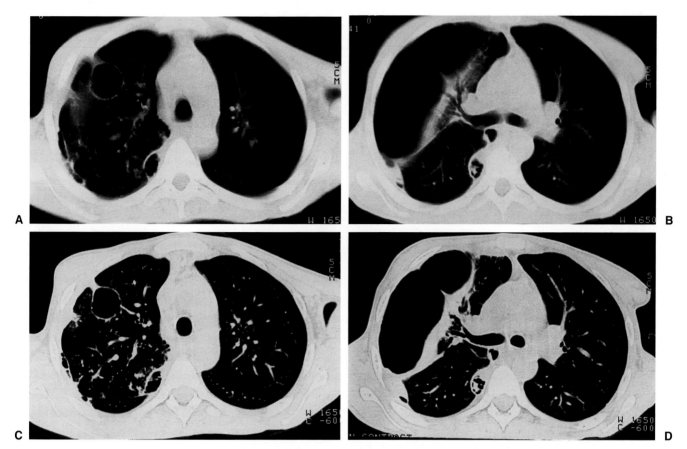

FIG. 5-29. (A–D) A comparison of spiral CT versus high-resolution CT **(C,D)**. **(A,B)** Spiral CT using an 8-mm collimation, pitch of 1, and reconstruction interval of 4 mm, kVp of 137, and mA of 110. **(C,D)** High-resolution CT scan in the same patient for comparison using 2-mm collimation, 8-mm table incrementation, kVp of 137, and mA of 255. Notice the slight blur evident on the spiral CT images and the sharper resolution of the HRCT scan **(C,D)**.

CONCLUSION

Spiral CT has greatly expanded the usefulness of CT in the evaluation of chest disorders. By combining the advantages of a single breath-hold acquisition with improved vascular contrast enhancement, and improved multiplanar and 3D reconstruction capabilities, spiral CT has become the imaging modality of choice for most chest diseases.

REFERENCES

1. Vock P, Soucek M, Daepp M, Kalender WA. Lung: spiral volumetric CT with single-breath-hold technique. *Radiology* 1990;176:864–867.
2. Kalender WA, Seissler W, Koltz E, Vock P. Spiral volumetric CT with single-breath-hold technique, continuous transport, and continuous scanner rotation. *Radiology* 1990;176:181–183.
3. Costello P, Thoracic helical CT. *Radiographics* 1994;14:913–918.
4. Costello P, Dupuy DE, Ecker CP, Tello R. Spiral CT of the thorax with reduced volume of contrast materials: A comparative study. *Radiology* 1992;183:663–666.
5. Zeman RK, Silverman PM, Vieco PT, Costello P. CT angiography. *AJR* 1995;165:1079–1088.
6. Polacin A, Kalender WA, Marchal G. Evaluation of section sensitivity profiles and image noise in spiral CT. *Radiology* 1992;185:29–35.
7. Brink KA, Heiken JP, Wang G, McEnery KW, Schlueter FJ, Vannier MW. Helical CT: principles and technical considerations. *Radiographics* 1994;14:887–893.
8. Kalender WA. Thin-section three-dimensional spiral CT: is isotropic imaging possible? *Radiology* 1995;197:578–580.
9. Kasales CJ, Hopper KD, Ariola DN, et al. Reconstructed helical CT scans: improvement in z-axis resolution compared with overlapped and nonoverlapped conventional CT scans. *AJR* 1995;164:1281–1284.
10. Tomiak MM, Foley WD, Jacobson DR. Variable-mode helical CT: imaging protocols. *AJR* 1995;164:1525–1531.
11. Foley WD, Oneson SR. Helical CT: clinical performance and imaging strategies. *Radiographics* 1994;14:894–904.
12. Korobkin M. Helical CT: principles, techniques, and clinical applications: introduction. *Radiographics* 1994;14:885–886.
13. Wright AR, Collie DA, Williams JR, Hashemi-Malayeri B, Stevenson AJM, Turnbull CM. Pulmonary nodules: effect on detection of spiral CT pitch. *Radiology* 1996;1996:837–841.
14. Rubin GD, Napel S. Increased scan pitch for vascular and thoracic spiral CT. *Radiology* 1995;197:315–316.
15. Brink JA, Heiken JP, Semenkovich J, Teefey SA, McClennan BL, Sagel SS. Abnormalities of the diaphragm and adjacent structures: findings on multiplanar spiral CT scans. *AJR* 1994;163:307–310.
16. Kalender WA, Polacin A, Suss C. A comparison of conventional and spiral CT: an experimental study on the detection of spherical lesions. *J Comput Assist Tomogr* 1994;18:167–176.
17. Costello P, Anderson W, Blume D. Pulmonary nodule: evaluation with spiral volumetric CT. *Radiology* 1991;179:875–876.
18. Heywang-Koebrunner S, Lommatzch B, Fink U, Mayr B. Comparison of spiral and conventional CT in the detection of pulmonary nodules. *Radiology* 1992;185(P):131(abst).

19. Remy-Jardin M, Remy J, Giraud F, Marquette CH. Pulmonary nodules: detection with thick-section spiral CT versus conventional CT. *Radiology* 1993;187:513–520.
20. Kalender WA, Polacin A. Physical performance characteristics of spiral CT scanning. *Med Phys* 1991;18:910–915.
21. Shaffer K, Pugatch RD. Small pulmonary nodules: dynamic CT with a single-breath technique. *Radiology* 1989;173:567–568.
22. Croisille P, Souto M, Cova M, et al. Pulmonary nodules: improved detection with vascular segmentation and extraction with spiral CT. *Radiology* 995;197:397–401.
23. Buckley JA, Scott WW, Siegelman SS, et al. Pulmonary nodules: effect of increased data sampling on detection with spiral CT and confidence in diagnosis. *Radiology* 1995;196:395–400.
24. Cann CE. Quantitative accuracy of spiral CT versus discrete volume CT scanning. *Radiology* 1992;185(P):126–127(abst).
25. Swenson SJ, Brown LR, Colby TV, Weaver AL. Pulmonary nodules: CT evaluation of enhancement with iodinated contrast material. *Radiology* 1995;194:393–398.
26. Park KJ, Kang DK, Suh JH. Small pulmonary masses: imaging pattern on two-phase enhanced spiral CT. 1996 ARRS, paper 147, p. 76 (abst).
27. Remy J, Remy-Jardin M, Giraud F, Wattinne L. Angioarchitecture of pulmonary arteriovenous malformations: clinical utility of three-dimensional helical CT. *Radiology* 1994;191:657–664.
28. Nadich DP. Helical computed tomography of the thorax. Clinical applications. *Radiol Clin North Am* 1994;32:759–774.
29. Seltzer SE, Judy PF, Adams DF, et al. Spiral CT of the chest: comparison of cine and film-based viewing. *Radiology* 1995;197:73–78.
30. Quint LE, Whyte RI, Kazerooni EA, et al. Stenosis of the central airways: evaluation by using helical CT with multiplanar reconstructions. *Radiology* 1995;194:871–877.
31. Silverman PM, Zeiberg AS, Sessions RB, Troost TR, Davros WJ, Zeman RK. Helical CT of the upper airway: normal and abnormal findings on three-dimensional reconstructed images. *AJR* 1995;165:541–546.
32. Zeiberg AS, Silverman PM, Sessions RB, Troost TR, Davros WJ, Zeman RK. Helical (spiral) CT of the upper airway with three-dimensional imaging: technique and clinical assessment. *AJR* 1996;166:293–299.
33. Vining DJ, Liu K, Choplin RH, Haponik EF. Virtual bronchoscopy: relationships of virtual reality endobronchial simulations to actual bronchoscopic findings. *Chest* 1996;109:549–553.
34. Ney DR, Kuhlman JE, Hruban RH, Ren H, Hutchins GM, Fishman EK. Three-dimensional CT-volumetric reconstruction and display of the bronchial tree. *Invest Radiol* 1990;25:736–742.
35. Rubin GD, Beaulieu CF, Argiro V, et al. Perspective volume rendering of CT and MR images: applications for endoscopic imaging. *Radiology* 1996;199:321–330.
36. Hopper KD. Questions and answers: with helical CT, is nonionic contrast a better choice than ionic contrast for rapid and large IV bolus injections? *AJR* 1996;166:715–719.
37. Silverman PM, Brown B, Wray H, et al. Optimal contrast enhancement of the liver using helical (spiral) CT: value of SmartPrep. *AJR* 1995;164:1169–1171.
38. Gefter WB, Davis SD, Gurney JW, et al. RSNA '95 meeting notes: thoracic radiology. *Radiology* 1996;198:926–931.
39. Costello P, Ecker CP, Tello R, Hartnell GG. Assessment of the thoracic aorta by spiral CT. *AJR* 1992;158:1127–1130.
40. Remy-Jardin M, Remy J, Wattinne L, Giraud F. Central pulmonary thromboembolism: diagnosis with spiral volumetric CT with the single breath hold technique—comparison with pulmonary angiography. *Radiology* 1992;185:381–387.
41. Remy-Jardin M, Remy J, Cauvain O, Petyt L, Wannebroucq J, Beregi JP. Diagnosis of central pulmonary embolism with helical CT: role of two-dimensional multiplanar reformations. *AJR* 1995;165:1131–1138.
42. Goodman LR, Curtin JJ, Mewissen MW, et al. Detection of pulmonary embolism in patients with unresolved clinical and scintigraphic diagnosis: helical CT versus angiography. *AJR* 1995;164:1369–1374.
43. Posniak HV, Olson MC, Demos TC. Aortic motion artifact simulating dissection on CT scans: elimination with reconstructive segmented images. *AJR* 1993;161:557–558.
44. Burns MA, Molina PL, Gutierrez IR, Sagel SS. Motion artifact simulating aortic dissection on CT. *AJR* 1991;157:465–467.
45. Remy-Jardin M, Duyck P, Remy J, et al. Hilar lymph nodes: identification with spiral CT and histologic correlation. *Radiology* 1995;196:387–394.
46. Padhani AR, Fishman EK, Heitmiller RF, Wang K, Wheeler JH, Kuhlman JE. Multiplanar display of spiral CT data of the pulmonary hila in patients with lung cancer: Preliminary observations. *Clin Imaging* 1996;20:60–62.
47. Kuriyama K, Tateishi R, Kumatani T, et al. Pleural invasion by peripheral bronchogenic carcinoma: assessment with three-dimensional helical CT. *Radiology* 1994;191:365–369.
48. Wang G, Vannier MW. Longitudinal resolution in volumetric x-ray computerized tomography: analytical comparison between conventional and helical computerized tomography. *Med Phys* 1994;21:429–433.

CHAPTER 6

Spiral CT of Lung Cancer

Anwar R. Padhani and Elliot K. Fishman

In the United States, lung cancer is the leading cause of cancer death in men and has surpassed breast cancer as the leading cause of cancer death in women since the late 1980s (1). The incidence of lung cancer deaths has risen from 5 to more than 70 per 100,000 (2), and in women from 3 to more than 20 per 100,000 (3). In 1992, there were 161,000 new cases and 146,000 deaths from this disease. Many researchers have emphasized the association of smoking with lung cancer. Kabat and Wynder, for example, studied 2,668 patients with lung cancer (4–5). They found that only 1.9% of men and 13% of women were nonsmokers, but the cause of lung cancer can be attributed to many factors, considering the fact that only 10% of heavy smokers ever get lung cancer. It has been estimated that lung cancer mortality attributed to smoking is 80% among men (about 65,000 deaths per year) and 75% among women (about 27,00 deaths) (6). Other causative factors include occupational exposure to carcinogens such as asbestos, radon gas, bis(chloromethyl)ether, polycyclic aromatic hydrocarbons, chromium, nickel, and inorganic arsenic compounds. A genetic predisposition is an area of active research, but to date there is no conclusive genetic abnormality defining the risk for lung cancer.

The most important distinction with regard to treatment lies between small-cell lung cancer (20% to 30% of all lung cancers) and non–small-cell lung cancer, which is broadly divided into squamous cell carcinoma (30–50%), adenocarcinoma (10–35%), and large cell carcinoma (10–15%). Currently, the best chance for cure in cases of non–small-cell lung cancer is surgical resection, although radiation therapy and chemotherapy also offer potential cure. Unfortunately, less than 20% to 30% of patients prove to be operable after staging investigations. Factors rendering lung cancer inoperable include locally extensive disease, distant metastases, poor lung function, and clinically related factors such as ischemic heart disease. Advanced age alone is not a bar to surgery, although the risks are higher in the elderly. Surgery may be considered for small-cell cancer, and there are long-

term survivors, but very few patients are found to be operable after careful staging.

Although radiation therapy is most commonly used for palliative purposes, its role as an adjuvant therapy prior to surgery has been shown to improve survival in stage III non–small-cell carcinoma. Laser therapy effectively destroys endobronchial tumors but is rarely curative for larger lesions. Its main role lies in its ability to clear the larger bronchi, permitting the expansion of collapsed lobes. Laser therapy is also used to facilitate brachytherapy and conventional radiation treatment. Chemotherapy has been successful in the treatment of small-cell lung cancer but is limited in the treatment of non–small-cell tumors. There is some evidence that neoadjuvant chemotherapy increases the successful resection of stage IIIA tumors and can make some stage IIIB tumors resectable (7).

ROLE OF IMAGING IN EVALUATING LUNG CANCER

Because of its low cost, availability, and sensitivity, chest radiography is the preferred initial diagnostic technique for patients with known or suspected lung cancer (8). Computed tomography (CT) can confirm abnormalities seen on plain radiographs and can often detect lesions that are not seen on radiographs or linear tomograms. Before discussing the role of spiral CT it is necessary to appreciate what information is required by surgeons to perform a successful resection. This includes the optimal means of obtaining histological diagnosis, lesion stage, operability, and technical difficulty. It should be appreciated that even well-performed CT disagrees with stage found at surgery in a significant proportion of patients (9,10). Imaging can be used to define the appropriate therapy and to choose the appropriate diagnostic study (percutaneous needle aspiration, bronchoscopy, or mediastinoscopy). Its role extends to guiding therapy, including surgical resection and/or nonsurgical therapies such as laser coagulation, brachytherapy, and radiation planing.

95

SPIRAL CT PROTOCOL OPTIMIZATION

Although specific scanning protocols will vary, depending on the capabilities of each scanner, certain basic principles still apply (Table 6-1). Collimation of about 5 mm is ideal for evaluating most oncologic processes in the chest. Although thinner collimation of about 2 mm can be used for defining fine detail of the bronchial tree, this tends to be reserved for a more focused examination. Similarly, slice collimation in the range of 2–3 mm is also the preferred selection in cases where 3D reconstruction is to be obtained to achieve the best data sets possible. A pitch of up to 2 can be used when imaging the vascular system in the chest, although typically a pitch of up to 1.6 is usually used in most thoracic applications. For example, in cases performed for evaluation of suspected lung metastasis a protocol of 5-mm-thick sections, 8-mm/s table speed (pitch of 1.6), and 5-mm reconstruction interval are satisfactory.

The timing of data acquisition and rate and volume of contrast injection will vary, depending on the application. Injection rates in the range of 3–4 mL are usually reserved for cases where 3D reconstruction is required. In these cases a properly timed study in the arterial or venous phase can be achieved as needed. In most cases of staging lung cancer a scan delay of 40–50 s is adequate. An injection rate of 2 mL/s of a contrast such as Omnipaque-300 or Omnipaque-350 (Nycomed Inc, Princeton, NJ) is satisfactory. More dilute contrast can also be used, which provides a cost savings and helps to decrease artifacts from contrast in the central veins.

Where the chest and abdomen are to be scanned in a single examination, several options are available. One technique is to scan from an inferior to a superior direction, thereby scanning the liver at an earlier phase and following this up with the examination of the chest. On the other hand, depending on what phase of liver enhancement is desirable (arterial or portal phase), the chest can be examined first. With current subsecond CT scanning it is fairly easy to scan the entire chest and abdomen in less than 40 s, which is ideal in most cases. We have had little problem with patients holding their breath for the required period of time.

EVALUATION OF THE PERIPHERAL LUNG MASS

Approximately 40% of lung cancers are peripheral (i.e., arise beyond the origin of a segmental bronchus), and in 30% a peripheral lung mass is the main x-ray abnormality. It was hoped that screening of high-risk populations by sputum cytology and plain radiographs would improve the identification of early-stage lung cancer. Several very-large-scale studies, including the NCI Cooperative Evaluation Lung Cancer Group (11,12), showed that lung cancers identified by screening were more often early-stage tumors (40% versus 15%), and patients detected by screening had an improved 5-year survival of 35% versus 13% for the general population. Despite this, screening intervention failed to alter overall mortality rates, and mass screening for lung cancer cannot be recommended. Recently, a reappraisal of lung cancer screening (13) has suggested an improved outcome for patients with screening-detected cancer, and many physicians continue to screen patients at high risk for developing lung cancer with annual chest x-rays. In Japan, where 70% of lung cancers are peripheral, a recent study has evaluated the role of low-dose spiral CT in screening a high-risk population (14). Spiral CT detected 15 cancers in 3,457 examinations, only four of which were detected at radiography. Fourteen cancers were stage I. The role and cost effectiveness of low-dose spiral CT as an alternative screening modality has yet to be fully evaluated.

Spiral CT scanning adds a new dimension, both for the detection and for the characterization of pulmonary nodules (15–18). Spiral CT is the method of choice for detecting

TABLE 6-1. *Spiral CT acquisition protocols for evaluation of lung cancer*

CT parameters	CT indication			
	Metastatic surveys (lungs)	Lung cancer staging (including abdomen)	Lung cancer staging (thorax only)	3D reconstruction (i.e., pre-op planning)
Rotation time (secs)	.75–1	.75–1	.75–1	.75–1
Slice thickness (mm)	5	5–8	3–5	2–3
Pitch	1–1.6	1–1.6	1–1.6	1–2
kVp	120–140	120–140	120–140	120–140
mAs	210–300	210–300	210–300	210–300
Scan duration	≤30 secs	≤40 secs	≤30 secs	≤40 secs
Reconstruction Index (mm)	5	5–8	5	1–3
Reconstruction algorithm	180 LI, High resolution or standard	180 LI, Standard	180 LI, Standard	180 LI, Standard
Scan direction	IS/SI	SI/IS	SI	SI
Respiration	Inspiration	Inspiration	Inspiration	Inspiration
Contrast enhancement	–	+	+	+

180 LI = 180 linear interpolation; + required, – not required; SI and IS = superoinferior and inferosuperior.

pulmonary nodules because of its ability to scan the entire volume of the lungs contiguously in a breath-hold without slice-to-slice misregistration. This is particularly valuable at the lung bases, where the potential for respiratory misregistration is greatest. Respiratory motion artifacts that occasionally degrade image quality in conventional CT studies and obscure lesions are also significantly reduced. Costello et al. (15) compared standard and spiral CT in 20 patients with suspected lung nodules of less than 1 cm. Spiral CT with overlapping sections (8 mm thick with 50% overlap) detected four of 22 nodules in 55 patients that were missed by standard CT due to respiratory misregistration. Similarly, Heywang-Koebrunner et al. (16) were able to detect 301 of 305 nodules with spiral CT; the four missed nodules measured less than 5 mm. In comparison, conventional CT missed 10% of nodules, mostly those that measured less than 10 mm. Similarly, Remy-Jardin et al. (19) compared

nonoverlapping but contiguous thick-sectioned spiral CT (10 mm) with conventional CT in 39 patients who had suspected pulmonary nodules. They found that the mean number of nodules per patient was significantly higher with spiral CT and that detection of small nodules (less than 5 mm) was improved. However, in only three patients with single nodules on conventional CT were multiple nodules with spiral CT detected. Furthermore, six additional nodules were not seen by spiral CT but were detected by surgery.

While spiral CT can consistently detect more lung lesions than conventional CT, the role of overlapping reconstructions is still somewhat controversial (Figs. 6-1, 6-2). Collie et al. (20) used 10-mm-thick slices constructed every 5 mm and showed no additional advantage to scans reconstructed every 10 mm. Buckley et al. (21), however, using 8-mm slices and reconstructions of 4–5 mm in 67 patients found that more nodules were detected with the use of overlapping

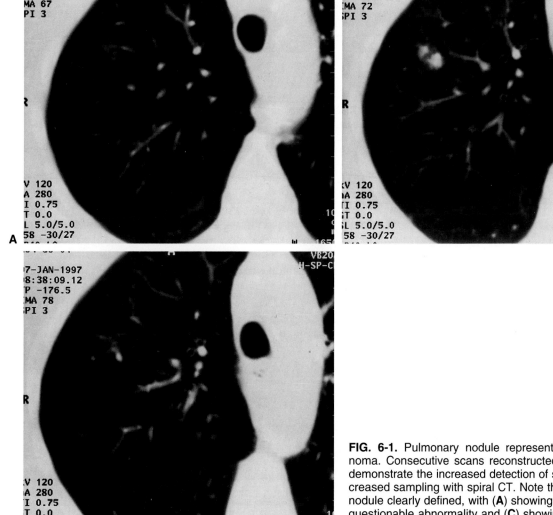

FIG. 6-1. Pulmonary nodule representing an adenocarcinoma. Consecutive scans reconstructed at 2-mm intervals demonstrate the increased detection of small nodules by increased sampling with spiral CT. Note that only in (**B**) is the nodule clearly defined, with (**A**) showing the suggestion of a questionable abnormality and (**C**) showing no suggestion of even a possible lesion. The increased sampling with spiral CT increases lesion detection by approximately 9%.

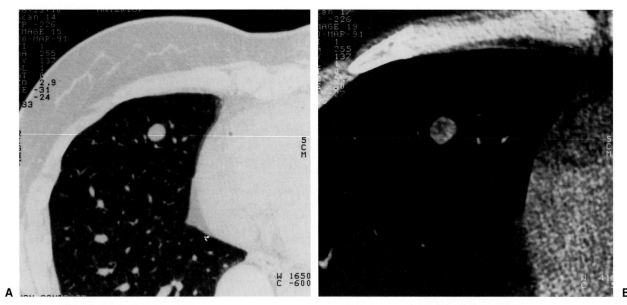

FIG. 6-2. Pulmonary hamartoma. Spiral CT (**A**) demonstrates a nodule in the right middle lobe that is well defined with sharp margins. On soft-tissue windows (**B**) evidence of fat within the lesion is seen consistent with a hamartoma.

scans (583 versus 566) and that there was a significant improvement in the confidence of interpreters, with more definite and less indeterminate nodules. Overlapping scans appeared to aid less experienced observers. The most important advantage of overlapping scans is a reduction of false-positive results. In the study by Buckley, 259 of 688 lesions identified were false positive, and whereas 94 nodules were reclassified using overlapping sections, a sizable number of false-positive results remained. In addition to standard film and console viewing of spiral CT images, Seltzer et al. (22) have evaluated the role of cine viewing of highly overlapped scans (10-mm slices reconstructed every 2 mm) and found an increased number of nodules detected with cine rather than film evaluation (mean 0.69 vs. 0.58 per patient; $p <$ 0.006).

The increased sensitivity of spiral CT in detecting pulmonary nodules is accompanied by decreased specificity. Small lesions are a real dilemma because they cannot be biopsied percutaneously and are not palpable at thoracotomy. The sensitivity and specificity of spiral CT has not been formally assessed in radiological–pathological studies. Palpation of the lungs for nodules is not a reliable standard (23). The specificity depends on the presence of extrathoracic malignancy and the frequency of benign entities in a population. Granulomas frequently due to histoplasmosis feature prominently in studies using conventional CT from the United States (24–26) but are less common in European countries (27,28).

Despite the increased sensitivity of spiral CT, it is still unclear whether all routine chest examinations for lung nodules require overlapping spiral CT. Overlapping reconstructions may be more time-consuming to generate on some scanners, and the cost of additional films and data storage is

important. Some institutions reserve the use of overlapping reconstructions for those patients in whom there is a high index of suspicion that nodules are present, and when detection of solitary or additional nodules is clinically significant. This includes patients who have lesions that are potentially resectable, because they have only one or a few pulmonary nodules (e.g., sarcoma and teratoma metastases). Other institutions routinely use spiral CT with overlapping reconstructions for all patients.

Spiral CT can be valuable for nodule characterization (evaluation of nodule density, structure and vascularity). Volumetric acquisition ensures that contiguous scans are obtained and the ability to retrospectively reconstruct slices at any given position, assures that at least one reconstructed slice falls through the center of a nodule. This reduces partial volume averaging and allows improved densitometry assessment of lesions. However, when the slice thickness is larger than the size of the nodule being evaluated, densitometry measures may still be erroneous due to partial volume averaging of aerated lung with the nodule. Densitometry seeks to evaluate nodules for the presence of calcium and fat in an attempt to characterize nodules as benign. It must be remembered, however, that 10% of cancers have evidence of calcification, and although the presence of fat in a nodule represents evidence of a hamartoma, this is present in less than 50% of cases (29) (see Fig. 6-2).

Spiral CT also allows a more precise morphological evaluation of pulmonary nodules than routine axial images. Morphological cues suggesting metastatic lesions include size and contour of lesions. A frequently observed sign is the connection of a metastatic nodule with an adjacent branch of the pulmonary artery (30). The ability to reliably demonstrate the relationship of vessels to pulmonary nodules has

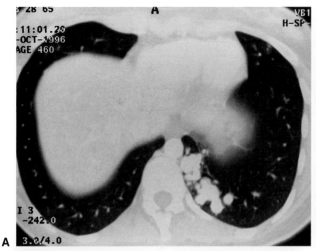

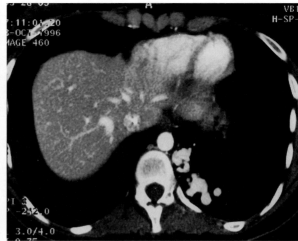

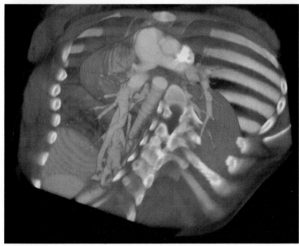

FIG. 6-3. Pulmonary arterial venous malformation (PAVM) (**A,B**). Spiral CT demonstrates a multilobular enhancing mass in the posterior portion of the left lower lung. The enhancement is equal to that of the aorta and is consistent with the pulmonary arterial venous malformation. (**C**) The 3D reconstruction clearly defines the full extent of the AVM. This was subsequently embolized.

also proved valuable in assessing patients with pulmonary arteriovenous malformations (AVMs). Remy et al. (31) showed that thin-section spiral CT is a sensitive, noninvasive means of detecting and localizing pulmonary AVMs (Fig. 6-3). Enhancement of pulmonary nodules following intravenous contrast increases the likelihood of a lesion being malignant (32,33). This represents an important new approach to nodule assessment and one in which spiral CT plays an important role. We recommend that thin sections be used (3–4 mm) with a pitch of 1 and standard reconstruction algorithms. Precontrast and postcontrast images at 1, 2, 3, and 4 min should be obtained from the onset of administration of 80–120 mL of intravenous contrast. The imaging parameters should be identical, and region-of-interest analysis should be performed through the center of lesions.

Spiral CT is also valuable in the assessment of the relationship of masses with adjacent airways (Fig. 6-4). Using thin sections, routine identification of sixth- and seventh-order airways even in the periphery of the lungs is possible (34). The ability to demonstrate the relationship of lung nodules to bronchial anatomy appears to correlate with the success of fibreoptic bronchoscopy diagnosis (34–36). Thus although the yield of bronchoscopy can be improved with

spiral CT, the accuracy of the overall procedure is more limited. In a prospective study by Naidich (34) the accuracy of bronchoscopy for 21 focal lesions in 18 patients was not improved compared with retrospective evaluations. However, Wang et al. (37) have demonstrated that when a bronchus is seen leading to a nodule of >2 cm, the use of transbronchial biopsy may improve the accuracy of fibreoptic bronchoscopy. This suggests a potential role for spiral CT in determining the optimal method for obtaining histological diagnosis. Spiral CT with multiplanar reconstructions is also of some value in performing needle-tip localizations when patients undergo CT-guided percutaneous needle aspiration or biopsy (38).

EVALUATION OF CENTRAL AIRWAYS

Conventional and spiral CT are useful for evaluating the central airways of patients with hemoptysis, particularly for the detection of endobronchial lesions (36,39). Volumetric imaging allows excellent multiplanar reconstructions with routine demonstration of all lobar and segmental airways, and provides improved depiction of airway involvement by lung cancer (Figs. 6-5, 6-6).

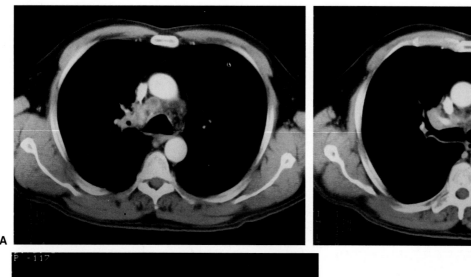

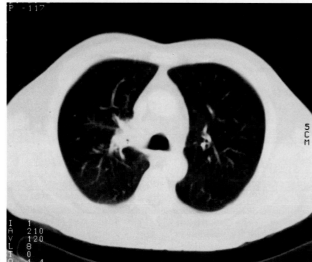

FIG. 6-4. Large cell undifferentiated carcinoma with encasement of right upper lung bronchus and mediastinal adenopathy. Sequence of images of soft-tissue window setting (**A,B**) demonstrates nodes in the pretracheal space extending into the right hilum with encasement around right upper lobe bronchus. Image at lung setting (**C**) demonstrates the encasement by tumor of the right upper lung bronchus that is now but a pinhole. The extension through the right wall of the trachea is also seen. Interestingly, this patient presented with a cerebellar metastasis.

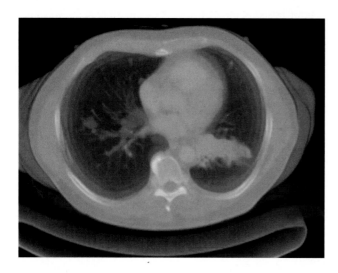

FIG. 6-5. Undifferentiated carcinoma with satellite lesions. A volumetric 3D reconstruction demonstrates the primary mass encasing the left lower lung bronchus. Satellite lesions are seen bilaterally.

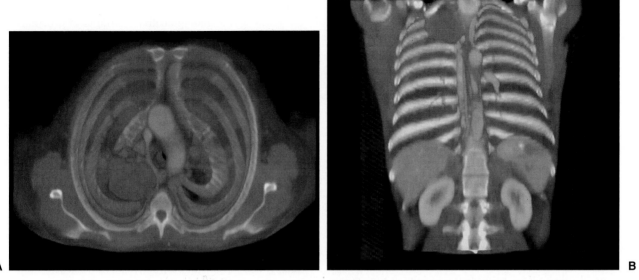

FIG. 6-6. (A,B) Pancoast tumor. Volumetric 3D reconstructions from different projections clearly define the extent of tumor. These images can be useful for preoperative planning and for radiation therapy simulation.

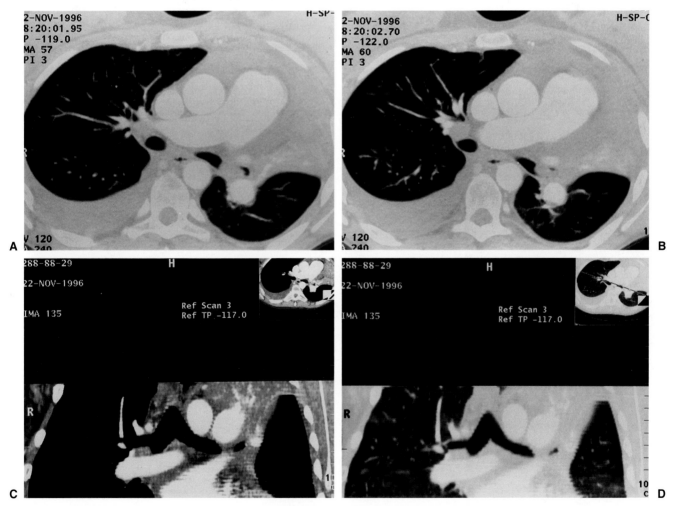

FIG. 6-7. Left upper lung collapse secondary to central mucous plug, simulating a central neoplasm. Spiral CT with contrast enhancement **(A,B)** demonstrates collapse of the left upper lung. Thin-section CT with multiplanar reconstructions **(C,D)** demonstrates an intraluminal mass. On bronchoscopy this was not a tumor but a mucous plug. The patient had a history of collagen vascular disease.

Although multiplanar reconstructions are useful for assessing airways, the utility of 3D reconstruction in evaluating central airways is unclear. Three-dimensional reconstructions demonstrate tracheal and bronchial lesions/stenoses better than conventional scans and can demonstrate airways beyond stenoses and therefore beyond the reach of the bronchoscope (40). Remy et al. (41) have shown that multiplanar reconstructions combined with 3D surface-shaded displays were better than conventional axial images, and provided information on the location and type of lesions within the tracheobronchial tree. When multiplanar reconstructions and 3D displays (Fig. 6-7) were compared with fibreoptic bronchoscopy appearances, concordance was demonstrated in 83% of cases, and multiplanar reconstructions and 3D images were superior in 17%, depicting airways changes that were either not seen or incompletely evaluated by fibreoptic bronchoscopy. Three-dimensional reconstructions are also helpful in the evaluation of the postoperative airway after lung or lobar resections and in patients with anastomotic complications after lung transplantation (42).

Another exciting area of bronchial tree visualization is virtual-reality bronchoscopy. Thin, highly overlapped spiral CT images of the airways are used in this computer simulation technique (43–49), which allows endobronchial visualization from the viewpoint of a bronchoscopist. Compared with axial images, multiplanar reconstructions, and conventional 3D techniques, virtual reality allows a unique perspective with free exploration within the 3D imaging volume (Fig. 6-8). The potential advantages of this technique include

noninvasive diagnosis; improved evaluation of the extent of pathology, including anatomy distal to obstructions; and planning of endoscopic procedures (45).

LUNG CANCER STAGING

Rationale for Staging Lung Cancer

The stage of lung cancer plays a pivotal role in directing therapy and predicting prognosis. Curative resection of non–small-cell lung cancer is possible if the disease is diagnosed early before mediastinal lymph node or systemic metastases occur. If lymph node metastases are present at the time of surgery, some studies have shown that only 8% of patients survive 5 years, whereas without nodal metastases, the 5-year survival approaches 50%. Because the morbidity and mortality may be substantial in some patients (e.g., the elderly and those with obstructive airway disease), emphasis has been placed on careful staging in these patients before surgery. If a patient has mediastinal lymph node metastases and is a high surgical risk, radiation and/or chemotherapy may be preferable. Similarly, histologically proven contralateral metastases contraindicate surgery even if the patient is otherwise healthy.

In 1997 the American Joint Committee on Cancer (AJCC), and the Union Internationale Contre Cancer (UICC), issued a revised worldwide tumor, node, metastasis (TNM) staging system (Table 6-2) (46,47). Using this system, *T* indicates the features of the primary tumor, *N* indicates the involvement of regional lymph nodes, and *M* refers

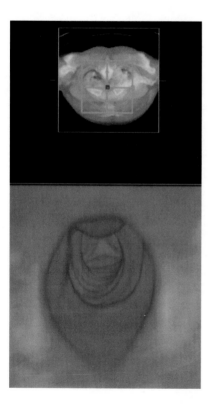

FIG. 6-8. Virtual bronchoscopy. Three-dimensional reconstruction looking down the trachea to the bifurcation in a virtual bronchoscopy presentation.

TABLE 6-2. *(1997) TNM staging systems for lung cancer*

T-Primary Tumor

T0 No evidence of primary tumor

Tx Tumor proved by the presence of malignant cells in bronchopulmonary secretions, but not visualized by x-ray or broncho-scopically, or any tumor that cannot be assessed as in a retreatment staging

Tis Carcinoma in situ

T1 A tumor 3 cm or less in size in greatest dimension, surrounded by lung or visceral pleura, and without evidence of invasion proximal to lobar bronchus at bronchoscopy*

T2 A tumor more than 3 cm in greatest dimension, or a tumor of any size that invades the visceral pleura or has associated atelectasis or obstructive pneumonitis extending to the hilar region. At bronchoscopy the proximal extent of the demonstrable tumor must be within a lobar bronchus or at least 2 cm distal to the carina. Any associated atelectasis or obstructive pneumonitis must involve less than the entire lung.

T3 A tumor of any size with direct extension into the chest wall (including superior sulcus tumors), diaphragm, or mediastinal pleura or pericardium without involving the heart, great vessels, trachea, esophagus or vertebral body or a tumor in the main bronchus within 2 cm of the carina without involvement of the carina.

T4 A tumor of any size with invasion of the mediastinum, heart, great vessels, trachea, esophagus, vertebral body, separate tumor nodule(s) in the same lobe carina; or presence of malignant pleural effusion.#

N-Regional Lymph Nodes

N0 No demonstrable metastasis to regional lymph nodes

N1 Metastasis to lymph nodes in the ipsilateral peribronchial and/or ipsilateral hilar region (including direct extension)

N2 Metastasis to ipsilateral mediastinal and/or subcarinal lymph node(s)

N3 Metastasis in contralateral mediastinal, contralateral hilar, ipsilateral or contralateral scalene or supraclavicular lymph node(s)

M-Distant Metastases

M0 No (known) distant metastases

M1 Distant metastasis present includes separate tumor nodule(s) on a different lobe (ipsilateral or contralateral)

* The uncommon superifical tumor of any size with its invasive component limited to the bronchial wall that may extend proximal to the left main bronchus is classified as T1

Most pleural effusions associated with lung cancer are due to tumor. There are, however, a few patients in whom cytopathological examination of the pleural fluid is negative for tumor; the fluid is non bloody and is not an exudate. In such cases where these elements and clinical judgment dictate that the effusion is not related to the tumor, the cancer should be staged T1, T2 or T3 excluding effusion as a staging element.

to the presence or absence of metastases. The primary tumor is subdivided into four T categories, depending on size, site, and local involvement (T1–T4). Lymph node spread has been divided into bronchopulmonary (N1), ipsilateral mediastinal (N2), and contralateral or supraclavicular disease (N3), and metastatic spread is absent or present (M0 or M1).

Four stages have been identified with significant differences in 5-year survival, depending on the stage at diagnosis (Table 6-3). Stage I consists of T1 or T2 lesions with no hilar or mediastinal lymph node and no distant metastases. These lesions are resectable, and T1 lesions have a better prognosis than T2 tumors in this group. Stage II tumors have peribronchial or hilar lymph node involvement and are

TABLE 6-3. *Staging descriptors and 5 year survivals*

Stage	Description	5 Year survival (%)
1	T1–2, N0, M0	60–80
2	T1–2, N1, M0	25–50
3a	T3, N0–1, M0	25–40
	T1–3, N2, M0	10–30
3b	T4, any N, M0; any T, N3, M0	<5
4	Any T, any N, M1	<5

resectable by lobectomy or pneumonectomy, with the hope of cure. Stage III has been divided into two groups; group IIIA is characterized by limited mediastinal, pericardial, and chest wall invasion and represents potentially resectable tumors, depending on patient selection, surgical skill, and patient fitness. Stage IIIB tumors are considered unresectable on the basis of extensive local spread or because of contralateral or supraclavicular nodal metastases. These patients are still localized in terms of radiation treatment planning.

In addition to redefining the stages, new descriptors were added to the TNM classification. T4 indicates lesions with extensive invasion into the mediastinum, chest wall, or diaphragm, or the presence of a malignant pleural effusion. T3 indicates localized invasion and is therefore potentially resectable. N3 disease indicates the involvement of supraclavicular or mediastinal or hilar nodes on the contralateral side of the tumor. This nodal involvement is associated with a worse prognosis than ipsilateral nodal involvement. When patients are staged using minimally invasive procedures, a significant percentage are understaged compared with the ultimate surgical and pathological stage. Despite this it is clinically relevant to stage patients before (clinical and imaging) and after therapy (surgical and pathological). This system is also used for small-cell lung cancer, although most oncologists divide small-cell lung cancer into limited and extensive disease, according to the Veterans Administration Lung Group. Limited disease is defined as tumor confined to one hemithorax and regional lymph nodes based on whether all detectable tumor can be encompassed within a tolerable radiotherapy port. Extensive disease is defined as that which exists beyond these bounds. Ipsilateral pleural effusion and varying degrees of supraclavicular node involvement have been considered consistent with limited or extensive stage (48). Regardless of the staging system used, spiral CT has the potential to provide a more accurate evaluation than other techniques used to date.

Evaluation of the Primary Tumor

Tumor Size

Maximal lesion size is one factor that distinguishes a T1 from a T2 lesion (≤3 cm). The maximal tumor diameter may not be in the axial plane and the size determined from spiral-generated multiplanar reconstructions may be more accurate. Spiral CT also allows accurate tumor volume estimations, which are important for planning radiotherapy and may be used for monitoring response of tumors to chemotherapy. The assessment of tumor boundaries in patients with central obstructing lung cancers with adjacent lung atelectasis or consolidation is often difficult. In such patients, spiral CT with intravenous contrast enhancement can occasionally allow differentiation of central enhancing vessels from adjacent tumor and occasionally tumor from adjacent enhancing collapsed lung (Fig. 6-9) (49).

Tracheobronchial Tree Invasion

Invasion of the main bronchus usually classifies the tumor as T2 (Fig. 6-10), although the uncommon superficial grow-ing tumor with an invasive component limited to the bronchial wall is still classified as T1. CT signs suggestive of bronchial involvement include abnormal soft tissue within the bronchus and/or a reduced caliber of the airway with irregular bronchial wall thickening. The proximal invasion of the tracheobronchial tree by tumor is important for staging and surgical resection. At bronchoscopy, a T2 tumor (resectable) must be confined to a lobar bronchus or must be at least 2 cm distal to the tracheal carina. Conventional CT has poor accuracy in predicting the proximal extent of bronchial involvement by central cancers. Surgeons frequently rely on bronchoscopy or on the findings during thoracotomy (50). The accuracy of axial CT in predicting the proximal extent of bronchial invasion is limited due to partial volume averaging and the axial plane of imaging. Submucosal extension by tumors may lead to false-negative findings both at CT and at bronchoscopy. Thin sections improve sensitivity of conventional CT (51) and thin-section spiral (≤ 4 mm) are helpful in evaluating the central airways optimally (52). The use of multiplanar reconstructions may facilitate the analysis of tumor invasion into adjacent structures. However, the accuracy in predicting the extent of tracheobronchial invasion by central lung cancers with surgical correlation has not been formally evaluated.

Chest Wall Invasion

Invasion of the parietal pleura, chest wall, or ribs constitutes T3 tumor (Fig. 6-11). The deeper the invasion, the worse the prognosis. Chest wall invasion does not preclude surgical resection because the tumor and chest wall can be removed en bloc with a clear margin followed by chest wall reconstruction. This procedure is associated with increased morbidity and mortality. Prognosis is related to the completeness of resection, with no patients surviving 5 years after incomplete resection.

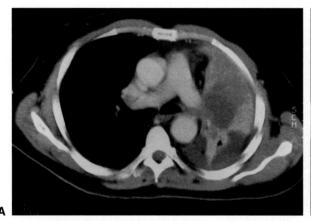
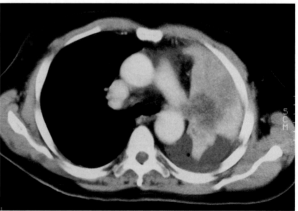

FIG. 6-9. (**A,B**) Non–small-cell carcinoma of the left lung with tumor margins demonstrated by differential enhancement. In this image the pulmonary artery and the aorta enhance, as does the atelectatic lung. The posterior pleural effusion is of lowered attenuation. The left hilar tumor is also clearly defined, based on a lower attenuation. This differential enhancement can be very valuable in designing accurate radiation therapy ports.

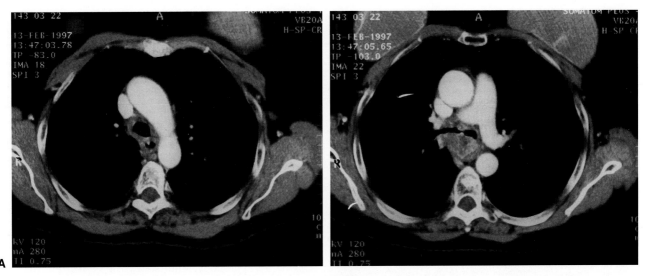

FIG. 6-10. (A,B) Invasion of the trachea by tumor. Carcinoma of the lung shows encasement of the tracheal bifurcation with narrowing of both right and left main stem bronchi. The patient also had tumor extension with secondary involvement of the esophagus, causing dysphagia.

Generally, the results of CT in predicting chest wall invasion have been disappointing, with local pain being as sensitive an indicator of invasion as CT (53). Sensitivities range from 38% to 87%, and specificities from 40% to 90% (54–58). A number of CT signs of invasion have been evaluated, including those depicting rib destruction, pleural thickening, obtuse angle between the mass and chest wall, and ≥3 cm contact between the mass and chest wall. Bone destruction and obvious chest wall invasion are the only reliable signs of chest wall invasion (Fig. 6-12) (54,55). Artificially induced pneumothorax has also been evaluated in a small number of patients to diagnose chest wall invasion (59,60). Problems occur when benign pleural adhesions are present, resulting in intermediate specificity for the technique and accuracy ranges of from 76% to 100%. Recently, studies have also evaluated the relative movement of the tumor mass in relation to the mediastinum or chest wall during a series of deep breath-holds (61,62). These investigators have found that the presence of movement with respiratory phase is a reliable indicator of the lack of parietal pleural invasion for tumors in the middle and lower lungs.

Another recent study has evaluated the role of 3D surface-shaded displays in predicting chest wall invasion (63). These investigators reviewed axial and 3D images in 42 patients with peripheral lung cancer. They found that 3D reconstructions were superior to axial images in assessing *visceral* pleural invasion and could predict visceral pleural invasion more accurately (92% versus 17%). They were also able to

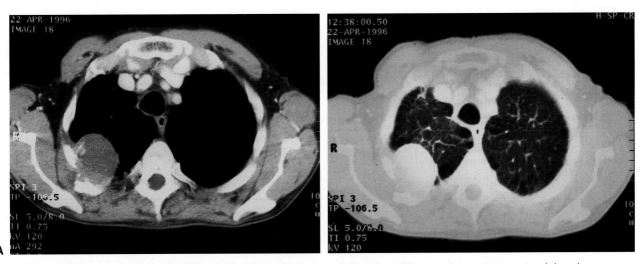

FIG. 6-11. (A,B) Carcinoma of the lung with chest wall invasion. CT scan demonstrates a peripheral carcinoma of the right upper lung with direct invasion of pleura and chest wall. Note the obvious rib destruction. The patient had underlying chronic obstructive pulmonary disease.

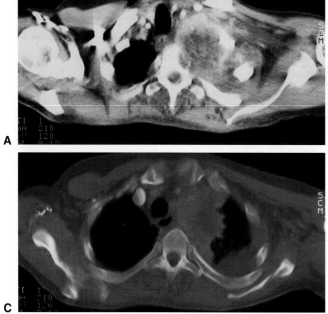

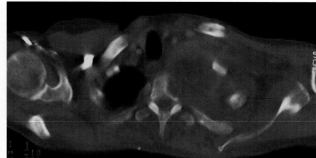

FIG. 6-12. (A–C) Pancoast tumor. Spiral CT scan demonstrates the large tumor in the left apex extending into the mediastinum. The tumor invades the spine at approximately the T2 level, with destruction of the thoracic vertebral body.

differentiate simple pleural tags from pleural invasion by tumor. Although their results are encouraging, false positives occurred with benign pleural fibrosis, adjacent lung atelectasis, and consolidation commonly found adjacent to tumors. In addition, the results are very dependent on the threshold chosen for reconstructions. Volume rendering of these data sets may prove useful in this group of patients (Fig. 6-13).

Multiple resonance imaging (MRI) has better contrast resolution and provides direct multiplanar imaging capability, making it potentially superior to conventional CT in predicting chest wall invasion (64–68). However, MRI frequently fails to show rib destruction, and CT is superior in this regard. Deschildre et al. (69) found that MRI and spiral CT had similar sensitivities for detecting rib involvement, but the specificity of spiral CT was higher. Furthermore, inflammatory change and tumor extension into the chest wall may

have similar appearances on MRI, which makes it difficult to distinguish between these two entities (66,67). Indeed, in the report of the Radiology Diagnostic Oncology Group (RDOG) trial involving 23 patients with surgical and pathological correlation, CT and MRI were found to be equivalent (68). More recently, the use of surface coil imaging with contrast enhancement has shown improved results. Padovani et al. (64), showed that in 34 patients with pathological proof and/or CT evidence of bony destruction near the tumor, MRI has a sensitivity of 90% and a specificity of 86%.

Superior Sulcus Tumors

Superior sulcus tumors (Pancoast tumor) involve the lung apex and invade the first rib, brachial plexus, and stellate ganglion, causing Pancoast syndrome (Fig. 6-14). Treatments include preoperative radiotherapy followed by en bloc resection of the lung, chest wall, and frequently the T1 nerve root. Residual disease is treated with postoperative radiotherapy. The overall survival is about 40%. Contraindications to surgery include T4 tumor (vertebral body invasion, subclavian artery, or venous invasion) or unresectable N2 nodal disease.

MRI is superior to CT in detecting chest wall invasion as well as in evaluating other structures, such as the brachial plexus, blood vessels, and vertebral body. The limitations of CT arise from the axial plane of imaging, the presence of beam-hardening artifacts from bony structures, and the poorer contrast resolution when compared with MRI. Anatomic relationships are better demonstrated in the sagittal and coronal planes and thus MRI is the favored technique. However, MRI frequently fails to demonstrate rib destruction and spiral CT–acquired multiplanar images may be

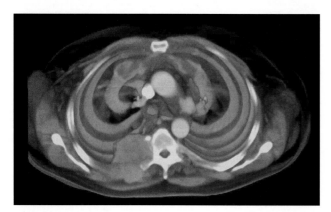

FIG. 6-13. Carcinoma of the lung with chest wall invasion. Volume-rendered 3D image defines tumor and associated rib destruction and chest wall extension.

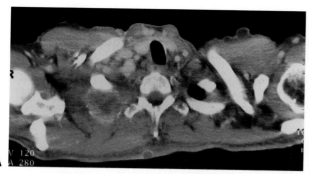
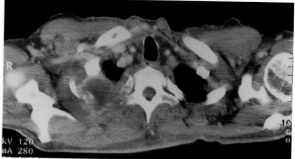

FIG. 6-14. (A,B) Pancoast tumor. CT using soft-tissue window demonstrates a mass in the right upper lung that is a classic Pancoast tumor. Note that the mass invades the spine with destruction of the T2 vertebral body and extension through the chest wall also noted at other levels.

more sensitive than MRI. Three-dimensional reconstructions can also be used in selective cases to clarify the complex relationships between chest wall and vascular structures at the thoracic inlet (70–72).

Mediastinal Pleura, Pericardium, and Diaphragm Invasion

Tumors that invade the mediastinal pleural fat or the pericardium and diaphragm are T3 tumors and are therefore potentially resectable (Fig. 6-15). Neither CT nor MRI has been valuable in diagnosing early mediastinal pleural invasion (73,74). Contiguity of tumor with pleura does not necessarily indicate invasion, and only with definite interdigitation by tumor of the mediastinum can invasion be confirmed. Similarly, continuity of tumor to pericardium and diaphragm does not necessarily indicate invasion. Lesions that abut the diaphragm are ideally suited for imaging in the coronal or sagittal plane. Spiral-generated multiplanar images are superior to MRI in this regard because suspended respiration results in sharp delineation of the diaphragm. Multiplanar recon-

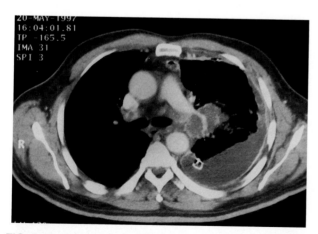

FIG. 6-15. Spiral CT of lung cancer with invasion of pulmonary artery. Spiral CT demonstrates central tumor with encasement of the left main pulmonary artery. A left pleural effusion is also seen. Postobstructive changes are noted, as well as narrowing of the left main stem bronchus.

structions are also helpful in determining the extent of peridiaphragmatic lesions.

Invasion of the Mediastinum, Heart, and Great Vessels

T4 cancers are either so extensive or so centrally located that surgical resection for cure is not an option. Involvement of mediastinal structures (esophagus, carina, trachea, heart, and great vessels and vertebral body) indicates advanced cancer, as does the presence of a malignant pleural effusion. Of patients with lung cancer, 5% to 10% have nonmalignant pleural effusions as a result of atelectasis, obstructive pneumonitis, lymphatic or venous obstruction, or pulmonary embolism. Such patients should be staged without effusion as a stage element. Despite effusions being nonmalignant, patients with pleural effusions form a poor diagnostic group, with 95% eventually turning out to be surgically unresectable.

Preoperative distinction of mediastinal invasion by tumor (T4) (Fig. 6-16) or its involved mediastinal lymph nodes (N2) can sometimes be difficult. Excellent vascular opacification is essential for the diagnosis of vascular invasion. Although the diagnosis can be made confidently using transaxial CT, most investigators believe that MRI is more sensitive than CT. However, the excellent vascular opacification together with thin cuts and the MPR and 3D capability of spiral CT should make it more sensitive than conventional CT. In addition, spiral CT should replace the occasional use of angiography in evaluating vascular involvement by lung cancer (75) (see Fig. 6-16; Figs. 6-17–6-18).

Evaluation of Regional Lymphadenopathy

Peribronchial and hilar nodes beyond the mediastinal pleural reflection at surgery constitute N1 lymphadenopathy (Fig. 6-19). These are generally resected at the time of lung resection. Surgery for N2 disease remains a controversial area in the surgical management of lung cancer. Involvement of ipsilateral mediastinal and subcarinal nodes implies a poorer prognosis, particularly if diagnosed preoperatively

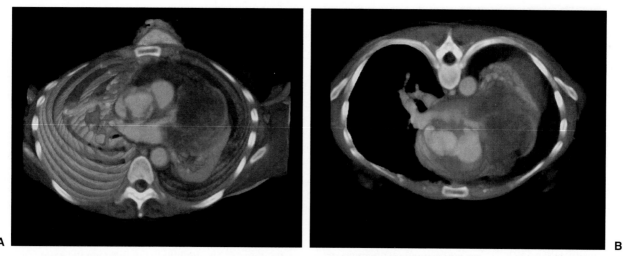

FIG. 6-16. (A,B) Invasion of the left atrium by a small-cell carcinoma. Three-dimensional reconstructions as viewed from below and above define tumor invading left atrium by direct extension.

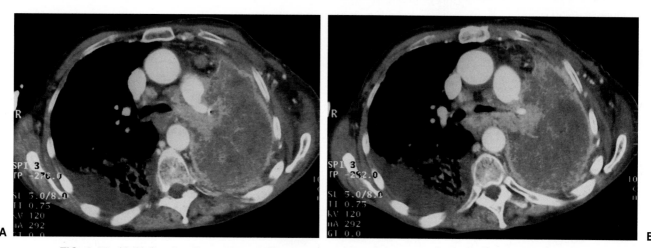

FIG. 6-17. (A,B) Small-cell carcinoma of the lung. Extensive tumor infiltration of the left hilum is seen with tumor extending to and encasing the left main pulmonary artery. Involvement of nodes in left hilum and subcarinal region are also seen on this study. Collapsed left upper lobe is also well defined with tumor encasement of the left main stem bronchus.

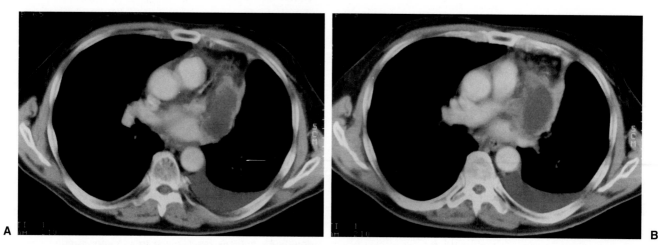

FIG. 6-18. (A,B) Small-cell carcinoma with invasion of left pulmonary artery and atrium. Small-cell carcinoma encases the left pulmonary artery with extension into the left atrium. The patient also has a left pleural effusion that was malignant. The encasement is well defined because of the ability to scan during optimal opacification of the vessels with spiral CT.

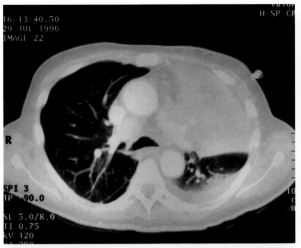

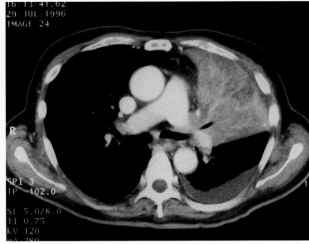

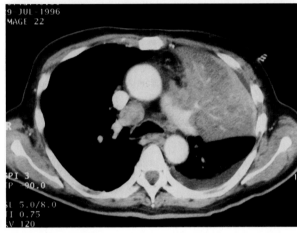

FIG. 6-19. (A,B) Non–small-cell lung cancer with extensive hilar and mediastinal disease. Spiral CT with rapid contrast infusion and early acquisition demonstrates the full extent of tumor with nodal disease seen in right pretracheal zone. The collapse of the left lung secondary to central tumor encasement is also seen, as is the invasion of the left pulmonary artery.

using invasive or noninvasive staging techniques. Less than 10% of patients survive 5 years. Patients with N2 disease should be considered for surgery, but patient selection is important. Adverse prognostic factors include multiple levels of N2 disease, multiple lymph nodes enlarged at one level, an adenocarcinoma histology, and extranodal spread of disease. More than 75% of patients with N2 disease are discovered to be in this category.

Minimal N2 Disease

Single-station nodal disease with microscopic foci of disease not clinically apparent on noninvasive staging constitutes this subset. Patients are usually discovered to have nodal disease at the time of thoracotomy or on mediastinoscopy. Five-year survival rates range from 10% to 20% but can be higher if these lymph nodes are completely resected. Few patients survive incomplete resection. The criteria for resection in patients with minimal N2 disease include a normal CT scan or mediastinoscopy identifying one station of lymph node involvement with only microscopic disease. These patients should have a complete mediastinal lymph node dissection at the time of surgical excision of the primary tumor. One retrospective study has suggested a dou-

bling of 5-year survival (16% versus 7%) when lymph nodal dissection is carried out in patients with this stage of disease (76).

Advanced N2 Disease

Patients with bulky N2 disease comprise the major part of stage IIIA disease. These patients are usually discovered preoperatively and are considered by most surgeons to be inoperable, with few patients surviving 5 years after surgical resection. This group of patients is usually treated with chemotherapy or chemoradiation.

Recently, both retrospective (77) and prospective (78) studies have demonstrated that induction chemotherapy improves resectability and long-term survival in patients with histologically proved N2 disease. Response to chemotherapy occurs in 50% of patients, and complete resection is possible in 50% to 60% of patients. In the study by Roth et al. (78) patients randomized with preoperative chemotherapy and surgery had a survival of 64 months, compared with 11 months for patients randomized to surgery alone.

From the preceding discussion it is apparent that the optimal surgical approach (surgery alone, induction chemotherapy and surgery, no surgery) depends on the location and disease status of mediastinal lymph nodal staging. The N staging can be performed invasively by surgical exploration or by imaging techniques. It should be noted that subaortic and aortopulmonary nodes cannot be reached by a cervical mediastinoscopy. These nodes can be sampled via a left anterior mediastinotomy. Thoracoscopy can sample paraesophageal nodes and pulmonary ligament nodes. Mediastinoscopy has a sensitivity of 85% to 90%, a specificity of 100%, and an accuracy of 66% to 90% (79).

Both CT and MRI define abnormality of mediastinal lymph nodes by site and size criteria, although morphological features such as the presence of lymph node calcification or hilar fat indicate benign features, and extracapsular soft tissue generally indicates malignant disease with poor prognosis (Fig. 6-20). There is no general agreement on the size of normal mediastinal lymph nodes or on whether long- or short-axis transverse diameter should be measured. In some cases MRI has advantages over CT: Signal void in vessels helps to differentiate nodes from vessels, and multiplanar imaging can allow optimal visualization of lymph nodes in the subcarinal and aortopulmonary window. However, the poorer spatial resolution of MRI overestimates lymph node size, and respiratory motion can cause blurring and can overestimate lymph node size. The failure of MRI to detect lymph node calcification can result in benign fully calcified lymph nodes being misdiagnosed as large malignant nodes. Spiral CT with optimal enhancement contrast injection makes it significantly easier to detect even the smallest of nodes.

Many studies have aroused controversy and confusion about the role of CT in staging mediastinal lymph node metastases in patients with lung cancer. Sensitivities range between 41% and 95%; specificities, between 25% and 99%; accuracy, between 53% and 94%. A detailed discussion of this is beyond the scope of this article, and the reader is directed toward many excellent review articles for more details (80–83). An important reason for this variation is related to the method of nodal measurement. Currently, the consensus is to measure the short axis diameter, as this is a more accurate predictor of nodal size (84) (Fig. 6-21).

Another variable is the size above which a node is considered malignant. It can be expected that a decrease in size will increase specificity but at the expense of sensitivity. Normal-sized regional lymph nodes may prove to have metastases at histology, and nodal enlargement can be due to reactive hyperplasia or other nonmalignant conditions. In general, normal-sized mediastinal lymph nodes may be more than 1 cm in maximal transverse diameter, but most are not. An enlarged lymph node (regardless of definition) need not have metastatic disease, and histopathological proof is required, particularly when a surgical option is being considered (81) (Fig. 6-22). CT and mediastinoscopy should be considered complementary procedures, and surgical candidates would be considered for both. Patients without enlarged lymph nodes (<1 cm) should proceed to surgery to detect the true pathological stage of the disease and should have a thorough mediastinal dissection. Metastases to these nodes are uncommon, occurring in approximately 7% of cases. It seems reasonable to proceed directly to surgery in these patients, with an expectation of 90% to 95% that no N2 disease will be found. Furthermore, patients with microscopic metastases noted at time of surgery have improved survival rates if the metastases and the primary tumor are all resected. In patients with enlarged lymph nodes by any criteria, a prethorocotomy staging procedure seems warranted (e.g., mediastinoscopy) because of the higher (20% to 35%) false-positive rate.

Spiral CT or MRI adds little in the differentiation of malignant and benign lymph nodes because size criteria are used by both imaging modalities. Positron emission tomography (PET) using fluor-2-deoxy-D-glucose (FDG) provides information on tumor metabolism, and there are strong indications that this technology may provide a solution to this common clinical problem. FDG–PET appears very sensitive

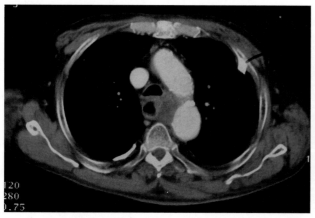
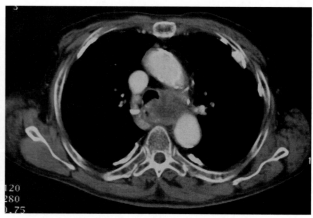

FIG. 6-20. **(A,B)** Carcinoma of the lung with tracheoesophageal (TE) fistula. Spiral CT demonstrates extensive carcinoma of the lung with invasion of the left main stem bronchus and esophagus consistent with a TE fistula. Based on this imaging alone it may be difficult to determine whether it is a primary lung tumor or an esophageal tumor.

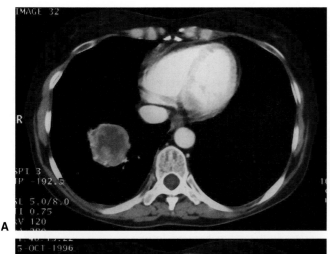

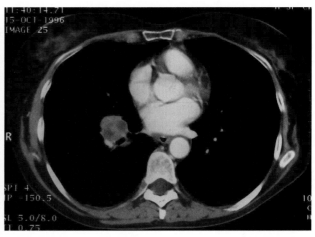

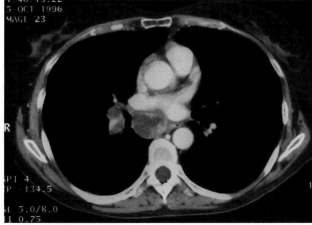

FIG. 6-21. (A-C) Adenocarcinoma of the lung. The patient had a carcinoma with a large necrotic mass in the right lower lung. The nodes in the hilum and subcarinal region were also necrotic, with a similar enhancement pattern as the primary tumor.

to the presence of metastases in normal and enlarged lymph nodes. In a recent report where PET was compared with CT, PET showed significantly better results (sensitivity 89% versus 57%, specificity 99% versus 94%, and accuracy 96% versus 57%) (85). Specificity is not perfect, because some reactive nodes also have increased FDG accumulation and

false-negative results occur because of the difficulty PET has in detecting tracer uptake in small nodes.

Currently, conventional CT demonstrates metastases to peribronchial and ipsilateral hilar lymph nodes (N1) poorly. This is attributable to several factors, including poor vascular opacification, longer scan times, and the axial imaging plane.

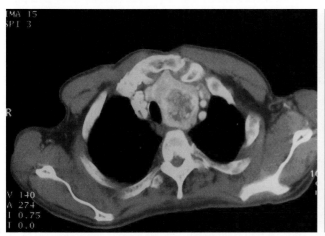

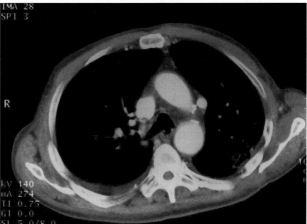

FIG. 6-22. (A,B) Normal variants simulating disease. The patient had a widened mediastinum and a chest CT was requested. The study defines two normal structures simulating disease that are substernal extensions of the thyroid and a persistent left superior vena cava.

Spiral CT images, because of their high level of vascular opacification and thin sections, consistently depict these nodes excellently. Multiplanar reconstructions show hilar nodes well and allow the differentiation of the right hilar pseudotumor from adenopathy, a well-known diagnostic pitfall in axial imaging (86). In addition, some lymph node groups are suboptimally visualized in the transaxial plane (e.g., in the aortopulmonary window and subcarinal area). Lymph nodes at these stations are best demonstrated in the coronal plane with the multiplanar reconstructions. Improved localization of lymph node groups according to American Thoracic Society (87) and AJCC classifications with accurate labeling of resected lymph nodes is likely to be critical in evaluating future treatment regimens.

METASTASES

Lung Metastases

In patients with lung cancer, the presence of nodules of uncertain significance may be important when surgery is

being considered, especially when located in an ipsilateral lobe or in the contralateral lung. A recent study documented a 16% prevalence of noncalcified nodules in patients undergoing lung cancer staging; the majority (70%) were benign (88). It can be difficult to differentiate a second primary lung cancer from a synchronous metastasis from a lung cancer. A second lung lesion should be considered a metastasis if the histology is identical to that of the primary tumor and occurs in the opposite lung or in a noncontiguous area of the ipsilateral lung. The presence of satellite nodules discovered at surgery with identical histological characteristics is a poor prognostic factor (89). Five-year survival for these patients is approximately 22%, compared with 44% if no nodules are present. The TNM staging classification fails to classify these synchronous lesions.

Other Metastases

Brain metastases constitute more than 25% of all observed recurrences in patients with resected non–small-cell lung

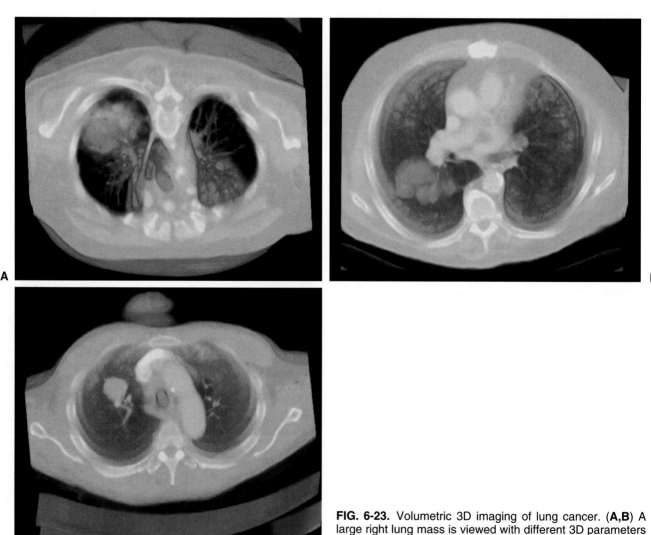

FIG. 6-23. Volumetric 3D imaging of lung cancer. **(A,B)** A large right lung mass is viewed with different 3D parameters from above and below the tumor. **(C)** Right upper lobe carcinoma seen with 3D rendering.

cancer and are seen with greater frequency at autopsy. Nearly half of patients with brain metastases have solitary lesions on CT scan. A solitary brain metastasis is best treated surgically, with 5-year survival ranging from 10% to 20%. Adrenal metastases from lung cancer are found in approximately one-third of patients at autopsy. Routine preoperative upper abdominal CT scanning reveals an adrenal mass in approximately 10% of patients (90). Approximately two-thirds of these are benign adrenal cortical adenomas.

CONCLUSION

Spiral CT is the imaging modality of choice for the evaluation of lung masses. The acquisition of volume data allows multiplanar reconstructions and 3D imaging, but the staging accuracy compared with conventional CT and other imaging techniques is largely undetermined (Fig. 6-23). Its advantages should lead to improved accuracy in local tumor staging, but the difficulties of assessing metastatic lymph node disease are likely to remain. Other imaging modalities (e.g., MRI and PET) are unlikely to replace spiral CT for the primary assessment of lung cancer and lung masses. The imaging protocol should always be tailored to answer questions posed by clinicians. The benefits of spiral CT in lung cancer evaluation include precise delineation of the tumor mass and its relationship to mediastinal structures and chest wall, superior detection and characterization of pulmonary nodules, improved demonstration of adrenal anatomy, and exact measurement of the volume of inoperable tumors. Spiral CT has an established role in directing the investigation most likely to lead to a histological diagnosis (e.g., mediastinoscopy, bronchoscopic biopsy, percutaneous aspiration). Virtual-reality applications may become routine in the long term for planning of bronchoscopic procedures. The data from spiral CT are also useful for surgical planning treatment (e.g., stent placement, laser coagulation) and for radiotherapy applications (e.g., brachytherapy and conformal radiotherapy planning).

REFERENCES

1. Epidemiology cancer statistics 1991. *CA* 1991;41:19–36.
2. Jett JR, Cortese DA, Fontana RS. Lung cancer: current concepts and prospects. *CA* 1983;33:74–86.
3. Silverberg E, Lubera J. Cancer statistics, 1987. *CA* 1987;37:2–19.
4. Wynder EL, Graham EA. Tobacco smoking as a possible etiologic factor in bronchogenic carcinoma: a study of six hundred and eighty four proved cases. *JAMA* 1950;143:329–336.
5. Kabat GC, Wynder EL. Lung cancer in nonsmokers. *Cancer* 1984;53: 1214–1221.
6. Ginsberg RJ, Kris MG, Armstrong JG. Cancer of the lung. In: DeVita VT, Hellman S, Rosenberg SA, eds. *Cancer: principles and practice of oncology*, 4th ed. Philadelphia: JB Lippincott; 1993:673–722.
7. Einhorn LH. Neoadjuvant therapy of stage III non–small cell lung cancer. *Ann Thorac Surg* 1988;46:362–365.
8. Heelan RT. Lung cancer imaging: primary diagnosis, staging, and local recurrence. *Semin Oncol* 1991;18:87–98.
9. Lahde S, Paivansalo M, Rainio P. CT for predicting the resectability of lung cancer: a prospective study. *Acta Radiol* 1991;32:449–454.
10. Lewis JW, Pearlberg JL, Beute GH, et al. Can computed tomography of the chest stage lung cancer? Yes and no. *Ann Thorac Surg* 1990; 49:591–595.
11. Berlin NI, Buncher CR, Fontana RS, et al. The National Cancer Institute cooperative early lung cancer detection programme. Results of initial screening (prevalence). *Am Rev Respir Dis* 1984;130:545–549.
12. Berlin NI, Buncher CR, Fontana RS, et al. Early lung cancer detection: summary and conclusions. *Am Rev Respir Dis* 1984;130:565–570.
13. Strauss GM, Gleason RE, Sugarbaker DJ. Chest x-ray screening improves outcome in lung cancer: a reappraisal of randomized trials on lung cancer screening. *Chest* 1995;107:270S–279S.
14. Kaneko M, Eguchi K, Ohmatsu H, et al. Peripheral lung cancer: screening and detection with low dose spiral CT versus radiography. *Radiology* 1996;201:798–802.
15. Costello P, Anderson W, Blume D. Pulmonary nodule: evaluation with spiral volumetric CT. *Radiology* 1991;179:875–876.
16. Heywang-Koebrunner SH, Lommatzsch B, Kloeppel R, et al. Comparison of conventional and spiral CT: detection of pulmonary nodules. *Radiology* 1993;189(P):263(abst).
17. Vock P, Soucek M. Spiral computed tomography in the assessment of focal lung and diffuse lung disease. *J Thorac Imaging* 1993;8:283–290.
18. Vock P, Soucek M, Daepp M, Kalender WA. Lung: spiral volumetric CT with single-breath-hold technique. *Radiology* 1990;176:864–867.
19. Remy-Jardin M, Remy J, Giraud F, Marquette CH. Pulmonary nodules: detection with thick-section spiral CT versus conventional CT. *Radiology* 1993;187:513–520.
20. Collie DA, Wright AR, Williams JR, Hashemi-Malayeri BS, Stevenson AJM, Turnbull CM. Comparison of spiral acquisition computed tomography and conventional computed tomography in the assessment of pulmonary metastatic disease. *Br J Radiol* 1994;67:436–444.
21. Buckley JA, Scott WW, Siegelman SS, et al. Pulmonary nodules: effect of increased data sampling on detection with spiral CT and confidence in diagnosis. *Radiology* 1995;196:395–400.
22. Seltzer SE, Judy PF, Adams DF, et al. Spiral CT of the chest: comparison of cine and film based viewing. *Radiology* 1995;197:73–78.
23. Schaner EG, Chang AE, Doppman JL, et al. Comparison of computed and conventional whole lung tomography in detecting pulmonary nodules: a prospective radiologic-pathologic study. *AJR* 1978;131:51–54.
24. Chang AE, Schaner EG, Conkle DM, et al. Evaluation of computed tomography in the detection of pulmonary metastases: a prospective study. *Cancer* 1979;23:913–916.
25. Lund G, Heilo A. Computed tomography of pulmonary metastases. *Acta Radiol Diagn* 1982;23:617–620.
26. Peuchot M. Libshitz HI. Pulmonary metastatic disease: radiologic-surgical correlation. *Radiology* 1987;164:719–722.
27. Husband JE, MacDonald JS, Peckham MJ. Computed tomography in testicular disease: a review. *J R Soc Med* 1981;74:441–447.
28. Vanel D, Henry-Amar M, Lumbroso J, et al. Pulmonary evaluation of patients with osteosarcoma: roles of standard radiography, tomography, CT, scintigraphy and tomoscintigraphy. *Am J Roentgenol* 1984;143: 519–523.
29. Siegelman SS, Khouri NF, Scott WW, et al. Pulmonary hamartoma: CT findings. *Radiology* 1986;160:313–317.
30. Meziane MA, Hruban RH, Zerhouni EA, et al. High resolution CT of the lung parenchyma with pathological correlation. *Radiographics* 1988;8:27–54.
31. Remy J, Remy-Jardin M, Wattinne L, Deffontaines C. Pulmonary arteriovenous malformations: evaluation with CT of the chest before and after treatment. *Radiology* 1992;182:809–816.
32. Swensen SJ, Brown LR, Colby TV, Weaver AL. Pulmonary nodules: CT evaluation of enhancement with iodinated contrast material. *Radiology* 1995;194:393–398.
33. Yamashita K, Matsunobe S, Tsuda T, et al. Solitary pulmonary nodule: preliminary study of evaluation with incremental dynamic CT. *Radiology* 1995;194:399–405.
34. Naidich DP, Harkin TJ, McGuinness G. Focal parenchymal disease: helical CT/bronchoscopic correlations. Presented at the 16th Annual Meeting of the Society of Computed Body Tomography and Magnetic Resonance Imaging, Orlando, 1993 (abst).
35. Gaeta M, Pandolfo I, Volta S, et al. Bronchus sign on CT in peripheral carcinoma of the lung: value in predicting results of transbronchial biopsy. *AJR* 1991;157:1181–1185.
36. Naidich DP, Sussman R, Kutcher WL, et al. Solitary pulmonary nodules: CT–bronchoscopic correlation. *Chest* 1988;93:595–598.
37. Wang KP, Haponik EF, Britt EJ, et al. Transbronchial needle aspiration of peripheral pulmonary nodules. *Chest* 1984;86:819–823.
38. Silverman SG, Bloom DA, Seltzer SE, et al. Needle tip localization

during CT-guided abdominal biopsy: comparison of conventional and spiral CT. *AJR* 1992;159:1095–1097.

39. Set PA, Flower CD, Smith IE, Chan AP, Twentyman OP, Shneerson JM. Hemoptysis: comparative study of the role of CT and fibreoptic bronchoscopy. *Radiology* 1993;189:677–680.

40. Adachi S, Kono M, Takemura T, et al. Evaluation of 3D spiral CT bronchoscopy in patients with lung cancer. *Radiology* 1993;189(P): 264.

41. Remy J, Remy-Jardin M, Petyt L, et al. Spiral CT tracheobronchography with multiplanar and 3-dimensional reformations. *Eur Radiol* 1995; 5[Suppl]:26(abst).

42. Schaefer CM, Prokop M, Zink C, Galanski M. Spiral CT of anastomotic complications after lung transplantation. *Radiology* 1993;189(P): 263(abst).

43. Vining DJ, Liu K, Choplin RH, Haponik EF. Virtual bronchoscopy: relationship of virtual reality endobronchial simulations to actual bronchoscopic findings. *Chest* 1996;109:549–553.

44. Rubin GD, Beaulieu CF, Argiro B, et al. Perspective volume rendering of CT and MR images: applications for endoscopic imaging. *Radiology* 1996;199:321–330.

45. Vining DJ. Virtual endoscopy: Is it reality? *Radiology* 1996;200:30–31.

46. Sobin LH, Wittekind CH (eds.). TNM classification of malignant tumours. Fifth edition. Wiley-Liss, New York 1997.

47. Fleming ID, Cooper JS, Henson DE, Hutter RVP, Kennedy BJ, Murphy GP, O'Sullivan B, Yarbro JW (eds.). J.B. Lippincott, Philadelphia 1977.

48. Ihde DC. Staging evaluation and prognostic factors in small cell lung cancer. In: Aisner J, ed. *Lung cancer*. New York: Churchill Livingstone; 1985:241–268.

49. Onitsuka H, Tsukuda M, Araki A, et al. Differentiation of central lung tumor from post obstructive lobar collapse by rapid sequence computed tomography. *J Thorac Imaging* 1991;6:28–31.

50. Quint LE, Glazer GM, Orringer MB. Central lung masses: prediction with CT of the need for pneumonectomy versus lobectomy. *Radiology* 1987;165:735–738.

51. Kwong JS, Muller NL, Miller RR. Diseases of the trachea and main stem bronchi: correlation with pathologic findings. *Radiographics* 1992;12:645–657.

52. Padhani AR, Fishman EK, Heitmiller RF, et al. Multiplanar display of spiral CT data of the pulmonary hila in patients with lung cancer: preliminary observations. *Clin Imaging* 1995;19:252–257.

53. Glazer HS, Duncan-Meyer J, Aronberg DJ, et al. Pleural and chest wall invasion in bronchogenic cancer: CT evaluation. *Radiology* 1985;157: 191–194.

54. Pennes DR, Glazer GM, Wimbish KJ, et al. Chest wall invasion by lung cancer: limitations of CT evaluation. *AJR* 1985;144:507–511.

55. Pearlberg JL, Sandler MA, Beute GH, et al. Limitation of CT in evaluation of neoplasm involving chest wall. *J Comput Assist Tomogr* 1987; 11:290–293.

56. Musset D, Grenier P, Carette MF, et al. Primary lung cancer staging: prospective comparative of MR imaging with CT. *Radiology* 1986; 160:607–611.

57. Rendina EA, Bognolo DA, Mineo TC, et al. Computed tomography for the evaluation of intrathoracic invasion by lung cancer. *J Cardiovasc Surg* 1987;94:57–63.

58. Ratto GB, Piacenza G, Frola C, et al. Chest wall involvement by lung cancer: computed tomographic detection and results of operation. *Ann Thorac Surg* 1991;51:182–188.

59. Watanabe A, Shimokata K, Saka H, et al. Chest CT combined with artificial pneumothorax: value in detecting origin and extent of tumor. *AJR* 1991;156:707–710.

60. Yokoi K, Mori K, Miyazawa N, et al. Tumor invasion of chest wall and mediastinum in lung cancer: evaluation with pneumothorax CT. *Radiology* 1991;181:147–152.

61. Murata T, Takuhashi M, Mori M, et al. Chest wall and mediastinal invasion by lung cancer: evaluation with multisection expiratory dynamic CT. *Radiology* 1994;191:251–255.

62. Shirakawa T, Fukuda K, Miyamoto Y, Tanabe H, Tada S. Parietal pleural invasion of lung masses: evaluation with CT performed during deep inspiration and expiration. *Radiology* 1994;192:809–811.

63. Kuriyama K, Tateishi R, Kumatami T, et al. Pleural invasion by peripheral bronchogenic carcinoma; assessment with three-dimensional helical CT. *Radiology* 1994;191:365–369.

64. Padovani B, Mouroux J, Seksik L, et al. Chest wall invasion by bronchogenic carcinoma: evaluation with MR imaging. *Radiology* 1993; 187:33–38.

65. Haggar AM, Pearlberg JL, Froelich JW, et al. Chest wall invasion by carcinoma of the lung: detection by MR imaging. *AJR* 1987;148: 1075–1078.

66. Webb WR, Gatsonis C, Zerhouni EA, et al. CT and MR imaging in staging non–small cell bronchogenic carcinoma. Report of the Radiologic Diagnostic Oncology Group. *Radiology* 1991;178:705–713.

67. Gefter WB. Magnetic resonance imaging in the evaluation of lung cancer. *Semin Roentgenol* 1990;25:73–84.

68. Webb WR, Sostman HD. MR imaging of thoracic disease: clinical uses. *Radiology* 1992;182:621–630.

69. Deschildre F, Petyt L, Remy-Jardin M, et al. Evaluation de la TDM par balayage spirale volumique (BSV) vs IRM dans le bilan d'extension pariétal des masses thoraciques. *Rev Im Med* 1994;6(S):188.

70. Rubin GD, Dake MD, Semba CP. Current status of three-dimensional spiral CT scanning for imaging the vasculature. *Radiol Clin North Am* 1995;33:51–70.

71. Tello R, Scholz E, Finn JP, Costello P. Subclavian vein thrombosis detected with spiral CT and three-dimensional reconstructions. *AJR* 1993;160:33–34.

72. Meier RA, Marianacci EB, Costello P, Fitzpatrick PJ, Hartnell GG. 3D image reconstruction of the right subclavian artery aneurysms. *J Comput Assist Tomogr* 1993;17:887–890.

73. Herman SJ, Winton TL, Weisbrod GL, et al. Mediastinal invasion by bronchogenic carcinoma: CT signs. *Radiology* 1994;190:841–846.

74. Grenier P, Dubray B, Carette MF, et al. Pre-operative thoracic staging of lung cancer: CT and MR evaluation. *Diagn Intervent Radiol* 1989; 1:23–28.

75. Miyamoto H, Hayakawa K, Hata E, et al. Preoperative evaluation of digital subtraction pulmonary angiography in primary lung cancer. *Kokyu To Junkan* 1989;37:1209–1214.

76. Naruke T, Goya T, Tsuchiya R, Suemasu K. The importance of surgery to non–small cell carcinoma of the lung with mediastinal lymph node metastases. *Ann Thorac Surg* 1988;46:603–610.

77. Martini N, Kris MG, Flehinger BJ, et al. Preoperative chemotherapy for stage 3A (N2) lung cancer: the Sloan-Kettering experience with 136 patients. *Ann Thorac Surg* 1993;55:1365–1373.

78. Roth JA, Fonsella F, Komaki R, et al. A randomized trial comparing perioperative chemotherapy and surgery with surgery alone in resectable stage 3A non–small cell lung cancer. *J Natl Cancer Inst* 1994; 86:650–651.

79. Patterson GA, Ginsberg RJ, Poon PY, et al. A prospective evaluation of magnetic resonance imaging, computed tomography and mediastinoscopy in the preoperative assessment of mediastinal node status in bronchogenic carcinoma. *J Thorac Cardiovasc Surg* 1987;94:679–684.

80. Aronchick JM. CT of mediastinal lymph nodes in patients with non–small cell lung carcinoma. *Radiol Clin North Am* 1990;28: 573–581.

81. Libshitz HI. Computed tomography in bronchogenic carcinoma. *Semin Roentgenol* 1990;25:64–72.

82. Grover FL. The role of CT and MRI in staging of the mediastinum. *Chest* 1994;106[Suppl]:391S–396S.

83. Quint LE, Francis IR, Wahl RL, Gross BH, Glazer GM. Preoperative staging of non–small cell carcinoma of the lung: imaging methods. *AJR* 1995;164:1349–1359.

84. Glazer GM, Gross BH, Quint LE, et al. Normal mediastinal lymph nodes: number and size according to the American Thoracic Society mapping. *AJR* 1985;144:261–265.

85. Steinert HC, Hauser M, Allemann F, et al. Non-small cell lung cancer: nodal mapping with FDG PET versus CT with correlative lymph node mapping and sampling. *Radiology* 1997;202:441–446.

86. Ashida C, Zerhouni EA, Fishman EK. CT demonstration of prominent right hilar soft tissue collections. *J Comput Assist Tomogr* 1987;11(1): 57–59.

87. Tisi GM, Friedman PJ, Peters RM, et al. Clinical staging of primary lung cancer: official statement of the American Thoracic Society. *Am Rev Respir Dis* 1983;127:659.

88. Keogan MT, Tung KT, Kaplan DK, et al. The significance of pulmonary nodules detection on CT staging for lung cancer. *Clin Radiol* 1993;48:94–96.

89. Deslauriers J, Brisson J, Cartier R, et al. Carcinoma of the lung: evaluation of satellite nodules as a factor influencing prognosis after resection. *J Thorac Cardiovasc Surg* 1989;97:504–512.

90. Allard P, Yankaskas BC, Fletcher RH, et al. Sensitivity and specificity of computed tomography for the detection of adrenal metastatic lesions among 91 autopsied lung cancer patients. *Cancer* 1990;66:457–462.

PART 3

Gastrointestinal Applications

CHAPTER 7

Spiral CT of Liver Tumors

David A. Bluemke and Elliot K. Fishman

The importance of computed tomography (CT) in the detection of hepatic tumors is well established. High-quality CT scanning requires rapid bolus infusion of iodinated contrast followed by rapid image acquisition. In addition, patient respiratory motion must be minimized. These requirements can be readily achieved when using spiral or helical CT techniques (1). Spiral CT scanning is continuous, resulting in acquisition of CT attenuation values that represent a true three-dimensional (3D) data set.

There are three advantages of spiral CT for the evaluation of hepatic tumors. First, because imaging with spiral CT is extremely rapid, hepatic scanning can be completed during the interval of peak hepatic contrast enhancement. Second, axial reconstructions can be obtained at arbitrarily determined intervals, so that consecutive, overlapping axial reconstructions are obtained. By obtaining reconstructions centered on focal lesions in the liver, partial volume averaging of small lesions with normal liver is reduced. This improves the accuracy of densitometry of small lesions. Finally, respiratory misregistration between adjacent scan slices is eliminated. This is because the liver can generally be imaged within a single breath-hold with spiral CT. These three factors combine to result in improved lesion *detection* in the liver.

Since the inception of CT, contrast enhancement of the liver has been one of the most intensively evaluated areas of CT investigation. These studies have led to a good understanding of the pharmacokinetics of intravenously delivered iodinated contrast media in the normal liver. Enhancement of the normal liver, discussed in Chapter 2, has been studied because an understanding of contrast dynamics closely impacts on liver tumor detection. In addition, recent studies suggest that spiral CT shows promise in improving not only tumor detection, but also *characterization*. This chapter reviews issues of liver contrast enhancement pertinent to tumor detection with spiral CT and discusses clinical applications to imaging of hepatic tumors.

SPIRAL SCANNING TECHNIQUE FOR THE LIVER

In this discussion we first discuss a typical protocol with established efficacy for hepatic tumor detection. This protocol can be adapted to different vendors' CT scanners, recognizing that small changes in various parameters (e.g., collimation or pitch) probably induce less change in overall CT accuracy compared with physiological variation among different patients. Subsequently, various elements of that protocol—including the contrast rate of injection and volume, delay time, and reconstruction interval—are discussed separately, with emphasis on the impact on hepatic tumor detection.

Scanning Protocol

For spiral CT of the liver, a routine protocol consists of 120 mL of iodinated contrast material (300 mg of iodine/mL, 36 g iodine) injected into a peripheral intravenous catheter at a rate of 2–3 mL/s (Table 7-1) (2,3). Spiral scanning begins immediately after completion of the contrast injection. A power injector should be used to control the injection rate and volume. The table incrementation speed is 8 mm/s, with 5-mm collimation. Smaller collimation intervals (e.g., 3 mm) can easily be accommodated on the most recently developed spiral scanners, but their increased efficacy has not yet been established. The entire liver can reliably be imaged within a 24-s spiral scan using an 8 mm/s table speed. This results in an approximately 19 cm scanned length along the long axis (z-axis) of the patient. After data acquisition, the rate of lesion detection is improved if reconstructions are performed every 5 mm (for 5-mm collimation) (discussed further later). Prior to starting the spiral scan, patients are instructed to hyperventilate for several breaths. This maneuver helps patients hold their breath during the image acquisition.

If necessary, multiplanar and 3D analysis may be performed online or with dedicated imaging workstations. Mul-

TABLE 7-1. *Spiral CT: routine liver imaging protocol*

X-ray tube	Spiral mode
Slice thickness	5 mm
Table incrementation	5–8 mm/s
Reconstruction interval	3–5 mm
Contrast	
Volume	120 mL
Rate	3 mL/s power injector
Delay	40–60-s delay prior to scan
Imaging time	24–40 s
Image volume length	20–32 cm

tiplanar imaging is useful to evaluate the relationship of hepatic tumors to major vascular structures. The porta hepatis is anatomically complex, and multiplanar display of reconstructed images may also be useful in this region.

The slice thickness and table speed need to be determined prior to the onset of spiral scanning (4). These parameters are chosen so that the entire region of interest is covered during the scan. Either a single spiral scan covering the length of the liver or several consecutive spiral scans may be performed. Consecutive spiral scans, or "clustered" scanning, have the potential disadvantage of respiratory misregistration between adjacent scans; the advantage, however, is that breath-hold times are reduced (5). Also, any delay between adjacent spiral scans must be considered when determining the contrast injection rate and volume. We routinely use a single breath-hold protocol in our clinical practice.

Pitch and Interpolation Algorithm

The pitch of the spiral scan is the ratio of the table speed (expressed in millimeters per second) to collimation thickness (expressed in millimeters) multiplied by the time to acquire 360 degrees of data (generally 1 s). For routine scanning, a pitch of 1 is often used (6). Current scanners allow the user to vary the pitch, usually up to a pitch of 2. This has been referred to as "extended" spiral scanning. With extended spiral scanning using a pitch of 2, twice the distance along the *z*-axis of the patient can be scanned in the same time using a pitch of 1. Extended spiral scanning ensures that the region of interest will be covered during the duration of the spiral scan. It is usually desirable to scan the lower abdomen and pelvis in conjunction with the liver. Extended spiral scanning can be used to accomplish this during a single spiral scan.

Linear 180-degree interpolation is used for image reconstruction on most current scanners (7,8). With linear 180-degree interpolation and a pitch of 1, the section sensitivity profile is nearly equal to the ideal rectangular slice profile. With extended spiral scanning (pitch >1), 180-degree algorithms are required to prevent excessive broadening of the slice profile. Because higher spatial resolution is available along the *z*-axis than with 360-degree reconstructions, 180-

degree algorithms are also very desirable for multiplanar reconstructions (9).

Contrast Injection

Three parameters that determine the degree of hepatic enhancement are controlled by the radiologist: the contrast volume and concentration, the rate of injection, and the time after the injection at which the liver is imaged (i.e., the delay time). Although each is discussed individually later, it is the combination of all three parameters that ultimately determines the degree of hepatic enhancement, and thus the relative difference in attenuation between the liver and tumor.

Contrast Volume

With dynamic CT, typically 150–180 mL of iodinated contrast is injected by peripheral venous access (10). In the 1980s, protocols for dynamic CT were developed to sustain high levels of enhancement over approximately 2 min. Since spiral CT scans are completed within 20–30 s, it is reasonable to consider the use of lower contrast doses with spiral CT than with dynamic CT. For example, in the chest, contrast volumes as low as 60 mL are effective for vascular opacification (11). In the abdomen, however, considerations for reduction of contrast involve not only the vasculature (aorta and portal vein), but also the liver parenchyma.

The minimum volume of intravenous contrast necessary for CT of the liver has commonly been taken as that which increases the attenuation of the liver by 40–50 Hounsfield units (HU). Alternatively, Heiken et al. have defined the *contrast enhancement index* (CEI) as the area under the hepatic enhancement curve above a desired enhancement level (e.g., above 30 HU) (12). Note that these definitions are somewhat arbitrary and do not discuss the relative attenuation of the liver compared with the tumor, nor the relative vascularity of the tumor. However, these measures make intuitive sense and can be used to compare different injection protocols.

With regard to the minimum volume of contrast material for spiral CT of the liver, investigations to date are somewhat contradictory. Two large patient studies by Brink et al. (13) and Freeny et al. (14) differ in their conclusions. The series by Brink indicates adequate enhancement with doses of 26–36 g of iodine (depending on patient weight), whereas Freeny cautions substantial reduction of hepatic contrast occurs at doses of 30–32 g of iodine. Similarly, Berland believes that 45 g iodine or more is required for adequate hepatic enhancement (15). Our own experience, correlating tumor detection at spiral CT with surgical findings (3), is consistent with the results of Brink et al., that modest reductions of contrast dose (see Table 7-1) may be used while still obtaining high sensitivity for tumor detection. Berland concurs that a small contrast dose reduction is reasonable when more expensive nonionic contrast agents are used (15). We believe that it is important to adjust the contrast volume for patient weight, as outlined by Brink et al. The minimum iodine load for patients of more than 183 lb (83 kg) was 38 g, whereas that for patients of less than 183 lb was 26 g.

Contrast Concentration

Iodinated contrast agents for CT range in concentration of iodine from approximately 240 mg I/mL to 350 mg I/mL. The primary determinant of hepatic enhancement is the total iodine load (13,16) (Fig. 7-1). The total iodine load (in grams of iodine) is calculated as the iodine concentration multiplied by the administered volume. Our approach to determining the concentration of nonionic contrast agents is to choose that which is priced most economically (17) and then to adjust the total volume administered to deliver approximately 36 g I (for patients of less than 183 lb).

Rate of Contrast Injection

Iodinated contrast may be injected at a single, constant rate (uniphasic injection), or the injection rate may be varied, using an initial high rate and then a slower rate for the second portion of the contrast dose (biphasic injection). Biphasic injections are desirable for dynamic CT, because the time until the onset of the equilibrium phase of enhancement (dis-

TABLE 7-2. *Peak hepatic enhancement versus rate of contrast injection*

	Rate of injection	
	2 mL/s	4 mL/s
Time to peak enhancement	90 s	61 s
Maximum hepatic enhancement	92 HU	98 HU

Adapted from Mitsuzaki K, Yamashita Y, Ogata I, Urata J, Takahashi M. Multiple-phase helical CT of the liver for detecting small hepatomas in patients with liver cirrhosis: contrast-injection protocol and optimal timing. *AJR* 1996;167:753.

cussed later) is prolonged (10). However, this appears to be unnecessary for spiral CT, with both uniphasic and biphasic injection protocols providing similar levels of hepatic enhancement (5), although not all authors agree (18). Our preference is for a uniphasic injection, because it is implemented more easily than a biphasic injection.

The rate of contrast material injection is a key determinant of the rate of hepatic enhancement; higher injection rates result in shorter times to peak enhancement (Table 7-2) (15). Interestingly, the maximum hepatic enhancement has been shown to be relatively insensitive to the injection rate, although peak enhancement of the aorta is achieved using relatively high injection rates of 4 mL/s or more (19,20). Typical injection rates are 2–3 mL/s, which can be achieved using a 20- or 22-gauge angiocatheter (21). We prefer a 20-gauge angiocatheter when injecting at rates of more than 3 mL/s.

Delay Time

The scan delay time refers to the time interval from the beginning of the contrast injection to the start of the helical scan. As a general rule, *peak hepatic enhancement occurs about 5–15 s after the end of the injection* using injection rates of 2–5 mL/s (15). As an example, for 125 mL of contrast injected at 2.5 mL/s, the injection duration is 50 s. Using these parameters, the appropriate delay time to image the liver during its peak enhancement would be approximately 60 s (22).

Computer-Aided Determination of Delay Time

From the preceding discussion it is clear that multiple combinations of contrast injection parameters influence hepatic enhancement. Furthermore, hepatic enhancement in a particular patient is influenced by factors intrinsic to the patient that determine circulation time, such as cardiac status, age, recent meal (e.g., mesenteric circulation changes due to oral contrast) or possible anxiety. Therefore despite extensive testing of a variety of contrast injection protocols on relatively large patient populations, radiologists still encounter patients whose peak hepatic enhancement occurs either before or after the spiral CT scan. Rather than trying to predict circulation times prior to scanning, it is now possible to monitor tissue enhancement in real time, using low-

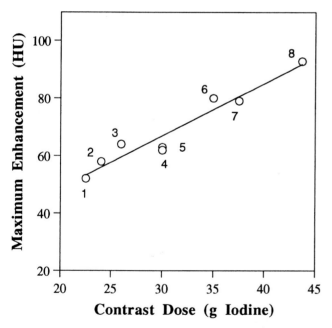

FIG. 7-1. Effect of concentration of contrast agent on hepatic enhancement. Average maximum enhancement (HU) is proportional to total iodine load. Eight different iodine concentrations and volumes: (1) +300 mg I/mL, 75 mL; (2) 240 mg I/mL, 100 mL; (3) 350 mg I/mL, 75 mL; (4) 300 mg I/mL, 100 mL; (5) 240 mg I/mL, 125 mL; (6) 350 mg I/mL, 100 mL; (7) 300 mg I/mL, 125 mL; (8) 350 mg I/mL, 125 mL. Data for patients of ≤183 lb. (Adapted from Brink JA, Heiken JP, Forman HP, Sagel SS, Molina PL, Brown PC. Hepatic spiral CT: reduction of dose of intravenous contrast material. *Radiology* 1995;197:83.)

radiation-dose scans (23,24). The initial application of this computer software by General Electric is termed *SmartPrep*, and the method allows delay times to be optimized for each patient based on the patient's physiological response to the contrast injection (25,26). Based on experience to date, SmartPrep appears to be an outstanding method for obtaining extremely high-quality spiral CT scans in nearly all patients. Other manufacturers have recently introduced similar products that have the ability to automatically trigger the spiral CT acquisition. The CARE bolus program from Siemens Medical Systems allows the user to monitor anatomic areas, such as the aorta, with scan initiation performed automatically when a threshold increase in attenuation has been reached. These techniques may be particularly valuable when arterial phase data acquisitions are required.

HEPATIC TUMORS: GENERAL CONSIDERATIONS

Principles of Tumor Visualization with Iodinated Contrast

The detection of a focal lesion in the liver depends on the relative difference in attenuation between the lesion and the normal liver. The size of a lesion also affects the relative attenuation (and thus detectability) of that lesion. For small lesions, more partial volume averaging will be present, so the attenuation difference between the lesion and liver will appear to be similar. The minimum necessary attenuation difference for lesion detection in the liver is felt to be about 10 HU (27,28) (Fig. 7-2A).

The CT detection of primary and metastatic lesions in the liver is improved with the use of iodinated contrast, because of an increased difference in x-ray attenuation between normal and diseased areas of hepatic parenchyma. The earliest contrast delivered to the liver is from branches of the hepatic artery. This *hepatic arterial phase* of liver enhancement begins approximately 20 s after peripheral intravenous contrast injection (Figs. 7-2B, 7-3). With helical CT, Frederick has recently determined that the end of the hepatic arterial phase is on average 44 s after the beginning of contrast injection (using 120 mL at 3 mL/s, then 55 mL at 2 mL/s) (29). Most tumors are supplied by the hepatic artery, but only about 20% to 30% of the blood supply to the liver occurs from the hepatic artery, with the remainder from the portal vein. Thus the relative attenuation between the liver and the tumor does not significantly change, and most tumors, having a relatively poor vascular supply, are not well detected during this phase. Such tumors, termed *hypovascular* tumors, are among the most common tumors metastatic to the liver, including, for example, adenocarcinomas from primary tumors such as colon, pancreas, and gastric carcinomas. A smaller subset of so-called hypervascular tumors in the liver behaves as though arterial blood supply of the tumors is greater than that of the liver. This subset of tumors (Table 7-3) includes both malignant and benign masses. Hypervascular tumors

TABLE 7-3. *Hypervascular liver tumors**

Malignant	Benign
Primary	
Hepatocellular carcinoma*	Focal nodular hyperplasia
Metastatic	Adenoma
Islet cell tumors	Hemangioma (≤ 1 cm)
Melanoma	
Breast cancer	
Renal cell carcinoma	
Carcinoid	
Leiomyosarcoma	
Thyroid medullary carcinoma	

* As tumors become larger (>2–3 cm), they tend to have mixed attenuation or hypoattenuation, rather than hyperattenuation, compared with the normal liver.

are seen best during the hepatic arterial phase of enhancement as hyperattenuating masses compared with the surrounding liver.

After blood (and intravenous contrast) circulates to the gut, it is delivered to the portal vein and the liver. The time at which contrast reaches the portal vein appears to be highly variable between patients, although the circulation time for any particular patient appears to be reproducible (30). Generally, the portal vein begins to enhance as early as 40–50 s following contrast injection. As blood is delivered to the liver from the portal vein, the attenuation of the liver begins to rise rapidly. For most tumors (i.e., hypovascular tumors) the difference in attenuation between the liver and the tumor is maximized during this portal phase of hepatic enhancement (also referred to as the hepatic parenchymal phase) (Fig. 7-2C). For helical CT, Silverman suggests that this maximum attenuation difference occurs at 75 s after contrast injection (of 150 mL at 3 mL/s) (31). Hypervascular tumors may be obscured during the portal phase, because the increased attenuation of the tumors is similar to that of the enhanced liver.

Eventually, contrast from the interstitial spaces of the liver diffuses into the liver tumor, which enhances (Fig. 7-2D). Also, the attenuation of the liver begins to decline over time, usually beginning 20–25 s after the end of the contrast injection. The combination of declining hepatic attenuation and increasing attenuation of the tumor mass may result in the tumor becoming nearly isoattenuating to the normal liver and not detectable. CT imaging during this phase of enhancement, termed the *equilibrium phase,* results in decreased tumor detection. Foley proposed an empirical method to determine the onset of the equilibrium phase: Hepatic equilibrium has been defined as that time when the slopes of the aortic and hepatic enhancement curves become parallel (10). Using this definition, the onset of the equilibrium phase is believed to occur 90–120 s after contrast injection. A basic principle of hepatic tumor detection is that CT imaging (using spiral or dynamic CT) should be completed before the onset of the equilibrium phase of enhancement. Because

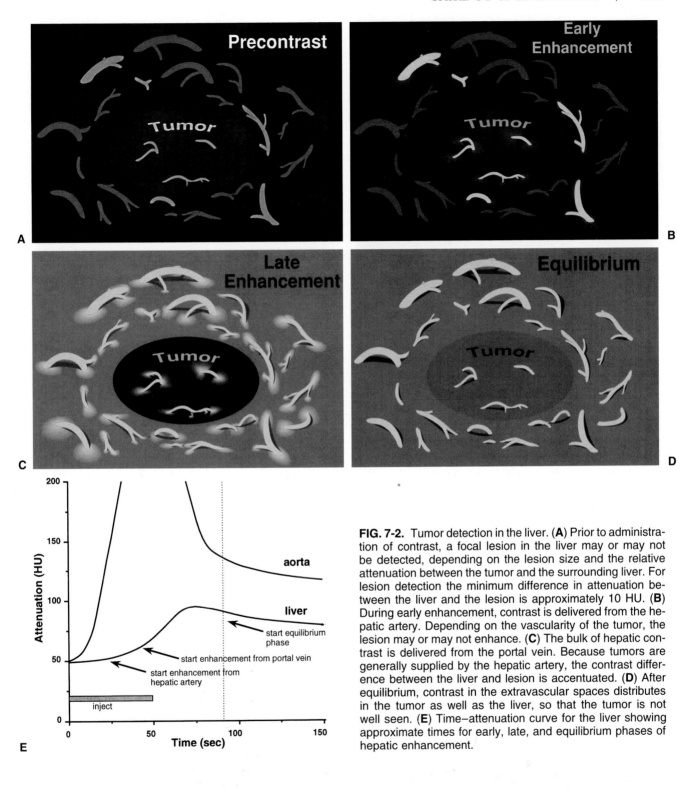

FIG. 7-2. Tumor detection in the liver. **(A)** Prior to administration of contrast, a focal lesion in the liver may or may not be detected, depending on the lesion size and the relative attenuation between the tumor and the surrounding liver. For lesion detection the minimum difference in attenuation between the liver and the lesion is approximately 10 HU. **(B)** During early enhancement, contrast is delivered from the hepatic artery. Depending on the vascularity of the tumor, the lesion may or may not enhance. **(C)** The bulk of hepatic contrast is delivered from the portal vein. Because tumors are generally supplied by the hepatic artery, the contrast difference between the liver and lesion is accentuated. **(D)** After equilibrium, contrast in the extravascular spaces distributes in the tumor as well as the liver, so that the tumor is not well seen. **(E)** Time–attenuation curve for the liver showing approximate times for early, late, and equilibrium phases of hepatic enhancement.

of its rapid speed of image acquisition, it is clear that spiral CT can easily accomplish this (Fig. 7-2E).

Data to determine the time of onset of the equilibrium phase have been determined using dynamic CT or spiral CT using multiple passes through the liver. (Multiple passes are necessary with spiral CT because only a short segment of the hepatic enhancement curve is captured with each spiral

CT scan [32].) Heiken et al. showed that for a uniphasic injection at 2.5 mL/s, a delay time of approximately 60 s is necessary to achieve an enhancement of 40 HU over baseline liver attenuation (12). Their data also indicate that the liver must then be scanned within about 31 s; otherwise the liver enhancement will fall below 40 HU. In addition, scanning is completed prior to the onset of the equilibrium phase of

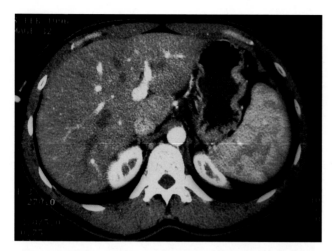

FIG. 7-3. Hepatic arterial-phase spiral CT scan of the liver. The CT scan was acquired 38 s after the start of contrast injection. Contrast has begun to enter the portal vein, but very little hepatic enhancement has occurred. The spleen shows (normal) inhomogeneous enhancement at this stage, and the hepatic veins are unenhanced.

hepatic enhancement. This 31-s time interval is clearly adequate to scan the liver using spiral CT (Fig. 7-4).

Multiple-Phase Spiral CT Scanning of the Liver

From the preceding discussion, the benefit of separately imaging the hepatic arterial and portal phases of hepatic enhancement is feasible with spiral CT, because each set of images through the liver requires only about 20 s. X-ray tubes with a very high capacity for continuous operation of up to 60 s or more have been developed for spiral CT, making multiple-phase scanning technically feasible (Fig. 7-5). The principal application of multiple-phase scanning is for

patients with suspected hepatocellular carcinoma, because small tumors (<3 cm) are frequently hypervascular, whereas larger tumors are hypovascular and more ideally imaged during the portal phase of enhancement. (This technique is also referred to as *dual-phase* scanning by some investigators). Presurgical planning may be an additional application of this technique; the arterial phase can be used not only for detection of hypervascular tumors, but also for distinct visualization of the hepatic arterial supply to the liver (e.g., replaced hepatic artery arising from the superior mesenteric artery). In imaging of the pancreas, arterial-phase scanning is helpful in the detection of pancreatic adenocarcinoma, but portal-phase scanning is better for detection of intrahepatic metastases. Finally, in addition to tumor detection, tumors may be better characterized (i.e., malignant versus benign) by analysis of their enhancement patterns over time, including noncontrast CT, arterial phase, portal phase, and delayed or equilibrium phase. Issues of multiple-phase spiral CT scanning specific to tumor detection and characterization are discussed further later. Dual-phase imaging of the liver is discussed in detail in Chapter 9.

Reconstruction Interval

A major advantage of spiral CT for imaging hepatic tumors is the use of small, overlapping reconstruction intervals. With spiral CT, overlapping cross-sectional reconstructions can be obtained without additional scanning time or radiation. For example, if the liver is scanned with 8-mm collimation, reconstruction intervals can be selected to be 4 mm. The advantage of this approach is illustrated in Fig. 7-6. It is important to note, however, that *the reconstructions that are obtained every 4 mm are still 8 mm thick.* Using this approach, the conspicuity of small lesions may be enhanced by centering of the lesion within the slice interval.

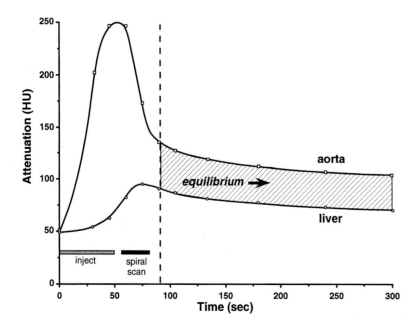

FIG. 7-4. Time–attenuation curves for the liver and aorta. Following the injection of iodinated contrast, the aorta rapidly shows increased attenuation, followed by an increase in attenuation of the liver. At approximately 90 s, the curves for the liver and aorta become parallel; this has been defined as the start of the equilibrium phase of enhancement. During equilibrium, small lesions may be isodense to normal liver parenchyma. Bars indicate the duration of the injection and the duration of a spiral CT scan of the liver. (Adapted from Heiken JP, Brink JA, McClennan BL, Sagel SS, Forman HP, DiCroce J. Dynamic contrast-enhanced CT of the liver: comparison of contrast medium injection rates and uniphasic and biphasic injection protocols. *Radiology* 1993;187:327.)

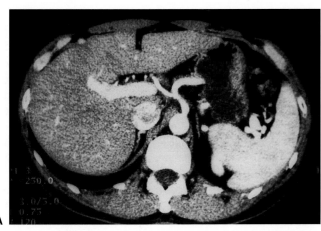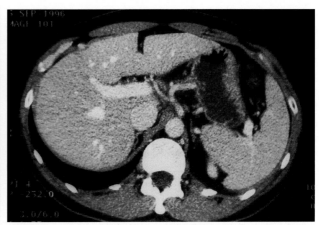

A   B

FIG. 7-5. Spiral CT showing (**A**) arterial- and (**B**) portal-phase scans of the liver, obtained at 32 and 78 s, respectively, after the start of contrast injection. In the arterial phase scan in (**A**), the celiac axis is densely opacified with contrast, and contrast has begun to enter the portal vein. The spleen shows marked enhancement. In the portal-phase scan (**B**), hepatic veins demonstrate enhancement, with similar attenuation of the liver and spleen.

With 5-mm scan collimation, a reasonable reconstruction would likely be 4–5 mm. Reconstruction of data at intervals of 2–3 mm is technically possible, but to date no increase in lesion detection has been documented in the literature. We currently reserve 2–3-mm reconstruction intervals for 3D reconstructions of the liver and hepatic vasculature.

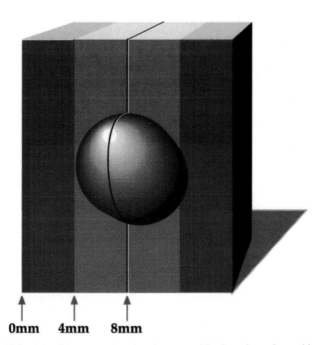

0mm   4mm   8mm

FIG. 7-6. Diagram showing improved lesion detection with 4-mm reconstruction intervals. The lesion, displayed as a sphere, would show significant partial volume averaging in the first 8-mm slice, beginning at position 0. A reconstruction beginning at position 4 and extending for 8 mm would contain the entire volume of the lesion, with less partial volume averaging.[2]

Tumor Detection with Spiral CT

Urban et al. evaluated the role of overlapping, 4-mm reconstruction intervals with spiral CT in the detection of hepatic lesions (33). In 42 consecutive patients with lesions of less than 4 cm, 10% more liver lesions were detected using 4-mm intervals than were found using 8-mm intervals (251 versus 229 lesions, respectively) (Table 7-4). Also, radiologists were able to detect lesions with a higher degree of confidence with 4-mm reconstruction intervals. Lesions that were considered "definite" were diagnosed 33% more frequently using 4-mm reconstruction intervals (191 versus 144 lesions).

Appropriately, no study directly comparing tumor detection with dynamic CT and that with spiral CT has been done. The superiority of spiral CT is intuitive, given its ability to provide overlapping reconstruction intervals, and such a study would therefore involve unnecessary radiation to the patient. To date, however, few studies have compared tumor detection with spiral CT with intravenous contrast with intraoperative findings and pathological examination. In a series of 21 patients, Kuszyk et al. have found that spiral CT detected 91% of tumors of more than 10 mm using portal-

TABLE 7-4. *Comparison of 4- and 8-mm interscan spacing with spiral CT: rate of lesion detection*

	Number of lesions			
	Definite	Probable	Possible	Total
4 mm	191	46	14	251
8 mm	144	60	25	229
Difference:	+47	−14	−11	+22
4–8 mm	(+33%)	(−23%)	(−44%)	(+10%)

Adapted from Urban BA, Fishman EK, Kuhlman JE, Kawashima A, Hennessey JG, Siegelman SS. Detection of focal hepatic lesions with spiral CT: comparison of 4- and 8-mm interscan spacing. *AJR* 1993; 160:783.

phase scanning, with 56% sensitivity for tumors of 10 mm or less, and 81% sensitivity overall (3). For comparison, the reported sensitivities for conventional CT range from 38% to 84%, with most series reporting between 60% and 75% sensitivity (34–36). Similarly, CT during arterial portography (CTAP) using dynamic CT has a reported sensitivity of 81% to 91% (34,37,38), so that spiral CT again compares favorably with this more invasive and expensive technique. In a series of 48 patients, Choi et al. included 15 patients who underwent surgical confirmation of CT findings and comparison to iodized-oil CT (39). Choi et al. reported an overall sensitivity of spiral CT of 92%.

Tumor Characterization with Spiral CT

It is clear that most of our knowledge to date regarding the use of spiral CT in hepatic tumor imaging is limited to tumor detection. However, as we begin to *detect* small tumors, one could argue that little is gained if the lesions cannot also be adequately *characterized*. Indeed, a study by Jones et al. puts the detection of small liver lesions in perspective: for small lesions ≤15 mm in diameter in 209 patients with a known malignancy, more than 50% of those small tumors were benign (40). In the preceding study by Kuszyk et al. (3), the false-positive rate for spiral CT was only 4%, compared with false-positive rates of 5% to 15%, which are typically associated with CT during arterial portography. This indicates good potential for spiral CT characterization as well as detection of tumors.

Conceivably, the specificity of CT for determining if a tumor is benign or malignant could be improved by evaluation of the contrast enhancement pattern of the tumor at multiple time points (multiple phases of enhancement). For example, very rapid dynamic CT has been helpful in characterizing both hepatocellular carcinoma and hemangioma (41,42). On the newest spiral CT scanners, multiple passes through the liver can be obtained, subject to the desire not to irradiate the patient unnecessarily. The enhancement characteristics of most tumors on arterial or portal-phase scans is already known from dynamic CT investigations.

Van Leeuwen et al. have classified the enhancement patterns of focal lesions using three-phase CT (approximately 25 s, 60 s and 8–10 min after injection of contrast material) (43). They observed 11 different patterns of tumor enhancement in 375 lesions (Table 7-5). Two of the enhancement patterns were nearly always due to malignant disease, and six of 11 patterns of enhancement were always due to benign disease. Benign lesions—including hemangioma, cyst, or focal nodular hyperplasia—were correctly characterized in 107 of 117 (91%) cases. Overall, these results suggest an important role for spiral CT in the characterization of hepatic tumors. Further studies are needed to determine the reproducibility of these results.

BENIGN HEPATIC LESIONS

Common benign tumors of the liver include hemangioma, simple hepatic cyst, focal nodular hyperplasia, and hepatic

TABLE 7-5. *Characterization of focal hepatic lesions using multiple-phase spiral CT*

Enhancement at various CT phases			Overall incidence (%)	Pathological diagnosis		Comments
Arterial	Portal	Delay		Number malignant (type)	Number benign (type)	
Hypo	Hypo	Hypo	36	94%, metastases (colon, thyroid, renal, breast, islet cell)	6%, fibrosed hemangioma	
Hypocyst	Hypocyst	Hypocyst	21	0	100% cyst	Well-circumscribed lesion, water attenuation
Rim	Hypo	Hypo	12	100%, metastases (colon, carcinoid, islet, islet cell)	No benign tumors	Hyperattenuation rim, but hypocenter at arterial phase
Hypo	Hypo	Hyper	3	62%, metastases (colon)	38%, hemangioma	
Mixed	Mixed	Mixed	11	28%, metastases (carcinoid, breast, colon)	0, benign	Mixed hyper- and hypoattenuation at all phases
Hyper	Hyper	Hyper	21	0%	100% hemangioma	Peripheral nodular attenuation, equal to adjacent arteries
Hyper	–	–	18	84% metastases (thyroid, renal)	16% adenoma or FNH	Less hyperattenuating than arteries; any pattern at portal and delayed phase

Adapted from Van Leeuwen MS, Noordzij J, Feldberg MAM, Hennipman AH, Doornewaard H. Focal liver lesions: characterization with triphasic spiral CT. *Radiology* 1996;201:327.

adenoma. Their significance is generally that they may be confused with metastatic disease in the liver. Differentiation of these tumors from malignant lesions is often critical to patient management. Together, hepatic cysts and hemangioma occur in more than 10% of patients; exclusion of these benign entities often results in a differential diagnosis of rare benign tumors versus malignant tumors.

Hemangioma

Hemangiomas are the most common liver tumor, occurring in about 4% to 7% of patients. They are somewhat more common in females and frequently occur in the posterior segment of the right lobe of the liver. They may be isolated or multiple. Because they are so common, distinguishing hemangiomas from metastasis is frequently encountered in the clinical setting.

Spiral CT cannot be considered the preferred CT method for hemangioma characterization. Hemangiomas are best evaluated with dynamic bolus CT by performing repeated scanning for 2–15 min at a single level in the liver (44,45). Most hemangiomas demonstrate a characteristic initial pattern of peripheral nodular enhancement that progresses to central enhancement. Eventually, most hemangiomas become isoattenuating on delayed scans. Of note, however, is that not all hemangiomas demonstrate this characteristic pattern. This is particularly true of giant cavernous hemangiomas. Central scarring and fibrosis may prevent complete enhancement of the central portion of large lesions.

On spiral CT using standard portal-phase imaging, hepatic hemangioma will most often have the appearance of a low-attenuation round lesion. Careful inspection reveals that the lesions frequently have areas of nodular, peripheral enhancement (Figs. 7-7–7-9). Foci of globular (nodular) enhance-

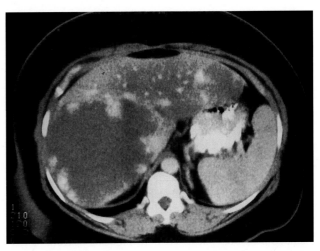

FIG. 7-8. Giant cavernous hemangioma. Spiral CT scan shows a large hypodense lesion greater than 5 cm in the right lobe of the liver. Multiple peripheral enhancing nodules characteristic of hemangioma are present.

ment within the hemangioma have previously been described with bolus dynamic CT (46). This effect is similar to pooling of contrast seen with hemangioma on hepatic angiograms. More than 90% of hemangiomas demonstrate peripheral, nodular enhancement; infrequently, however, a similar pattern can be seen in metastatic liver lesions. Nevertheless, this feature is useful and highly suggestive of hemangioma in the correct clinical setting. Additional criteria that should suggest hemangioma include an isolated lesion in a patient without a known malignancy, location in the posterior segment of the right lobe, isodensity to hepatic vessels on the delayed scan. Because peripheral, nodular enhancement and isodensity to hepatic vessels on delayed scans are

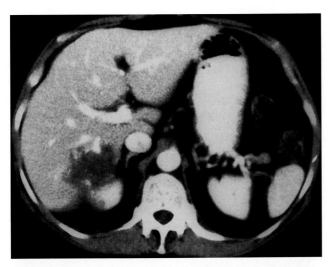

FIG. 7-7. Hemangioma. Spiral CT scan shows a hypodense lesion in the right lobe of the liver during the portal phase of hepatic enhancement. Nodular, peripheral enhancement is present, characteristic of hemangioma.

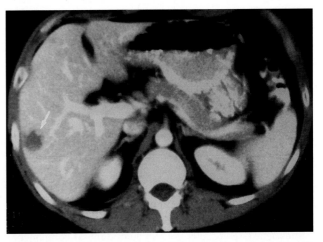

FIG. 7-9. Hemangioma. Spiral CT scan shows 2-cm low-attenuation lesion in the right lobe of the liver. A small focus of globular enhancement is seen peripherally (*arrow*), characteristic of hemangioma. (Reprinted with permission from Zeman RK, Fox SH, Silverman PM, et al. Helical [spiral] CT of the abdomen. *AJR* 1993;160:719.)

not 100% specific for this diagnosis, further work-up of the lesion (tagged red cell scan, MRI, or dedicated CT study) is frequently required.

Hanafusa et al. have described the appearance of hemangioma at multiple-phase imaging (axial liver imaging at 30 and 55 s following 120 mL contrast at 3 mL/s) (41). Sixty-two percent of hemangiomas showed what can be considered to be a "typical" appearance: low or peripheral nodular enhancement at 30 s, progressing to peripheral or high homogeneous attenuation at 55 s. *Atypical* enhancement patterns included low–low (8%), high–iso (14%), or high–high (16%) enhancement on 30- and 55-s scans, respectively. Atypical enhancement patterns are most common with small hemangiomas (less than 15 mm). Hemangiomas that are low attenuation on both phases are indistinguishable from typical "hypovascular" metastases, whereas those that have a high–iso pattern are indistinct from small hepatocellular carcinoma or hypervascular metastases. Using three-phase spiral CT (i.e., adding a delayed phase) may help increase spiral CT specificity, although approximately 8% of hemangiomas will remain low attenuation on all phases (43).

Hepatic Cyst

Hepatic cysts are a common benign lesion in the liver, similar in frequency to hemangioma. The incidence of hepatic cysts is approximately 2% to 7% of the general population. Half of patients with polycystic liver disease have associated polycystic kidneys, whereas approximately 25% of patients with polycystic kidney disease have associated cystic disease of the liver.

Like other cysts, the criteria for diagnosis of hepatic cyst include sharp margins with no definable walls (Figs. 7-10, 7-11). The CT attenuation is usually water density (<20 HU). After contrast administration, cysts do not enhance. For small lesions of 15 mm or less, a small increase in attenuation on contrast-enhanced scans is probably due to partial volume averaging with normal enhancing liver. Using spiral CT, accurate densitometry can be obtained more easily by selecting reconstruction intervals to center the lesion in a single slice. Multiphase spiral CT imaging—including pre- and postcontrast phases, or portal phase and delayed phase—is 100% specific for hepatic cyst (Fig. 7-12).

The differential diagnosis of a hepatic cyst includes cystic metastases, such as GI stromal tumors or some ovarian metastases. Also, with spiral CT, there is often marked increase in the attenuation of the liver of the contrast administration; in these cases, improper window width and level settings can make noncystic lesions appear very dark, or cystlike, relative to the brightly enhanced liver. Unlike simple cysts, cystic metastases usually contain a solid mural component. Biliary cystadenoma and cystadenocarcinoma are rare primary cystic neoplasms of the biliary duct system (Fig. 7-13). Hepatic pyogenic abscesses often have a thick wall, numerous locules, and internal debris, and may contain air (Fig. 7-14). Ecchinococcal cysts are usually multiloculated

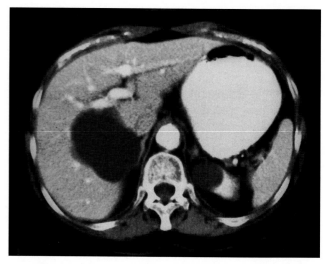

FIG. 7-10. Hepatic cyst. Spiral CT shows well-defined 6-cm water attenuation mass with no perceptible wall thickness.

(*Echinococcus granulosa*) with internal daughter cysts and rim calcification.

Focal Nodular Hyperplasia

Focal nodular hyperplasia (FNH) is a benign tumor that occurs most commonly in young adult females and may be incidentally discovered, although 10% to 20% of lesions occur in men. Occasionally, patients may present with right upper pain. These lesions must be differentiated from adenoma, because the two types of tumor occur in a similar patient populations. FNH has no malignant potential and is unlikely to hemorrhage; adenomas are often resected because of the potential for hemorrhage and malignant degeneration. On sulfur colloid scan, 60% of FNH lesions will have characteristic uniform uptake of radiotracer; this is very

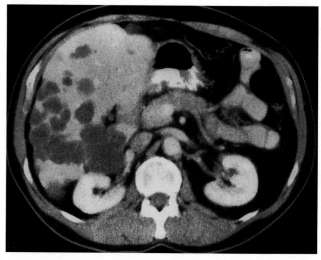

FIG. 7-11. Polycystic liver disease. Multiple well-defined low-attenuation lesions are seen throughout the liver.

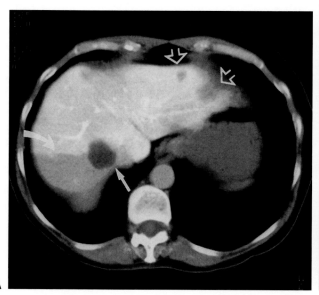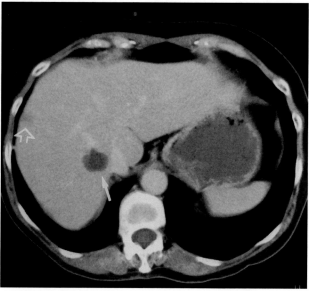

A   B

FIG. 7-12. Hepatic cyst in a patient with multifocal hepatocellular carcinoma. **(A)** Spiral CT scan during arterial portography shows a water density lesion in the right lobe of the liver (*solid arrow*). Several low-density lesions in the left lobe of the liver due to hepatocellular carcinoma are present (*open arrows*). A linear area of decreased density is present in the right lobe (*curved arrow*). This is a perfusion defect due to centrally obstructing tumor at a more inferior level in the liver. **(B)** Delayed scan obtained 10 min later showing that the cyst in the right lobe does not enhance (*solid arrow*). A low-attenuation lesion due to hepatocellular carcinoma is visible in the lateral portion of the liver (*open arrow*). (Reprinted with permission from Bluemke DA, Fishman EK. Spiral CT of the liver. *AJR* 1993;160:787.)

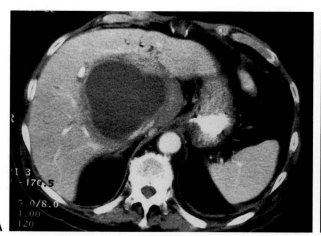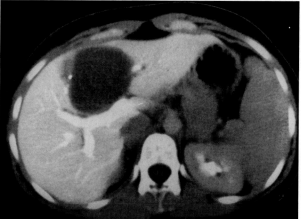

A   B

FIG. 7-13. Spiral CT of complex cystic masses. **(A)** Water attenuation mass with a thick rim of enhancing tissue, due to pyogenic abscess following abdominal surgery. The peripheral rim is distinguishes the lesion from a simple cyst. **(B)** Recurrent biliary cystadenoma. Spiral CT scan shows a water density lesion in the porta hepatis that is similar in appearance to a simple cyst. A surgical clip is present at the site of previous resection.

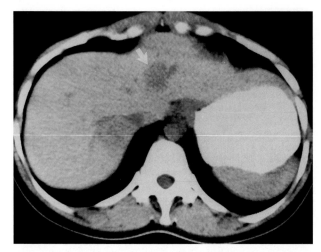

FIG. 7-14. Focal nodular hyperplasia. Noncontrast CT is non-specific, demonstrating a low-attenuation mass near the dome of the liver capsule (*arrow*).

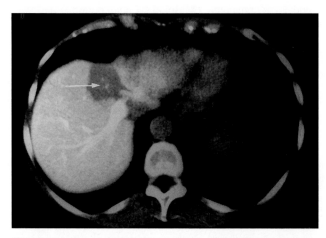

FIG. 7-15. Focal nodular hyperplasia. Spiral CT during arterial portography shows low-attenuation mass with a central, enhancing blood supply (*arrow*). Surgical resection revealed focal nodular hyperplasia.

infrequent with adenomas. Using trimethylbromoimino-diacetic acid (TBIDA) hepatobiliary scanning, the sensitivity for FNH has been reported to be 92% (47). FNH is a hypervascular lesion, with a prominent arterial blood supply. In our experience, small FNH lesions are detected more frequently with spiral CT than with dynamic CT. This is because arterial-phase images are more readily obtained with spiral CT; FNH lesions are frequently isoattenuating to normal liver (and thus undetected) on dynamic CT images obtained during the portal phase of hepatic enhancement.

Noncontrast CT of FNH demonstrates a nonspecific low-density lesion, often located adjacent to the liver capsule (see Fig. 7-14). A central scar may be present. FNH is highly vascular and has a central blood supply (Fig. 7-15). Because of its prominent vascularity, FNH is frequently hyperattenuating to the surrounding liver on spiral CT during the arterial phase of enhancement, and a central cleft may be present (Figs. 7-16, 7-17). On portal-phase images, the appearance of FNH is extremely variable and depends on the lesion size, although a central cleft should again be searched for to suggest FNH.

Hepatic Adenoma

In 95% of cases, hepatic adenomas are found in young adult women and are associated with oral contraceptive use. Patients may present with hepatomegaly as well as acute onset of abdominal pain secondary to spontaneous hemorrhage.

The appearance of hepatic adenoma on spiral CT is that of an enhancing lesion during the arterial phase of contrast enhancement. Large tumors may not enhance homogeneously (Fig. 7-18), but these may have bled and can show increased attenuation on noncontrast CT. Hepatic adenomas demonstrate rapid, early, and transient enhancement after contrast administration, so that the portal and delayed phases

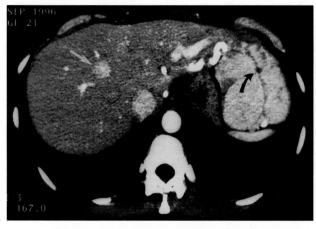

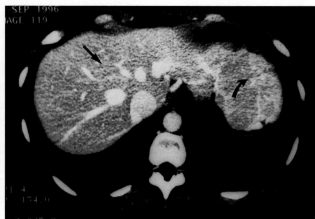

FIG. 7-16. (**A**) Arterial-phase spiral CT scan shows a large mass related to the left lobe of the liver. The mass is hyperattenuating compared with the liver, and a central scar is evident (*curved arrow*). A second lesion due to focal nodular hyperplasia is present in the right lobe (*straight arrow*). (**B**) During the portal phase, both masses are isoattenuating compared with the liver. This pattern of enhancement is typical of focal nodular hyperplasia.

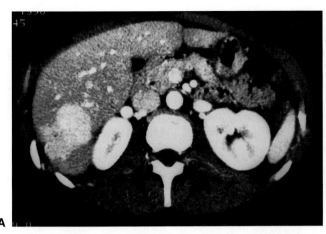
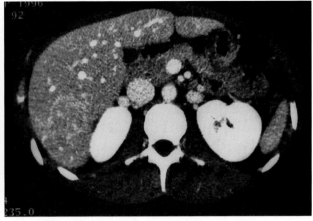

FIG. 7-17. Focal nodular hyperplasia. (**A**) Arterial phase spiral CT shows a 4-cm hyperattenuating mass in the inferior tip of the right lobe of the liver. (**B**) Portal-phase spiral CT shows the mass is nearly isoattenuating to the adjacent liver.

appear differently. Unlike FNH, no central cleft is typically present. Areas of calcification may be identified on noncontrast CT.

Other Benign Lesions

Fatty Infiltration

Fatty infiltration of the liver is associated with obesity, malnutrition, chemotherapy, total parenteral nutrition, steroid administration, alcohol consumption, and pregnancy (48,49). In diffuse infiltration, the liver appears lower in attenuation than nonenhanced hepatic blood vessels (50). Focal infiltration commonly occurs adjacent to the falciform ligament or near the gallbladder fossa (51). CT demonstrates low attenuation of the hepatic parenchyma, often in a geographic distribution. Focal fatty deposits, without adequate

bolus contrast administration, can be confused with parenchymal mass lesions (Fig. 7-19) (52,53). The demonstration of normal-caliber vessels coursing through a hypodense lesion on spiral CT is characteristic of fatty infiltration, although this rarely occurs with malignant tumors (12). Typically, these focal fat accumulations do not have an associated mass effect. Recognition of focal fatty infiltration can avoid the need to perform additional imaging exams.

Focal fatty infiltration may represent a diagnostic dilemma in two circumstances. First, focal steatosis of the liver may simulate a mass lesion. With spiral CT, a good-contrast bolus will demonstrate normal vessels coursing through the area of focal fat, essentially excluding a mass lesion. Second, focal *sparing* of fatty infiltration occasionally appears as a high-density mass in an otherwise low-attenuation liver. Again, lack of mass effect favors fatty infiltration. *Diffuse*

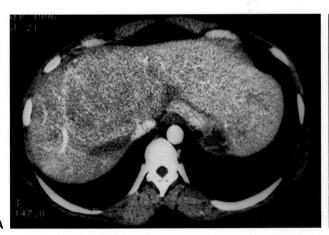
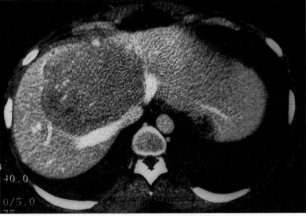

FIG. 7-18. Hepatic adenoma, 26-year-old woman with a history of oral contraceptive use. (**A**) Arterial-phase spiral CT scan shows displacement of vascular structures due to a centrally located 10-cm mass, nearly isointense to liver due to early enhancement. (**B**) Portal-phase spiral CT scan better demonstrates displacement of the right and middle hepatic veins by mass, which now appears hypoattenuating to liver. Smaller adenomas frequently demonstrate hyperenhancement on arterial-phase images.

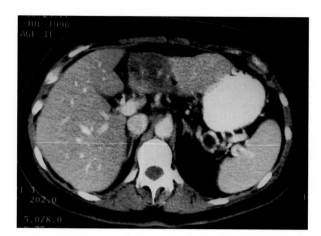

FIG. 7-19. Focal fatty infiltration of the liver simulating a mass. Note that there are internal vessels within the lesion (*arrowheads*), which would be unusual for a tumor of this size.

fatty infiltration is most reliably diagnosed using noncontrast CT demonstrating a spleen–liver difference of attenuation of more than 10 HU.

Hepatic Perfusion Abnormalities

Both focal and diffuse, or geographic, perfusion defects tend to be highlighted on spiral CT scans as a result of rapid scanning (Fig. 7-20). Focal perfusion abnormalities, or transient hepatic attenuation differences (THAD), may be due to tumors, areas of hyperemia, small areas of steatosis, or fibrosis (Fig. 7-21), but occasionally no pathological abnormality may be detected (43). Typically, focal perfusion abnormalities are hypointense to the liver and are poorly seen during the late portal phase or on equilibrium-phase images. Patients with portal hypertension and portal–systemic shunts have reduced hepatic enhancement, and detection of focal

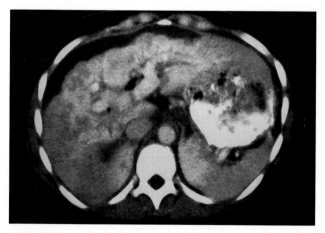

FIG. 7-20. Diffusely inhomogeneous enhancement of the liver during spiral CT in a patient with long-standing sclerosing cholangitis. Perfusion defects in this patient are due to areas of underlying cirrhosis and small-vessel obstruction in the portal triads.

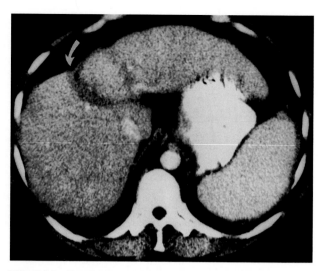

FIG. 7-21. Focal area of decreased enhancement (*arrow*) in a patient with severe cirrhosis. The linear band of decreased signal is due to confluent fibrosis.

hepatic lesions is reduced (Fig. 7-22). Geographic areas of hyperattenuation may be seen in lesions with arterial–portal shunting, including hepatocellular carcinoma and hemangioma (41), or distal to a central tumor mass (Figs. 7-23, 7-24). A focal area of hyperattenuation in segment 4 of the liver anterior to the porta hepatis has been described and is probably due to a site of aberrant venous drainage from the stomach (54).

MALIGNANT HEPATIC TUMORS

Hepatocellular Carcinoma

Hepatocellular carcinoma is more prevalent in Asia and Africa than in Europe and North America. In Asian populations, most cases are associated with cirrhosis secondary to hepatitis B. In the United States, most patients have associated alcoholic cirrhosis or no known underlying parenchymal disease. The clinical presentation in the United States is often with pain, weight loss, and palpable hepatic mass with elevated alpha-fetoprotein. In patients with underlying cirrhosis, dynamic CT detects 60% to 70% of hepatocellular carcinomas (35), with smaller lesions frequently missed.

There are three CT patterns of hepatocellular carcinoma: a solitary mass (see Fig. 7-24), a dominant mass with smaller satellite lesions (i.e., multifocal hepatocellular carcinoma, 20% of cases), and rarely, diffuse involvement. Diffuse involvement is more common in patients with cirrhosis. Hepatocellular carcinomas are highly vascular lesions and may infrequently present with spontaneous hemorrhage. In some patients, lesions are well circumscribed and have the appearance of a well-defined "capsule" (Fig. 7-25). Contrast enhancement is usually intense but transient, with internal areas of low attenuation and vascular channels (Figs. 7-26, 7-27), referred to as a "mosaic" pattern.

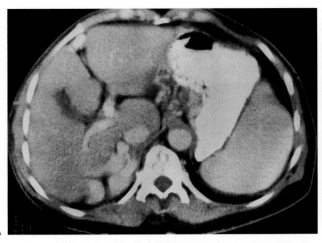 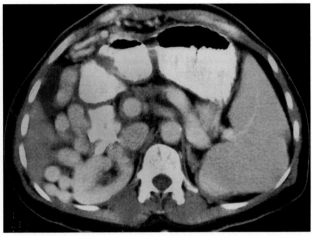

A   B

FIG. 7-22. (A,B) Portal hypertension with enlarged porto-systemic collateral vessels. Intravenous contrast that is normally delivered to the liver from the portal vein is shunted away to the systemic circulation in this patient, resulting in reduced hepatic enhancement.

Fibrolamellar hepatocellular carcinoma is a distinctive clinical and pathological type of hepatocellular carcinoma that occurs in younger patients (mean age of 20 years) with no underlying parenchymal disease. Although it is a malignant lesion, the prognosis is better than typical hepatocellular carcinoma, with 25% of patients having resectable lesions. Alpha-fetoprotein levels are usually not elevated. Fibrolamellar hepatocellular carcinoma is typically a well-circumscribed lesion showing uniform contrast enhancement. Central calcifications are present in one-third of lesions. Associated capsular retraction has been reported (55). The differential diagnosis includes adenoma or focal nodular hyperplasia.

Hepatocellular carcinomas have a tendency to invade the portal vein (in one-third of cases) as well as the inferior vena cava (IVC), hepatic arteries, and veins. Portal venous invasion or compression results in obstruction of blood flow to the involved segment. Wedge-shaped areas of decreased attenuation may result. These changes are particularly prom-

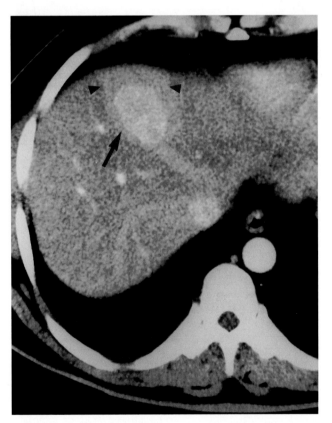

FIG. 7-24. Small hepatocellular carcinoma. Spiral CT during the arterial phase of hepatic enhancement demonstrates a hyperenhancing lesion (*arrow*) due to hepatocellular carcinoma. Distal to the the mass, a small area of hyperperfusion is present (*arrowhead*), probably due to arterial–portal shunting of blood flow.

FIG. 7-23. Focal hyperperfusion abnormality on spiral CT. Arterial-phase image of the liver demonstrates a focal hyperenhancing lesion (*arrowhead*) in the anterior portion of the liver. No underlying lesions were found.

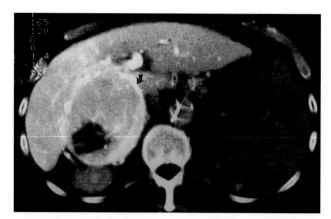

FIG. 7-25. Hepatocellular carcinoma. Spiral CT during arterial portography shows a well-defined lesion arising from the caudate lobe of the liver. The capsule is hypervascular, showing marked enhancement (*arrow*). Necrosis is present centrally in the lesion. (Reprinted with permission from Bluemke DA, Fishman EK. Spiral CT of the liver. *AJR* 1993;160:787.)

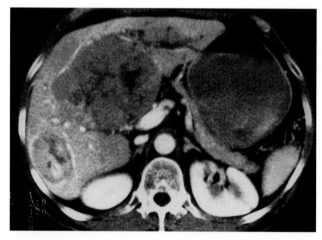

FIG. 7-26. Hepatocellular carcinoma. Spiral CT shows two masses, with hyperattenuation of the small mass in the right lobe compared with the surrounding liver. Larger masses tend to demonstrate less enhancement than smaller hepatocellular carcinoma.

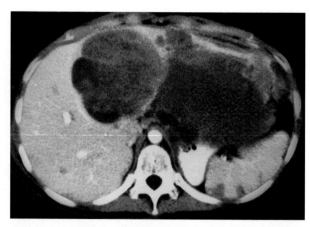

FIG. 7-27. Hepatocellular carcinoma. Spiral CT during the portal phase of hepatic enhancement shows a large, partially cystic and solid mass. Small intrahepatic metastases are present in the right lobe.

inent when using CT with arterial portography (discussed further later). Arterial–portal shunts within the tumors result in variable areas of increased attenuation and dilated intrahepatic vessels.

Ohashi et al. first demonstrated the use of multiphase dynamic CT scanning for improved detection of hepatocellular carcinoma (42). The detection of small hepatocellular carcinoma using multiple-phase helical CT has since been the subject of several investigations (20,56–58). The focus of studies to date has been to compare the arterial versus the portal phase of hepatic enhancement for tumor detection, so that the true sensitivity and specificity are not known. However, studies to date consistently show that *arterial-phase scans identify 15% to 30% more tumors than portal-phase images* (Table 7-6). The largest differences in sensitivity are for small tumors (less than 2–3 cm in size) that may be missed on portal-phase scans. Delayed-phase images at 5 min after injection appear to add further to the arterial- and portal-phase images, with an additional nearly 10% of lesions detected only on delayed images (58). In patients with cirrhosis or suspected hepatocellular carcinoma, early arterial-phase scans are strongly recommended for optimal tumor detection (see Fig. 7-24; Fig 7-28).

TABLE 7-6. *Detection of hepatocellular carcinoma: arterial-versus portal-phase spiral CT*

Study	Injection protocol*	Arterial-phase sensitivity	Portal-phase sensitivity	Study size
Baron et al. (Ref. 56)	150 mL @2.5–5 mL/s, 20 s, 60 s	95%	82%	66 patients, 326 tumors
Yamashita et al. (Ref. 81)	2 mL/kg @4 mL/s, 25 s, 60 s	64%	28%	50 patients, 72 tumors
Hwang et al. (Ref. 58)	2 mL/kg @3 mL/s, 25 s, 60 s	83%	57%	45 patients, 81 tumors
Mitsuzaki et al. (Ref. 20)	2 mL/kg @2–4 mL/s, 20 s, 60 s	95%	59%	217 patients, 109 tumors

* Injection of intravenous contrast, specified as contrast volume at injection rate, delay time of arterial-phase helical scan, delay time of portal-phase helical scan. In studies in which the time of the helical scans varied, only the earliest delay time is indicated.

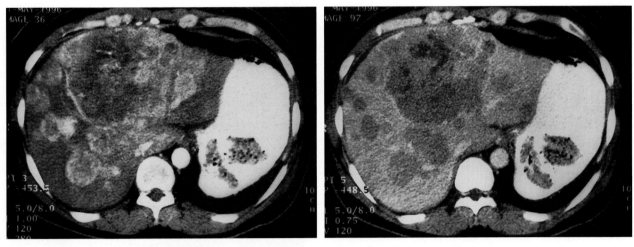

FIG. 7-28. Dual-phase spiral CT of hepatocellular carcinoma. **(A)** The arterial-phase scan demonstrates many small lesions with increased attenuation compared with the liver. **(B)** During the portal phase, most tumors are hypo- or isoattenuating compared with the liver.

Cholangiocarcinoma

Cholangiocarcinoma is the second most common primary hepatic tumor and is a malignancy arising from the bile ducts. Cholangiocarcinoma is associated with chronic bile duct inflammation. Patients typically present with painless jaundice. Cholangiocarcinoma is associated with liver fluke infestation, biliary papillomas, ulcerative colitis complicated with sclerosing cholangitis, cholelithiasis, and choledochal cysts. Half of tumors arise at the common duct bifurcation or in the distal bile duct. The so-called Klatskin tumor is an

infiltrating cholangiocarcinoma arising at the junction of the left and right hepatic ducts. These tumors produce bilobar biliary duct obstruction and are nearly always unresectable. There may be little evidence of an associated hepatic mass, as a thin sheet of tumor invades the bile duct. The differential diagnosis includes central metastasis or possibly lymphoma. Peripheral cholangiocarcinoma may occasionally be resectable when it does not involve the IVC or caudate lobe.

A common CT feature of cholangiocarcinoma is intrahepatic biliary dilatation (Fig. 7-29). Morphological changes may occur late in the disease process, with atrophy of the

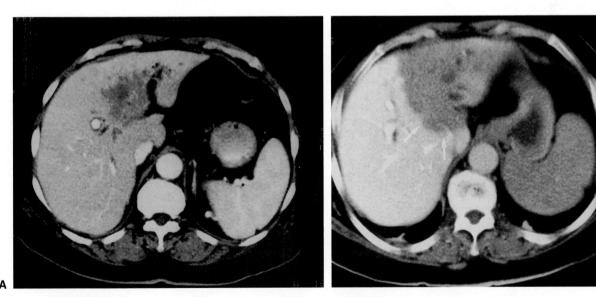

FIG. 7-29. Cholangiocarcinoma. **(A)** CT performed 1 week before **(A)** with peripheral intravenous contrast shows biliary duct dilatation with a central hypodense mass. (Reprinted with permission from Bluemke DA, Fishman EK. Spiral CT of the liver. *AJR* 1993;160:787.) **(B)** Spiral CT during arterial portography shows a low-attenuation lesion that involves the entire left lobe of the liver. The right border of the lesion is linear because of vascular invasion by the tumor. The rounded apex of the hypoattenuating lesion represents the central portion of the tumor.

left lobe of the liver compared with the right lobe. The left-sided hepatic ducts may be more dilated than those in the right lobe. With spiral CT, early imaging after bolus contrast injection is more likely to demonstrate a central mass of decreased attenuation. Vascular invasion and portal nodes should be carefully searched for, because these findings preclude resection of the tumor. Solitary peripheral masses appear similar to hepatocellular carcinoma or hepatic metastases.

Hepatic Metastasis

Metastatic disease to the liver is approximately 20 times more common than primary hepatic neoplasms. The most common metastatic tumors to the liver are colon, breast, lung, pancreas, melanoma, and sarcoma. Metastatic disease in the liver usually appears as focal, discrete lesions, but diffuse infiltrative involvement of the liver may be seen in breast cancer or lymphoma, and rarely, with colon or lung primaries.

Most common metastatic tumors in the liver are hypovascular and appear as low-density lesions (Figs. 7-30, 7-31). If fatty infiltration of the liver is present, metastases may show attenuation that is similar to or even higher than that of the liver (Fig. 7-32). In these cases, rapid bolus of intravenous contrast combined with spiral CT scanning frequently results in peripheral rim enhancement, improving lesion detection. Some tumors may have metastases to the liver that are hypervascular—that is, that demonstrate early arterial-phase enhancement following contrast injection (see Table 7-3) (Figs. 7-33, 7-34). These hypervascular metastases may be obscured during the portal phase of enhancement or with delayed scanning. Hypervascular metastases were thought to be isodense to normal liver, with dynamic CT in 25% to 39% of cases (59,60), indicating that nonenhanced scans should be performed additionally when evaluating patients

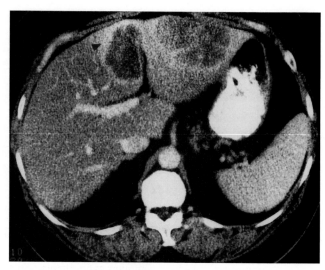

FIG. 7-31. Hypoattenuating masses in the left lobe of the liver due to metastatic colon cancer. Small areas of hyperperfusion are present distal to the medial mass (*arrowhead*).

with suspected hypervascular metastases. However, a recent study by Patten et al. indicated that nonenhanced CT did not aid in the detection of hypervascular metastases when optimal CT technique was utilized, including a power injector and biphasic contrast injection (61). Nevertheless, these hypervascular tumors frequently appear hypoattenuating on dynamic CT (61). With arterial-phase spiral scanning, the same lesions, particularly small tumors, are hyperattenuating to the liver.

The sensitivity of spiral CT for metastatic disease compared with dynamic CT has been discussed. The overall sensitivity of portal-phase spiral CT is 81% for metastatic disease (3). However, two important categories of lesions

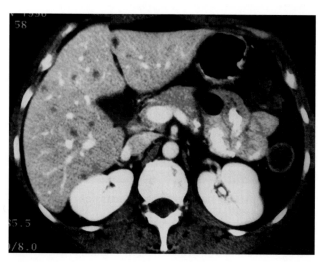

FIG. 7-30. Spiral CT demonstrating multiple small, intrahepatic metastases of less than 1 cm.

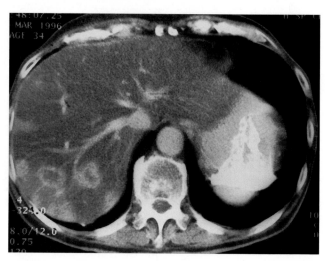

FIG. 7-32. Spiral CT of metastatic colon cancer with fatty infiltration of the liver. Peripheral masses in the right lobe have areas of hyper- and hypoattenuation, relative to the low-attenuation liver.

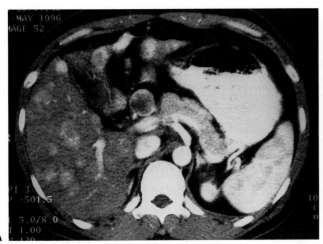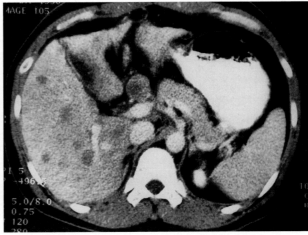

FIG. 7-33. **(A)** Dual-phase spiral CT of the liver demonstrates hyperattenuating masses in the right lobe during the arterial phases of enhancement. **(B)** During the portal phase the masses are hypoattenuating. A primary colon cancer was found following the CT scan.

appear to be more successfully evaluated with spiral CT than with dynamic CT. First, small tumors (5–20 mm) show an increased rate of detection on spiral CT, because of consistently high degrees of contrast enhancement in the normal liver, and overlapping reconstruction intervals. The detection of small tumors is important for presurgical planning, because more than four intrahepatic metastases traditionally contraindicates attempted surgical resection. The second category of tumors for which spiral CT is superior consists of small hypervascular metastases (see Table 7-3). Hollett et al. indicate that lesions of less than 15 mm were better detected on arterial-phase scans in approximately one-third of cases, but tumors of more than 15 mm were identified on portal-phase scans as well.

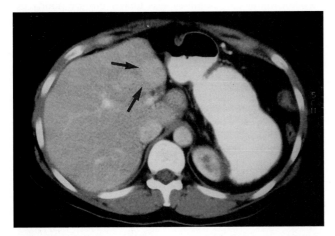

FIG. 7-34. Metastatic islet cell recurrence following partial hepatectomy. A focus of hyperattenuation (*arrows*) is present at the surgical margin due to proven recurrence. Islet cell tumors typically present as "hypervascular" hepatic metastases. Earlier-phase imaging would result in improved lesion detection.

SPIRAL CT WITH ARTERIAL PORTOGRAPHY

Background

Partial hepatic resection of metastases can improve survival of patients with certain types of primary neoplasms, such as hepatocellular carcinoma and colorectal cancer (62). Careful preoperative evaluation of these patients is essential to determine the precise location and number of metastatic lesions for accurate surgical planning (63–65).

Spiral CT during arterial portography (CTAP) is a particularly exciting application of spiral CT technology to the evaluation of hepatic disease (66–68). One reason it is especially attractive is that it is extremely effective for tumor detection compared with conventional CT techniques. With spiral CTAP, tumors of 5 mm or less can be routinely imaged, and the overall sensitivity of the technique for tumor detection is greater than 90%. By comparison, dynamic or spiral CT with intravenous contrast detects only about 70% to 80% of intrahepatic tumors and less than 50% of tumors of less than 1 cm. Spiral CTAP provides the radiologist and clinician with an effective means of detecting these small liver lesions.

CT during arterial portography maximizes the conspicuity of intrahepatic lesions by selectively delivering high levels of iodinated contrast material from the portal vein to the normal liver. Intrahepatic tumors receive relatively little contrast agent, because their blood supply is predominantly from the hepatic artery (69,70). As a result, the attenuation difference between normal and abnormal hepatic tissue dramatically increases. Intrahepatic tumors that are smaller than the effective collimation, typically about 7–8 mm, can be readily detected despite partial volume averaging effects. There is, however, an important "requirement" for CT during arterial portography studies: Imaging of the liver should be completed very rapidly, ideally within 20–30 s. After this time, there is distribution of iodinated contrast material from the hepatic veins back to the systemic arterial circulation and eventually to the hepatic artery; this results in enhancement of the tumor, potentially decreasing lesion conspicuity. Thus spiral CT technology is extremely well suited to meet this technical demand of CTAP for rapid scanning. A further benefit of spiral CT is that a 3D data set is obtained (71). Volumetric reconstruction of the liver with spiral CT is an important asset to the surgeon for preoperative planning of partial hepatic resections. Thus spiral CTAP is preferred over CTAP using a nonspiral acquisition.

Technique

Prior to spiral CTAP, superior mesenteric artery (SMA) and celiac angiography is performed for catheter placement as well as to evaluate for variant hepatic arterial supply. Contrast dose from visceral angiography is kept to a minimum. The catheter tip is placed in the proximal SMA, but beyond the origin of hepatic arteries arising from the SMA. Alternatively, the catheter can be placed in the splenic artery, with perfusion of the portal vein via the splenic vein. Splenic arterial injection has been argued to result in greater liver enhancement with fewer perfusion abnormalities than superior mesenteric artery injection (72), although this result has not been replicated by others.

Different CT laboratories have used a variety of protocols for contrast injection and timing of the spiral CTAP study following contrast injection (Table 7-7). Although these various laboratories utilize different injection protocols, spiral CT scanning is generally begun just after the end of the contrast injection. Because the spiral acquisition is so rapid, if the spiral scan is started before the contrast injection has ended, there is insufficient time for the remaining contrast bolus to circulate to and enhance the liver parenchyma.

The optimal delay time from the beginning of the injection to the start of spiral acquisition is quite variable between various published protocols. In theory it would seem that the spiral CT scan should be initiated and completed prior to distribution of contrast to the systemic circulation (i.e., before about 60 s). Using a 66-s delay time, Freeny et al. documented systemic recirculation and enhancement of in-trahepatic tumors by an average of 25%, which would seem to be deleterious to tumor detection (73). Surprisingly, Freeny et al. found better sensitivity for tumor detection when they scanned between 66 and 93 s after the beginning of the contrast injection, compared with before 60 s. These results reflect the complexity of the hepatic circulation and indicate that it is not simply one parameter, such as the delay time, that determines the quality of the spiral CTAP examination. Rather, the delay times must be chosen in conjunction with an appropriate injection rate and iodine dose. The implementation of a spiral CTAP protocol should take into account the limitations or advantages of the CT equipment at hand. Finally, indirect measures of scan quality, such as maximum hepatic enhancement, are insufficient to predict the success of the protocol for lesion detection. Instead, sensitivity and specificity should be determined to validate the scanning protocol.

Clinical Applications

Using spiral CTAP, hepatic imaging is generally completed prior to significant circulation of contrast to the abdominal aorta, so that excellent liver-to-lesion contrast is obtained (Fig. 7-35). Lesions less than 1 cm is routinely imaged (Figs. 7-36, 7-37). Excellent enhancement of the hepatic veins is important for preoperative localization of metastases and determining their relationship to major venous structures. Spiral CTAP studies result in high-quality 3D reconstructions because of lack of respiratory motion.

The sensitivity of spiral CTAP in the evaluation of colorectal cancer is 94% (74), reported in a series of 23 patients, with two tumor nodules of 4 and 5 mm not being detected. The false-positive rate in the same patient population was approximately 15%. In patients with parenchymal liver disease, the sensitivity of spiral CTAP is significantly less (72%) (75). In particular, primary malignant tumors such as hepatocellular carcinoma of less than 1 cm are poorly detected with spiral CTAP (sensitivity, 25%). Technical failures of spiral CTAP technique are likely in this patient population in the presence of spontaneous portal–systemic shunts (67), so that noninvasive preoperative evaluation should be

TABLE 7-7. *Spiral CT during arterial portography: protocols*

Study	Contrast volume (mL)	Iodine concentration (mg I/mL)	Total iodine dose (g)	Injection rate (mL/s)	Injection duration (s)	Delay time to start of scan (s)	Injection site
Bluemke et al., Soyer et al. (Refs. 66, 74, 75, 78)	150	150	22.5	3	50	35	SMA
Graf et al. (Ref. 68)	80	300	24	5	16	20	SMA
Freeney et al. (Ref. 73)	200	300	60	3	66	60–66	SMA
Lupetin et al. (Ref. 82)	150	300	45	3	50	30	Splenic artery or superior mesenteric artery

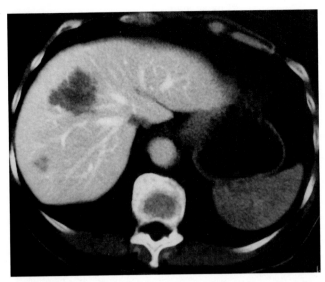

FIG. 7-35. Spiral CTAP of metastatic carcinoid tumor. Two low-attenuation lesions are present in the liver. Note that the spleen shows no contrast enhancement, because the injection was performed in the superior mesenteric artery. (Reprinted with permission from Zeman RK, Fox SH, Silverman PM, et al. Helical [spiral] CT of the abdomen. *AJR* 1993;160: 719.)

performed to evaluate the degree of portal hypertension. CT angiography, with direct contrast injection in the hepatic artery, is likely to be more beneficial in these cases.

Diagnostic Pitfalls

Although the sensitivity of CTAP methods for detection of tumor is very high, the appearance of intrahepatic lesions is nonspecific with regard to their etiology (i.e., benign vs. malignant). On both CTAP and spiral CTAP examinations, liver lesions are detected because they have a different de-

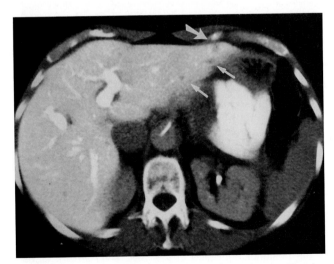

FIG. 7-36. Spiral CTAP of metastatic colon cancer. Two lesions, one of 5 mm and another of 8 mm, are present in the left lobe of the liver (*arrows*).

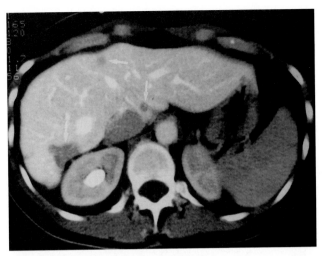

FIG. 7-37. Spiral CTAP of metastatic colon cancer. Two lesions of less than 1 cm are present in the left lobe of the liver as well as a larger lesion in the posterior segment of the right lobe (*arrows*).

gree of perfusion relative to the surrounding liver. *Nontumorous* perfusion defects are frequently present on CTAP studies. These nontumorous perfusion defects mimic the appearance of tumors, and their incorrect recognition and interpretation may deny an otherwise good surgical candidate the benefit of operative therapy. A common diagnostic problem is a hypodense defect in the medial segment of the left hepatic lobe anterior to the porta hepatis (Figs. 7-38, 7-39).

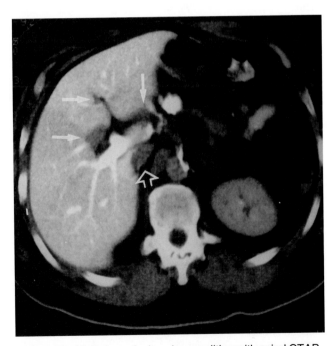

FIG. 7-38. Multiple perfusion abnormalities with spiral CTAP. Three hypoperfusion defects are present near the porta hepatis and along the falciform ligament (*solid arrow*). Their location is typical of hypoperfusion defect, rather than tumor. A fourth hypodense lesion is present in the caudate lobe (*open arrow*) and is due to metastatic colon cancer.

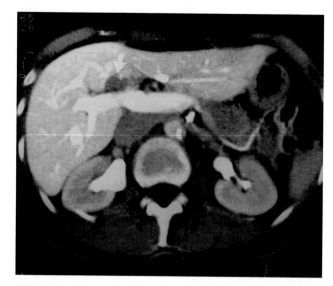

FIG. 7-39. Central perfusion abnormality with spiral CTAP. This perfusion abnormality is not due to tumor. It is recognized by its characteristic location and appearance (*arrow*). (Reprinted with permission from Zeman RK, Fox SH, Silverman PM, et al. Helical [spiral] CT of the abdomen. *AJR* 1993;160: 719.)

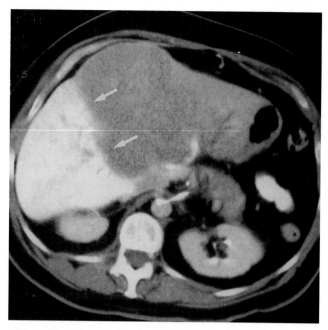

FIG. 7-40. "Straight-line" sign during spiral CTAP. A large hypoattenuation lesion is present in the left lobe of the liver due to metastatic leiomyosarcoma. Note the linear border of the nonenhancing lesion (*arrows*). A linear border is characteristic of a perfusion defect and is not typically seen with tumors.

Hypoattenuation in this region may be due to blood supply primarily from the hepatic artery rather than from the portal vein. Delayed scans or MRI will show this pseudolesion to be isodense or isointense to normal parenchyma. The typical appearances of hepatic pseudolesions have been well documented (Table 7-8) (76,77), so that with experience, nontumorous perfusion defects generally can be identified as such (78). In indeterminant cases, other modalities, including delayed CT and MRI, may be helpful for interpretation. By using longer delay times of 66 s after the start of the injection, Freeny et al. were able to reduce the rate of nontumorous perfusion abnormalities by 50% (73), using a protocol with a large contrast volume (200 mL at 3 mL/s).

The "straight-line" sign consists of a well-defined area of hypoattenuation radiating from a central neoplasm to the

periphery of the liver (Fig. 7-40). The hypoattenuating area is larger than the tumor and is due to tumor invasion or occlusion of proximal portal venous branches. Delayed images are essential to ascertain the true size of the lesion. Large lesions may also cause ill-defined perfusion abnormalities (Fig. 7-41). These are recognized as being adjacent to

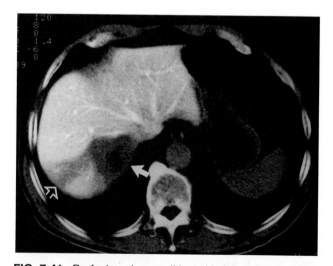

FIG. 7-41. Perfusion abnormalities with spiral CTAP. A low-attenuation lesion due to metastatic colon cancer is present in the posterior right lobe of the liver (*solid arrow*). Linear perfusion abnormalities are present peripherally to the tumor (*open arrow*). (Reprinted with permission Bluemke DA, Fishman EK. Spiral CT of the liver. *AJR* 1993;160:787.)

TABLE 7-8. *Prevalence of focal nontumorous perfusion defects detected on helical CT during arterial portography (CTAP) in 89 patients*

Location of defect	Percentage of patients*
Adjacent to gallbladder fossa	39
Porta hepatis	38
Subcapsular	15
Adjacent to falciform ligament	13
Hepatic surface, adjacent to rib	2
Posterior portion, segment 2	1

* Percentages do not add to 100 because some patients had more than one defect.
Adapted from Bluemke DA, Soyer P, Fishman EK. Nontumorous low-attenuation defects in the liver on helical CT during arterial portography—frequency, location, and appearance. *AJR* 1995;164:1141.

or extending from a central hepatic lesion. Benign lesions such as hemangioma also mimic the appearance of metastatic disease. In some cases, a delayed scan will suggest the diagnosis, so that further preoperative evaluation can be performed.

Role of Spiral CTAP

An important area of concern is the detection of hepatocellular carcinoma in the presence of underlying cirrhosis. In a carefully performed study, Miller et al. showed that the sensitivity of conventional CT with and without intravenous contrast in the detection of hepatocellular carcinoma in cirrhotic livers is only 63% and 68%, respectively (35). Spiral CTAP is unlikely to offer significant benefit in patients with portal hypertension (75,79). With portal hypertension, there is diminished delivery of contrast medium to the liver from the portal vein, resulting in substantially decreased hepatic enhancement. As an alternative, CT arteriography with or without portography may be of benefit for these patients (80).

With the implementation of multiphase spiral CT using peripheral intravenous injection of contrast, the need for CTAP studies may be reduced for several reasons: (a) Lesion detection appears to be excellent using spiral CT with peripheral intravenous contrast. (Initial results using spiral CT with intravenous contrast have demonstrated an overall sensitivity of 81%, and 91% for tumors greater than 1 cm.) Dual-phase spiral scanning further improves detection of small tumors, defines arterial anatomy, and offers the potential for improved specificity. (b) CTAP is expensive; the patient charge for CTAP is approximately four to five times greater than that of MRI, and eight to nine times that of conventional CT. (c) Improved surgical techniques—including cryotherapy, intraoperative ultrasound, and laparoscopy—have altered practice patterns of surgeons in managing patients with liver metastases. In clinical practice, there may be fewer cases available for spiral CTAP because of indeterminant noninvasive imaging. The combined results of multiple-phase spiral CT scanning with intravenous contrast, MRI, and ultrasound may approach the accuracy of spiral CTAP. Nevertheless, spiral CTAP may benefit both the patient and the surgeon as a problem-solving modality that provides a very high sensitivity for tumor detection in the noncirrhotic liver. Spiral CTAP should continue to be evaluated and used as a standard by which other imaging modalities may be measured.[81,82]

REFERENCES

1. Kalender WA, Seissler W, Klotz E, Vock P. Spiral volumetric CT with single-breath-hold technique, continuous transport, and continuous scanner rotation. *Radiology* 1990;176:181.
2. Bluemke DA, Fishman EK. Spiral CT of the liver. *AJR* 1993;160:787.
3. Kuszyk BS, Bluemke DA, Urban BA, et al. Portal-phase contrast-enhanced helical CT for the detection of malignant hepatic tumors: sensitivity based on comparison with intraoperative and pathologic findings. *AJR* 1996;166:9.
4. Zeman RK, Fox SH, Silverman PM, et al. Helical (spiral) CT of the abdomen. *AJR* 1993;160:719.
5. Foley WD, Hoffmann RG, Quiroz FA, Kahn C Jr., Perret RS. Hepatic helical CT: contrast material injection protocol. *Radiology* 1994;192:367.
6. Rigauts H, Marchal G, Baert AL, et al. Initial experience with volume CT scanning. *J Comput Assist Tomogr* 1990;14:675.
7. Crawford CR, King KF. Computed tomography scanning with simultaneous patient translation. *Med Phys* 1990;17:967.
8. Polacin A, Kalender WA, Marchal G. Evaluation of section sensitivity profiles and image noise in spiral CT. *Radiology* 1992;185:29.
9. Brink JA, Heiken JP, Balfe DM, Sagel SS, DiCroce J, Vannier MW. Spiral CT: decreased spatial resolution in vivo due to broadening of section-sensitivity profile. *Radiology* 1992;185:469.
10. Foley WD. Dynamic hepatic CT. *Radiology* 1989;170:617.
11. Costello P, Dupuy DE, Ecker CP, Tello R. Spiral CT of the thorax with reduced volume of contrast material: a comparative study. *Radiology* 1992;183:663.
12. Heiken JP, Brink JA, McClennan BL, Sagel SS, Forman HP, DiCroce J. Dynamic contrast-enhanced CT of the liver: comparison of contrast medium injection rates and uniphasic and biphasic injection protocols. *Radiology* 1993;187:327.
13. Brink JA, Heiken JP, Forman HP, Sagel SS, Molina PL, Brown PC. Hepatic spiral CT: reduction of dose of intravenous contrast material. *Radiology* 1995;197:83.
14. Freeny PC, Gardner JC, von Ingersleben G, Heyano S, Nghiem HV, Winter TC. Hepatic helical CT: effect of reduction of iodine dose of intravenous contrast material on hepatic contrast enhancement. *Radiology* 1995;197:89.
15. Berland LL. Slip-ring and conventional dynamic hepatic CT: contrast material and timing considerations. *Radiology* 1995;195:1.
16. Berland LL, Lee JY. Comparison of contrast media injection rates and volumes for dynamic incremented computed tomography. *Invest Radiol* 1988;23:918.
17. Baker ME, Beam C, Leder R, Gulliver D, Paine SS, Dunnick NR. Contrast material for combined abdominal and pelvic CT: can cost be reduced by increasing the concentration and decreasing the volume? *AJR* 1993;160:637.
18. Birnbaum BA, Jacobs JE, Yin D. Hepatic enhancement during helical CT: a comparison of moderate rate uniphasic and biphasic contrast injection protocols. *AJR* 1995;165:853.
19. Garcia PA, Bonaldi VM, Bret PM, Liang L, Reinhold C, Atri M. Effect of rate of contrast medium injection on hepatic enhancement at CT. *Radiology* 1996;199:185.
20. Mitsuzaki K, Yamashita Y, Ogata I, Urata J, Takahashi M. Multiple-phase helical CT of the liver for detecting small hepatomas in patients with liver cirrhosis: contrast-injection protocol and optimal timing. *AJR* 1996;167:753.
21. McCarthy S, Moss AA. The use of a flow rate injector for contrast-enhanced computed tomography. *Radiology* 1984;151:800.
22. Herts BR, Paushter DM, Einstein DM, Zepp R, Friedman RA, Obuchowski N. Use of contrast material for spiral CT of the abdomen: comparison of hepatic enhancement and vascular attenuation for three different contrast media at two different delay times. *AJR* 1995;164:327.
23. Kopka L, Funke M, Fischer U, Vosshenrich R, Oestmann JW, Grabbe E. Parenchymal liver enhancement with bolus-triggered helical CT: preliminary clinical results. *Radiology* 1995;195:282.
24. Silverman PM, Roberts S, Tefft MC, et al. Helical CT of the liver: clinical application of an automated computer technique, SmartPrep, for obtaining images with optimal contrast enhancement. *AJR* 1995;165:73.
25. Silverman PM, Brown B, Wray H, et al. Optimal contrast enhancement of the liver using helical (spiral) CT: value of SmartPrep. *AJR* 1995;164:1169.
26. Silverman PM, Roberts SC, Ducic I, et al. Assessment of a technology that permits individualized scan delays on helical hepatic CT: a technique to improve efficiency in use of contrast material. *AJR* 1996;167:79.

27. Alpern MB, Lawson TL, Foley WD, et al. Focal hepatic masses and fatty infiltration detected by enhanced dynamic CT. *Radiology* 1986; 158:45.

28. Foley WD, Berland LL, Lawson TL, Smith DF, Thorsen MK. Contrast enhancement technique for dynamic hepatic computed tomographic scanning. *Radiology* 1983;147:797.

29. Frederick MG, McElaney BL, Singer A, et al. Timing of parenchymal enhancement on dual-phase dynamic helical CT of the liver: how long does the hepatic arterial phase predominate? *AJR* 1996;166:1305.

30. Chambers TP, Baron RL, Lush RM, Dodd GD, Miller WJ, Confer SR. Hepatic enhancement: a method to demonstrate reproducibility. *Radiology* 1993;188:627.

31. Silverman PM, O'Malley J, Tefft MC, Cooper C, Zeman RK. Conspicuity of hepatic metastases on helical CT: effect of different time delays between contrast administration and scanning. *AJR* 1995;164: 619.

32. Small WC, Nelson RC, Bernardino ME, Brummer LT. Contrast-enhanced spiral CT of the liver: effect of different amounts and injection rates of contrast material on early contrast enhancement. *AJR* 1994; 163:87.

33. Urban BA, Fishman EK, Kuhlman JE, Kawashima A, Hennessey JG, Siegelman SS. Detection of focal hepatic lesions with spiral CT: comparison of 4- and 8-mm interscan spacing. *AJR* 1993;160:783.

34. Matsui O, Takashima T, Kadoya M, et al. Liver metastases from colorectal cancer: detection with CT during arterial portography. *Radiology* 1987;165:65.

35. Miller WJ, Baron RL, Dodd III GD, Federle MP. Malignancies in patients with cirrhosis: CT sensitivity and specificity in 200 consecutive transplant patients. *Radiology* 1994;193:645.

36. Wernecke K, Rummeny E, Bongartz G, et al. Detection of hepatic masses in patients with carcinoma: comparative sensitivities of sonography, CT, and MR imaging. *AJR* 1991;157:731.

37. Soyer P, Levesque M, Elias D, Zeitoun G, Roche A. Detection of liver metastases from colorectal cancer: comparison of intraoperative US and CT during arterial portography. *Radiology* 1992;183:541.

38. Soyer P, Roche A, Gad M, et al. Preoperative segmental localization of hepatic metastases: utility of three-dimensional CT during arterial portography. *Radiology* 1991;180:653.

39. Choi BI, Lee JH, Han JK, Choi DS, Seo JB, Han MC. Detection of hypervascular nodular hepatocellular carcinomas: value of triphasic helical CT compared with iodized-oil CT. *AJR* 1997;168:219.

40. Jones EC, Chezmar JL, Nelson RC, Bernardino ME. The frequency and significance of small (≤15 mm) hepatic lesions detected by CT. *AJR* 1992;158:535.

41. Hanafusa K, Ohashi I, Himeno Y, Suzuki S, Shibuya H. Hepatic hemangioma: findings with two-phase CT. *Radiology* 1995;196:465.

42. Ohashi I, Hanafusa K, Yoshida T. Small hepatocellular carcinomas: two-phase dynamic incremental CT in detection and evaluation. *Radiology* 1993;1989:851.

43. van Leeuwen MS, Noordzij J, Feldberg MAM, Hennipman AH, Doornewaard H. Focal liver lesions: characterization with triphasic spiral CT. *Radiology* 1996;201:327.

44. Ashida C, Fishman EK, Zerhouni EA, et al. Computed tomography of hepatic cavernous hemangioma. *J Comput Assist Tomogr* 1987;11:455.

45. Freeny PC, Marks WM. Hepatic hemangioma: dynamic bolus CT. *AJR* 1986;147:711.

46. Quinn SF, Benjamin GG. Hepatic cavernous hemangiomas: simple diagnostic sign with dynamic bolus CT. *Radiology* 1992;182:545.

47. Boulahdour H, Cherqui D, Charlotte F, et al. The hot spot hepatobiliary scan in focal nodular hyperplasia. *J Nucl Med* 1993;34:2105.

48. McKee CM, Weir PE, Foster JH, Murnaghan GA, Callender ME. Acute fatty liver of pregnancy and diagnosis by computed tomography. *Br Med J* 1986;292:291.

49. Nomura F, Ohnishi K, Ochiai T, Okuda K. Obesity-related nonalcoholic fatty liver: CT features and follow-up studies after low-calorie diet. *Radiology* 1987;162:845.

50. Halvorsen RA, Korobkin M, Ram PC, et al. CT appearance of focal fatty infiltration of the liver. *AJR* 1982;139:277.

51. Yoshikawa J, Matsui O, Takashima T, et al. Focal fatty change of the liver adjacent to the falciform ligament: CT and sonographic findings in five surgically confirmed cases. *AJR* 1987;149:491.

52. Adkins MC, Halvorsen R Jr, du Cret RP. CT evaluation of atypical hepatic fatty metamorphosis. *J Comput Assist Tomogr* 1990;14:1013.

53. Kawashima A, Suehiro S, Murayama S, Russell WJ. Focal fatty infiltration of the liver mimicking a tumor: sonographic and CT features. *J Comput Assist Tomogr* 1986;10:329.

54. Matsui O, Takahashi S, Kadoya M, et al. Pseudolesion in segment IV of the liver at CT during arterial portography: correlation with aberrant gastric venous drainage. *Radiology* 1994;193:31.

55. Soyer P, Bluemke DA, Vissuzaine C, Beers BV, Barge J, Levesque M. CT of hepatic tumors: prevalence and specificity of retraction of the adjacent liver capsule. *AJR* 1994;162:1119.

56. Baron RL, Oliver JH, Dodd GD, Nalesnik M, Holbert BL, Carr B. Hepatocellular carcinoma: evaluation with biphasic, contrast-enhanced, helical CT. *Radiology* 1996;199:505.

57. Hollett MD, Jeffrey RB Jr, Nino-Murcia M, Jorgensen MJ, Harris DP. Dual-phase helical CT of the liver: value of arterial phase scans in the detection of small (≤1.5 cm) malignant hepatic neoplasms. *AJR* 1995; 164:879.

58. Hwang GJ, Kim M-J, Yoo HS, Lee JT. Nodular hepatocellular carcinomas: detection with arterial; portal; and delayed phase images at spiral CT. *Radiology* 1997;202:383.

59. Bressler EL, Alpern MB, Glazer GM, Francis IR, Ensminger WD. Hypervascular hepatic metastasis. *Radiology* 1987;162:49.

60. DuBrow RA, David CL, Libshitz HI, Lorigan JG. Detection of hepatic metastases in breast cancer: the role of nonenhanced and enhanced CT scanning. *J Comput Assist Tomogr* 1990;14:366.

61. Patten RM, Byun JY, Freeny PC. CT of hypervascular hepatic tumors: are unenhanced scans necessary for diagnosis? *AJR* 1993;161:979.

62. Soyer P, Bluemke DA, Fishman EK. CT during arterial portography for the preoperative evaluation of hepatic tumors: how, when, and why? *AJR* 1994;163:1325.

63. Small WC, Mehard WB, Langmo LS, et al. Preoperative determination of the resectability of hepatic tumors: efficacy of CT during arterial portography. *AJR* 1993;161:319.

64. Soyer P, Bluemke DA, Bliss DF, Woodhouse CE, Fishman EK. Surgical segmental anatomy of the liver: demonstration with spiral CT during arterial portography and multiplanar reconstruction. *AJR* 1994;163:99.

65. Soyer P, Levesque M, Elias D, Zeitoun G, Roche A. Preoperative assessment of resectability of hepatic metastases from colonic carcinoma: CT portography vs sonography and dynamic CT. *AJR* 1992; 159:741.

66. Bluemke DA, Fishman EK. Spiral CT arterial portography of the liver. *Radiology* 1993;186:576.

67. Bluemke DA, Soyer P, Chan B, Bliss D, Calhoun P, Fishman EK. Spiral CT during arterial portography: techniques and applications. *Radiographics* 1995;15:623.

68. Graf O, Dock WI, Lammer J, et al. Determination of optimal time window for liver scanning with CT during arterial portography. *Radiology* 1994;190:43.

69. Greenway CV, Stark RD. Hepatic vascular bed. *Physiol Rev* 1971;51: 23.

70. Matsui O, Kadoya M, Kameyama T, et al. Benign and malignant nodules in cirrhotic livers: distinction based on blood supply. *Radiology* 1991;178:493.

71. Heath DG, Soyer PA, Kuszyk BS, et al. Three-dimensional spiral CTAP: comparison of three rendering techniques. *Radiographics* 1995; 15:1001.

72. Little AF, Baron RL, Peterson MS, et al. Optimizing CT portography: a prospective comparison of injection into the splenic verus superior mesenteric artery. *Radiology* 1994;193:651.

73. Freeny PC, Nghiem HV, Winter TC. Helical CT during arterial portography: optimization of contrast enhancement and scanning parameters. *Radiology* 1995;194:83.

74. Soyer P, Bluemke DA, Hruban RH, Sitzmann JV, Fishman EK. Hepatic metastases from colorectal cancer: detection and false-positive findings with helical CT during arterial portography. *Radiology* 1994;193:71.

75. Soyer P, Bluemke DA, Hruban RH, Sitzmann JV, Fishman EK. Primary malignant neoplasms of the liver: detection with helical CT during arterial portography. *Radiology* 1994;192:389.

76. Nelson RC, Thompson GH, Chezmar JL, Harned Jr RK, Fernandez MP. CT during arterial portography: diagnostic pitfalls. *Radiographics* 1992;12:705.

77. Peterson MS, Baron RL, Dodd III GD, et al. Hepatic parenchymal perfusion defects detected with CTAP: imaging-pathologic correlation. *Radiology* 1992;185:149.

78. Bluemke DA, Soyer P, Fishman EK. Nontumorous low-attenuation defects in the liver on helical CT during arterial portography: frequency, location, and appearance. *AJR* 1995;164:1141.
79. Oliver III JH, Baron RL, Dodd III GD, Peterson MS, Carr BI. Does advanced cirrhosis with portosystemic shunting affect the value of CT arterial portography in the evaluation of the liver? *AJR* 1995;164:333.
80. Chezman JL, Bernardino ME, Kaufman SH, Nelson RC. Combined CT arterial portography and CT hepatic angiography for evaluation of the hepatic resection candidate. *Radiology* 1993;189:407.
81. Yamashita Y, Mitsuzaki K, Yi T, et al. Small hepatocellular carcinoma in patients with chronic liver damage—prospective comparison of detection with dynamic MR imaging and helical CT of the whole liver. *Radiology* 1996;200:79.
82. Lupetin AR, Cammisa BA, Beckman I, et al. Spiral CT during arterial portography. *Radiographics* 1996;16:723.

CHAPTER 8

Spiral CT of Hepatic Parenchymal Disease

Bruce A. Urban and Elliot K. Fishman

Spiral CT is the preferred modality for routine evaluation of the liver (1–3). The unique advantage of spiral CT as compared with conventional CT is an ability to perform single-breath-hold imaging during peak contrast enhancement (4–6). This minimizes data misregistration and motion artifact, resulting in a uniformly high level of contrast enhancement. Furthermore, the entire liver can be scanned in 20–30 s, avoiding equilibrium and thus improving lesion detection and characterization. A wide spectrum of hepatic parenchymal disease can also be accurately diagnosed and characterized with spiral CT (3,7–9). This chapter provides an overview of the advantages of spiral scanning in the evaluation of parenchymal liver disease.

DIFFUSE PARENCHYMAL DISEASE

Cirrhosis

Cirrhosis represents chronic fibrosis caused by hepatic injury from a wide spectrum of disease processes (10). The most common etiologies include alcoholic liver disease and chronic viral hepatitis. Cirrhosis is usually a chronic and progressive disorder. Parenchymal nodules develop from cell regeneration and scar formation. Portal hypertension with ascites, portosystemic shunts, and splenomegaly often ensue.

Characteristic imaging features have been well described with conventional CT. Often there is a decrease in size of the right hepatic lobe and medial segment of the left lobe, with compensatory enlargement of the lateral segment of the left lobe and caudate lobe (11). The liver demonstrates an irregular surface contour. A ratio comparing the sizes of the caudate lobe and the right lobe may be helpful in determining subtle cases of cirrhosis: the caudate lobe is measured from medial to lateral at the level of the portal vein; the right lobe is measured from the lateral liver edge to the lateral edge of the portal vein. If the caudate-to-right-lobe ratio is greater than 0.65, cirrhosis is likely with a 96% confidence (11).

Because it allows for scanning during peak vascular en-

hancement, spiral CT is excellent in evaluation of the altered blood flow and distribution commonly seen in patients with cirrhosis (12–14). Regenerating nodules, in combination with periportal and perisinusoidal fibrosis, can divert splanchnic venous drainage. In addition, microcirculatory shunts that form between the portal venous and hepatic venous systems result in inhomogeneous decreased flow to the liver (13–16). Together these factors can produce a mottled enhancement pattern (Fig. 8-1). Fatty infiltration and inflammatory hepatitis can also contribute to this inhomogeneous enhancement pattern (17). In some cases, abnormal parenchymal enhancement may be the only spiral CT abnormality demonstrated in the cirrhotic liver. Spiral scanning can also provide reliable demonstration of the hepatic vasculature into the outer third of the normal liver parenchyma. In patients with cirrhosis, however, the peripheral intrahepatic vasculature is often attenuated (Fig. 8-2). This results in a "pruned tree" appearance similar to that described in the lung for patients with pulmonary hypertension.

Heterogeneous enhancement caused by fibrosis and regeneration in the cirrhotic liver makes it difficult to detect underlying neoplasia. The importance of this problem is accentuated by the high prevalence of primary liver tumors in patients with cirrhosis. Conventional CT has been relatively insensitive for detection of neoplasms in the cirrhotic liver (18). Dual-phase spiral CT examination will likely improve tumor detection in patients with known cirrhosis. Dual-phase scanning maximizes the detection of small, often hypervascular hepatocellular carcinomas that can complicate cirrhosis by acquiring an arterial-phase scan in addition to the subsequent portal venous-phase scan (19). Often hypervascular tumors are detectable only during the first scan obtained during the arterial phase (2). In one study, tumors of 1.5 cm or less were only visible or were more conspicuous on the arterial-phase images in 37% of patients who had at least one small malignant hepatic neoplasm (20). Another study demonstrated an 8% increase in the detection of focal liver lesions using dual-phase imaging (19).

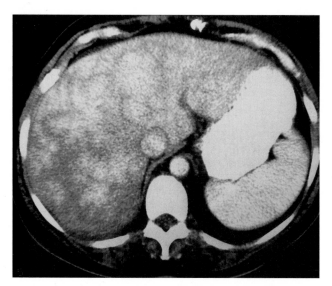

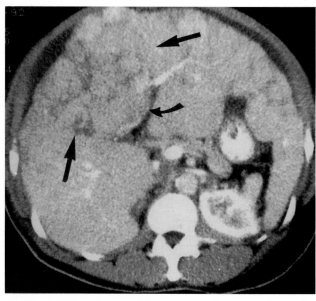

FIG. 8-1. Cirrhosis in 50-year-old female. Spiral CT reveals nodular, inhomogeneous parenchymal enhancement. This is the only clue to the patient's underlying liver disease. This pattern of contrast enhancement is similar to that of patients with heart failure and passive congestion of the liver.

FIG. 8-3. Hepatoma complicating cirrhosis in 69-year-old male. The inhomogeneously enhancing tumor mass (*straight arrows*) can be seen centrally, invading the portal vein (*curved arrow*).

At times, it may be difficult to differentiate the abnormal parenchymal enhancement of cirrhosis from diffuse or multifocal hepatoma, as well as from multiple regenerating nodules. It is important to recognize flow abnormalities due to cirrhosis that might otherwise lead to selection of an inappropriate location for biopsy, or an overestimation of tumor size. Clues to the diagnosis of an underlying tumor in a cirrhotic liver include focal contour abnormality, mass effect upon the hepatic vasculature, and vascular invasion or thrombosis (Fig. 8-3). Spiral CT with bolus contrast en-

hancement can provide a reliable, and perhaps more importantly, reproducible method for follow-up in these difficult cases.

Portal hypertension is a frequent complication of cirrhosis. It is related to increased resistance to vascular outflow. Spiral scanning can readily demonstrate varices and portosystemic collateral pathways. These dilated and tortuous vessels appear as brightly enhancing tubular structures. Common locations include the lower esophagus, gastrohepatic ligament, and splenic hilum. Esophageal varices are by far

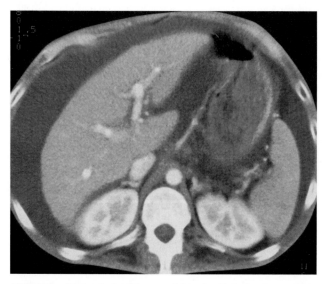

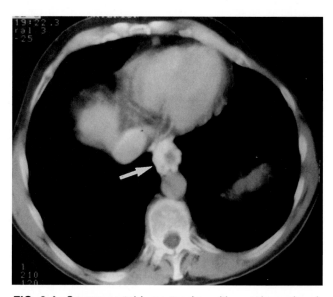

FIG. 8-2. Cirrhosis in 37-year-old male. Spiral scan reveals a small liver and ascites. The distal intrahepatic vasculature is attenuated.

FIG. 8-4. Severe portal hypertension with esophageal varices. Peak enhancement allows for detection of varices in the lower esophagus (*arrow*).

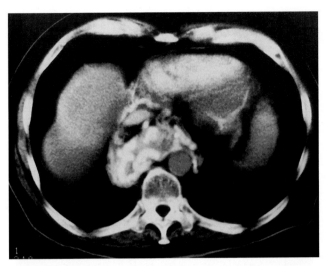

FIG. 8-5. Extensive esophageal varices in 70-year-old male. Many dilated varices are seen surrounding the esophagus in the lower chest.

the most important finding clinically, present in about 65% of patients with advanced cirrhosis (Figs. 8-4–8-6). They are a cause of massive hematemesis and death in half of these patients (10). If the diagnosis of cirrhosis is suspected prior to scanning, beginning the spiral scan slightly cephalad to the dome of the liver will help detect distal esophageal varices. Some cases of portal hypertension result in recanalization of the paraumbilical veins. These can be identified in the region of the falciform ligament, before extending medial and inferiorly to the umbilicus (Fig. 8-7). Retroperitoneal and mesenteric collaterals can be demonstrated in cases of severe portal hypertension (Fig. 8-8). The ability to scan the entire liver during peak contrast enhancement can significantly improve detection of vascular collaterals that may otherwise be mistaken for lymph nodes. This is especially true in the gastrohepatic ligament, mesenteric root, and para-

aortic regions (Figs. 8-9, 8-10). Furthermore, multiplanar reconstruction of the spiral data set results in exquisite display of the portosystemic collaterals, free from respiratory misregistration seen with conventional dynamic CT (14–17).

Fatty Infiltration

Fatty liver results from the reversible accumulation of triglycerides. Common etiologies include obesity, excessive alcohol consumption, starvation, steroid administration, total parenteral nutrition, pregnancy, chemotherapeutic agents, and a multitude of other causes (10). Fatty infiltration of the liver occurs in various distributions: generalized, lobar, segmental, subsegmental, and focal. In diffuse infiltration (Fig. 8-11), the liver appears lower in density than the nonenhanced hepatic blood vessels (21,22). Focal fatty infiltration results in a geographic region of low attenuation. Focal deposits can be confused with parenchymal mass lesions. This commonly occurs adjacent to the falciform ligament or near the gallbladder fossa, probably reflecting a separate vascular supply to these areas (Fig. 8-12) (22–25). Fatty change likely occurs here because of regional tissue hypoxia (23). Because scanning is performed during peak vascular enhancement, spiral CT can readily demonstrate normal-caliber vessels coursing through a hypodense lesion (Fig. 8-13). This can confidently establish the diagnosis of fatty infiltration in most cases, and avert the need to perform additional confirmatory studies with ultrasound or magnetic resonance imaging (MRI). Note should be made of the very rare case of malignancy that infiltrates the liver parenchyma while preserving the underlying hepatic vascular architecture (26).

Focal fatty sparing—"normal" liver that appears hyperdense against the diffusely infiltrated liver—can be seen in irradiated hepatic parenchyma that has resistance to fatty infiltration, or in parenchyma that lacks portal venous flow

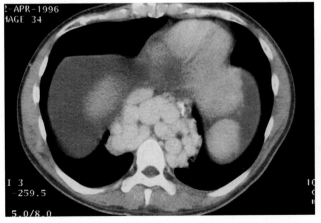

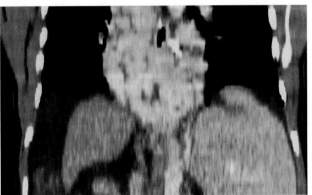

FIG. 8-6. Marked esophageal varices in 29-year-old male with cirrhosis. **(A)** Large varices are demonstrated. Nonspiral, unenhanced outside CT scan had mistakenly diagnosed adenopathy. **(B)** Multiplanar coronal reconstruction nicely demonstrates the extensive nature of the varices.

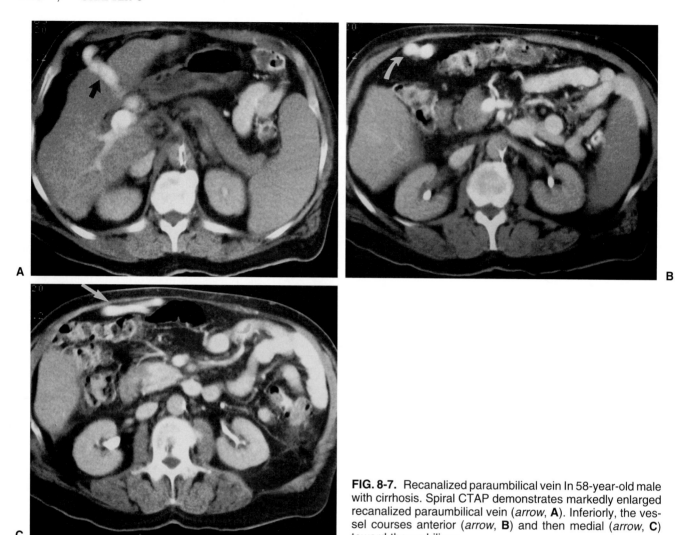

A

B

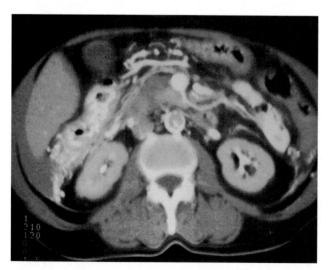

C

FIG. 8-7. Recanalized paraumbilical vein In 58-year-old male with cirrhosis. Spiral CTAP demonstrates markedly enlarged recanalized paraumbilical vein (*arrow*, **A**). Inferiorly, the vessel courses anterior (*arrow*, **B**) and then medial (*arrow*, **C**) toward the umbilicus.

FIG. 8-8. Severe portal hypertension with retroperitoneal collaterals. Excellent contrast enhancement allows visualization of marked collaterals in the retroperitoneum and mesentery.

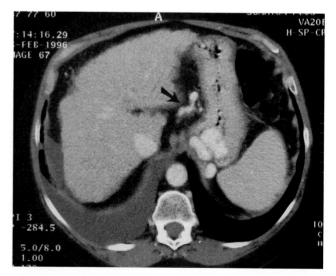

FIG. 8-9. Varices in patient with portal vein and splenic vein thrombosis. Large varices are seen in the stomach and gastrohepatic ligament. *Arrow* = coronary vein.

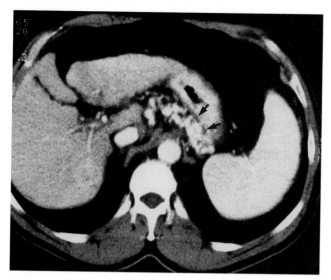

FIG. 8-10. Cirrhosis with varices in 57-year-old male. The liver is small. Spiral CT nicely demonstrates multiple varices posterior to the stomach (*arrows*).

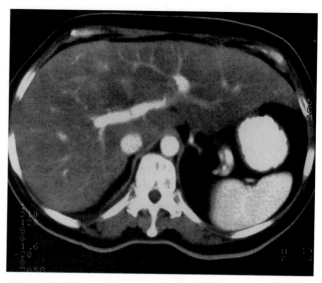

FIG. 8-11. Fatty infiltration in 57-year-old female. Normal vessels are seen coursing through a predominantly fatty replaced liver.

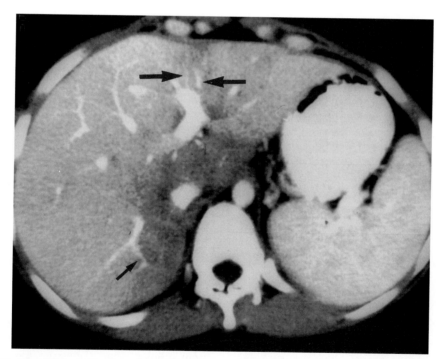

FIG. 8-12. Focal fatty infiltration. Geographic regions of low attenuation are seen in the region of the falciform ligament and ports hepatis. Normal-caliber vessels (*arrows*) course through these areas, confirming fatty infiltration.

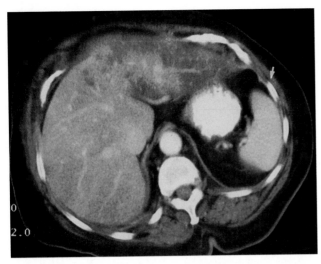

FIG. 8-13. Focal fatty infiltration in 63-year-old female with breast cancer. A geographic region of decreased attenuation is demonstrated in the left lobe of the liver. The hepatic vasculature (*arrows*) is seen coursing undisturbed through the left lobe.

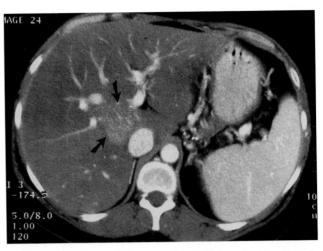

FIG. 8-15. Fatty sparing in 45-year-old female. The liver is fat infiltrated, with a focal area of sparing seen centrally near the porta hepatis (*arrows*). Small vessels course through the spared area, helping differentiate it from a mass lesion.

(27,28). Focal regions of fatty sparing in a vascular distribution, such as can occur with peripheral portal venous occlusion from small tumors or thrombi, should raise the specter for an underlying mass lesion (Fig. 8-14). In such cases, the liver parenchyma distal to the occluded vessel does not "see" the milieu of nutrients responsible for the fatty infiltration. Most commonly, however, fatty sparing is an incidental benign finding, seen in areas of aberrant vascularity near the gallbladder fossa or centrally in the porta hepatis (Fig. 8-15).

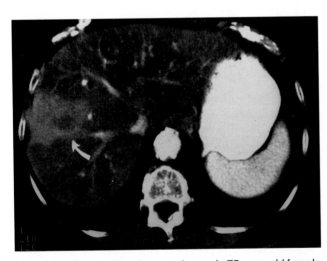

FIG. 8-14. Metastatic adenocarcinoma in 75-year-old female following Whipple surgery. Focal fatty sparing is demonstrated in the periphery of the right lobe of the liver. A subtle mass lesion is seen at the apex of the lesion (*arrow*). Biopsy revealed solitary metastasis from known ampullary adenocarcinoma. Fatty sparing results from peripheral portal venous occlusion.

Hepatitis

Viral hepatitis is a common disease with a spectrum of clinical findings ranging from minor symptoms to fulminant hepatic failure. Chronic hepatitis exists when clinical or biochemical evidence of hepatic inflammation is present for at least 3–6 months. Chronic active hepatitis (CAH) is a severe form that often leads to cirrhosis and liver failure. In fulminant hepatic necrosis associated with acute hepatitis, collapse of the periportal reticulin framework, as well as bile duct proliferation, results in enlarged periportal spaces. These widened spaces can be seen on CT as diffuse periportal low attenuation (29). This finding can also be seen in patients with hepatic trauma, congestive heart failure, liver transplant, cirrhosis, or malignant periportal or retroperitoneal adenopathy (29,30–33). In these conditions, periportal hypodensity reflects either the presence of blood, dilated lymphatics, or portal inflammation (29). Spiral CT accentuates the periportal low attenuation because of peak contrast enhancement in the portal venous system. Some patients with hepatitis demonstrate subtle, irregular parenchymal enhancement following bolus injection. This is different from the more coarse enhancement seen in patients with cirrhosis, and probably reflects diffuse parenchymal swelling resulting from cellular edema. However, a similar inhomogeneous pattern can also be seen in patients with heart failure and hepatic congestion, and correlation with serum titers is recommended in the appropriate clinical setting. We have also seen early cases of fulminant hepatic necrosis demonstrate a spiral CT appearance indistinguishable from that of hepatitis (Figs. 8-16, 8-17).

Radiation hepatitis typically has an onset 2–6 weeks after the completion of radiotherapy and consists of symptoms of hepatomegaly, ascites, and jaundice. The threshold dose is in the range of 3,000–5,500 rad. Patients typically demonstrate sharply defined, geographic regions of low attenuation that

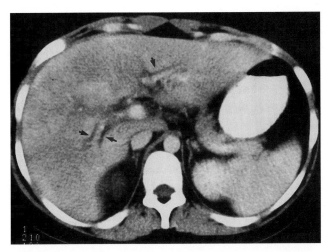

FIG. 8-16. Hepatic necrosis in 30-year-old female following bone marrow transplant. The liver enhances inhomogeneously. A periportal collar of low attenuation is demonstrated (*small arrows*). The spiral CT appearance is most suggestive of hepatitis; biopsy confirmed fulminant hepatic necrosis.

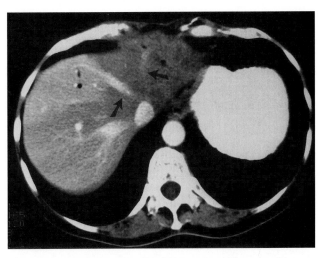

FIG. 8-18. Radiation hepatitis in 55-year-old female with pancreatic cancer. A geographic region of low attenuation is seen in the left lobe of the liver, corresponding to radiation therapy port. Normal-caliber, nondisplaced vessels (*arrow*) course through the lesion, excluding a mass. Air is seen in the biliary tree from prior sphincterotomy.

correspond to the radiation port (34). The low attenuation corresponds to increased water content (35). Spiral CT can demonstrate normal-caliber vessels coursing through the low-attenuation lesion, much like that seen with focal fatty infiltration (Fig. 8-18). The irradiated area shrinks over time, with the remaining liver undergoing compensatory hypertrophy.

Budd-Chiari Syndrome

Budd-Chiari syndrome results from hepatic vein occlusion. Etiologies include neoplasm, hypercoagulable states,

medications, and trauma (10). Many cases are idiopathic. Spiral CT demonstrates nonopacification of the hepatic veins, with inhomogeneous parenchymal enhancement, enhanced lobules of the liver, and hepatomegaly (Fig. 8-19) (36–39). The caudate lobe is enlarged in chronic cases and often demonstrates increased (probably "normal") enhancement compared with the periphery of the liver. This is due to the preservation of normal venous drainage of the caudate lobe directly in the inferior vena cava. The persistence of patchy peripheral enhancement 45–60 s after injection results from stagnant venous outflow (Figs. 8-20, 8-21) (39). Some caution must be used in making the diagnosis of Budd-Chiari syndrome with spiral CT, as nonopacification of the hepatic veins occasionally occurs if scanning is performed

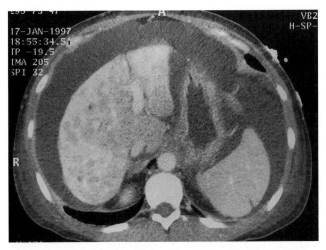

FIG. 8-17. Subacute autoimmune hepatitis and cirrhosis in 47-year-old female. Spiral CT scan reveals a small liver with heterogeneous enhancement. Extensive ascites is present. The patient soon expired. Autopsy revealed cirrhosis with chronic inflammatory infiltrate and secondary massive hepatic necrosis.

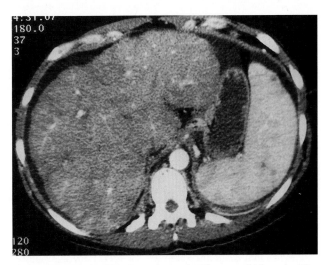

FIG. 8-19. Budd-Chiari syndrome in 42-year-old female. The liver is enlarged and shows diffuse heterogeneous enhancement. The main hepatic veins are not identified.

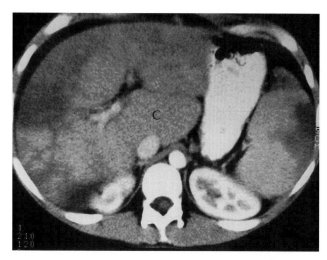

FIG. 8-20. Budd-Chiari syndrome in a 19-year-old female. Patchy peripheral enhancement is demonstrated. Normal enhancement is seen in the caudate lobe (C). Infarcts are noted in the spleen.

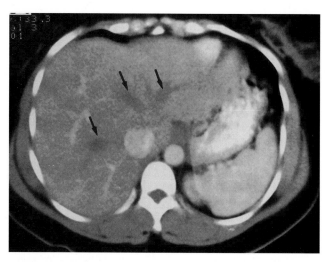

FIG. 8-22. Normal nonopacification of the hepatic veins. Spiral scan soon after injection reveals low density in the nonfilled hepatic veins (*arrows*). This should not be confused with thrombus.

in patients with poor cardiac output or heart failure (Fig. 8-22). In these patients, hepatic venous opacification may yet to have reached adequate levels while scanning is performed. Inhomogeneous parenchymal enhancement is an essential finding for the diagnosis of Budd-Chiari syndrome.

Venous Congestion

Passive hepatic congestion is a possible cause of mottled hepatic enhancement. The intrahepatic vascular hemodynamics become altered, resulting in relative stasis of blood in the hepatic sinusoids (40–42). Spiral CT, with rapid scan acquisition and peak contrast opacification, can reliably de-

tect this transient inhomogeneity (Fig. 8-23). Linear and curvilinear regions of decreased enhancement correspond to delayed enhancement in regions of small and medium-sized hepatic veins (43). With more severe congestion, larger areas of delayed enhancement can be seen in the liver periphery. Differential diagnosis includes cirrhosis, Budd-Chiari syndrome, diffuse malignancy, fatty infiltration, and hepatitis. Confusion can be avoided by noting secondary signs of heart failure, such as dilatation of the inferior vena cava and hepatic veins, cardiomegaly, a periportal collar of low-attenuation fluid, and lack of hepatic venous opacification detected during the spiral scan. These findings reflect decreased cardiac output and/or right heart failure (Fig. 8-24).

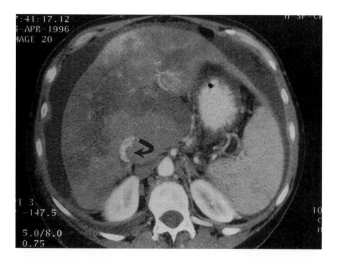

FIG. 8-21. Budd-Chiari syndrome secondary to polycythemia rubra vera in a 67-year-old female. Spiral CT reveals patchy areas of decreased enhancement, most pronounced in the periphery of the liver. The enlarged caudate lobe compresses the inferior vena cava (*arrow*).

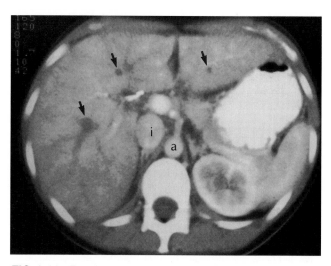

FIG. 8-23. Passive hepatic congestion in elderly patient. The liver shows irregular parenchymal enhancement. Nonfilling of the hepatic veins (*arrows*) and enlargement of the inferior vena cava (i) reflect the patient's underlying heart failure. Aorta = a.

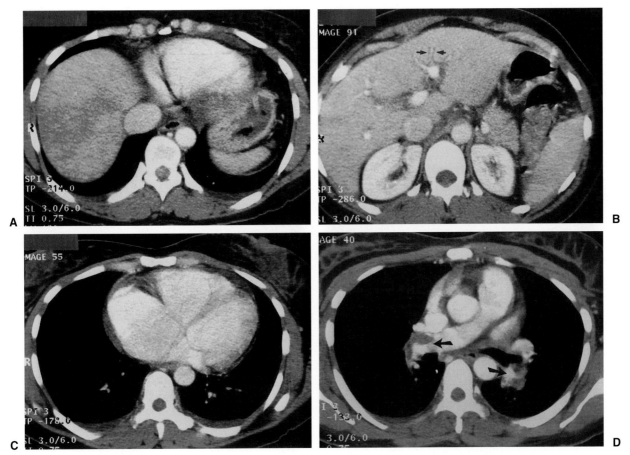

FIG. 8-24. Hepatic congestion due to secondary right heart failure in a 36-year-old female with pulmonary embolism. (**A**) The liver enhances inhomogeneously, reflecting passive congestion. (**B**) Inferiorly, a periportal collar of edema is seen (*small arrows*). (**C**) The right heart (RV) is enlarged, reflecting pulmonary hypertension from the extensive pulmonary embolism (**D**) (*large arrows*).

Other Diffuse Diseases

A variety of other diffuse parenchymal diseases can affect the liver. These include glycogen storage disease, hemachromatosis, cystic fibrosis, amiodarone toxicity, Wilson's disease, and Thorotrast deposition (Fig. 8-25) (44). Patients with glycogen storage disease and Thorotrast exposure should be monitored for the development of malignancy. Spiral evaluation in these disorders will likely add little to findings demonstrated on conventional CT, except in cases of coexistent malignancy where tumor detection and vascularity can be reliably assessed.

FOCAL PARENCHYMAL DISEASE

Abscess

Bacterial infection can affect the liver through either direct extension from the biliary tract in patients with cholangitis or cholecystitis or hematogenous seeding via the portal venous system in patients with diverticulitis, appendicitis, or inflammatory bowel disease. Another common predisposing factor

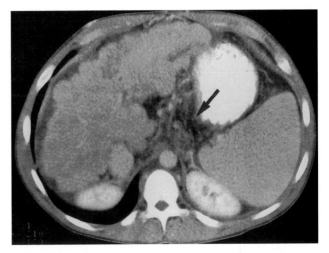

FIG. 8-25. Cirrhosis in 26-year-old male with cystic fibrosis. The liver demonstrates a nodular contour and inhomogeneous enhancement. Note is made of splenomegaly, and a fatty-replaced pancreas (*arrow*).

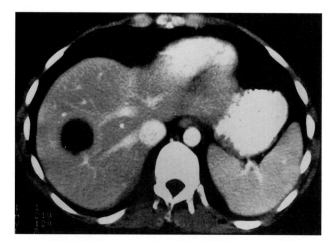

FIG. 8-26. Liver abscess in 31-year-old HIV-positive male. The low-attenuation abscess demonstrates a subtle enhancing capsule, differentiating this lesion from a cyst. Aspiration yielded aspergillus.

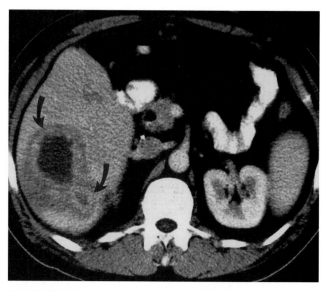

FIG. 8-28. Multiple liver abscesses in 52-year-old male. Spiral scan reveals several foci of infection. Note the enhancing rims (*arrows*).

is prior abdominal surgery. A characteristic CT finding in bacterial abscess is a central area of low attenuation with contrast enhancement of a peripheral rim or capsule (Figs. 8-26–8-28) (45). Many abscesses have sharp external margins. Improved contrast enhancement with spiral CT can help define these characteristics. Furthermore, the virtual elimination of partial volume averaging provided by spiral scanning can aid in the detection of smaller lesions and in the demonstration of gas bubbles, which are seen with conventional CT in approximately 20% of cases (Fig. 8-29) (44).

Fungal microabscesses, usually due to candidiasis, can be seen in immunocompromised hosts. Systemic candidiasis has also been described in patients following hyperalimentation or during pregnancy. The liver and spleen are usually involved because of hematogenous spread from other organs, especially the lungs. CT demonstrates multiple, very

small lesions throughout the liver and spleen (46–49). Because of peak contrast enhancement and contiguous data acquisition, spiral CT can depict lesions as small as 2 mm.

Hepatic Infarcts

Causes of hepatic infarction include hypercoagulable states, neoplasm, trauma, and interarterial chemotherapy. Infarction can be focal or diffuse. Focal infarcts classically demonstrate sharp, peripheral wedge-shaped hypodense lesions that reflect their vascular etiology, although rounded or centrally located lesions can be seen (Fig. 8-30) (50).

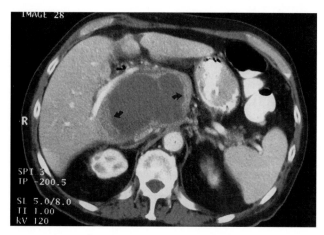

FIG. 8-27. Large abscess in 80-year-old male. The collection has a thick, enhancing rim (*arrows*). The appearance is indistinguishable from a necrotic or cystic neoplasm. Aspiration revealed purulent material.

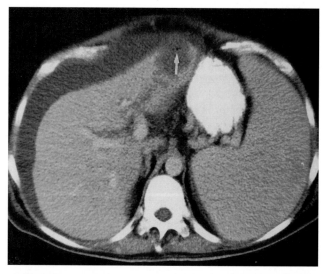

FIG. 8-29. Liver abscess in HIV-positive patient. Spiral CT helps detect a very small bubble of air in the lesion (*arrow*), suggesting infection.

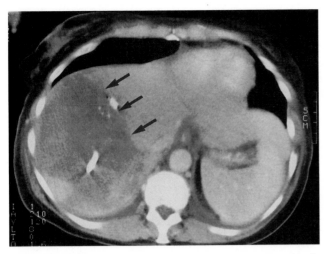

FIG. 8-30. Large hepatic infarct following aneurysm embolization in a 57-year-old female. Note the "straight-line" sign (*arrows*), reflecting the vascular etiology of the lesion.

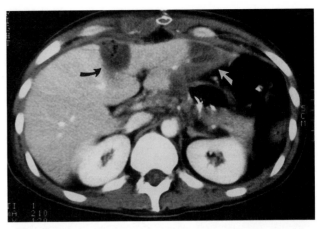

FIG. 8-32. Cryolesion and liver infarct in a 30-year-old male following resection of gastric leiomyosarcoma. The lateral segment of the liver is infarcted, likely resulting from aggressive surgical retraction (*straight arrow*). The cryoablated liver metastasis (*curved arrow*) demonstrates characteristic wedge-shaped configuration with some central foci of air. This lesion should not be confused with abscess.

Infarcts can also contain gas (Fig. 8-31). Following liver transplantation, partial or complete occlusion of the hepatic artery can occur. This is a rare but catastrophic outcome. Spiral CT can help in evaluation of the liver transplant patient by reliably demonstrating the central and peripheral portions of the hepatic artery in most normal patients (51,52). Spiral CT with maximum-intensity projection is also highly accurate in identifying hepatic artery thrombosis following liver transplant. In a study by Legmann et al., 30 liver transplant patients underwent Doppler sonography and spiral CT with maximum-intensity projection (MIP) to evaluate the hepatic parenchyma and hepatic vessels (53). Both Doppler sonography and spiral CT were 100% sensitive to the presence of hepatic artery occlusion in the five patients with

confirmed occlusion. Doppler sonography proved minimally more specific for vascular patency (96% vs. 92%).

The normal postoperative appearance of the liver in patients following cryoablation surgery for hepatic metastases can mimic the appearance of hepatic abscess or infarct (54,55). Hepatic cryolesions typically demonstrate extension to the liver capsule, often containing foci of air (Fig. 8-32). Hemorrhage is seen within the vast majority of lesions (54). More than half of these lesions can demonstrate peripheral enhancement following bolus contrast enhancement (54). Careful attention to the surgical history of the patient is essential for accurate diagnosis.

Perfusion Defects Associated with Portal Vein Thrombosis

Portal vein thrombosis can complicate cirrhosis, infection, tumors, or trauma. It can be seen in patients with a hypercoagulable state due to polycythemia, underlying malignant neoplasm, use of birth control pills, and so on, or can result from direct extrinsic compression due to adjacent or invading tumor (44). Spiral CT can frequently help detect the underlying cause of the portal venous thrombosis. Patients with cirrhosis and portal hypertension without hepatoma may also have portal venous thrombosis; this does not necessarily imply the presence of an underlying tumor.

The CT appearance of thrombosis of the portal venous system has been well described (56). The portal vein demonstrates a central intraluminal filling defect of lower-density tumoral or nontumoral thrombus (Figs. 8-33–8-35). Vessel wall enhancement is also likely present but is obscured by the luminal contrast (56). Uniform, peak-contrast opacification makes spiral CT very useful not only in demonstration of main portal venous thrombosis, but also in detection of

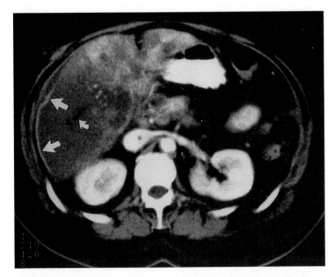

FIG. 8-31. Hepatic infarct in a 54-year-old female. The infarcted liver demonstrates capsular enhancement (*straight arrows*). Note the foci of air within the infarcted tissue (*curved arrow*).

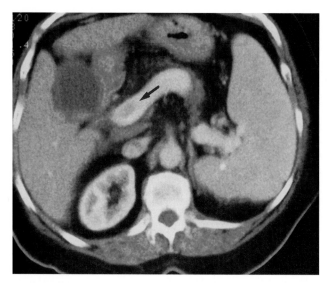

FIG. 8-33. Portal vein thrombosis. Thrombus is demonstrated in the main portal vein (*arrow*). Splenomegaly and splenic varices result from portal hypertension.

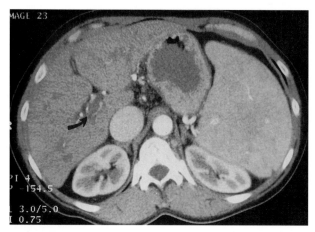

FIG. 8-34. Portal vein thrombosis in 48-year-old female. Arterial-phase spiral CT scan nicely demonstrates small hepatic arterioles surrounding the large portal vein clot (*arrow*).

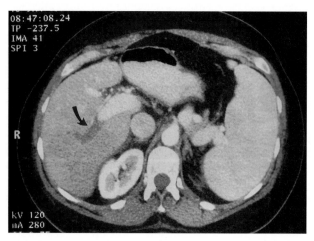

FIG. 8-35. Portal vein thrombosis in a 41-year-old female. Spiral CT scan demonstrates an isolated clot in the right portal vein (*arrow*). The enlarged main portal vein is patent.

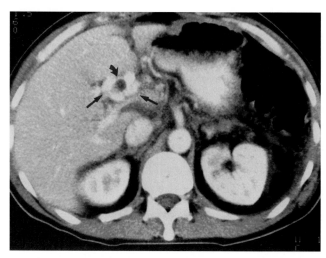

FIG. 8-36. Portal vein thrombosis. Central thrombus is demonstrated in the portal vein (*curved arrow*), with dense opacification of large periportal collaterals (*straight arrows*). (Used with permission from Bluemke DA, Fishman EK. Spiral CT of the liver. *AJR* 1993;160:787–792.)

small, dilated periportal collateral vessels, the so-called cavernous transformation (Fig. 8-36). Excellent contrast enhancement has also increased our ability to detect previously unsuspected, relatively small thrombi in the portal vein and major mesenteric veins (Fig. 8-37). Similar capabilities with spiral CT have been demonstrated in the evaluation of pulmonary emboli (57,58). The significance of these small portal thrombi has yet to be clinically determined.

In patients with portal vein thrombosis, transient increased enhancement with straight borders can be demonstrated in portions of the liver deprived of portal venous flow (56,59). This transient phenomenon is especially well appreciated

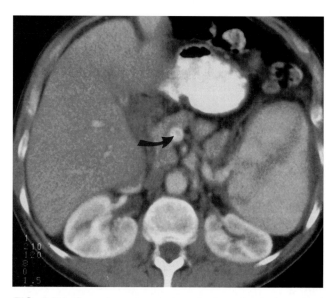

FIG. 8-37. Superior mesenteric vein thrombosis in patient with cirrhosis. Spiral scan detects a small thrombus in the superior mesenteric vein (*arrow*).

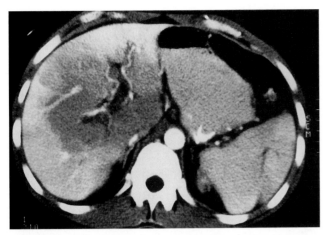

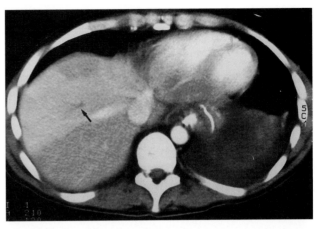

FIG. 8-38. Portal vein thrombosis with peripheral hyperattenuation in 44-year-old male. There is extensive thrombosis of the portal vein with cavernous transformation. The peripheral liver shows transient hyperattenuation, reflecting the collateral supply to the inner liver from the central cavernoma.

FIG. 8-40. Transient hyperattenuation difference from peripheral portal vein thrombosis. The characteristic wedge-shaped difference is seen in the distribution of a peripherally thrombosed portal venous branch (*arrow*).

during the arterial phase of a dual-phase spiral CT scan. The involved liver is relatively enhanced compared with the "normal" liver, because of a combination of compensatory hepatic arterial hyperemia and lack of enhancement from relatively contrast-dilute portal venous blood. In cases of extensive cavernous transformation of the main portal vein, this relative increased enhancement occurs peripherally, because the cavernoma provides only adequate flow to the central portions of the liver (Fig. 8-38) (56). With segmental portal venous occlusion, the hyperattenuating differences are often wedge-shaped and extend to the periphery of the liver, reflecting the vascular distribution of the involved vessel (Figs. 8-39, 8-40) (60). At times, subtle hyperattenuation differences may be the only sign of an underlying segmental thrombosis. It is important to remember that not every focal

alteration of hepatic enhancement is due to portal venous thrombosis: hepatic vein occlusion (61), cirrhosis, and nodular regeneration can produce similar findings. More importantly, tumors can result in a transient hyperattenuation defect from compression or occlusion of portal flow. Typically, the responsible lesion is present at the apex of the defect. A careful search for any underlying mass is of paramount importance when evaluating any wedge-shaped flow-related abnormality; spiral CT is very useful for the detection of any underlying lesions.

Other Perfusion Defects

Numerous authors have described nonlobar, nonsegmental perfusion abnormalities with CTAP (28,62–66). These

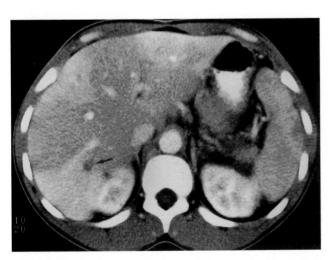

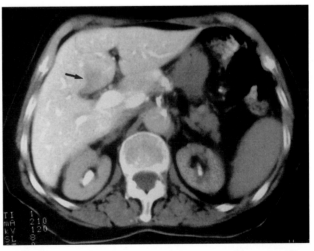

FIG. 8-39. Peripheral portal vein thrombosis in 30-year-old male. Several wedge-shaped transient hyperattenuation differences are seen in the liver. Underlying peripheral portal venous thrombosis is demonstrated (*arrow*).

FIG. 8-41. Flow-related pseudolesion on CTAP. The geographic nature and characteristic location of the lesion (*arrow*), anterior to the porta hepatis, are clues to the correct diagnosis.

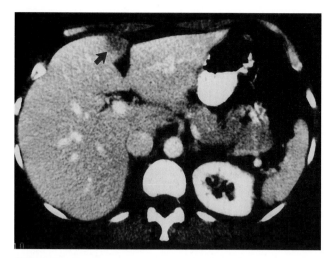

FIG. 8-42. Pseudolesion in 45-year-old female. Transient hypoattenuation (*arrow*) is seen in a characteristic location near the fissure for the ligamentum teres. This is also a common area of focal fatty infiltration. This should not be mistaken for a mass lesion.

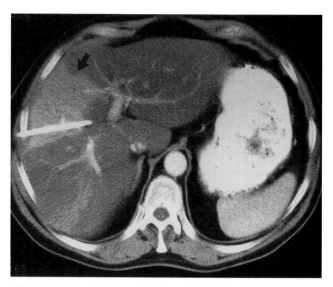

FIG. 8-44. Focal hyperattenuation in 68-year-old male with percutaneous biliary drainage catheter. The liver is predominantly fatty infiltrated. Relative focal hyperattenuation (*arrow*) is seen adjacent to the biliary tube.

lesions are typically located in the medial segment of the left lobe immediately anterior to the porta hepatis (Fig. 8-41) and in the medial or lateral segment of the left lobe adjacent to the fissure for the ligamentum teres (Fig. 8-42). At helical CT, pseudolesions are also seen with increased frequency. The sooner the liver is scanned after bolus injection, the more probable that pseudolesions will be detected. One study found the prevalence of pseudolesions in the left lobe near the fissure for the ligamentum teres at helical CT to be 14% overall (67). Familiarity with these pseudolesions is important because these defects are the result of aberrant vascularity and are not caused by tumors or thrombosis

(65,68). Similarly, these areas may be the site of focal fatty sparing or fatty infiltration (65,68).

Obstruction of the superior vena cava can result in a unique hyperperfusion defect (69). Characteristically, one of the collateral vessels enters the left lobe of the liver, and can usually be seen anterior to the lateral segment of the left lobe of the liver. Following bolus contrast enhancement, a wedge-shaped hyperattenuation area in the anterior part of the medial segment is seen (Fig. 8-43).

We have seen several cases of focal increased attenuation adjacent to recently placed percutaneous biliary catheters (Figs. 8-44, 8-45). Similar areas of hepatic hyperattenuation

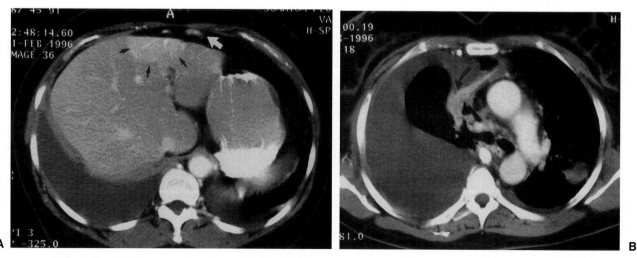

FIG. 8-43. "Hot spot" in the liver associated with superior vena cava occlusion in 54-year-old female with lung cancer. **(A)** Collateral vessels (*straight arrow*) enter the medial segment of the left lobe of the liver (*small arrows*), with relative hyperperfusion demonstrated. **(B)** Superiorly, the superior vena cava is occluded from tumor (*curved arrow*),

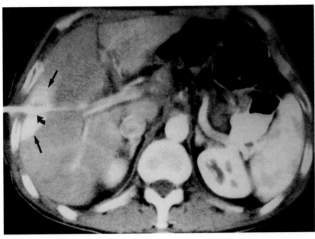 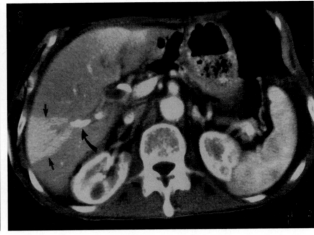

FIG. 8-45. Focal hyperattenuation adjacent to biliary tube. Two patients (**A** and **B**) demonstrate increased attenuation (*straight arrows*) at catheter insertion site (*curved arrows*).

can be seen adjacent to subcapsular fluid collections (Fig. 8-46), or adjacent to the gallbladder in patients with acute cholecystitis (70). This phenomenon likely represents a combination of relative hyperattenuation due to focal compressive effects upon the hepatic parenchyma, post-traumatic or inflammatory hyperemia, and/or peripheral portal venous occlusion. Early venous drainage can also contribute to the transient hyperattenuation, especially near an inflamed gallbladder (70). The ability of spiral CT to scan the entire liver during maximum contrast enhancement has increased our ability to detect these very subtle regions of abnormal perfusion, and care must be taken in not confusing them with true hepatic pathology. Their geographic and focal nature are the clues to accurate diagnosis.

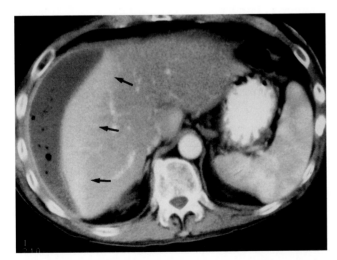

FIG. 8-46. Infected biloma in 5-year-old male following cholecystectomy. Infected subcapsular fluid collection is seen compressing the underlying liver, which demonstrates focal hyperattenuation (*arrows*).

REFERENCES

1. Zeman RK, Zeiberg AS, Davros WJ, et al. Routine helical CT of the abdomen: image quality considerations. *Radiology* 1993;189:395–400.
2. Tomiak MM, Foley WD, Jacobson DR. Variable-mode helical CT: imaging protocols. *AJR* 1995;164:1525–1531.
3. Bluemke DA, Fishman EK. Spiral CT of the liver. *AJR* 1993;160: 787–792.
4. Kalender WA, Polacin A. Physical performance characteristics of spiral CT scanning. *Med Phys* 1991;18:910–915.
5. Kalender WA, Seissler W, Klotz E, Vock P. Spiral volumetric CT with single-hold-technique, continuous transport, and continuous scanner rotation. *Radiology* 1990;176:181–183.
6. Vock P, Soucek M, Daepp M, Kalender WA. Lung: spiral volumetric CT with single-breath-hold technique. *Radiology* 1990;176:864–867.
7. Zeman RK, Fox SH, Silverman PM, et al. Helical (spiral) CT of the abdomen. *AJR* 1993;160:719–725.
8. Urban BA, Fishman EK, Kuhlman JE, Kawashima A, Hennessey JG, Siegelman SS. Detection of focal hepatic lesions with spiral CT: comparison of 4- and 8-mm interscan spacing. *AJR* 1993;160:783–785.
9. Bluemke DA, Fishman EK. Spiral CT arterial portography of the liver. *Radiology* 1993;186:576–579.
10. Robbins SL, Cotran RS, Kumar V. *Pathologic basis of disease*, 3rd ed. Philadelphia: WB Saunders; 1984:884–942.
11. Harbin WP, Robert NJ, Ferrucci JT. Diagnosis of cirrhosis based on regional changes in hepatic morphology. *Radiology* 1980;135: 273–283.
12. Popper H, Elias H, Petty DE. Vascular pattern of cirrhotic liver. *Am J Clin Pathol* 1952;22:717–729.
13. Popper H. Pathologic aspects of cirrhosis. A review. *Am J Pathol* 1977; 87:228–264.
14. Huet PM, DuReau A, Marleau D. Arterial and portal blood supply in cirrhosis: a functional evaluation. *Gut* 1979;20:792–796.
15. Huet PM, Marleau D, Lavole P, Viallet A. Extraction of I-125 albumin microaggregates from portal blood: an index of functional portal blood supply in cirrhotics. *Gastroenterology* 1976;70:74–81.
16. Groszman RJ, Kravetz D, Parysow O. Intrahepatic arteriovenous shunting in cirrhosis of the liver. *Gastroenterology* 1977;73:201–204.
17. Mulhern CB, Arger PH, Coleman BG, et al. Nonuniform attenuation in computed tomography study of the cirrhotic liver. *Radiology* 1979; 132:399–402.
18. Miller WJ, Baron RL, Dodd III GD, Federle MP. Malignancies in patients with cirrhosis: CT sensitivity and specificity in 200 consecutive transplant patients. *Radiology* 1994;193:645–650.
19. Bonaldi VM, Bret PM, Reinhold C, Atri M. Helical CT of the liver: value of an early hepatic arterial phase. *Radiology* 1995;197:357–363.
20. Hollet MD, Jeffrey Jr RB, Nino-Murcia M, Jorgensen MJ, Harris DP.

Dual-phase helical CT of the liver: value of arterial phase scans in the detection of small (<1.5 cm) malignant hepatic neoplasms. *AJR* 1995; 164:879–884.

21. Halvorsen RA, Korobkin M, Ram PC, et al. CT appearance of focal fatty infiltration of the liver. *AJR* 1982;139:277–281.

22. Adkins MC, Halvorsen RA, duCret RP. CT evaluation of atypical fatty metamorphosis. *J Comput Assist Tomogr* 1990;14:1013–1015.

23. Yoshikawa J, Matsui O, Takashima T, et al. Focal fatty change of the liver adjacent to the falciform ligament: CT and sonographic findings in five surgically confirmed cases. *AJR* 1987;149:491–494.

24. Brawer MK, Austin GE, Lewin KJ. Focal fatty change of the liver, a hitherto poorly recognized entity. *Gastroenterology* 1980;78:247–252.

25. Kawashima A, Suehiro S, Murayama S, Russel WJ. Focal fatty infiltration of the liver mimicking a tumor: sonographic and CT features. *J Comput Assist Tomogr* 1986;10:329–331.

26. Apecella PL, Mirowitz SA, Weinreb JC. Extension of vessels through hepatic neoplasms: MR and CT findings. *Radiology* 1994;191: 135–136.

27. Cutillo DP, Swayne LC, Fasciano MG, Schwarz JR. Absence of fatty replacement in radiation damaged liver: CT demonstration. *J Comput Assist Tomogr* 1989;13:259–261.

28. Arai K, Matsui O, Takashima T, et al. Focal spared areas in fatty liver caused by regional decreased portal flow. *AJR* 1988;151:300–302.

29. Siegel MJ, Herman TE. Periportal low attenuation at CT in childhood. *Radiology* 1992;183:685–688.

30. Marincek B, Barbier PA, Becker CD, et al. Appearance of impaired lymphatic drainage in liver transplants. *AJR* 1986;147:519–523.

31. Dupuy D, Costello P, Lewis, D, et al. Abdominal CT findings after liver transplantation in 66 patients. *AJR* 1991;156:1167–1170.

32. Aspetrand F, Schrumpf E, Jacobsen M, Hanssen L, Endresen K. Increased lymphatic flow from the liver in different intra- and extrahepatic diseases demonstrated by CT. *J Comput Assist Tomogr* 1991;15: 550–554.

33. Koslin DB, Stanley RJ, Berland LL, Shin MS, Dalton SC. Hepatic perivascular lymphedema: CT appearance. *AJR* 1988;150:11–113.

34. Jeffrey RB, Moss A, Quivey JM, et al. CT of radiation-induced hepatic injury. *AJR* 1980;135:445–448.

35. Unger EC, Lee JKT, Weyman PJ. CT and MR imaging of radiation hepatitis. *J Comput Assist Tomogr* 1987;11:264–268.

36. Rossi P, Sposito M, Simonetti G, Sposato S, Cusumano G. CT diagnosis of Budd-Chiari syndrome. *J Comput Assist Tomogr* 1981;5:366–369.

37. Harter LP, Gross BH, Hilaire JS, Filly RA, Goldberg HI. CT and sonographic appearance of hepatic vein obstruction. *AJR* 1982;139: 176–178.

38. Vogelzang RL, Anschuetz SL, Gore RM. Budd-Chiari syndrome: CT observations. *Radiology* 1987;163:329–333.

39. Mathieu D, Vasile N, Menu Y, et al. Budd-Chiari syndrome: dynamic CT. *Radiology* 1987;165:409–413.

40. Mauro MA, Stackhouse DJ, Parker LA, Schiebler ML. Computed tomography of hepatic venous hypertension: the reticulated-mosaic pattern. *Gastrointest Radiol* 1990;15:35–38.

41. Holley HC, Koslin DB, Berland LL, et al. Inhomogeneous enhancement of liver parenchyma secondary to passive congestion: contrast-enhanced CT. *Radiology* 1989;170:795–800.

42. Moulton JS, Miller BL, Dodd III GD. Passive hepatic congestion in heart failure: CT abnormalities. *AJR* 1988;151:939–942.

43. Gore RM, Mathieu DG, White EM, Ghahremani GG, Panella JS, Rochester D. Passive hepatic congestion: cross-sectional imaging features. *AJR* 1994;162:71–75.

44. Lee JKT, Sagel SS, Stanley RJ. *Computed body tomography with MRI correlation*, 2nd ed. New York: Raven Press; 1989:627–639.

45. Terrier F, Becker CD, Triller JK. Morphologic aspects of hepatic abscesses at computed tomography and ultrasound. *Acta Radiol Diagn* 1983;24:129–137.

46. Pastakia B, Shawker TH, Thaler M, O'Leary T, Pizzo PA. Hepatosplenic candidiasis: wheels within wheels. *Radiology* 1988;166: 417–421.

47. Shirkhoda A. CT findings in hepatosplenic and renal candidiasis. *J Comput Assist Tomogr* 1987;11:795–798.

48. Ho B, Cooperberg PL, Li DKB, Mack L, Naiman SC, Grossman L. Ultrasonography and computed tomography of hepatic candidiasis in the immunocompromised patient. *J Ultrasound Med* 1982;1:157–159.

49. Callen PW, Filly RA, Marcus FS. Ultrasonography and computed tomography in the evaluation of hepatic microabscesses in the immunocompromised patient. *Radiology* 1980;136:433–434.

50. Kev-Toaff AS, Friedman AC, Cohen LM, Radecki PD, Caroline DF. Hepatic infarcts: new observations by CT and sonography. *AJR* 1987; 149:87–90.

51. Rubin GD, Dake MD, Napel SA, McDonnell CH, Jeffrey RB. Three-dimensional spiral CT angiography of the abdomen: initial clinical experience. *Radiology* 1993;186:147–152.

52. Ney DR, Fishman EK, Niederhuber JE. Three-dimensional display of hepatic venous anatomy generated from spiral computed tomography data: preliminary results. *J Digit Imaging* 1992;5:242–245.

53. Legmann P, Costes V, Tudoret L, et al. Hepatic artery thrombosis after liver transplantation: diagnosis with spiral CT. *AJR* 1995;164:97–101.

54. Kuszyk BS, Choti MA, Urban BA, et al. Hepatic tumors treated by cryosurgery: normal CT appearance. *AJR* 1996;166:363–367.

55. McLoughlin RF, Saliken JF, McKinnon G, Wiseman D, Temple W. CT of the liver after cryotherapy of hepatic metastases: imaging findings. *AJR* 1995;165:329–332.

56. Mathieu D, Vasile N, Grenier P. Portal thrombosis: dynamic CT features and course. *Radiology* 1985;154:737–741.

57. Vogelsang RL, Gore RM, Anschuetz SL, Blei AT. Thrombosis of the splanchnic veins: CT diagnosis. *AJR* 1988;150:93–96.

58. Remy-Jardin M, Remy J, Wattinne L, Giraud F. Central pulmonary thromboembolism: diagnosis with spiral volumetric CT with the single-breath-hold technique: comparison with pulmonary angiography. *Radiology* 1992;185:381–387.

59. Mathieu D, Vasile N, Dibie C, Grenier P. Portal cavernoma: dynamic CT features and transient differences in hepatic attenuation. *Radiology* 1985;154:743–748.

60. Marn CS, Francis IR. CT of portal venous occlusion. *AJR* 1992:159: 717–726.

61. Murata S, Itai Y, Asato M, et al. Effect of temporary occlusion of the hepatic vein on dual blood supply in the liver: evaluation with spiral CT. *Radiology* 1995;197:351–356.

62. Fernandea MP, Bernardino ME. Hepatic pseudolesion: appearance of focal low attenuation in the medial segment of the left lobe at CT arterial portography. *Radiology* 1991;181:809–812.

63. Nelson RC, Thompson GH, Chezmar JL, Harned RK Jr, Fernandez MP. CT during arterial portography: diagnostic pitfalls. *Radiographics* 1992;12:705–718.

64. Peterson MS, Baron RL, Dodd GD III, et al. Hepatic parenchymal perfusion defects detected with CTAP: imaging-pathologic correlation. *Radiology* 1992;185:149–155.

65. Matsui O, Takahashi S, Kadoya M, et al. Pseudolesion in segment IV of the liver at CT during arterial portography: correlation with aberrant gastric venous drainage. *Radiology* 1994;193:31–35.

66. Bluemke DA, Soyer P, Fishman EK. Nontumorous low-attenuation defects in the liver on helical CT during arterial portography: frequency, location, and appearance. *AJR* 1995;164:1141–1145.

67. Ohashi I, Ina H, Gomi N, et al. Hepatic pseudolesion in the left lobe around the falciform ligament at helical CT. *Radiology* 1995;196: 245–249.

68. Matsui O, Kadoya M, Takahashi S, et al. Focal sparing of segment IV in fatty livers shown by sonography and CT: correlation with aberrant gastric venous drainage. *AJR* 1995;164:1137–1140.

69. Ishikawa T, Clark RA, Tokuda M, Ashida H. Focal contrast enhancement on hepatic CT in superior vena caval and brachiocephalic vein obstruction. *AJR* 1983;140:337–338.

70. Yamashita K, Jin MJ, Hirose Y, et al. CT finding of transient focal increased attenuation of the liver adjacent to the gallbladder in acute cholecystitis. *AJR* 1995;164:343–346.

CHAPTER 9

Dual-Phase Spiral CT of the Liver and Pancreas

R. Brooke Jeffrey, Jr.

The ability to perform back-to-back spiral CT acquisitions with a relatively short interscan delay represents an important technical advance for abdominal imaging. When combined with a rapid intravenous bolus of contrast, it is possible the first time to view images of the upper abdomen in both arterial and venous phases. Dual-phase (also referred to as biphasic or double-pass) spiral CT has important implications for the diagnosis and characterization of hepatic and pancreatic lesions. This chapter will focus on technical aspects and image interpretation of dual-phase spiral CT of the liver and pancreas.

DUAL-PHASE TECHNIQUE

Dual-phase examinations of the liver and pancreas are performed with back-to-back breath-held spiral acquisitions (Fig. 9-1). An initial digital scout radiograph is first performed during a breath-hold to outline the target volume to be scanned. For hepatic imaging, a 5–8-mm collimation is generally used for both arterial and venous acquisitions. For pancreatic imaging, the initial arterial-phase images of the pancreas are performed at 3-m collimation and then venous-phase images of the liver and upper abdomen are performed with 5–8-mm collimation. Depending on the size of the patient, a pitch of 1–1.5 is utilized. When using a pitch greater than 1, the data set must be reconstructed at the beam collimation interval to avoid misregistration artifacts.

For all dual-phase studies a rapid intravenous bolus is performed with an injection rate of 4–5 mL/s of 60% nonionic contrast for a total of 150 mL of contrast. This injection can be readily accomplished through a 20-gauge catheter placed within an antecubital fossa vein. The patient is first hyperventilated prior to the arterial-phase acquisition. The arterial-phase images are then obtained after a delay of 25–30 s. After completion of a 25–30-s breath-held acquisition during the arterial phase, the patient is repositioned and

hyperventilated and a second 30-s acquisition is performed during the venous phase, which begins approximately 60–70 s after the initiation of the contrast bolus.

DUAL-PHASE SPIRAL CT OF THE LIVER: INDICATIONS

The normal liver obtains approximately 80% of its blood supply from the portal vein and only 20% from the hepatic artery (1,2). A high percentage of hepatic neoplasms, however, derives their vascular supply from the hepatic artery (3). Hypervascular hepatic neoplasms, therefore, are often most conspicuous on images during the predominant arterial phase of hepatic enhancement prior to the circulation of contrast through the portal venous system.

The main indications for dual-phase spiral CT of the liver include evaluation of suspected hepatocellular carcinoma or hypervascular liver metastases (3,4). These metastases are typically from renal cell carcinoma, neuroendocrine tumors, melanoma, sarcoma, thyroid carcinoma, and breast carcinoma (3,4). In addition to the preceding malignant hepatic tumors, arterial-phase images may aid in the detection and characterization of benign hypervascular lesions such as focal nodular hyperplasia, hepatic adenomas, and confluent hepatic fibrosis (3,5). To date, no increased sensitivity has been demonstrated with dual-phase spiral CT in the detection of hypovascular lesions such as carcinomas of the gastrointestinal tract, pancreas, or lung (6). In some cases, however, the identification of a uniformly enhancing peripheral rim on arterial-phase images may aid in the characterization of small lesions (4). This finding strongly suggests metastatic disease rather than a benign lesion such as a hepatic cyst or hemangioma.

When compared with portal venous-phase scans, hepatic arterial-phase images improve the sensitivity of detection of both hepatocellular carcinomas and hypervascular liver

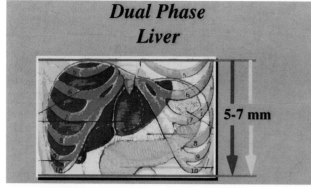

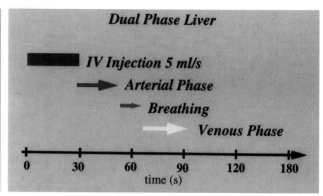

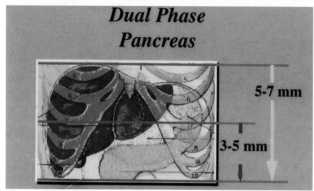

FIG. 9-1. Technique for dual-phase spiral CT of the liver and pancreas. For evaluation of the liver (**A**) slice collimation is 5–7 mm. (**B**) The injection protocol for both dual-phase liver and pancreas studies. Note that the initial arterial-phase spiral begins 25–30 s after the initiation of the intravenous contrast bolus. For pancreatic studies (**C**) the initial arterial-phase spiral acquisition is performed at 3-m collimation. The venous-phase acquisition is then performed through the liver and upper abdomen at 5–7 mm.

metastases. Baron et al. noted that hepatocellular carcinoma was only detected on arterial-phase images in 11% of patients (7). In the same study, additional tumor nodules of hepatocellular carcinoma were detected in 33% of patients with hepatocellular carcinoma diagnosed on portal venous-phase images (7). Similar results have been obtained in the evaluation of hypervascular metastases, particularly neuroendocrine tumors such as pancreatic islet cell tumors (4). Hollett et al. demonstrated that 11% of small (<1.5 cm) hypervascular lesions were more conspicuous on arterial-phase images (4).

Dual-phase imaging can also be used for vascular mapping of liver transplant recipients and for planning hepatic resection in the oncology patient. These applications are discussed in detail in Chapter 17.

ANALYSIS OF HEPATIC LESIONS WITH ARTERIAL-PHASE IMAGING

On arterial-phase images of the normal liver, there is little opacification of the hepatic veins (3). The spleen has a characteristic mottled appearance due to the difference in perfu-

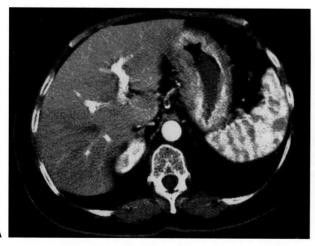

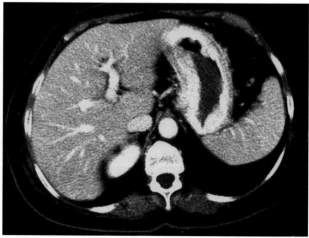

FIG. 9-2. Normal dual-phase spiral CT of the liver and spleen. In (**A**) note the mottled appearance of the spleen during the arterial phase. In (**B**) the spleen has a much more homogeneous appearance during the venous phase.

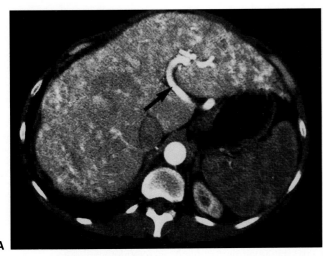
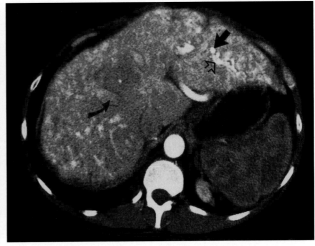

FIG. 9-3. Hepatic arteriovenous malformation from Osler-Weber-Rendu disease. **(A,B)** Arterial-phase scans from a dual-phase spiral CT. Note in **(A)** the hypertrophied replaced left hepatic artery (*arrow*). The liver demonstrates mottled enhancement due to small arteriovenous malformations. In **(B)** note the hypertrophied arterial branches in the left lobe (*arrow*) and the early visualization of the left portal vein (*open arrow*). There is also early opacification of the hepatic veins (*curved arrow*) due to the arteriovenous malformation.

sion between red pulp (vascular lakes) and white pulp (lymphatic follicles and reticuloendothelial cells) (Fig. 9-2). The first-order branches of the proper hepatic artery can typically be identified on rapid bolus arterial-phase images. A small amount of contrast may be noted in the proximal portal veins.

Arteriovenous shunting due to either an arteriovenous malformation or a hepatic tumor such as hepatocellular carcinoma has a characteristic appearance on arterial-phase images (Figs. 9-3, 9-4). Early venous enhancement, particularly of the hepatic veins, is characteristic. Hepatic arterial en-

largement is typical of arteriovenous malformations. Early venous enhancement in association with a hypervascular mass strongly suggests the diagnosis of hepatocellular carcinoma. This finding is rarely seen with metastatic disease (4).

Several distinct arterial-phase patterns of enhancement can be recognized that correspond to specific hepatic tumors. As previously noted, a uniformly enhancing rim on the periphery of a lesion strongly suggests metastatic disease (Figs. 9-5, 9-6). This finding is also present with hepatic abscesses, although the clinical presentation of the two entities will be

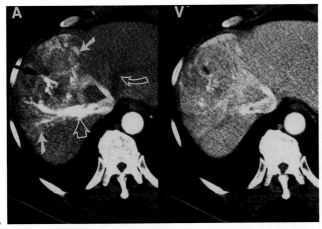
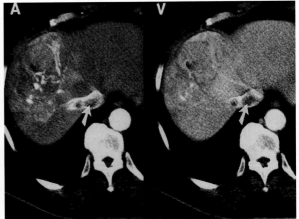

FIG. 9-4. Arteriovenous AV shunting due to hepatocellular carcinoma. **(A)** A side-by-side comparison of the arterial (A) and venous phases (V). Note the hypervascular mass that is well seen during the arterial phase (*white arrows*) and is much less conspicuous on the venous phase. Note the visualization of abnormal vessels within the tumor mass (*black arrow*). AV results in early visualization and enlargement of the right hepatic vein (*open arrow*). Note that there is no visualization of the normal left hepatic vein (*curved arrow*). In **(B)** both the arterial- and venous-phase images demonstrate tumor thrombus within the right hepatic vein and the IVC (*arrows*). Note the enhancement of the tumor thrombus on the arterial-phase image.

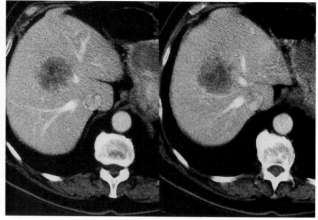

FIG. 9-5. Metastatic colon cancer. In (**A**), which is an arterial-phase acquisition, note the uniform peripheral rim enhancement (*arrow*). Venous-phase images (**B**) demonstrate a nonspecific hypodense abnormality.

quite different. Intense homogeneous arterial-phase enhancement is characteristic of hepatocellular carcinoma, focal nodular hyperplasia, hepatic adenomas, and hypervascular metastases (Figs. 9-7–9-12). These lesions are typically rounded or oval in configuration and exhibit mass effect on adjacent portal or hepatic veins on the venous phase. These hypervascular lesions do not have the straight margins or the wedge-shaped configuration of hepatic flow phenomena.

A nodular pattern of peripheral enhancement that is discontinuous is characteristic of cavernous hemangioma (Fig. 9-13). Depending on the timing of enhancement, small hemangiomas (<1.5 cm) may demonstrate a uniform diffuse enhancement when they are completely "filled in," and this may mimic hypervascular neoplasms. Hanafusa et al. reported that 29% of small hemangiomas demonstrated a uni-

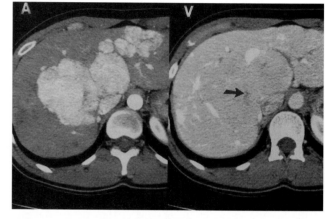

FIG. 9-7. Focal nodular hyperplasia. The arterial-phase images (A) demonstrate multiple rounded hypervascular lesions. Note that on the venous phase (V) these lesions are virtually isoattenuating with the remainder of the liver. Note the small hypodense central scar on the venous phase (*arrow*).

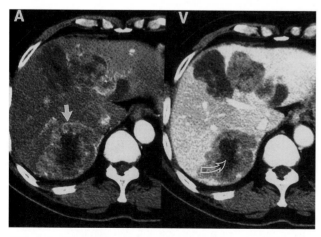

FIG. 9-6. Metastatic adenocarcinoma of the lung. A uniform rim of enhancement is seen on the periphery of the lesion during the arterial phase (*arrow*, A). During the venous phase (V) note the central necrosis within the lesion in the posterior segment of the right lobe (*curved arrow*).

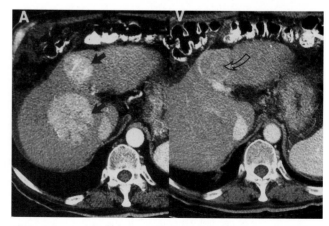

FIG. 9-8. Hepatocellular carcinoma best seen on arterial-phase images. On the arterial phase (A) note two large hypervascular tumor nodules (*arrows*). On the venous phase (V) only the more anterior lesion is identified (*open arrow*).

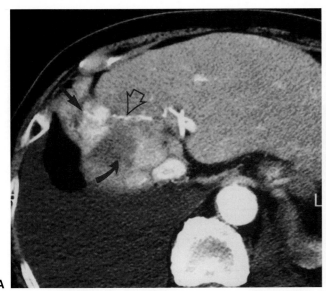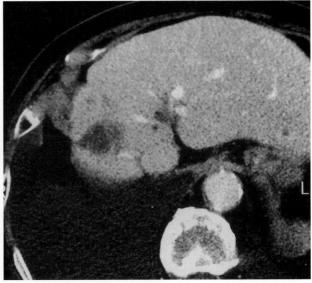

FIG. 9-9. Recurrent hepatocellular carcinoma only seen on arterial-phase images. Patient is status post right lobectomy for hepatocellular carcinoma. Now presents with rising alpha fetoprotein. In (**A**) (arterial-phase image) a hypervascular tumor mass (*arrow*) is noted with feeding hepatic artery (*open arrow*). This proved to be hepatocellular carcinoma on fine-needle aspiration biopsy. There is an adjacent hypodense area related to prior alcohol injection (*curved arrow*). Note that in (**B**) (venous phase) the lesion is not identified. Incidentally noted in a large right pleural effusion.

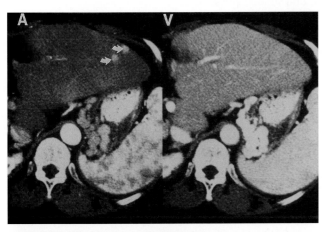

FIG. 9-10. Recurrent hepatocellular carcinoma seen only on arterial-phase images. Arterial-phase image (A) demonstrates two hypervascular nodules in the lateral segment of the left lobe (*arrows*). These lesions are not seen on the venous phase (V).

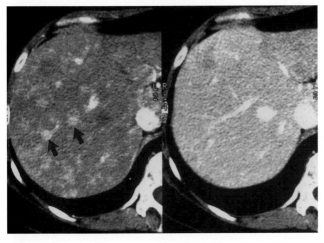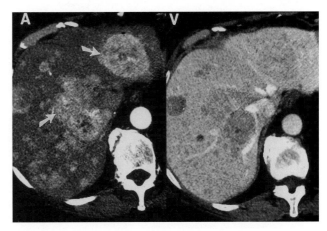

FIG. 9-11. Hypervascular metastases from breast carcinoma best seen on arterial-phase images. In the arterial phase (A) note multiple hypervascular metastases (*arrows*) that are poorly seen on the venous phase (V). Autopsy revealed metastatic breast carcinoma.

FIG. 9-12. Hypervascular metastases from small bowel carcinoid best seen on arterial-phase images. Arterial-phase images (A) demonstrate multiple large hypervascular lesions (*arrows*). Note that these are poorly defined on the venous phase (V).

163

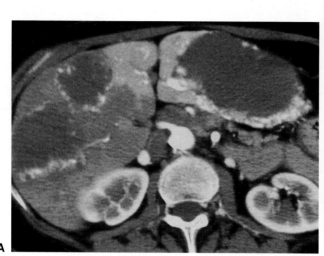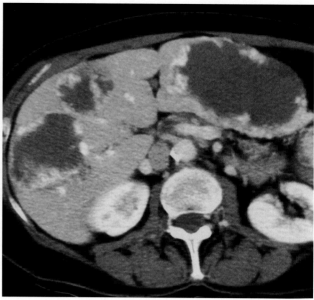

FIG. 9-13. Multiple cavernous hemangiomas. In (**A**) and (**B**) note multiple large hemangiomas involving the right and left lobes. There is a characteristic pattern of nodular peripheral enhancement that is discontinuous. This is identified both on the arterial (**A**) and venous phase (**B**).

formly enhancing pattern on arterial-phase image (8). One feature suggesting that the small "hypervascular" lesion on the arterial-phase images may be a hemangioma is that the contrast enhancement persists in the high-attenuation focus in the venous phase without the "washout" of contrast typical of a malignant hypervascular lesion (3).

Two other arterial-phase patterns are typically associated with hepatocellular carcinoma. One is a "mosaic pattern" (Fig. 9-14) with alternating areas of hyperintense enhancement and areas of necrosis. These lesions may demonstrate a peripherally enhancing pseudocapsule, often best visual-

ized on the venous phase. This second is an infiltrating hypervascular mass (Fig. 9-15) with multiple enlarged tumor vessels. Necrotic lesions, regardless of their histology, will demonstrate poor arterial-phase enhancement. They are best evaluated with venous-phase images.

HEPATIC PSEUDOLESIONS AND PITFALLS

Transient hepatic attenuation differences (THAD) are lobar or segmental hypervascular areas on arterial-phase images (9,10). The most common cause of a THAD is extrinsic

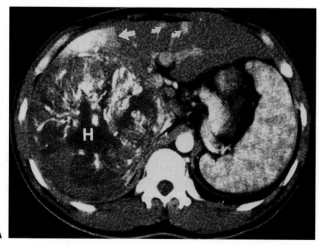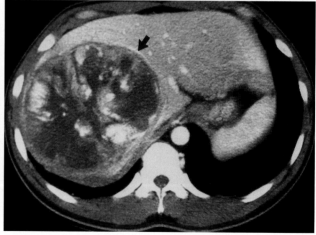

FIG. 9-14. Mosaic pattern of hepatocellular carcinoma. Note in (**A**) the large heterogeneous hepatocellular carcinoma (H) with low-attenuation areas of necrosis and hypervascular foci within the tumor. Adjacent increased attenuation is noted from a perilesional flow phenomena (*straight arrow*). Two satellite lesions are noted in the left lobe (*curved arrows*). In the venous phase (**B**) an enhancing peripheral pseudocapsule is evident (*arrow*).

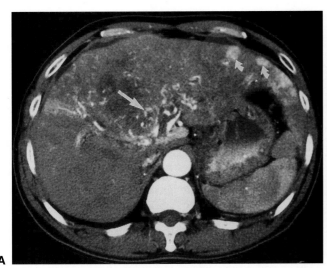
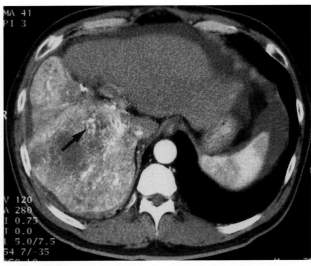

FIG. 9-15. Diffusely infiltrating hepatocellular carcinomas. Arterial-phase images in two patients (**A,B**) demonstrate enlarged tortuous tumor vessels (*arrows*) within a hypervascular mass consistent with hepatocellular carcinoma. Note in (**A**) the adjacent small satellite lesions (*curved arrow*).

compression or occlusion of a portal vein segment by an adjacent tumor (Fig. 9-16). This results in compensatory increased flow in the hepatic artery to the involved lobar or segment. Occasionally, THADs are identified in the absence of a tumor and may be due to arterioportal shunting or an anomalous portal venous circulation (9,10) (Fig. 9-17). THADs have a characteristic peripheral location and are typically wedge-shaped with straight margins. They may not

be identifiable on venous-phase images. One other potential pitfall to keep in mind is that purely vascular lesions such as hepatic artery aneurysms or pseudoaneurysms may have an appearance similar to a hypervascular ''mass.''

A relative contraindication to dual-phase imaging of the liver is poor cardiac output. It is very difficult in these patients to accurately determine the timing delay for the arterial phase of the scan acquisition. Radiation exposure and tube

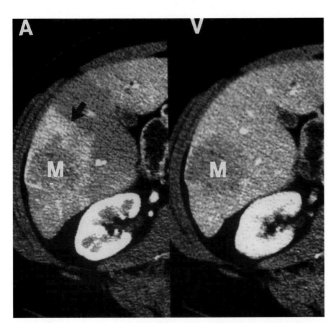

FIG. 9-16. Appearance of transient hepatic attenuation differences (THAD) due to colonic carcinoma. Note on the arterial phase (A) there is a hypervascular region with straight margins (*arrow*) surrounding a hypodense metastasis. This is no longer evident on the venous phase (V). The increased flow phenomenon in (A) represents a THAD.

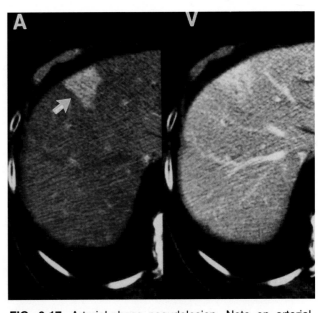

FIG. 9-17. Arterial-phase pseudolesion. Note on arterial-phase (A) there is a peripheral wedge-shaped hypervascular area. This lesion is relatively inconspicuous on the venous-phase (V). Clinical follow-up over 2 years and negative MRI suggests that this is a pseudolesion.

cooling considerations limit the number of scanning sequences that can be obtained by CT. In a patient with known cardiac disease, dynamic magnetic resonance imaging (MRI) with gadolinium is often the hepatic imaging technique of choice because it is not limited by the number of scanning acquisitions.

DUAL-PHASE SPIRAL CT OF THE PANCREAS: INDICATIONS

Dual-phase spiral CT of the pancreas may be a valuable technique for evaluating patients with a suspected pancreatic adenocarcinoma or neuroendocrine tumors. During the arterial phase of the injection, the normal pancreatic parenchyma enhances intensely. This improves the conspicuity of hypovascular lesions such as adenocarcinoma. The arterial phase is also excellent for identifying vascular encasement and tumor infiltration at the root of the mesentery. The portal venous phase, however, is essential for a complete assessment of resectability for pancreatic carcinoma as hepatic metastases are often best demonstrated during this portion of the injection. In addition, splenic vein occlusion and the development of perisplenic varices may only be imaged during the venous phase. Hypervascular pancreatic lesions, such as neuroendocrine tumors, are often best visualized with arterial-phase images. In addition, liver metastases from neuroendocrine tumors are most conspicuous during the arterial phase.

ANALYSIS OF PANCREATIC NEOPLASMS WITH ARTERIAL-PHASE IMAGING

Unlike the liver, which is largely perfused by venous blood, the normal pancreas is exclusively supplied by arterial inflow. Therefore the normal pancreas enhances intensely during the arterial phase, when a rapid contrast injection (5 mL/s) is utilized. Hollett et al. noted that the mean pancreatic enhancement during the arterial phase was 82 HU and that it decreased to 62 HU during the portal venous phase (11). This represents a highly significant difference, as there is nearly a 25% diminution in the pancreatic parenchymal enhancement during the portal venous phase. The avid enhancement of the normal pancreas during the arterial phase increases the conspicuity of ductal adenocarcinoma, which is hypovascular (Fig. 9-18). Lu et al. evaluated dual-phase spiral CT for pancreatic tumors and found that the attenuation differences between adenocarcinoma and normal pancreas was greatest during the early arterial-phase images (12). Small ductal adenocarcinomas may be identified with greater confidence on arterial-phase images. Arterial-phase images also improve detection of anatomic variations in the head of the pancreas that may simulate masses (13) (Fig. 9-19). In addition, subtle alterations in the dimension of the main pancreatic duct are better appreciated with thin collimation (3 mm) and rapid injection arterial-phase images.

One important clue to an underlying pancreatic parenchymal mass is the interrupted duct sign (Fig. 9-20). This sign refers to segmental dilatation of the pancreatic duct by an underlying mass lesion obstructing the duct (11). In some lesions of the body and tail of the pancreas, the interrupted duct sign may be the most conspicuous feature of an underlying pancreatic carcinoma. Dilatation and discontinuity of the pancreatic duct should always raise the possibility of pancreatic mass rather than chronic pancreatitis. Chronic pancreatitis should only be diagnosed with confidence if there is dilatation of the pancreatic duct throughout its entire length of the pancreas in association with intraductal calculi.

In addition to improving conspicuity of the primary pan-

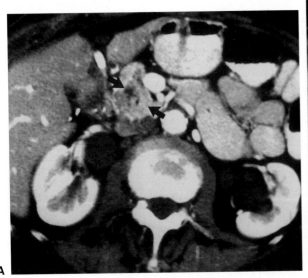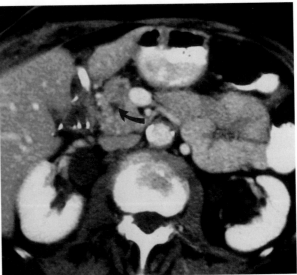

A   B

FIG. 9-18. Improved visualization of a pancreatic carcinoma on arterial-phase images. The arterial-phase image (**A**) demonstrates a hypodense mass in the pancreas (*arrows*) on the venous phase (**B**). Only the central area of necrosis is identified (*curved arrow*).

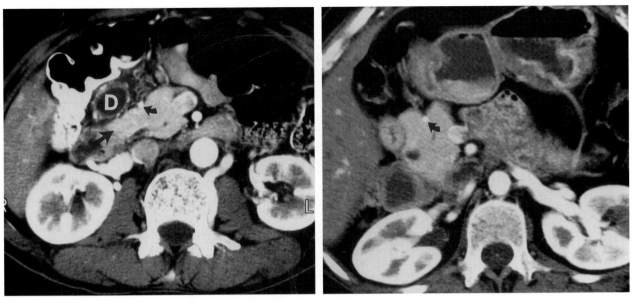

A   B

FIG. 9-19. Anatomic variations in the head of the pancreas are best seen on arterial-phase images. In (**A**) note a posterior lobule of the normal pancreatic head (*arrow*) adjacent to the fluid-filled duodenum (D). The anterior superior pancreaticoduodenal artery is clearly identified (*curved arrow*). In another patient (**B**) note the pancreatic notch for the anterior superior pancreaticoduodenal artery (*curved arrow*).

creatic lesion, arterial-phase images are of considerable value in assessing the extent of local invasion and potential for resection of pancreatic carcinoma. Arterial encasement of the splanchnic vasculature is an unequivocal sign of unresectability (14–16) (Fig. 9-21). This is often demonstrated on CT as subtle soft-tissue thickening along the splenic, hepatic, celiac, or superior mesenteric arteries. Caution must be exercised in patients scanned soon after ERCP as peripancreatic inflammatory changes may be misdiagnosed as tumor encasement (Fig. 9-22) (13). Intense enhancement of the celiac axis and splanchnic vasculature during the arterial

phase greatly facilitates diagnosis of tumor encasement of these vessels (Fig. 9-23). Tumor infiltration around very tiny mesenteric vessels, such as branches of the jejunal arteries, may also be readily diagnosed with this technique.

Although portal venous-phase images are essential for de-

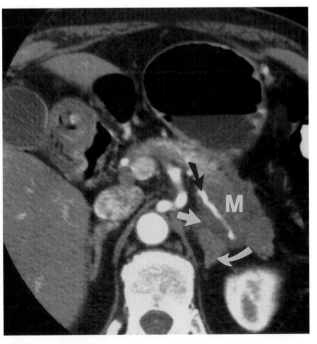

FIG. 9-21. Arterial encasement by pancreatic carcinoma. There is a large hypodense mass (M) in the tail of the pancreas that encases the splenic artery (*black arrow*). The tumor extends posterior to the splenic artery (*white arrow*) and infiltrates the fat around the left adrenal (*curved arrow*).

FIG. 9-20. Interrupted duct sign from pancreatic carcinoma. Note hypodense pancreatic mass (M) obstructing pancreatic duct (*curved arrow*). There is extensive encasement of the SMA (*black arrow*).

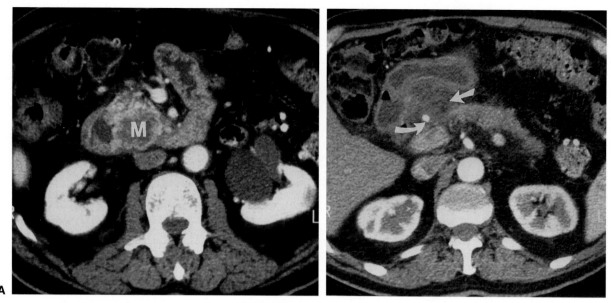

FIG. 9-22. Perivascular soft-tissue infiltration due to post-ERCP pancreatitis. In (**A**) note hypodense mass in the uncinate process of the pancreas (M) that invades the duodenum. In (**B**) there is hazy soft-tissue infiltration (*arrow*) around the gastroduodenal artery (*curved arrow*) that at surgery was not involved with tumor. The patient had had a difficult ERCP 24 hours previously.

tection of metastatic lesions from pancreatic carcinoma, arterial-phase images may be of value in improving the specificity of hepatic metastases by demonstrating peripheral rim enhancement around the lesion. Often small (<1.5 cm) hypodense lesions seen on the portal venous phase are nonspecific and, particularly when necrotic, may mimic benign hepatic cysts. The demonstration of peripheral enhancement around the hypodense lesion strongly suggests metastases in the absence of clinical signs indicating an abscess (4). Hepatic cysts do not demonstrate this peripheral rim enhancement.

Arterial-phase images of the pancreas may also greatly aid in the diagnosis of hypervascular pancreatic neoplasms such as neuroendocrine tumors and hypervascular pancreatic metastases (chiefly renal cell carcinoma and sarcomas) (17) (Figs. 9-24–9-26). Although most functioning islet cell tumors are clinically discovered on the basis of laboratory abnormalities and specific symptoms, many nonfunctioning islet cell tumors present with only vague symptomatology due to mass effect. The prognosis of most neuroendocrine tumors of the pancreas is significantly better than ductal adenocarcinoma; therefore an attempt should be made to

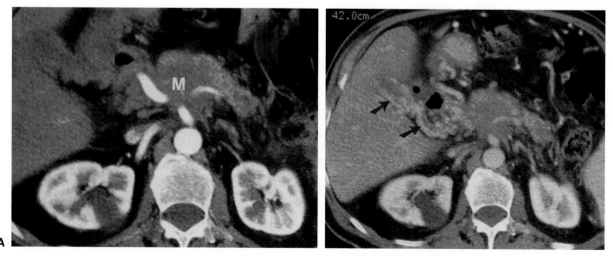

FIG. 9-23. Locally advanced pancreatic carcinoma. Arterial-phase images (**A**) demonstrate a pancreatic mass (M) encasing the celiac axis. On the venous phase (**B**) note the periportal and gallbladder wall varices from portal vein occlusion (*arrows*).

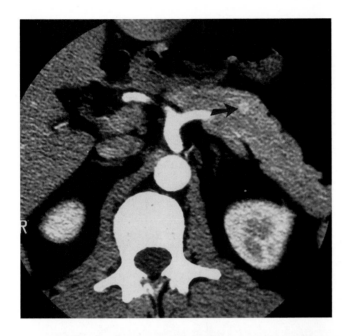

FIG. 9-24. Small insulinoma detected only on the arterial-phase images. Note small hypervascular mass seen in the body of the pancreas (*arrow*). This was not visible on venous-phase images.

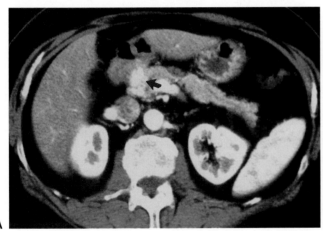

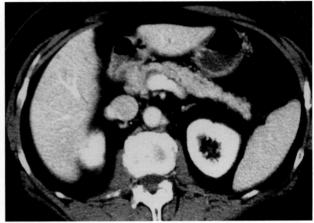

A   B

FIG. 9-25. Islet cell tumor visible only on the arterial-phase images. In (**A**) note the hypervascular mass in the region of the neck of the pancreas (*arrow*). Venous-phase images failed to demonstrate the lesion (**B**).

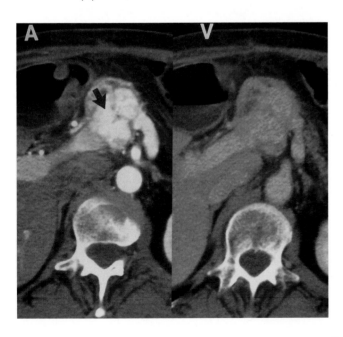

FIG. 9-26. Pancreatic metastasis from renal cell carcinoma. Note the hypervascular mass in the neck of the pancreas seen on the arterial phase (A, *arrow*). The lesion appears as a nonspecific soft-tissue mass on the venous phase.

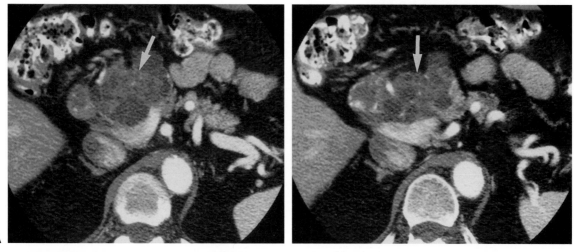

A
B

FIG. 9-27. Microcystic adenoma. **(A,B)** Arterial-phase images clearly demonstrate the thin enhancing septae within the benign cystic neoplasm (*arrows*).

resect the lesion whenever possible. The current evaluation for both functioning and nonfunctioning islet cell tumors is to perform dual-phase spiral CT of the pancreas followed by careful intraoperative sonography. Invasive studies such as selective angiography and venous sampling are no longer essential for accurate diagnosis. In patients who are unable to receive intravenous contrast, MRI (particularly using fat-suppressed T1-weighted images), and gadolinium-enhanced gradient recalled images are also of clear value in identifying these small tumors. Van Hoe et al. reported an 82% sensitivity for the CT detection of islet cell tumors of the pancreas in 10 patients with tumors (17). On two patients lesions were easier to detect on arterial-phase images (17).

In selected patients with cystic pancreatic neoplasms, arterial-phase images may add additional diagnostic value. The thin enhancing septae of a microcystic adenoma are often best visualized using narrow collimation (3 mm) and rapid bolus arterial-phase images (Fig. 9-27). The solid mural tissue and septal nodules present within mucinous cystic neoplasms may also be clearly shown to enhance on arterial-phase scans (Fig. 9-28).

REFERENCES

1. Greenway CV, Stark RD. Hepatic vascular bed. *Physiol Rev* 1971;51: 23–45.
2. Chaudhuri TK, Fink S. Physiological considerations in imaging liver metastases from colorectal carcinoma. *Am J Physiol Imaging* 1991;6: 150–60.
3. Oliver JH III, Baron RL. Helical biphasic contrast-enhanced CT of the liver: technique, indications, interpretation, and pitfalls. *Radiology* 1996;20:1–14.
4. Hollett MD, Jeffrey RB Jr, Nino MM, Jorgensen MJ, Harris DP. Dual-phase helical CT of the liver: value of arterial phase scans in the detection of small (≤1.5 cm) malignant hepatic neoplasms. *AJR* 1995;164: 879–884.
5. Ohtomo K, Baron RL, Dodd GD III, et al. Confluent hepatic fibrosis in advanced cirrhosis: appearance at CT. *Radiology* 1993;188:31–35.
6. Ch'en IY, Katz DS, Jeffrey RB Jr, et al. Do arterial phase helical CT images improve detection or characterization of colorectal liver metastases? *J Comput Assist Tomogr* 1997;21:391–397.
7. Baron RL, Oliver JH III, Dodd GD III, Nalesnik M, Holbert BL, Carr B. Hepatocellular carcinoma: evaluation with biphasic, contrast-enhanced, helical CT. *Radiology* 1996;199:505–511.
8. Hanafusa K, Ohashi I, Himeno Y, Suzuki S, Shibuya H. Hepatic hemangioma: findings with two-phase CT. *Radiology* 1995;196:465–469.
9. Itai Y, Moss AA, Goldberg HI. Transient hepatic attenuation difference of lobar or segmental distribution detected by dynamic computed tomography. *Radiology* 1982;144:835–839.
10. Itai Y, Hachiya J, Makita K, Ohtomo K, Kokubo T, Yamauchi T. Transient hepatic attenuation differences on dynamic computed tomography. *J Comput Assist Tomogr* 1987;11:461–465.
11. Hollett MD, Jorgensen MJ, Jeffrey RB Jr. Quantitative evaluation of pancreatic enhancement during dual-phase helical CT. *Radiology* 1995; 195:359–361.
12. Lu DS, Vedantham S, Krasny RM, Kadell B, Berger WL, Reber HA. Two-phase helical CT for pancreatic tumors: pancreatic versus hepatic

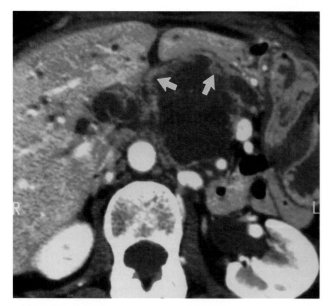

FIG. 9-28. Malignant mucinous cystic neoplasm. Note the enhancing mural tissue on the arterial-phase images. A malignant mucinous adenocarcinoma was found at surgery.

phase enhancement of tumor, pancreas, and vascular structures. *Radiology* 1996;199:697–701.

13. Ross BA, Jeffrey RB Jr, Mindelzun RE. Normal variations in the lateral contour of the head and neck of the pancreas mimicking neoplasm: evaluation with dual-phase helical CT. *AJR* 1996;166:799–801.

14. Thoeni RF, Blankenberg F. Pancreatic imaging: computed tomography and magnetic resonance imaging. *Radiol Clin North Am* 1993;31: 1085–1113.

15. Freeny PC, Traverso LW, Ryan JA. Diagnosis and staging of pancreatic adenocarcinoma with dynamic computed tomography. *Am J Surg* 1993; 165:600–606.

16. Hosoki T. Dynamic CT of pancreatic tumors. *AJR* 1983;140:959–965.

17. Van Hoe L, Gryspeerdt S, Marchal G, Baert AL, Mertens L. Helical CT for the preoperative localization of islet cell tumors of the pancreas: value of arterial and parenchymal phase images. *AJR* 1995;165: 1437–1439.

CHAPTER 10

Spiral CT Evaluation of the Pancreas

Elliot K. Fishman

Spiral CT technology now represents the state of the art in evaluation of known or suspected pancreatic pathology (1–5). Spiral CT capitalizes on those basic principles that are essential for optimal pancreatic imaging, including 3–5-mm thin-section scans at narrow interscan increments and scanning during the phase of maximum vascular opacification by iodinated intravenous contrast material. Furthermore, for both neoplastic and inflammatory diseases of the pancreas, spiral CT offers many unique advantages over conventional dynamic CT scanning.

In contrast to conventional dynamic CT scanning, in which a slice is obtained, followed by table incrementation (with a 4–8-s interscan delay) and then another slice is obtained, spiral CT is a continuous acquisition of data that typically lasts between 24 and 40 s as the patient travels through the gantry. This capability of obtaining a series of contiguous scans in a matter of a few seconds provides the following distinct advantages: (a) scanning during the phase of maximum vascular enhancement (either with single- or dual-phase arterial- and/or portal-phase imaging), with improved visualization of the superior mesenteric and gastro-duodenal arteries, and the superior mesenteric, splenic, and portal veins; (b) multiple thin sections through the area of interest during this phase of peak enhancement; (c) lack of misregistration of data because a volume data set is rapidly acquired during a single breath-hold (which typically eliminates patient motion); and (d) ability to view these data as axial slices, as a multiplanar (coronal and sagittal) display or as three-dimensional (3D) images (1–10).

TECHNIQUE

Patients should receive adequate oral contrast (e.g., 750 mL of 3% Hypaque, Nycomed, Inc., Princeton, NJ) over a 30-min period prior to their examination. In cases where 3D imaging with vascular mapping is contemplated, a positive oral contrast agent is not given and gastric and bowel distention is achieved by giving the patients an equal amount of water. After a topogram, a single unenhanced scan is obtained to center the image field. A total of 100–120 mL of intravenous (IV) contrast material (e.g., Omnipaque 300 or 350) is administered at a rate of 2–3 mL/s. For purposes of pancreatic evaluation, contrast is generally administered via a peripheral venous access route using a power injector. Data acquisition typically begins 30 s after the initiation of injection of contrast material for arterial-phase imaging and at 50 s for portal-phase imaging.

Scanning parameters will vary on the scanner used, but on a Siemens Plus-4 system (Siemens Medical Systems, Iselin, NJ) we use 0.75-s scan times, 120 kVp, and 280 mA with a slice thickness of 3 or 5 mm. We routinely hyperventilate the patient just prior to scanning and then have them hold their breath throughout the entire study. The total scanning time is in the 24–40-s range, depending on the specific case and questions to be answered. The spiral protocol uses a table incrementation of 3–8 mm, depending on whether 3D imaging is done.

Although early spiral scanners had a problem with adequate coverage due to limitations in pitch selection (i.e., pitch of only 1 available) and length of the spiral acquisition (only 24 s), current scanners allow the pitch to be varied, usually up to a pitch of 2. The increased pitch coupled with subsecond scanning (0.75 s or a gantry rotation of 80 cycles per minute) and its one-third increase in coverage now allows routine imaging of the entire liver and pancreas without compromising evaluation of either organ.

After acquisition, scans are reconstructed in about 4 s per image and may be sent via Ethernet to a free-standing workstation for further analysis. Three-dimensional display and interactive review of the data are then possible (6,7).

APPLICATIONS: PANCREATIC NEOPLASMS

CT has clearly become the mainstay of evaluation of pancreatic neoplasms and remains the single modality most capable of directly addressing the significant clinical issues.

CT is extremely accurate in both confirming or excluding the presence of a suspected pancreatic mass and in assessing tumor resectability. In both instances, spiral CT has improved the confidence with which we can make these determinations. Furthermore, in the patient referred for evaluation of jaundice, spiral CT findings will, in most cases, accurately differentiate between the various etiologies of biliary tract obstruction. With spiral CT we can not only identify the level of obstruction, but also confidently diagnose whether distal obstruction is due to a common duct calculus or neoplasm, or to a mass in the pancreatic head.

Adenocarcinoma

Pancreatic adenocarcinoma is most frequently manifest on CT as a mass distorting the gland, with approximately 60% of such masses found in the head region (10). With dynamic contrast-enhanced technique, these tumors have generally been described as focal regions of hypoattenuation as compared with the normal pancreas. This finding likely reflects the desmoplastic quality of these neoplasms, which also explains their propensity for vascular encasement (Figs. 10-1, 10-2). Additional CT findings that support a diagnosis of adenocarcinoma include (a) atrophy of the distal gland, with (b) dilatation of the pancreatic duct behind the obstructing lesion (which is particularly suggestive of carcinoma in the absence of pancreatic calculi), and (c) biliary ductal dilatation, particularly with abrupt termination of the duct. Pancreatic ductal dilatation tends to be smooth or beaded in cases of carcinoma (11–15) (Figs. 10-3, 10-4).

CT evidence of tumor extension may be manifest by lymphadenopathy, invasion of adjacent arterial and venous structures, invasion of adjacent organs, or metastases to the liver and peritoneum. Detecting metastatic spread is particularly useful when findings of pancreatic cancer and pancre-

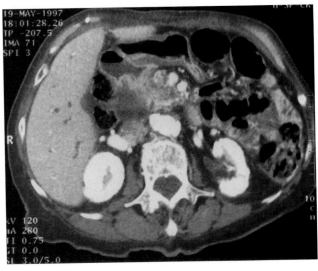

FIG. 10-2. Adenocarcinoma of the pancreas with early encasement of the SMV. Spiral CT scan demonstrates encasement of the SMV by a tumor involving the head of the pancreas.

atitis overlap, a problem encountered not frequently. An accurate assessment of vascular invasion is of critical importance, as it represents a contraindication to attempted surgical resection (16–21). A clear advantage of spiral CT is that it may demonstrate subtle adventitial involvement by tumor that may be missed at angiography. With dynamic scanning, the involved vessels have been described as either thickened or obscured by a focus of soft tissue with obliteration of perivascular fat. Spiral CT angiography with 3D reconstruction should increase the accuracy of defining vascular encasement when the difficulty is distinguishing between early tumor encasement and simply tumor adjacent to vessel without invasion (Figs. 10-5, 10-6).

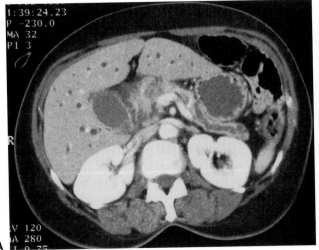
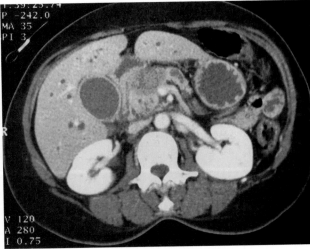

FIG. 10-1. (A,B) Carcinoma of the pancreas. Spiral CT demonstrates a mass in the pancreatic head. The mass is of lower CT attenuation than the rest of the pancreatic parenchyma consistent with carcinoma. Dilatation of the distal pancreatic duct is seen.

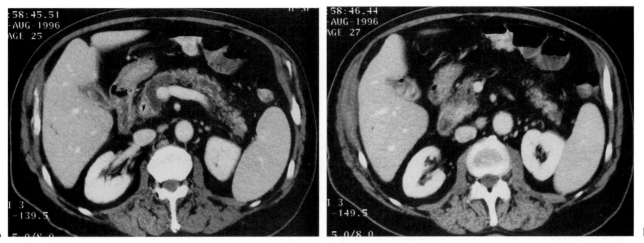

FIG. 10-3. (A,B) Adenocarcinoma of the pancreas with dilated pancreatic duct but no local invasion. Sequence of images demonstrates a dilated pancreatic duct with a mass seen in the head of the pancreas. The vascular structures appear well defined and this was a local tumor and was resectable at time of surgery.

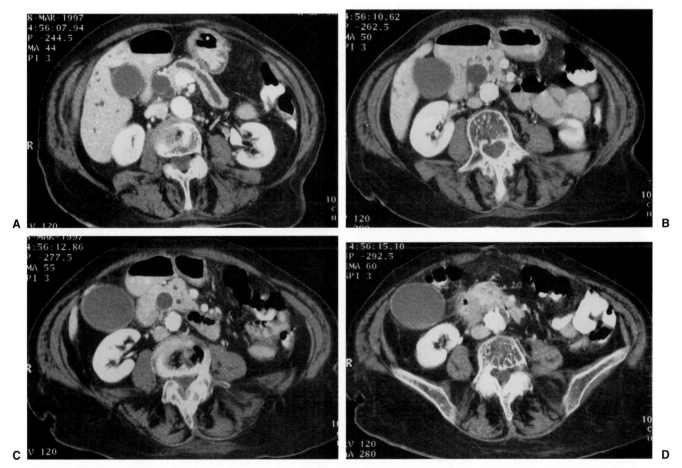

FIG. 10-4. (A–D) Adenocarcinoma of the pancreas with a dilated common bile duct and pancreatic duct. Sequential images demonstrate a dilated common duct as well as pancreatic duct. The site of obstruction and transition zone is well defined. Spiral CT excels by allowing precise definition of the site of obstruction, which in this case was in the pancreas with local spread of tumor. Note the differential enhancement of the mass relative to adjacent normal pancreas.

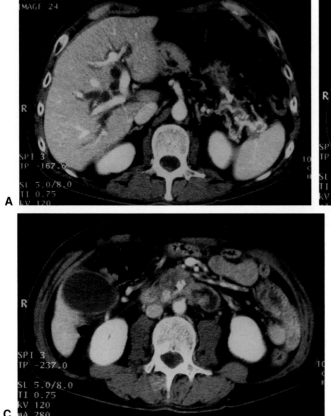

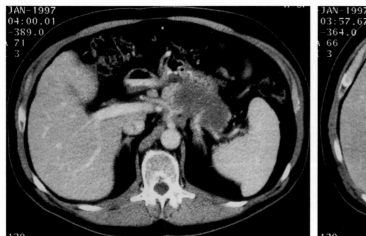

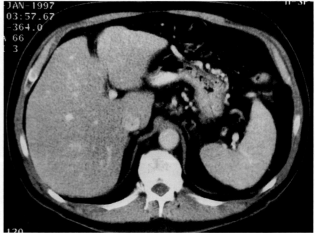

FIG. 10-5. (A–C) Pancreatic carcinoma in a patient with chronic pancreatitis. Spiral CT demonstrates evidence of chronic pancreatitis with dense calcification in the pancreatic head and body. A low-density zone is seen adjacent to the calcification in the pancreatic head consistent with carcinoma. Up to 5% of patients with carcinoma will also have CT evidence of prior pancreatitis.

Therefore, as addressed by Megibow (13), the key components of an adequate evaluation of the pancreas for suspected adenocarcinoma include proper administration of intravenous contrast, rapid acquisition of data, and appropriate thin sections through the pancreas. Critical attention to technique with spiral CT increases the conspicuity between a pancreatic neoplasm and adjacent normal parenchyma.

Compared with conventional scanning, spiral CT offers many unique advantages in the evaluation of pancreatic ductal adenocarcinoma. Although the normal pancreas shows only minimal enhancement with routine dynamic scanning, the optimal contrast enhancement achieved with spiral CT helps to accentuate the difference between normal pancreatic parenchyma and tumor (see Figs. 10-1–10-3) (1). Hollett et

FIG. 10-6. (A,B) Carcinoma of the pancreas with vessel encasement and nodes. Spiral CT demonstrates encasement of the patient's celiac axis. Collateral vessels are seen around the stomach. Tumor infiltrates tissue planes and is unresectable based on CT criteria.

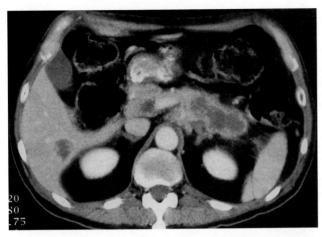

FIG. 10-7. Carcinoma infiltrating the body and tail of the pancreas. Spiral CT demonstrates extensive tumor, which is necrotic. Local infiltration of the vascular structures as well as distant liver metastasis is seen.

al. (3) demonstrated that with a spiral CT technique of 5 mL/s injection of 150 mL of iohexol (Omnipaque-300, Nycomed, Princeton, NJ) and acquisition of data beginning at 20 s (arterial phase) that the normal pancreas would enhance 82 ± 3 Hounsfield units (HU). The enhancement at the portal venous phase (49–71 s) was 62 ± 2 HU. Bonaldi et al. (4) also addressed the issue of pancreatic enhancement to determine the effect of high (6 mL/s) and low rates (2 mL/s) of contrast injection as well as to compare image quality between spiral and dynamic CT of the pancreas. The mean pancreatic enhancement was higher in the spiral CT group (61 ± 17 HU versus 54 ± 17 HU), although peak enhancement was similar (74 ± 19 HU versus 74 ± 17 HU). The time to peak enhancement in the spiral group was earlier,

with the higher injection rate (39 versus 71 s), although the optimal scanning interval was decreased (13 versus 21 s).

Clearly, an essential role of CT in the overall picture of this disease is that of detection of very small neoplasms at the earliest possible stage, since survival may be related to tumor size and extent (19). Spiral technique also provides for excellent parenchymal enhancement of the liver, which in turn improves detection of hepatic metastases (Figs. 10-7, 10-8) (22,23). The increased data sampling protocols through the liver have increased lesion detection, especially for lesions in the 1-cm range. Although dual-phase imaging of the liver is typically performed in the evaluation of the pancreas cancer, there are no published data to suggest that the arterial phase shows an increased incidence of liver lesion detection in cases of adenocarcinoma of the pancreas.

Furthermore, spiral CT enables superior opacification of the peripancreatic vasculature. Contrast opacification of these peripancreatic vessels provides critical information regarding vascular encasement or invasion, which in turn will determine tumor resectability (Figs. 10-9–10-12). Indeed, major peripancreatic arteries and veins are involved in up to 84% of cases of pancreatic carcinoma (12). When either displacement and compression or frank invasion of the portal vein results in portal vein occlusion, collateral vessels are exquisitely demonstrated with spiral CT scanning. Although the demonstration of venous collaterals on routine dynamic scanning often implies the existence of venous encasement, the actual site of vascular invasion may now be directly visualized with spiral technique, increasing the confidence with which we offer both a diagnosis of cancer and the stage of disease. Similarly, pancreatic tail masses may show invasion of the splenic vein with consequent venous collateral formation or even splenic infarction.

Several recent articles have addressed the role of CT in

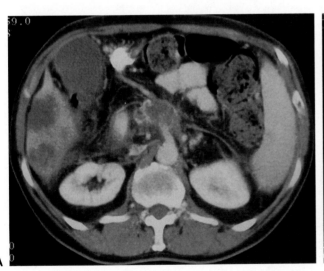

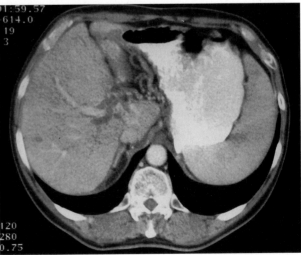

A   B

FIG. 10-8. **(A,B)** Carcinoma of the pancreas with spread around the celiac axis and portal vein thrombosis. Spiral CT clearly demonstrates the encasement of the celiac axis just past its origin. The tumor encases the vessel with local spread of tumor. Tumor involves the portal vein with collateral vessels in the porta hepatis seen. The patient has multiple liver metastasis.

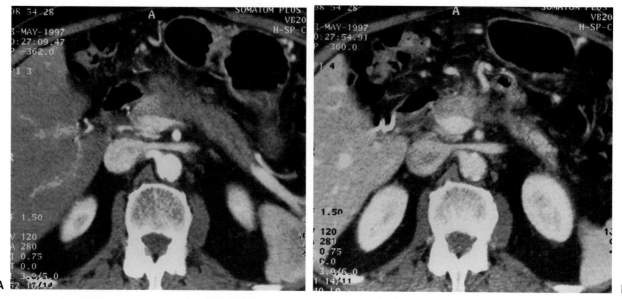

FIG. 10-9. (A,B) Carcinoma of the body of the pancreas with subtle encasement of the portal vein. Spiral CT in late arterial phase demonstrates a large low-density mass in the pancreas with extension around the portal vein. Note the shape of the portal vein due to tumor encasement. This was unresectable pancreatic cancer.

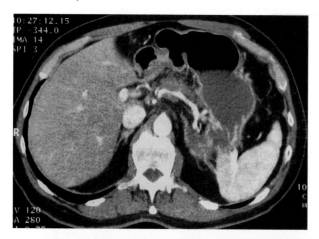

FIG. 10-10. Invasive adenocarcinoma of the body of the pancreas. Invasive infiltrating carcinoma of the body of the pancreas encases and invades the splenic artery at its origin off the celiac axis.

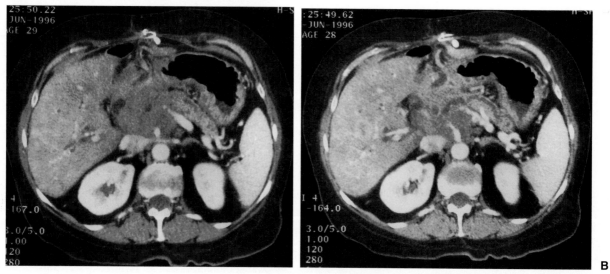

FIG. 10-11. (A,B) Adenocarcinoma of the pancreas with diffuse tumor spread. Spiral CT with arterial-phase injection demonstrates a large mass in the pancreatic head. The pancreatic mass is of lower CT attenuation than normal pancreas. The pancreatic duct is dilated. Encasement of the SMA is seen, and on select views both the portal vein and splenic vein were in part thrombosed.

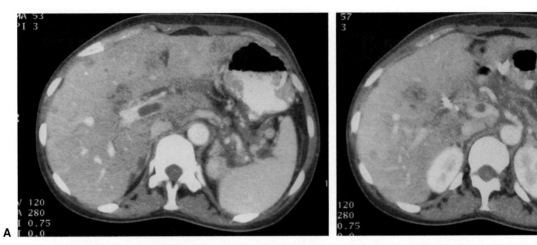

FIG. 10-12. (A,B) Carcinoma of the pancreas with portal vein thrombosis. Spiral CT demonstrates a tumor in the head of the pancreas that extends into and involves the portal vein with portal vein thrombosis seen. A dilated pancreatic duct is also seen. Multiple liver metastases also noted.

the evaluation of the peripancreatic vessels and the impact on staging pancreatic cancer. Sim et al. (9) demonstrated that thin-section (3-mm) spiral CT could reliably demonstrate the small pancreatic arteries such as the gastroduodenal, anterior and posterior superior pancreaticoduodenal, and right gastroepiploic arteries. A similar article by Graf et al.[24] demonstrated that with axial and volume-rendered CT venograms, spiral CT could clearly define the SMV, including variations in branching of this vessel.

Hommeyer et al. (18) specifically addressed the problem further by determining if dilatation of the pancreaticoduodenal veins would improve staging in pancreatic adenocarcinoma. By defining vessel size as normal gastrocolic venous trunk as ≤7 mm, anterior superior pancreaticoduodenal vein ≤4 mm, and posterior superior pancreaticoduodenal vein ≤4 mm, the authors found that dilatation of these veins was a highly accurate sign of unresectability even in patients without signs of unresectability. Loyer et al.[25] classified vascular involvement in pancreatic carcinoma into a six-stage classification ranging from type A (fat plane separates the tumor and/or normal pancreas from adjacent vessels) to type F (tumor occludes the vessel) and found that thin-section CT was a good predictor of resectability. Kaneko et al. (16) compared spiral CT and angiography and found that although angiography was better at defining small-vessel en-

casement (posterior pancreaticoduodenal arcades and other small arteries), there was little difference in determining resectability between the two studies. Finally, Raptopoulos et al. (17) used CT angiography in addition to transaxial spiral CT and found that the use of this 3D technique improved the radiologist's ability to determine resectability. The negative predictive value of a resectable tumor was 96% for CT angiography and spiral axial CT compared with 70% for axial spiral CT alone.

The work of Raptopoulos et al. (17) defining the added value of 3D CT angiography and that of Novick et al. (6) clearly show that spiral CT will benefit from the use of multiplanar reconstruction and 3D reconstructions for determining resectability of pancreatic tumors (Figs. 10-13–10-16). Multidimensional display of spiral CT scans of a lesion helps to define its relationship to adjacent organs and vessels. This is particularly useful for the accurate staging of pancreatic neoplasms and the involvement of the superior mesenteric artery (SMA) and the superior mesenteric vein (SMV). Although axial scans can nicely demonstrate encasement of the SMV, sagittal views are preferable for displaying the SMA, because it arises from the aorta at a 90-degree angle (see Fig. 10-13). Coronal scans are then helpful in assessing tumor involvement of the adjacent stomach or duodenum (Fig. 10-17).

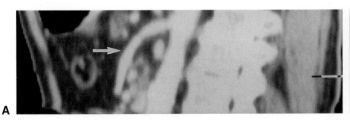
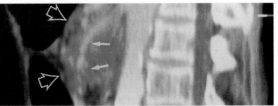

FIG. 10-13. Sagittal views of SMA. **(A)** Sagittal reconstruction demonstrates normal SMA (*arrow*) with renal vein coursing beneath the SMA. **(B)** Spiral CT demonstrates tumor encasement of the SMA (*arrow*) by a pancreatic carcinoma (*open arrows*).

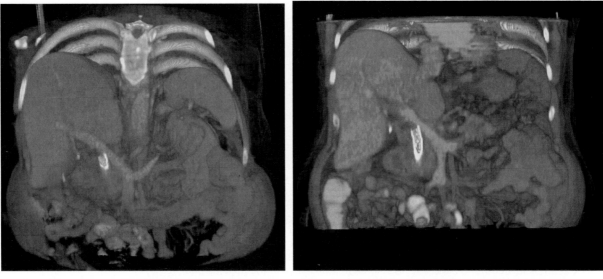

FIG. 10-14. (A,B) Adenocarcinoma of the head of the pancreas with no evidence of local spread. On routine transaxial CT images there was a suggestion of encasement of the SMV and portal vein at the confluence. Three-dimensional reconstructions demonstrate that the portal vein and SMV appear normal. Note the stent in place. At surgery there was no evidence of vascular encasement.

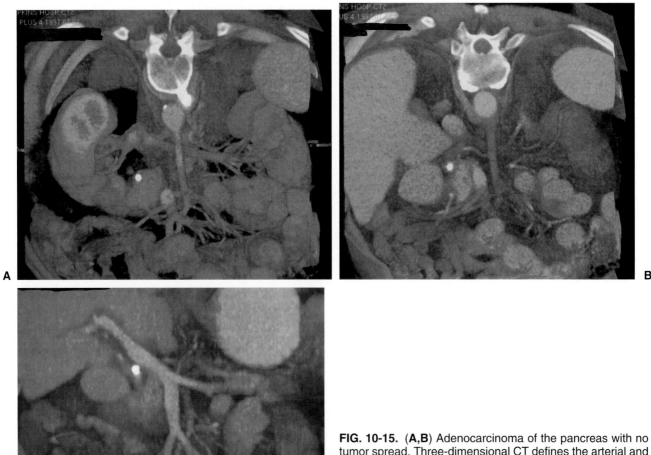

FIG. 10-15. (A,B) Adenocarcinoma of the pancreas with no tumor spread. Three-dimensional CT defines the arterial and venous vascular map, including an accessory right hepatic artery arising from the SMA. The study demonstrates no evidence of disease spread and the patient was resectable.

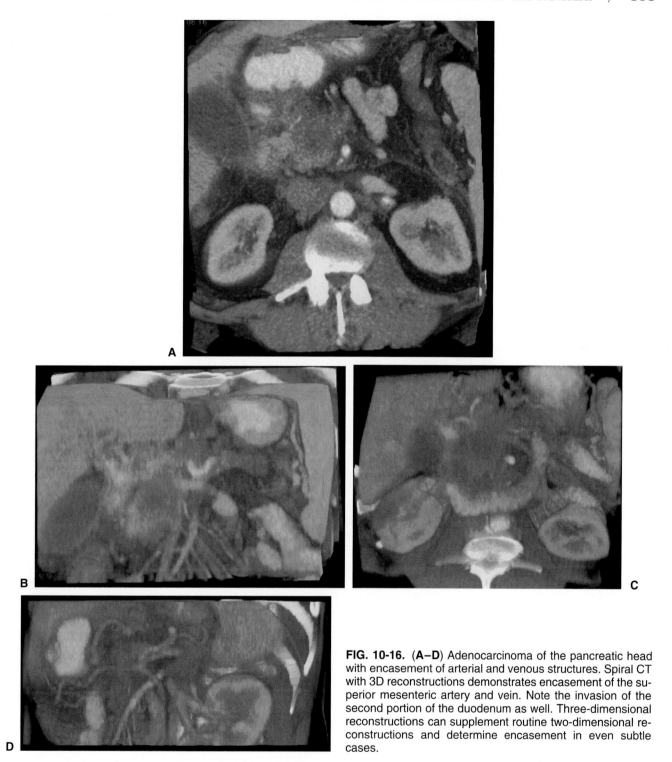

FIG. 10-16. (A–D) Adenocarcinoma of the pancreatic head with encasement of arterial and venous structures. Spiral CT with 3D reconstructions demonstrates encasement of the superior mesenteric artery and vein. Note the invasion of the second portion of the duodenum as well. Three-dimensional reconstructions can supplement routine two-dimensional reconstructions and determine encasement in even subtle cases.

In the first edition of this book we suggested that in the future, 3D spiral CT angiography could play a crucial role in defining vascular anatomy and may eventually replace angiography (20). This has indeed developed as we suspected. As defined by Raptopoulos et al. (17), the negative predictive value for determining resectability increased from 70% to 96% (p = .021) by adding CT angiography. Our experience has been very similar. In cases where there is an obvious fat plane between vessel and tumor mass or where invasion is obvious, the role of CT angiography is limited. However, in indeterminate cases the 3D vascular maps created from spiral CT data sets can be critical in distinguishing early invasion from simple poor tissue planes between the mesenteric vessels and the tumor. We have found that a dual-

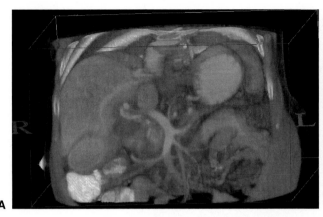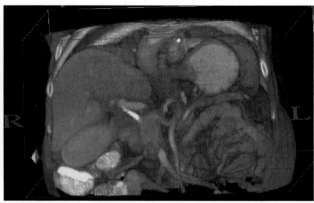

A

B

FIG. 10-17. (A,B) Carcinoma of the pancreatic head with encasement of an aberrant right hepatic artery. Three-dimensional reconstructions demonstrate encasement of aberrant right hepatic artery that arises off the SMA. Note the excellent detail of the arterial as well as venous anatomy. The portal vein and SMV confluence were normal.

phase spiral CT scan is optimal in this situation. The early phase (25–30 s) arterial-phase acquisition is best for defining SMA or celiac artery invasion. The portal-phase images (50–60 s) are best for defining SMV or portal vein involvement.

The Jaundiced Patient

One of the more important roles of spiral CT is the evaluation of the jaundiced patient. In most patients, spiral CT can determine the etiology of biliary tract obstruction. This is primarily due to the excellent parenchymal enhancement of both the liver and pancreas, and to the very thin sections with lack of spatial misregistration afforded by spiral technique. Obstruction can be localized to levels such as the distal intrahepatic ducts, porta hepatis, mid-common bile duct, or ampulla/pancreatic head (24–26).

When obstruction is at the level of the distal common bile duct, spiral CT findings often permit an accurate specific diagnosis. The differential diagnosis includes choledocholithiasis, primary cholangiocarcinoma of the distal duct, ampullary carcinoma, and pancreatic adenocarcinoma. The ability to differentiate a common duct calculus from a neoplastic process is of critical importance in the clinical management of a jaundiced patient (Fig. 10-18). Most common duct calculi are of soft-tissue density, with only a minority (approximately 20%) demonstrating homogeneous high attenuation; therefore these stones require meticulous technique for visualization. With spiral CT, the stone is frequently visualized as a focal increase in intraluminal attenuation within the duct, generally with a sharp zone of density transition with the normal low-density bile duct. A rim of low-attenuation bile producing either a "target" or "crescent" appearance of the duct may also be noted, and the duct wall itself may appear thickened (26). In general, neoplastic processes that involve the distal common duct will produce a less abrupt transition zone from a dilated duct

to a normal duct or normal parenchyma of the pancreatic head. Although ampullary carcinomas may be suggested on the basis of their characteristic location, spiral CT is also very sensitive in detecting additional findings such as porta hepatis adenopathy, indicating a neoplastic etiology.

Cystic Neoplasms

Cystic tumors of the pancreas are generally either microcystic adenomas or macrocystic cystadenomas or cystadenocarcinomas (previously serous or mucinous cystic tumors of the pancreas). Microcystic tumors have no malignant potential and are about 5 cm in size (Figs. 10-19, 10-20). The lesions are predominantly in the pancreatic head and may vary in appearance from a solid mass to multiple small cysts to a multilocular mass. A central scar with stellate calcifications may be present. Macrocystic tumors, on the other hand, are all considered to have malignant potential. They are generally on the order of 10 cm and are predominantly in the pancreatic body or tail. These lesions tend to be multiloculated with larger cysts and thicker septae. Calcification and/or mural nodules may be evident (26).

Because of excellent pancreatic enhancement, spiral CT can clearly define tumor spread and tumor margins within the gland. These tumors may show displacement or invasion of neighboring structures and vessels, which is exquisitely evaluated with spiral technique (Fig. 10-21). Spiral CT facilitates surgical planning for cystic pancreatic neoplasms as well as improved characterization of nonneoplastic pancreatic cysts. Finally, uncommon cystic tumors such as Hamoudi tumors may also be recognized with spiral CT (Fig. 10-22).

Islet Cell Tumors

Differentiation of an islet cell tumor from a pancreatic adenocarcinoma is of considerable clinical importance, as

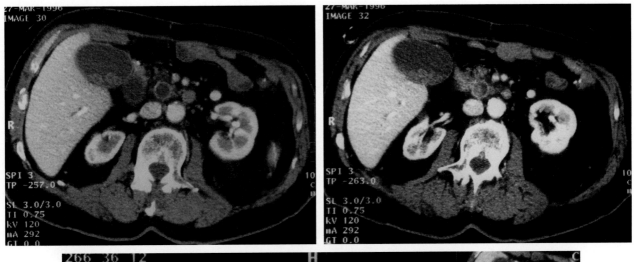

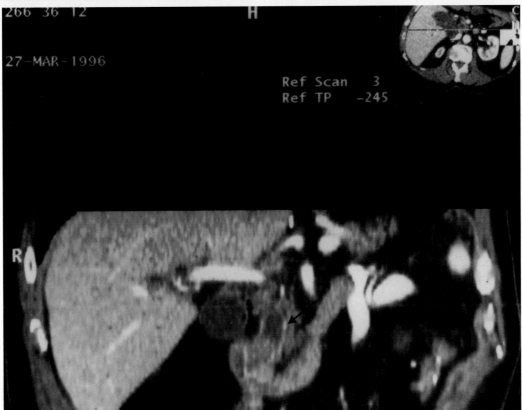

FIG. 10-18. **(A–C)** Biliary obstruction due to impacted stone in distal common duct. Spiral CT demonstrates multiple gallstones in the gallbladder. The common duct is dilated. Thin-section CT down to the level of obstruction demonstrates an impacted stone in the distal common duct. Coronal reconstructions clearly define the dilated duct and site of obstruction. Spiral CT with thin sections and sequential imaging can define the true course and cause of common duct obstruction.

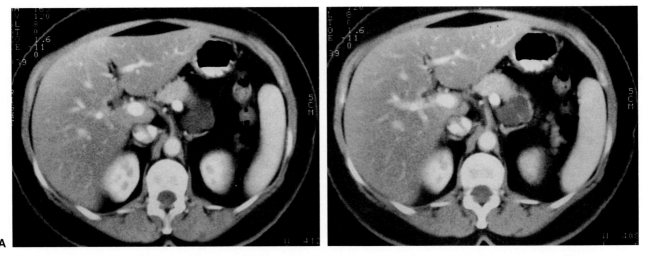

FIG. 10-19. (A,B) Cystadenoma of the pancreas. Cystic lesion involves the tail of the pancreas. The lesion has several septations. The patient had a history of pancreatitis, and this was surgically proved to be a cystadenoma.

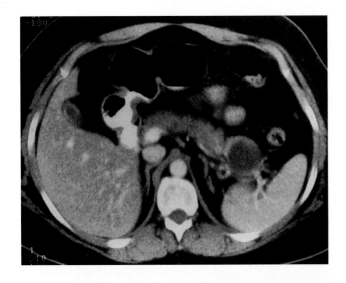

FIG. 10-20. Cystadenoma of the pancreas. Cystic lesion in pancreatic tail is seen in a patient with a history of pancreatitis. This was surgically removed and was a cystadenoma.

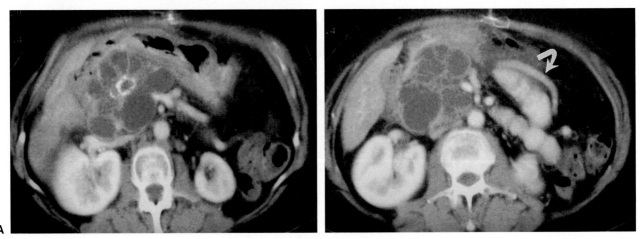

FIG. 10-21. Cystadenocarcinoma of the pancreatic head. (**A**) There is invasion of the portal vein by a large multiloculated cystic mass with characteristic central calcification. (**B**) Prominent venous collateral vessels are nicely demonstrated with spiral CT technique (*curved arrow*).

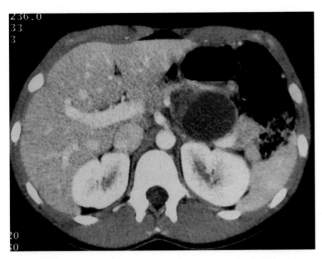

FIG. 10-22. Solid and cystic papillary epithelial neoplasm of the pancreas (Hamoudi tumor). Twenty-five-year-old female with a cystic and solid mass in the tail of the pancreas. No local invasion was seen. This was an unusual tumor, called a Hamoudi tumor.

deform the pancreatic contour, administration of adequate intravenous contrast is critical for detection of these tumors. Because of the high level of contrast enhancement afforded by spiral CT, this technique excels in detecting very small, hypervascular tumors. Spiral CT also utilizes contiguous, thin sections, which are critical for detection of such small lesions. Overlapping reconstructions (i.e., 3-mm collimation with reconstructions at 2-mm intervals) are especially valuable in these patients.

Van Hoe et al (29). reviewed a series of 10 patients with 11 surgically proven islet cell tumors. Spiral CT studies were performed with 5-mm collimation and overlapping reconstructions at 2-mm intervals in both the arterial and parenchymal phases. Nine of the 11 tumors could be detected (sensitivity of 82%), with the lesions missed being under 5 mm. Interestingly, two tumors in one patient were easier to see on the parenchymal-phase study, and in one case the tumor was seen only in this phase. In two patients tumor conspicuity was better on the arterial-phase images. The authors concluded that dual-phase CT imaging could yield improved detection rates for islet cell tumors (Fig. 10-25).

islet cell tumors have a more favorable response to chemotherapy. Unlike ductal adenocarcinomas, islet cell tumors (and their hepatic metastases) are characteristically hypervascular (see Fig. 10-22). CT may demonstrate calcification within the mass in up to 20% of patients. There is generally a lack of central necrosis or vascular invasion, features typical of ductal adenocarcinoma. Although most islet cell tumors (60%) occur in the body and tail of the pancreas, location is not a reliable discriminator (28).

These tumors tend to be of two types, depending on whether they are hormonally active (Fig. 10-23). Nonfunctional tumors are typically large lesions, on the order of 10 cm (Fig. 10-24). Functioning tumors are usually less than 2 cm (see Fig. 10-24). Because such small lesions will not

Other Neoplasms

Acinar cell neoplasms, lymphoma, metastases, and even peripancreatic masses may all mimic adenocarcinoma on CT (Fig. 10-26). Metastatic disease and lymphoma may involve the lymph nodes in the hepatoduodenal ligament and porta hepatis, and extend into the pancreas, making differentiation from a primary parenchymal mass difficult. Differential contrast enhancement permits clear delineation of pancreatic parenchyma and lymph nodes by defining intact fat planes between the pancreas and nodes (30). Similarly, peripancreatic masses may be more confidently distinguished from primary pancreatic neoplasms when sharp tissue planes of differential enhancement are delineated on spiral CT.

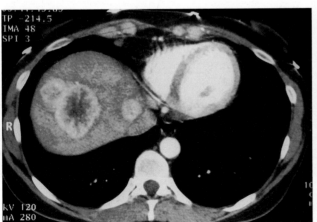
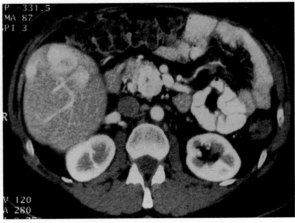

FIG. 10-23. (A,B) Islet cell tumor of the pancreas. Spiral CT demonstrates multiple vascular lesions in the liver consistent with metastatic islet cell tumor. Note the enhancing lesion in the pancreatic head consistent with the primary tumor.

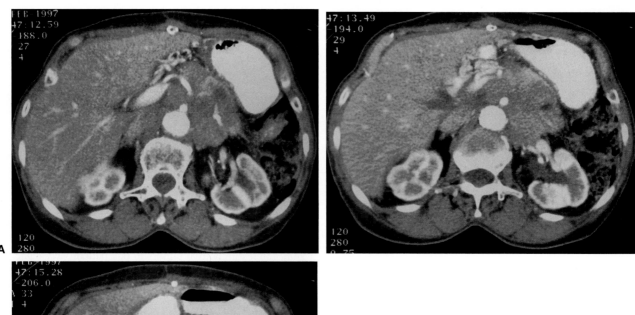

FIG. 10-24. (A–C) Nonfunctioning islet cell tumor of the pancreas. Large mass involving the body and tail of the pancreas was an unresectable nonfunctioning islet cell tumor. Note the differential enhancement of normal pancreas and mass. In this case the mass was of lower CT attenuation than the normal pancreas. Note the excellent definition of the vascular encasement of celiac axis.

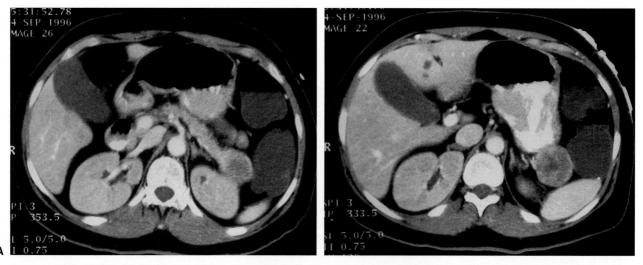

FIG. 10-25. (A,B) Vipoma of the pancreatic tail. The patient has a necrotic mass measuring about 3 cm involving the pancreatic tail. The patient presented with secretory diarrhea. (Note the excessive fluid in the bowel.) This was resected and was a Vipoma. Liver metastases are also seen.

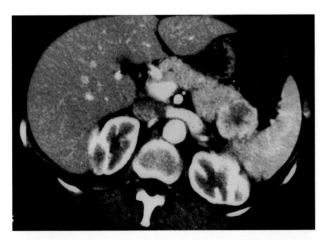

FIG. 10-26. Metastatic sarcoma to the pancreas. Hypervascular mass is seen involving the pancreatic tail. This was a metastatic lesion. The most common origin of sites of metastasis to the pancreas include renal cell carcinoma and melanoma.

Postsurgical Evaluation

CT is clearly the study of choice for follow-up evaluation of the patient who has undergone a Whipple procedure for pancreatic cancer (31–32). In this setting, spiral CT technique, with thin collimation, allows excellent visualization of the surgical bed. Spiral CT is quite sensitive for detection of small recurrent lesions (Figs. 10-27, 10-28). It has been shown that adjuvant radiotherapy can lead to thickening of the gastric antrum and proximal duodenum, which, in turn, may simulate recurrent tumor on CT. In these cases, spiral CT offers improved visualization of the porta hepatis and hepatic parenchyma for assessment of metastases to lymph nodes and the liver, respectively. Adequate opacification of anastomotic bowel loops in the porta hepatis is essential for accurate diagnosis (32).

APPLICATIONS/PANCREATIC INFLAMMATORY DISEASE

Contrast CT has greatly contributed to the current understanding of the morphological abnormalities in pancreatic inflammatory disease. CT remains the modality of choice for the imaging diagnosis of pancreatitis and its complications. The clinical severity of pancreatitis correlates well with the extent of pancreatic necrosis evident on CT. Thus CT can often predict expected clinical outcome (33–35). Early recognition of the complications of pancreatitis is essential for prompt, appropriate intervention.

Acute Pancreatitis

In up to one-third of patients with acute pancreatitis, CT demonstrates a normal pancreas. More often, CT findings in acute pancreatitis will include glandular enlargement due to interstitial parenchymal edema (Figs. 10-29–10-31). This glandular enlargement is most commonly diffuse, but when it is focal, findings may be indistinguishable from a neoplasm. In acute pancreatitis, the pancreatic contour may be irregular with focal hypodense regions likely representing focal necrosis or edema. The peripancreatic tissues will usually demonstrate inflammatory changes, resulting in an increase in density of the peripancreatic fat. One notable exception is the preservation of a rim of normal fat around the SMA and SMV. This finding, although not inviolate, may help to distinguish pancreatitis from a neoplastic process (13). Acute edematous pancreatitis may progress to a necrotizing pancreatitis with extensive phlegmon formation, peripancreatic fluid, hemorrhage, and extraglandular fat necrosis. Serial CT scans are essential to evaluate serial disease progression and diagnose complications early.

Pancreatic exudate and phlegmon tend to collect most often in the anterior pararenal space, the lesser sac, and eventually, in the greater peritoneal cavity. Spread of inflamma-

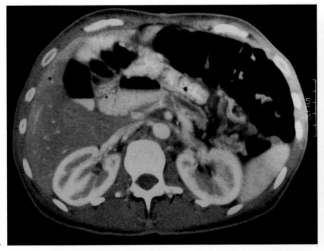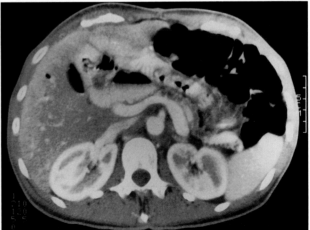

A
B

FIG. 10-27. **(A,B)** Normal post-Whipple's procedure CT scan. Spiral CT demonstrates excellent opacification of both bowel and vasculature. There is no evidence of tumor recurrence in this patient. Note the small atrophic pancreatic tail with dilated pancreatic duct.

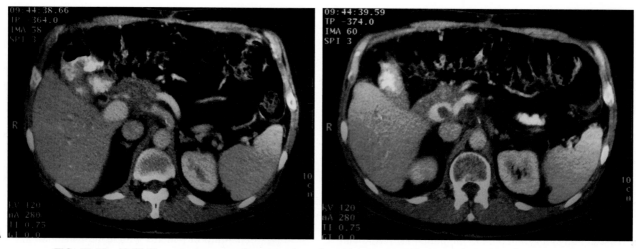

FIG. 10-28. (A,B) Recurrent pancreatic cancer invading portal vein. Follow-up CT scan in patient status after Whipple's procedure demonstrates recurrence in pancreatic bed. Tumor now invades the portal vein and SMA.

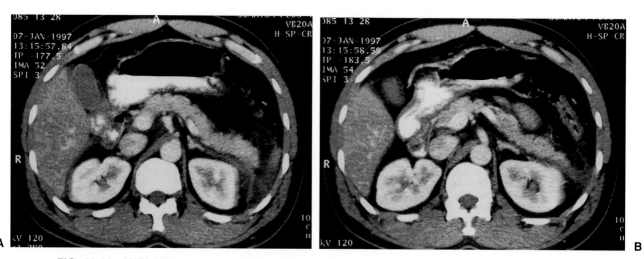

FIG. 10-29. (A,B) Mild acute pancreatitis. CT scan demonstrates minimal inflammation around pancreatic tail with fluid in the left anterior pararenal space.

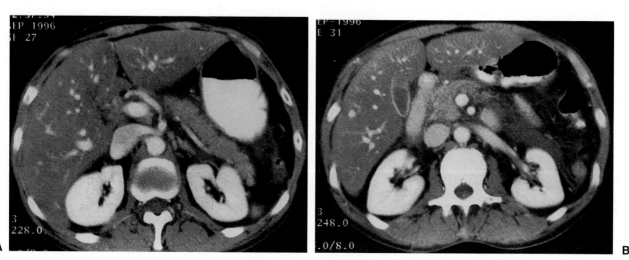

FIG. 10-30. (A,B) Acute pancreatitis. Spiral CT scan demonstrates pancreatitis with more extensive inflammation around the inferior border of the pancreas. There was normal enhancement of pancreas.

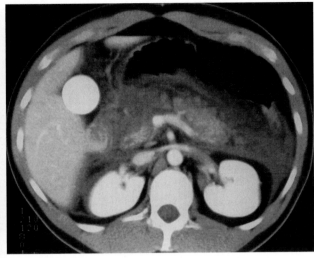

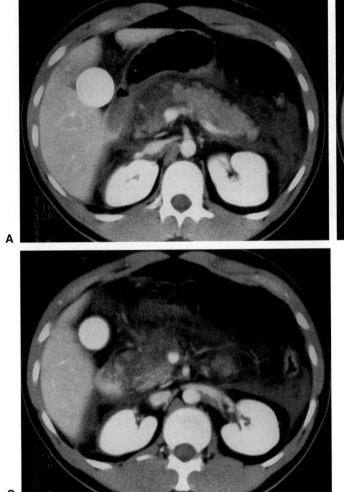

FIG. 10-31. (**A–C**) Acute pancreatitis following ERCP. Spiral CT demonstrates extensive pancreatitis with areas of minimal lack of glandular enhancement in the region of the pancreatic head. Inflammation involves mesentery as well as pararenal spaces.

tion typically occurs along the transverse mesocolon and root of the mesentery, as well as the gastrosplenic, gastrohepatic, and gastrocolic ligaments (36). Pancreatic phlegmons typically have higher attenuation values than pancreatic fluid collections and may appear heterogeneous due to blood, fat, and necrotic tissue components. Peripancreatic fluid collections may demonstrate regions of increased attenuation due to hemorrhage within the gland itself or to erosion of a nearby vascular structure.

Spiral CT offers several unique advantages in the evaluation of patients with acute pancreatitis. It can readily establish the presence of necrosis or hemorrhage within the gland. The diagnosis of pancreatic necrosis is of major clinical importance, as it directly affects patient prognosis. Areas of pancreatic necrosis are avascular with contrast-enhanced spiral CT. In patients with necrosis of greater than 50% of the pancreas, Balthazar et al. demonstrated that the morbidity and mortality increase substantially (33). Patients with significant pancreatic necrosis should be followed at close intervals with spiral CT to detect early abscess formation. CT-guided needle aspiration may be helpful in selected patients to document infected peripancreatic fluid (37).

Spiral CT is also valuable in diagnosing vascular complications of pancreatitis such as unsuspected pseudoaneurysm (most commonly of the gastroduodenal artery or splenic artery). Rupture of a peripancreatic pseudoaneurysm may lead to life-threatening hemorrhage. (Figs. 10-32, 10-33) (38). Inflammatory exudate encasing the splenic vein or portal vein with resultant venous thrombosis and collateral vessel formation is also well demonstrated on spiral CT (see Fig. 10-41).

Pancreatic Abscess

Pancreatic abscesses may develop in the setting of superinfection of a pancreatic phlegmon or of a pancreatic/peripancreatic fluid collection. This dreaded complication of acute pancreatitis contributes significantly to mortality with this disease. Attenuation of these collections tend to be higher than those of sterile exudates. Gas within a collection is very suggestive of abscess formation, although it may not be present (Figs. 10-34–10-36). Furthermore, this finding may also indicate communication with the bowel lumen, either from surgical drainage or from spontaneous fistulae (10).

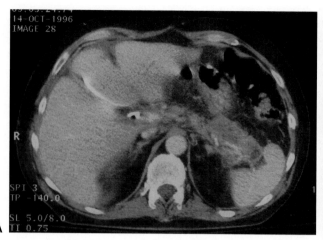

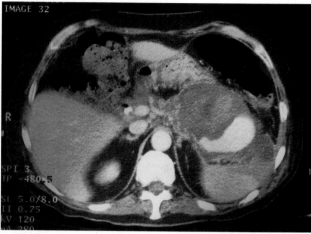

FIG. 10-32. **(A,B)** Splenic artery aneurysm secondary to prior pancreatitis. **(A)** CT scan demonstrates inflammation of the pancreas in a patient who has had repeat episodes of pancreatitis. The patient was discharged several days after the CT scan. **(B)** Two weeks later the patient had increasing abdominal pain and spiral CT scan was done, which demonstrated a 10-cm enhancing mass in the left upper quadrant. This was consistent with a splenic artery pseudoaneurysm. It was subsequently embolized.

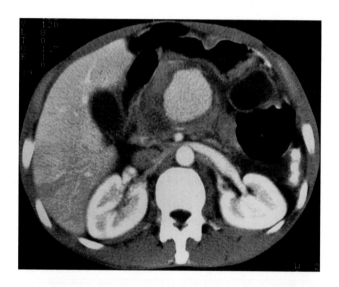

FIG. 10-33. Pseudoaneurysm of left gastric artery. Spiral CT demonstrates an enhancing lesion in the body of the pancreas. The patient was referred for drainage of a pseudocyst. This was a left gastric artery pseudoaneurysm rather than a pseudocyst as suspected.

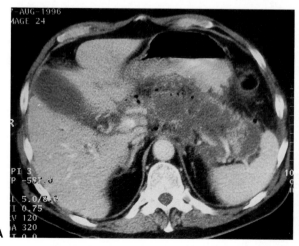

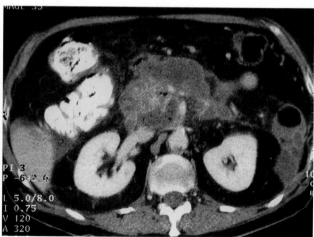

FIG. 10-34. **(A,B)** Pancreatic necrosis with pancreatic abscess. Spiral CT demonstrates diffuse inflammation of pancreas with lack of normal pancreatic enhancement. Several air bubbles are seen within the pancreas consistent with pancreatic abscess.

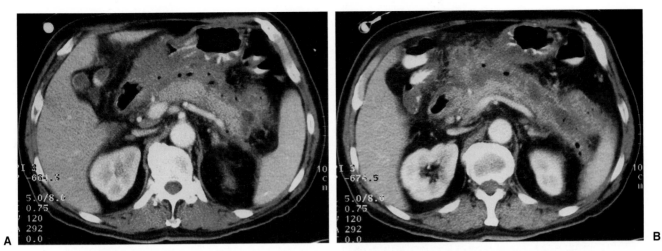

FIG. 10-35. (A,B) Pancreatic abscess. Spiral CT demonstrates lack of normal glandular enhancement consistent with pancreatic necrosis. Air bubbles are seen in and near gland consistent with infection and pancreatic abscess.

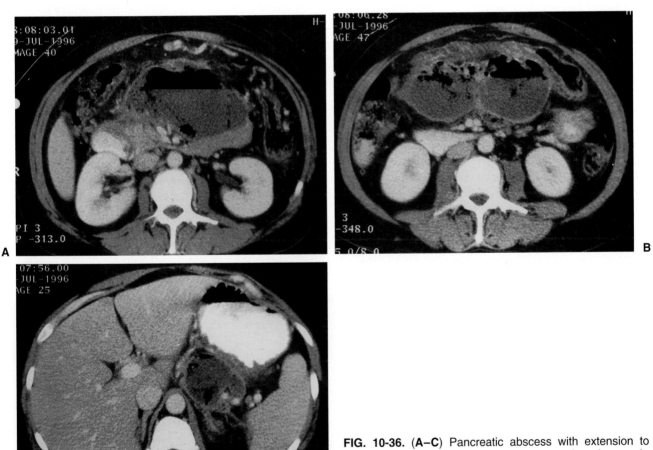

FIG. 10-36. (A–C) Pancreatic abscess with extension to lesser sac. Spiral CT demonstrates extensive abscess in body of pancreas with extension into lesser sac. Pancreatic abscesses can dissect through soft-tissue planes similar to pseudocysts.

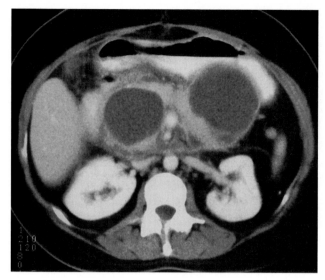

FIG. 10-37. Pancreatic pseudocyst following episode of acute pancreatitis. Pseudocysts are seen involving the head and tail of the pancreas. They are well defined and consistent with simple pseudocysts.

Pseudocysts

Approximately 30% to 50% of acute pancreatic fluid collections become encapsulated and evolve into true pseudocysts (35). In contrast to the dynamic fluid collections of acute pancreatitis, pseudocysts have defined fibrous pseudocapsules and typically occur in the setting of subacute or chronic pancreatitis. The fluid in pseudocysts is usually of homogeneously low attenuation, near that of water (Figs. 10-37, 10-38). When pseudocyst contents exhibit heterogeneously increased attenuation, this raises the possibility of superimposed hemorrhage or infection.

Spiral CT with multiplanar imaging can clearly define the location and extent of pancreatic pseudocysts. This information can then be used for planning surgical management or percutaneous drainage (Fig. 10-39). Pseudocysts may dis-

place or encase vascular structures adjacent to the pancreas, such as the portal or splenic veins. This may lead to extrinsic venous compression or even obstruction. Venous thrombosis in this setting may result in collateral varices or mesenteric thrombosis. Pseudocysts may erode into pancreatic or peripancreatic arteries with resultant acute hemorrhage (Fig. 10-40). Pseudoaneurysms may develop in the fibrous wall of the pseudocyst or involve adjacent vessels such as the splenic or gastroduodenal artery. Potentially life-threatening pseudoaneurysms are often first suspected on the basis of a spiral CT scan (34). Other complications include obstruction of the biliary or gastrointestinal tracts, or spontaneous rupture into the peritoneum, retroperitoneum, or bowel lumen (Figs. 10-41, 10-42). Spiral CT is clearly a very sensitive means for detecting the presence of such complications (35,36,38,39).

Chronic Pancreatitis

Chronic pancreatitis is a distinct clinical and pathological entity resulting from repeated bouts of acute pancreatitis. A variety of CT features may be evident in patients with chronic pancreatitis, including an atrophic gland, possibly with fatty replacement; dilatation of the pancreatic duct; pancreatic calculi; biliary ductal dilatation; pseudocyst formation; and focal pancreatic enlargement (Figs. 10-43, 10-44) (39).

An important diagnostic advantage of contrast-enhanced spiral CT is the increased conspicuity of the low-attenuation pancreatic and biliary ducts against the markedly enhanced parenchyma. Certain characteristics of the pancreatic duct suggest a benign versus malignant process. With chronic pancreatitis, the dilated pancreatic duct will appear beaded and irregular (i.e., chain of lakes), whereas a smooth pattern of dilatation tends to suggest carcinoma. The presence of intraductal calculi clearly favors the diagnosis of chronic pancreatitis. In addition, a ratio of pancreatic duct diameter to pancreatic gland greater than 0.5 favors carcinoma, whereas a ratio of less than 0.5 favors chronic pancreatitis (39). Not infrequently, the previously described changes of

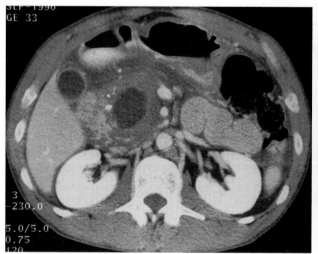
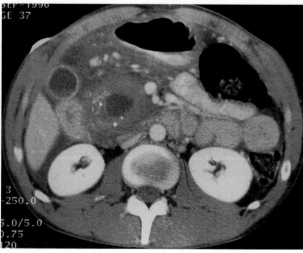

FIG. 10-38. (A,B) Acute and chronic pancreatitis with pseudocyst formation. Spiral CT demonstrates pseudocyst in the head of the pancreas. Evidence of subtle calcification in pancreatic head is seen. Diffuse inflammation of parapancreatic soft-tissue planes is also seen.

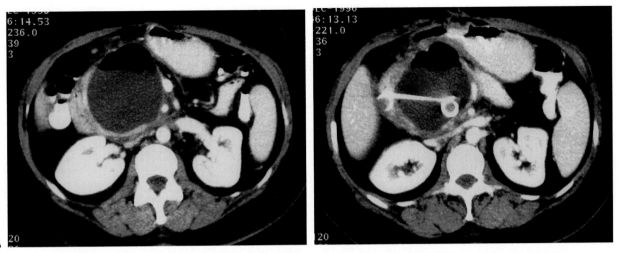

FIG. 10-39. **(A,B)** Unsuccessful drainage of pancreatic pseudocyst. Spiral CT demonstrates a pseudocyst in the pancreatic head. In this case an attempt was made to drain the pseudocyst endoscopically through the duodenum, which was unsuccessful.

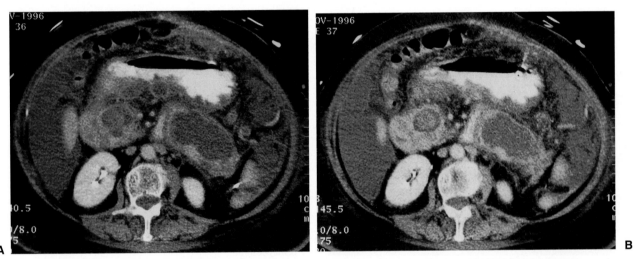

FIG. 10-40. **(A,B)** Hemorrhagic pancreatitis with hemorrhage into pseudocyst. Spiral CT demonstrates multiple pseudocysts and extensive pancreatitis with mesenteric inflammation. In the region of the pancreatic head the pseudocyst has increased attenuation consistent with hemorrhagic pancreatitis.

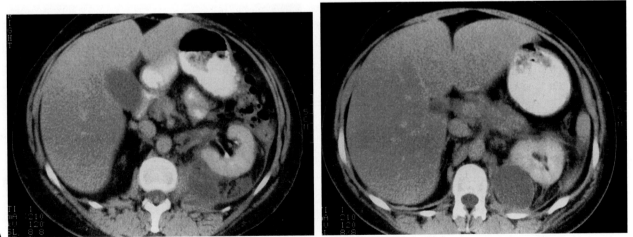

FIG. 10-41. **(A,B)** Pancreatitis with extension into left posterior pararenal space. Involvement of adjacent organs is not uncommon with pancreatitis. In this case the inflammation involved the left posterior pararenal space. Pseudocysts can dissect into the renal capsule.

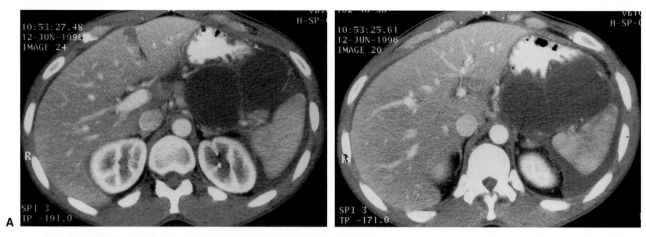

FIG. 10-42. **(A,B)** Pancreatic pseudocysts involving tail of the pancreas and extension into lesser sac. Pseudocysts involve the region of the lesser sac and spleen, which results in parenchymal enhancement irregularity. Splenic involvement by pancreatitis is not uncommon.

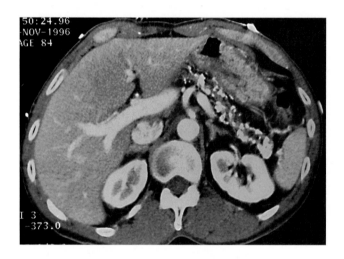

FIG. 10-43. Chronic pancreatitis with diffuse pancreatic calcification. Spiral CT demonstrates extensive pancreatic calcification of the pancreas. This is consistent with chronic atrophic pancreatitis.

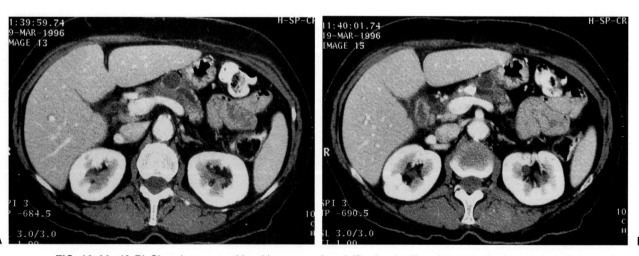

FIG. 10-44. **(A,B)** Chronic pancreatitis with pancreatic calcification in dilated pancreatic duct and small pseudocyst. Spiral CT scan demonstrates atrophic pancreas with calcification in the pancreatic duct consistent with chronic pancreatitis. A small pseudocyst is also seen.

acute pancreatitis will be superimposed on underlying chronic pancreatitis.

One remaining problematic area is that of the patient with a focal pancreatic mass secondary to chronic pancreatitis. Biopsy, ERCP, and/or close serial follow-up with spiral CT are often required to help differentiate focal pancreatitis from carcinoma.

FUTURE DIRECTIONS

In the first edition of this book we predicted that future advances in spiral CT technology would allow for longer spiral scans at higher milliampere settings. These higher milliampere settings (a result in great part of better tube heat-cooling capacities) are now available and allow for better resolution at narrow collimation, as well as decreased image noise, especially noticeable in the larger patient ($>$200 lb). Three-dimensional vascular imaging using either volume-rendering technique or maximum-intensity projection (MIP) now helps create vascular maps for the surgeon, which, in turn, are proving helpful in the more accurate staging of pancreatic cancer (40–41). Finally, the sensitivity and specificity of spiral CT compared with standard dynamic CT in terms of both pancreatitis and pancreatic cancer are no longer in doubt. Spiral CT represents the gold standard in the evaluation of known or suspected pancreatic pathology. We look forward to continuing advances in the years to come.

REFERENCES

1. Fishman EK, Wyatt SH, Ney DR, et al. Spiral CT of the pancreas with multiplanar display. *AJR* 1992;159:1209–1215.
2. Dupuy DE, Costello P, Ecker CP. Spiral CT of the pancreas. *Radiology* 1992;183:815–818.
3. Hollett MD, Jorgensen MJ, Jeffrey Jr RB. Quantitative evaluation of pancreatic enhancement during dual phase helical CT. *Radiology* 1995;195:359–361.
4. Bonaldi VM, Bret PM, Atri M, Garcia P, Reinhold C. A comparison of two injection protocols using helical and dynamic acquisitions in CT examinations of the pancreas. *AJR* 1996;167:49–55.
5. Zeman RK, Fox SH, Silverman PM, et al. Helical (spiral) CT of the abdomen. *AJR* 1993;160:719–725.
6. Novick SL, Fishman EK. 3D spiral CT angiography of pancreatic carcinoma: role in staging extent of disease. *AJR* 1998;170:139–143.
7. Novick SL, Fishman EK. Portal vein thrombosis: spectrum of helical CT angiographic findings. *Abdom Imaging* 1998;170:139–143.
8. Johnson PT, Heath DG, Kuszyk BS, Fishman EK. CT angiography with volume rendering: advantages and applications in splanchnic vascular imaging. *Radiology* 1996;200:564–568.
9. Sim JS, Choi BI, Han JK et al. Helical CT anatomy of pancreatic arteries. *Abdom Imaging* 1996;21:517–521.
10. Stanley RJ, Koslin DB, Lee JKT. Pancreas. In Lee JKT, Sagel SS, Stanley RJ, et al., eds. *Computed body tomography,* 2nd ed. New York: Raven Press; 1989:549–583.
11. Ward EM, Stephens DN, Sheedy PF Jr. Computed tomographic characteristics of pancreatic carcinoma: an analysis of 100 cases. *Radiographics* 1983;3:547–565.
12. Freeny PC, Marks WM, Ryan JA, et al. Pancreatic ductal adenocarcinoma: diagnosis and staging with dynamic CT. *Radiology* 1988;166:125–134.
13. Megibow AJ, Bosniak MA, Ambos MA, et al. Thickening of the celiac axis and/or superior mesenteric artery: a sign of pancreatic carcinoma on computed tomography. *Radiology* 1982;144:131–135.
14. Schulte SJ, Baron RL, Freeny PC, et al. Root of the superior mesenteric artery in pancreatitis and pancreatic carcinoma: evaluation with CT. *Radiology* 1991;180:659–662.
15. Megibow AJ. Pancreatic adenocarcinoma: designing the examination to evaluate the clinical questions. *Radiology* 1992;183:297–303.
16. Kaneko K, Honda H, Hayashi T, et al. Helical CT evaluation of arterial invasion in pancreatic tumors: comparison with angiography. *Abdom Imaging* 1997;22:204–207.
17. Raptopoulos V, Steer ML, Sheiman RG, Vrachliotis TG, Gougoutas CA, Movson JS. The use of helical CT and CT angiography to predict vascular involvement from pancreatic cancer: correlation with findings at surgery. *AJR* 1997;168:971–977.
18. Hommeyer SC, Freeny PC, Crabo LG. Carcinoma of the head of the pancreas: evaluation of the pancreaticoduodenal veins with dynamic CT: potential for improved accuracy in staging. *Radiology* 1995;196:233–238.
19. Bluemke DA, Cameron JL, Hruban RH, et al. Potentially resectable pancreatic adenocarcinoma: spiral CT assessment with surgical and pathologic correlation. *Radiology* 1995;197:381–385.
20. Wyatt SH, Fishman EK. Spiral CT of the pancreas (in) spiral CT: principles, techniques and clinical applications. In: Fishman EK, Jeffrey RB Jr, eds. *Spiral CT: principles, techniques and clinical applications.* New York: Raven Press; 1995:57–77.
21. Sheiman RG, Raptopoulos V. Delayed intravenous contrast medium washout from the small bowel in patients with pancreatic carcinoma and splanchnic venous invasion. *J Comput Assist Tomogr* 20(6):924–929.
22. Bluemke DA, Fishman EK. Spiral CT of the liver. *AJR* 1993;160:787–792.
23. Urban BA, Fishman EK, Kuhlman JE, et al. Detection of focal hepatic lesions with spiral CT: comparison of 4- and 8-mm interscan spacing. *AJR* 1993;160:783–785.
24. Graf O, Boland GW, Warshaw AL, Fernandez-del-Castillo C, Hahn PF, Mueller PR. Arterial versus portal venous helical CT for revealing pancreatic adenocarcinoma: Conspicuity of tumor and critical vascular anatomy. *AJR* 1997;169:119–123.
25. Loyer EM, David CL, Dubrow RA, Evans DB, Charnsargavej C. Vascular involvement in pancreatic adenocarcinoma: reassessment by thin-section CT. *Abdom Imaging* 1996;21:202–206.
26. Baron RL. Common bile duct stones: reassessment of criteria for CT diagnosis. *Radiology* 1987;162:419–424.
27. Itai Y, Moss AA, Ohtomo K. Computed tomography of cystadenoma and cystadenocarcinoma of the pancreas. *Radiology* 1982;145:419–425.
28. Eelkema EA, Stephens DH, Ward EM, et al. CT features of nonfunctioning islet call carcinoma. *AJR* 1984;143:943–948.
29. Van Hoe LV, Gryspeerdt S, Marchal G, Baert AL, Merter SL. Helical CT for the preoperative localization of islet cell tumors of the pancreas: value of arterial and parenchymal phase images. *AJR* 1995;165:1437–1439.
30. Rumancik WM, Megibow AJ, Bosniak MA, et al. Metastatic disease to the pancreas: evaluation by computed tomography. *J Comput Assist Tomogr* 1984;8:829–834.
31. Bluemke DA, Fishman EK, Kuhlman JE. CT evaluation following Whipple procedure: potential pitfalls in interpretation. *J Comput Assist Tomogr* 1992;16(5):704–708.
32. Bluemke DA, Abrams R, Yeo C, Cameron JL, Fishman EK. Recurrent pancreatic adenocarcinomas: spiral CT evaluation following the Whipple procedure. *Radiographics* 1997;17:303–313.
33. Balthazar EJ, Robinson DL, Megibow AJ, et al. Acute pancreatitis: value of CT in establishing prognosis. *Radiology* 1990;174:331–336.
34. Balthazar EJ. CT diagnosis and staging of acute pancreatitis. *Radiol Clin North Am* 1989;27:19–37.
35. Balthazar EJ, Ranson JHC, Naidich DP, et al. Acute pancreatitis: prognostic value of CT. *Radiology* 1985;156:767–772.
36. Donovan PJ, Sanders RC, Siegelman SS. Collections of fluid after pancreatitis: evaluation by computed tomography and ultrasonography. *Radiol Clin North Am* 1982;20:653–566.
37. Yeo CJ, Bastidas JA, Lynch-Nyhan A, et al. The natural history of pancreatic pseudocysts documented by computed tomography. *Surg Gynecol Obstet* 1990;170:411–417.
38. Burke JW, Erickson SJ, Kellum CD, et al. Pseudoaneurysms complicating pancreatitis: detection by CT. *Radiology* 1986;161:447–450.
39. Neff CC, Simeone JF, Wittenberg J. Inflammatory pancreatic masses: problems in differentiating focal pancreatitis from carcinoma. *Radiology* 1984;150:35–38.
40. Dillon EH, van Leeuwen MS, Fernandez MA, et al. Spiral CT angiography. *AJR* 1993;160:1273–1278.
41. Napel S, Marks MP, Rubin GD, et al. CT angiography with spiral CT and maximum intensity projection. *Radiology* 1992;185:607–610.

CHAPTER 11

Spiral CT Evaluation of the Spleen

Bruce A. Urban and Elliot K. Fishman

CT has long been recognized as the gold standard of splenic imaging (1–3). More recently, spiral (helical) CT has become accepted as the state-of-the-art modality for evaluation of the upper abdomen, especially the liver and pancreas (4,5). The unique advantage of spiral CT as compared with conventional CT is the ability to scan during a single breath-hold during peak contrast enhancement. This eliminates data misregistration, minimizes motion artifact, and results in a uniformly high level of contrast enhancement. Together, these factors also improve evaluation of the spleen, especially in the detection of subtle parenchymal disease and vascular pathology. This chapter will discuss the many advantages that spiral CT scanning offers in evaluating the spleen.

SPIRAL TECHNIQUE: SPLEEN

In most cases, evaluation of the spleen is done in conjunction with the liver and pancreas. The spleen is usually imaged utilizing the same parameters as described for the liver. Typically, 120 mL of nonionic contrast is administered at a rate of 2–3 mL/s. Scanning begins at the termination of injection. Individual scanning parameters vary depending on the manufacturer of the CT scanner. Ideally, thin collimation (5–7 mm) is preferred. Pitch can be increased to approximately 1.6 without significant image compromise. Reconstructed images are routinely reformatted using 4- or 5-mm incrementation. In select cases where directed evaluation of a known splenic process is desired, decreasing the collimation, pitch, and reconstruction interval can improve image quality. Delayed scans (5 min after injection) may be useful in cases of confusing splenic pathology or to help differentiate a normal inhomogeneously enhancing spleen from an abnormal spleen.

Software packages on most spiral CT machines allow for the convenient multiplanar reconstruction of an acquired volumetric data set within minutes. The subsequent images can be reviewed in real time utilizing an interactive display format. We have found multiplanar reconstructions to be very helpful in the demonstration of splenic and perisplenic processes. Coronal and sagittal views often help clarify confusing cases where the origin of a particular mass or lesion is uncertain. Certain processes, such as splenic infarcts and lacerations, are at times better demonstrated with additional views (Fig. 11-1).

THE NORMAL SPLEEN

The spleen consists of a network of lymphatic follicles and reticuloendothelial cells (the white pulp), with interspersed vascular lakes (the red pulp). Unlike the liver, the normal spleen enhances inhomogeneously. This is because blood, as it traverses the red pulp, takes two routes to reach the splenic veins (6,7). Some of the flow is through the "open circulation," reaching the splenic veins after traversing the splenic cords. The remaining flow is through the "closed circuit," directly reaching the splenic veins without intervening flow through the splenic cords. The latter is the more rapid course. In combination, this differential flow results in irregular enhancement. At least 50% of normal spleens demonstrate inhomogeneous enhancement on dynamic CT (8), with up to 66% of cases demonstrated on angiography (9). This inhomogeneous enhancement is particularly pronounced on spiral CT due to high levels of bolus contrast opacification, and in our experience it is seen on most spiral scans. Inhomogeneous enhancement is more pronounced with faster injection rates or when scanning begins soon after initiation of contrast administration (Fig. 11-2).

The pattern of normal splenic enhancement can vary greatly from patient to patient. We have encountered several distinct patterns in our clinical practice. Most commonly, a serpentine, cordlike distribution of enhancement is seen homogeneously throughout the splenic tissue. This has been termed an arciform or "Moire" pattern (Fig. 11-3). Another form of normal enhancement demonstrates peripheral opacification of the spleen with relative sparing of the central

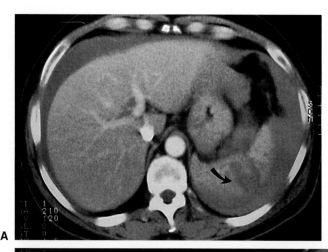

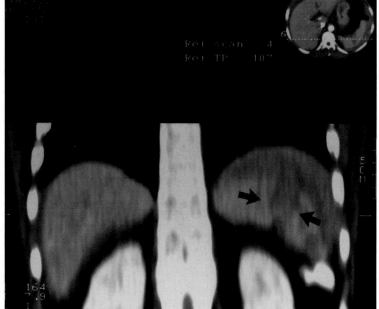

FIG. 11-1. Value of multiplanar reconstructions. **(A)** Axial scan from spiral CT demonstrates a laceration through the spleen (*curved arrow*), with moderate perisplenic hematoma. **(B)** The coronal reconstruction nicely conveys the severity of the injury in an additional plane. Complete transection is appreciated through the mid-portion of the spleen (*small arrows*).

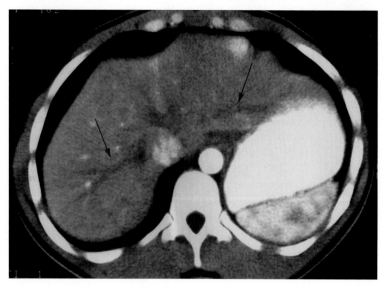

FIG. 11-2. Normal spleen in a 25-year-old male. Spiral acquisition soon after the initiation of contrast administration exaggerates the normal inhomogeneous pattern of splenic enhancement. Note lack of opacification of the hepatic veins (*arrows*).

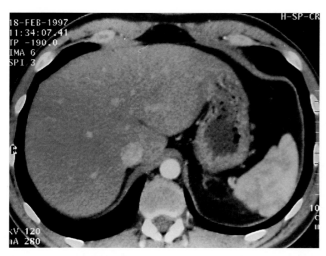

FIG. 11-3. Normal spleen in a 33-year-old male. Normal inhomogeneous splenic enhancement results from differential flow through the red pulp. Serpentine enhancement, as in this case, is the most common pattern.

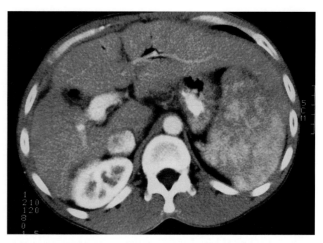

FIG. 11-5. Normal spleen in a 45-year-old male. Irregular enhancement is demonstrated throughout the spleen. The homogeneous distribution of the enhancement favors a diagnosis of normal.

splenic tissue (Fig. 11-4). Often we have seen this particular pattern of splenic enhancement in patients with portal hypertension. And at times, the spleen enhances irregularly in a manner that defies characterization (Fig. 11-5). However, if the pattern is homogeneously distributed, then in all likelihood one is dealing with a variation of normal enhancement. Whenever uncertainty arises, delayed images of the spleen are very helpful; diffuse forms of normal splenic inhomoge-

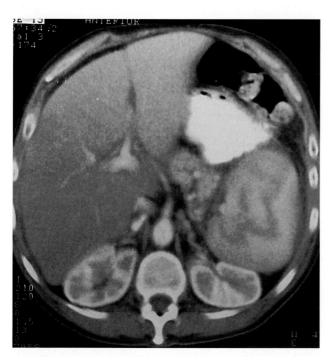

FIG. 11-4. Normal spleen in a 42-year-old male with cirrhosis. The spleen demonstrates prominent peripheral enhancement. This pattern is sometimes encountered in patients with portal hypertension.

neity are transient and disappear on delayed imaging (Fig. 11-6).

Normal inhomogeneous splenic enhancement can be marked in patients with decreased cardiac output or heart failure, primarily due to delayed transient time through the red pulp. Secondary delayed transit can result from splenic vein occlusion, portal hypertension, and/or portal vein thrombosis. All the preceding factors should be considered in patients with exaggerated variations of normal splenic enhancement (Fig. 11-7).

Focal regions of inhomogeneous splenic enhancement are invariably abnormal and represent true splenic pathology. Punctate foci are always abnormal and commonly result from an inflammatory or infectious insult. Often foci of involvement as small as 2 mm in diameter can be detected with spiral scanning (Fig. 11-8). Other patterns of abnormal enhancement are characterized as regional or geographic and typically present as focal decreased areas of enhancement on spiral CT following bolus contrast administration. Etiologies include infections, neoplasms, and infarction (Figs. 11-9, 11-10). In some of these patients, just as in those with normal variations of inhomogeneous splenic enhancement, delayed scans may appear normal. The focal or punctate nature of the initial splenic enhancement inhomogeneity is the key differential point in diagnosing the pattern as abnormal (Fig. 11-11).

NEOPLASM

Lymphoma

Lymphoma is the most common malignancy to involve the spleen, found at staging laparotomy in approximately one-third of patients with previously untreated disease (10,11). Splenomegaly is the most common CT finding; however, this is absent in up to one-third of patients with

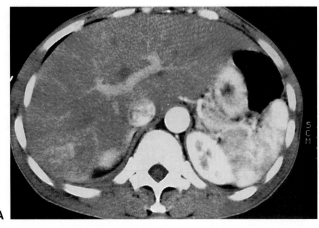
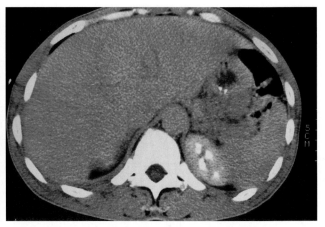

FIG. 11-6. Normal spleen in a 48-year-old male. **(A)** Spiral scan demonstrates diffuse inhomogeneous enhancement following bolus contrast administration. **(B)** Delayed scan reveals a homogeneous spleen. Diffuse, nonpunctate inhomogeneity that "disappears" on delayed views is usually normal.

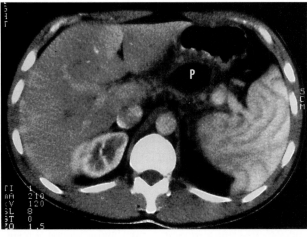

FIG. 11-7. Normal spleen in a 31-year-old male with pancreatitis and pseudocyst. The normal serpentine enhancement pattern is exaggerated due to splenic vein occlusion from the pseudocyst (P), which delays transit of contrast through the red pulp of the spleen.

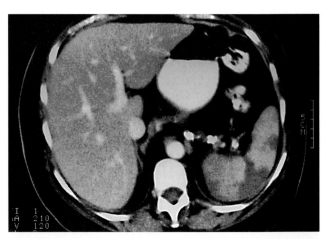

FIG. 11-9. Splenic infarcts in a 58-year-old female following splenic artery pseudoaneurysm embolization. Wedge-shaped regions of decreased enhancement are demonstrated, characteristic of infarction.

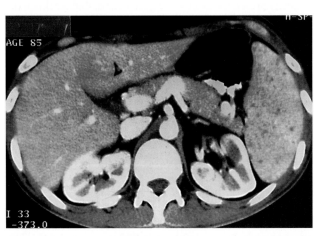

FIG. 11-8. *Pneumocystis carinii* infection in a 29-year-old male. Multiple, punctate foci of low attenuation are demonstrated in the spleen. This appearance is nonspecific but usually implies an infectious etiology.

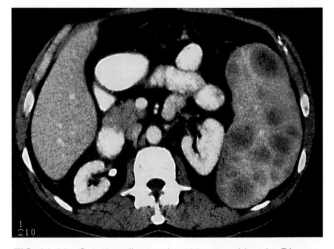

FIG. 11-10. Gaucher disease in a 60-year-old male. Discrete areas of decreased enhancement correspond to local deposits of glucocerebroside within the reticuloendothelial cells of the spleen. This appearance can also be seen with lymphoma or metastases.

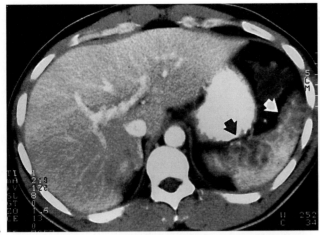
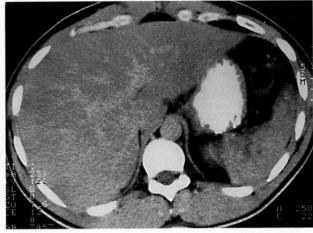

FIG. 11-11. MAI infection in an HIV-positive male. **(A)** Spiral scan reveals focal inhomogeneous enhancement in the anterior portion of the spleen (*arrows*). **(B)** Delayed scan shows persistent hypoattenuation anteriorly, confirming the abnormal nature of the enhancement pattern.

lymphomatous involvement. Moreover, in up to 30% of patients with lymphoma, splenic enlargement is due not to lymphoma but to reactive hyperplasia or congestion (12). Diffuse infiltrative involvement is difficult to detect with CT. When demonstrated, typical findings consist of one or several nodules, each usually measuring less than 1 cm (Fig. 11-12). The lesions are of lower attenuation than the normal spleen. Spiral scanning, by eliminating data misregistration with a single breath-hold acquisition, can improve detection of these smaller lesions. Larger lesions can present as cyst-like masses or can have cystic components within them.

Leukemia

In patients with leukemia, the spleen often demonstrates marked enlargement. However, the spleen will usually maintain a homogeneous enhancement pattern. No difference has been noted in the CT appearance among the various forms of leukemia. Patients with splenomegaly from leukemic involvement are more prone to spontaneous infarction and rupture.

Primary Tumors

Primary malignant splenic tumors are very rare. Most are of vascular origin, such as angiosarcoma and hemangioendothelioma (13). Angiosarcoma can be multiple and mimic the appearance of splenic abscesses. Patients can present with fever, malaise, ascites, and hepatosplenomegaly. A major advantage of spiral scanning is consistent and reliable demonstration of increased tumor vascularity, which can help distinguish them from benign tumors.

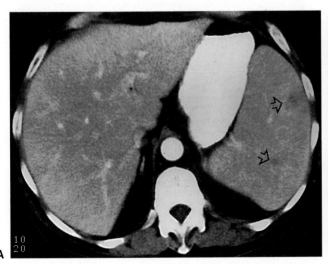
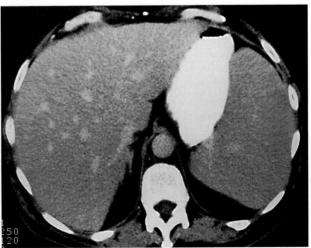

FIG. 11-12. Lymphoma in a patient status-post liver transplant. **(A)** Focal lymphomatous deposits (*arrows*) are seen in an enlarged spleen. **(B)** The lesions are not apparent on delayed imaging. Spiral CT with bolus contrast enhancement aids in the detection of focal splenic lesions.

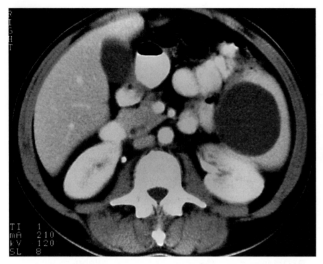

FIG. 11-13. Benign simple splenic cyst in a 58-year-old male. The low-density cyst demonstrates a sharp interface with the normal splenic tissue. There is no evidence of enhancement.

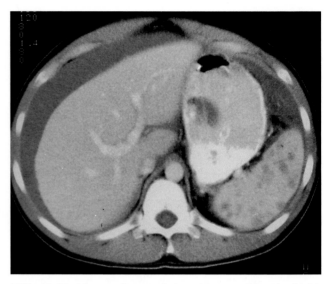

FIG. 11-15. Hemangiomatosis in a 34-year-old male. Multiple small, low-density lesions are demonstrated in the spleen. The patient presented with recurrent gastrointestinal bleeding. Surgery revealed multiple small hemangiomas.

Benign splenic tumors include splenic cysts, hemangiomas, lymphangiomas, and hamartomas. Splenic cysts are well-defined, low-density lesions (Fig. 11-13). The borders are sharply defined and lack appreciable contrast enhancement following bolus contrast administration. Many times a calcified wall is identified, often the result of prior hemorrhage (Fig. 11-14). Splenic hemangiomas are relatively common, second only to simple cysts as the most common benign splenic tumor. Hemangiomas can be multiple in cases of Klippel-Trenauney-Weber syndrome (14,15). Lesions can vary in size from a few millimeters to several centimeters. Spiral CT can demonstrate low-density lesions with peripheral enhancement, reflecting the vascular nature of these lesions (Figs. 11-15 and 11-16). The splenic hemangioma, however, may not necessarily demonstrate the typical "filling-in" seen with hepatic hemangiomas (15).

Metastases

Metastatic lesions to the spleen are far more common than primary splenic tumors; however, they remain relatively rare. Although usually present in cases of widespread metastases (16), cases of isolated splenic metastasis have been reported. Common metastatic tumors to the spleen include malignant melanoma, and carcinoma of the lung, breast, ovary, and stomach. Splenic metastases are typically small. The spleen may or may not be enlarged. Metastases can present as necrotic, low-density masses (11). Differentiation

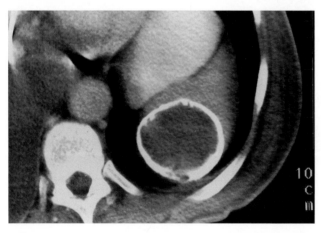

FIG. 11-14. Benign cyst with calcified wall in a 53-year-old male. Calcified cysts often result from prior trauma with hemorrhage.

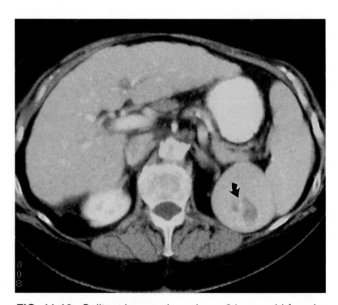

FIG. 11-16. Solitary hemangioma in an 84-year-old female. A 2-cm lesion is noted in the spleen (*arrow*). The periphery of the lesion is hypervascular, characteristic of hemangioma.

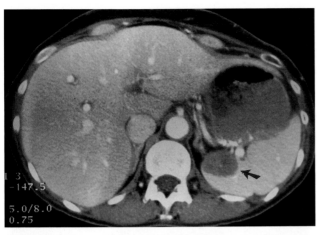

FIG. 11-17. Metastatic colon cancer in a 59-year-old female. The lesion (*arrow*) demonstrates central enhancement, confirming the solid nature of the metastasis.

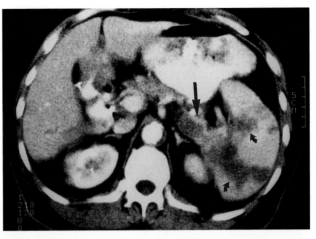

FIG. 11-19. Splenic invasion from pancreatic carcinoma in a 66-year-old male. The tumor has invaded the splenic hilum (*large arrow*), secondarily infarcting the splenic parenchyma (*curved arrows*).

of a cystic splenic metastasis from a benign cyst is often difficult. Spiral CT is helpful in evaluating for any enhancing components of the lesion that favor a diagnosis of malignancy (Fig. 11-17). Direct invasion into the splenic hilum can occur with pancreatic or gastric malignancies (Figs. 11-18, 11-19).

INFECTION

Splenic abscess is a rare yet potentially lethal disease process. The high morbidity is in part due to vague clinical symptoms, which often lead to a delay in diagnosis. CT has proven to be an accurate means for the early diagnosis of

abscesses, especially in the immunocompromised host. Early detection with CT can often alter and direct appropriate clinical management (17). Splenic abscesses are typically focal, hypodense, and slightly lobulated in shape. An enhancing capsule may be seen (Fig. 11-20). The spiral CT appearance is often similar to that of splenic infarction or chronic intrasplenic hemorrhage. Air within the abscess is seen in approximately 20% of cases and can be a helpful differential finding (11). The virtual elimination of partial volume averaging provided by spiral scanning can aid in the detection of small gas bubbles. CT can also demonstrate an air–fluid or fluid–fluid level (17).

The pattern of infection in the immunocompromised host

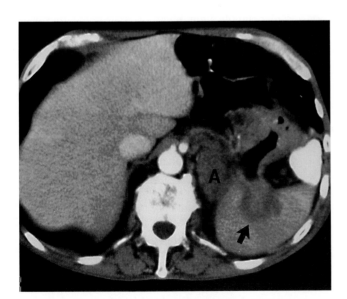

FIG. 11-18. Splenic invasion from gastric lymphoma in 72-year-old male. A large gastric lymphoma extends posteriorly to invade the splenic hilum (*arrow*). The adrenal gland (A) is also involved with tumor.

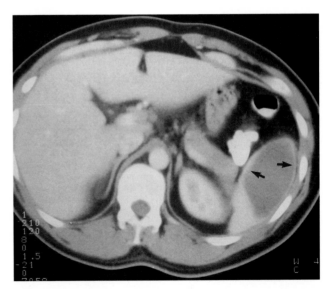

FIG. 11-20. Splenic abscess in 28-year-old male with endocarditis. A slightly hyperdense, rounded lesion is seen in the spleen. Note the enhancing rim of the abscess capsule (*arrows*), helping differentiate this lesion from a cyst or infarct.

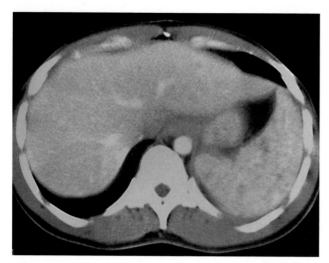

FIG. 11-21. Presumed *Pneumocystis carinii* infection in a 30-year-old HIV-positive male. The enlarged spleen reveals multiple low-density foci of infection. Peak contrast enhancement enhances detection of small splenic lesions.

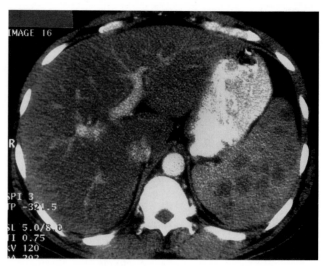

FIG. 11-23. Splenic tuberculosis in a 41-year-old HIV-positive male. Foci of infection have coalesced to form multiple masses within the spleen.

can have a specific appearance: Multiple, small, 2–5-mm low-density lesions can suggest the diagnosis of fungal microabscesses, usually due to candidiasis (18–20). Occasionally, a central focus of high attenuation can be seen. Individuals with acquired immunodeficiency syndrome (AIDS) can develop similar hypodense lesions, usually the result of *Pneumocystis carinii* infection (Fig. 11-21), disseminated tuberculosis (21,22), or *mycobacterium avium intracellulare* infection. Because of dynamic contrast enhancement and continuous data acquisition, spiral CT enhances the detection of these smaller lesions. Liver involvement is often apparent as well. Diffuse calcifications may appear in the spleen following therapy for *P. carinii* infection. Low-density adenop-

athy with peripheral rim enhancement is a supportive finding for tuberculosis (Fig. 11-22) (23,24). At times, infectious deposits can coalesce into larger areas of splenic involvement (Fig. 11-23).

Certain viral illnesses, such as mononucleosis, can result in splenomegaly without frank abscess formation. Spiral CT in such cases usually reveals nonspecific splenic enlargement. Occasionally, intrasplenic hemorrhage results.

INFARCTION

Spiral CT scanning is ideally suited for the evaluation of vascular pathology. Focal splenic infarction is a very common vascular complication. Many cases are clinically silent. Causes of focal infarction include bacterial endocarditis, sickle cell anemia, and lymphoma (11). Focal infarcts typically demonstrate wedge-shaped zones of decreased attenuation that extend to the surface of the spleen (Fig. 11-24). Splenomegaly itself can result in infarction due to relative ischemia (Fig. 11-25). Risk of infarction is further increased in patients with portal hypertension (Fig. 11-26). In our experience, focal infarcts can reliably be differentiated through the normal inhomogeneous pattern of enhancement (Fig. 11-27). Infarct appearance can vary, depending on age, usually becoming less dense and more well defined with time (25).

Global infarction can result in diffuse splenic hypodensity and can mimic splenic abscess or tumor (Fig. 11-28). The ability of spiral CT to scan during peak contrast enhancement allows reliable demonstration of the splenic artery and vein, which may be helpful in differentiating extensive abscess or tumor from global infarction. Some cases of global infarction maintain enhancement of the splenic periphery due to perfusion from capsular vessels (Fig. 11-29).

The most common cause of splenic vascular occlusion is pancreatic disease, usually due to pancreatitis or pancreatic

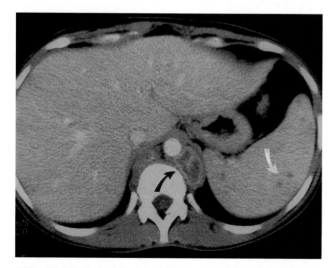

FIG. 11-22. Splenic tuberculosis in a 33-year-old female. Multiple, small low-density lesions are demonstrated in the spleen (*white arrow*). Retrocrural low-density adenopathy with an enhancing rim (*black arrow*) is typical in tuberculosis.

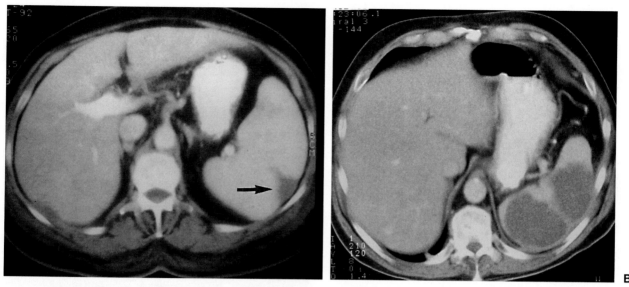

FIG. 11-24. Focal splenic infarcts. **(A)** A well-defined wedge-shaped defect is seen extending to the surface of the spleen (*arrow*). **(B)** Another patient demonstrates two focal infarcts in the spleen.

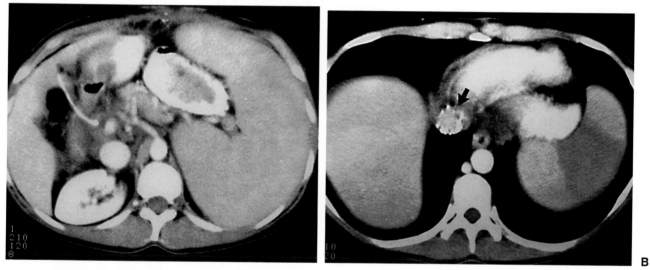

FIG. 11-25. Polycythemia vera with splenic infarct in a 31-year-old female. **(A)** There is marked spleno-megaly. **(B)** Superiorly, the spleen demonstrates a characteristic, wedge-shaped infarct. Note pericaval ring from liver transplant (*arrow*).

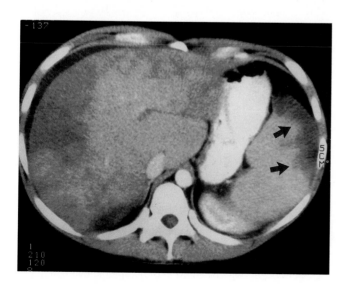

FIG. 11-26. Budd-Chiari syndrome with splenic infarcts in a 19-year-old male. Infarcts in the subcapsular portion of the spleen (*arrows*) result from splenomegaly due to portal hyper-tension. The caudate lobe is enlarged, with patchy peripheral liver enhancement, which is characteristic of Budd-Chiari syn-drome.

205

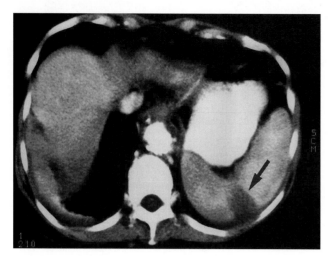

FIG. 11-27. Splenic infarct in a 69-year-old female. The infarct (*arrow*) is easily appreciated against the irregular enhancement of the normal splenic tissue.

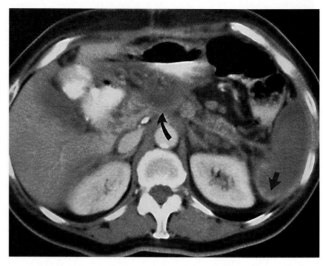

FIG. 11-29. Pancreatic carcinoma and global splenic infarction. A low-density mass (*curved arrow*) has occluded the splenic artery, resulting in global splenic infarction. Note the presence of peripheral enhancement (*straight arrow*) through preserved capsular branches.

carcinoma. Spiral scanning is routinely used in all patients with suspected pancreatic pathology. It is especially useful in the preoperative staging of pancreatic cancer. Because of the data continuity provided by spiral CT, improved multiplanar reconstruction is obtainable and can be very helpful in demonstrating vascular encasement or occlusion (26). It is also very useful in detecting splenic artery pseudoaneurysms, a relatively common complication of pancreatitis. Peak contrast enhancement allows for detection of pseudoaneurysms as small as 1–2 cm in diameter. Severe cases of pancreatitis can develop large pseudocysts that can track into the splenic hilum, resulting in vascular occlusion and infarction (Figs. 11-30, 11-31). Some pseudocysts track through the splenorenal ligament to become intrasplenic (27).

TRAUMA

The spleen is the most frequently injured organ in blunt abdominal trauma. CT scanning is extremely sensitive in the detection of splenic injury (28–30). Immediately following injury, a laceration or hematoma is often demonstrated (Figs. 11-32, 11-33). Lacerations appear as linear or geographic low-attenuating defects. Hyperdense, perisplenic clotted blood can be seen at times near the site of injury, often referred to as the ''sentinel clot'' sign (31). In select patients, active arterial extravasation may be seen as a focus of very high attenuation isodense with major visceral arteries. A subcapsular hematoma can subsequently form, appearing as a

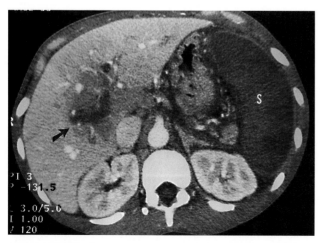

FIG. 11-28. Portal vein thrombosis with global splenic infarction in a 32-year-old male. The spleen is completely infarcted (S). Large portal vein thrombus (*arrow*) is seen with many small periportal collaterals.

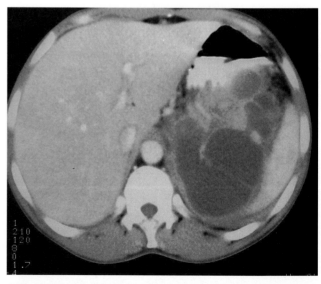

FIG. 11-30. Pancreatitis in a 38-year-old male. A large, septated pseudocyst has dissected into the splenic hilum.

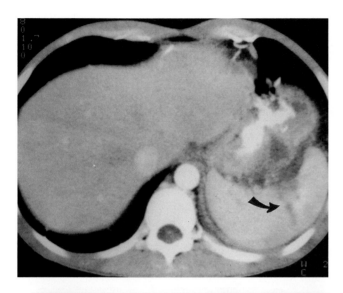

FIG. 11-31. Pancreatitis and splenic infarct. Extensive inflammatory changes have extended into the splenic hilum, resulting in focal splenic infarction (*arrow*).

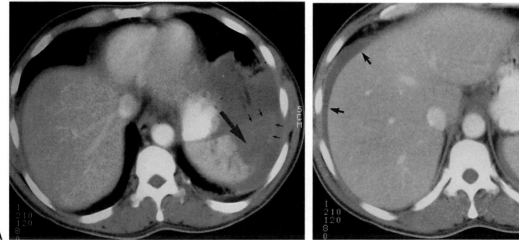

A   B

FIG. 11-32. Splenic laceration following motor vehicle accident. (**A,B**) The lateral aspect of the spleen is macerated, demonstrating heterogeneous decreased enhancement (*large arrows*). Note the preserved capsular enhancement (*small arrows,* **A**). Hemorrhagic ascites is collecting around the liver edge (*small arrows,* **B**).

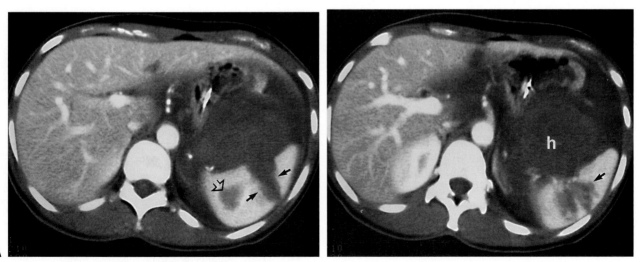

A   B

FIG. 11-33. Splenic laceration following motor vehicle accident. Superiorly, the spleen is transected (*arrows*). Normal inhomogeneous enhancement is seen medially (*arrowhead*). A large perisplenic hematoma (h) displaces the stomach anteriorly.

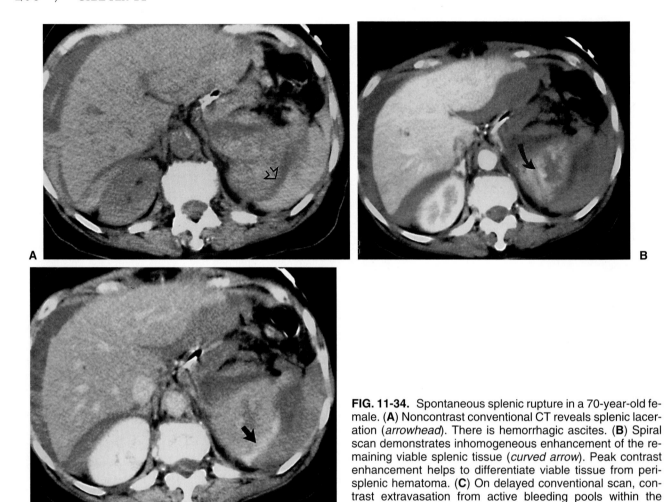

FIG. 11-34. Spontaneous splenic rupture in a 70-year-old female. **(A)** Noncontrast conventional CT reveals splenic laceration (*arrowhead*). There is hemorrhagic ascites. **(B)** Spiral scan demonstrates inhomogeneous enhancement of the remaining viable splenic tissue (*curved arrow*). Peak contrast enhancement helps to differentiate viable tissue from perisplenic hematoma. **(C)** On delayed conventional scan, contrast extravasation from active bleeding pools within the splenic laceration (*arrow*).

crescentic collection along the margin of the spleen that flattens the normally convex margin.

Optimal contrast enhancement with spiral scanning increases conspicuity of splenic injuries. Because the normal spleen enhances brightly against the injured tissue, lacerations and hematomas are more apparent with bolus contrast enhancement. Viable splenic tissue can be easily differentiated from surrounding clot (Fig. 11-34). Furthermore, single breath-hold acquisition using spiral CT markedly diminishes data misregistration, which is problematic with conventional CT due to variable diaphragmatic excursions in the upper abdomen. Spiral CT ensures continuous coverage of the entire spleen free from breathing artifact, enhancing detection of small splenic lacerations (Fig. 11-35).

The normal mottled appearance of the enhanced spleen should not be mistaken for splenic trauma. In our experience, dynamic enhancement with spiral scanning does not create diagnostic difficulty (32). Furthermore, in the setting of the acutely ill or injured patient, the benefits of spiral scanning far outweigh this potential pitfall. If uncertainty persists, delayed scans of the spleen can always be performed following the spiral acquisition.

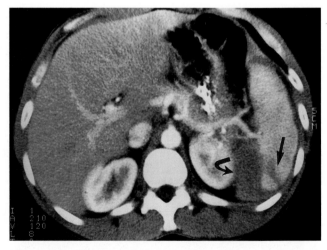

FIG. 11-35. Splenic laceration following motor vehicle accident in a 36-year-old male. A small laceration (*straight arrow*) is seen in the inferior tip of the spleen. Minimal perisplenic hematoma is seen near the site of injury (*curved arrow*).

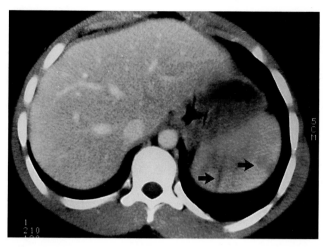

FIG. 11-36. Splenic laceration following motor vehicle accident in a 14-year-old male. Spiral scan detects subtle lacerations (*arrows*) in the superior aspect of the spleen.

Delayed splenic rupture is a well-defined clinical entity, often occurring more than 48 hours after trauma. The reported prevalence of delayed rupture is from 0.3% to 20% (33). Many of these cases likely represent small splenic lacerations without subcapsular hemorrhage, undetected at the initial time of trauma. Spiral scanning is very useful in detecting very subtle splenic lacerations and in our experience has been helpful in identifying those patients with subtle injuries who are at increased risk for delayed rupture (Fig. 11-36). In these patients careful hemodynamic monitoring is warranted.

REFERENCES

1. Piekarski J, Federle MP, Moss M, London SS. Computed tomography of the spleen. *Radiology* 1980;135:683–689.
2. Freeman JL, Jafri SZH, Roberts JL, Mezwa DG, Shirkhoda A. CT of congenital and acquired abnormalities of the spleen. *Radiographics* 1993;13:597–610.
3. Rabushka LS, Kawashima A, Fishman EK. Imaging of the spleen: CT with supplemental MR examination. *Radiographics* 1994;14:307–332.
4. Zeman RK, Fox SH, Silverman PM, et al. Helical (spiral) CT of the abdomen. *AJR* 1993;160:719–725.
5. Zeman RK, Zeiberg AS, Davros WJ, et al. Routine helical CT of the abdomen: image quality considerations. *Radiology* 1993;189:395–400.
6. Robbins SL, Cotran RS, Kumar V. *Pathologic basis of disease*, 3rd ed. Philadelphia: WB Saunders; 1984:884–942.
7. Miles KA, McPherson SJ, Hayball MP. Transient splenic inhomogeneity with contrast-enhanced CT: mechanism and effect of liver disease. *Radiology* 1995;194:91–95.
8. Glazer GM, Axel L, Goldberg HI, Moss AA. Dynamic CT of the normal spleen. *AJR* 1981;137:343–346.
9. Castellino R, Silverman J, Glatstein E, Blank N, Wexler L. Splenic arteriography in Hodgkin's disease: a roentgenologic-pathologic study in 33 consecutive untreated patients. *AJR* 1972;114:574–582.
10. Shirkhoda A, Ros R, Farah J, et al. Lymphoma of the solid abdominal viscera. *Radiol Clin North Am* 1990;155:805–810.
11. Lee JKT, Sagel SS, Stanley RJ. *Computed body tomography with MRI correlation*, 2nd ed. New York: Raven Press; 1989:521–541.
12. Kadin M, Glatstein E, Dorfman R. Clinicopathologic studies of 117 untreated patients subjected to laparotomy for the staging of Hodgkin's disease. *Cancer* 1971;27:1277–1294.
13. Kishikawa T, Numaguchi Y, Tokunaga M, Matsuura K. Hemangiosarcoma of the spleen with liver metastases: angiographic manifestations. *Radiology* 1977;123:31–35.
14. Moss CN, van Dyke JA, Koehler RE, Smedberg CT. Multiple cavernous hemangiomas of the spleen. *J Comput Assist Tomogr* 1986;10: 338–340.
15. Pakter RL, Fishman EK, Nussbaum A, Giargiana FA, Zerhouni EA. CT findings in splenic hemangiomas in the Klippel-Trenaunay-Weber syndrome. *J Comput Assist Tomogr* 1987;11:88–91.
16. Marymont J Jr, Gross S. Patterns of metastatic cancer in the spleen. *Am J Clin Pathol* 1963;40:58–66.
17. Van der Laan RT, Verbeeten B, Smits NJ, Lubbers MJ. Computed tomography in the diagnosis and treatment of solitary splenic abscesses. *J Comput Assist Tomogr* 1989;13:71–74.
18. Miller JH, Greenfield LD, Wald BR. Candidiasis of the liver and spleen in childhood. *Radiology* 1982;142:375–380.
19. Shirkhoda A. CT findings in hepatosplenic and renal candidiasis. *J Comput Assist Tomogr* 1987;11:795–798.
20. Pastakia B, Shawker TH, Thaler M, O'Leary T, Pizzo PA. Hepatosplenic candidiasis: wheels within wheels. *Radiology* 1988;166: 417–421.
21. Choi BI, Im JG, Han MC, Lee HS. Hepatosplenic tuberculosis with hypersplenism: CT evaluation. *Gastrointest Radiol* 1989;14:265–267.
22. Hulnick DH, Megibow AJ, Naidich DP, Hilton S, Cho KC, Balthazar EJ. Abdominal tuberculosis: CT evaluation. *Radiology* 1985;157: 199–204.
23. Epstein BM, Mann JH. CT of abdominal tuberculosis. *AJR* 1982;139: 861–866.
24. Im JG, Song KS, Kang HS, et al. Mediastinal tuberculous lymphadenitis: CT manifestations. *Radiology* 1987;164:115–119.
25. Balcar I, Seltzer SE, Davis S, Geller S. CT patterns of splenic infarction: a clinical and experimental study. *Radiology* 1984;151:723–729.
26. Fishman EK, Wyatt SH, Ney DR, Kuhlman JE, Siegelman SS. Spiral CT of the pancreas with multiplanar display. *AJR* 1992;159: 1209–1215.
27. Fishman EK, Soyer P, Bliss DF, Bluemke DA, Devine N. Splenic involvement in pancreatitis: spectrum of CT findings. *AJR* 1995;164: 631–635.
28. Federle MP, Griffiths B, Minagi H, Jeffrey RB. Splenic trauma: evaluation with CT. *Radiology* 1987;162:69–71.
29. Jeffrey RB, Laing FC, Federle MP, Goodman PC. Computed tomography of splenic trauma. *Radiology* 1981;141:729–732.
30. Wing VW, Federle MP, Morris JA, Jeffrey RB, Bluth R. The clinical impact of CT for blunt abdominal trauma. *AJR* 1985;14:1191–1194.
31. Orwig D, Federle MP. Localized clotted blood as evidence of visceral trauma on CT: the sentinel clot sign. *AJR* 1989;153:747–749.
32. Fishman EK. Spiral CT: applications in the emergency patient. *Radiographics* 1996;16:943–948.
33. Leppaniemi A, Haapiainen R, Standertskjod-Nordenstam CG, Taavitsainen M, Hastbacka J. Delayed presentation of blunt splenic injury. *Am J Surg* 1988;155:745–749.

CHAPTER 12

Spiral CT of the Esophagus and Stomach

Karen M. Horton and Elliot K. Fishman

Spiral computed tomography (CT) represents the latest advancement in gastrointestinal tract imaging by combining rapid contrast infusion, fast scanning, narrow collimation, and close interscan spacing. These distinct advantages over conventional CT, along with three-dimensional (3D) data manipulation and display capabilities, have made spiral CT an important adjunct to endoscopy and barium studies for the evaluation of many gastrointestinal diseases. In particular, spiral CT has come to play a valuable role in imaging both benign and malignant disease of the esophagus and stomach.

ESOPHAGUS

Although endoscopy and barium studies are often considered to be the diagnostic modalities of choice for evaluation of benign and malignant diseases of the esophagus, they only image the mucosa, providing little information about intramural or extraluminal spread of disease. Therefore CT has come to play an important role in evaluation of esophageal pathology due to its unique ability to accurately visualize the lumen, wall, adjacent structures, lymphadenopathy, and distant metastases. Although the accuracy of CT has been debated in the past, spiral CT has specific advantages that can overcome many of the prior limitations. We will discuss the role of spiral CT in evaluation of the esophagus, with particular emphasis on esophageal carcinoma.

Exam Technique

Accurate imaging of the esophagus requires the administration of both oral and intravenous contrast with careful attention to technique.

For esophageal imaging, 500 mL of a 3% oral Hypaque (Hypaque; Nycomed, Princeton, NJ) solution is routinely administered approximately 30 min prior to the scan to fully distend the stomach and proximal small bowel loops. An

additional 250 mL of oral contrast is given immediately prior to scanning to ensure maximal distention of the stomach. Once the patient is positioned on the scanning table, a low-density esophageal paste is administered immediately before the start of the intravenous injection. The paste (Esoph-o-CAT, E-Z-M Co., Westbury, NY) allows good opacification of the esophagus without creating streak artifacts.

The administration of intravenous contrast is essential for complete evaluation of esophageal disease, especially if extraluminal extension of disease is to be accurately evaluated. An intravenous injection of 120 mL of Omnipaque 300 or 100 mL of Omnipaque 350 is administered at a rate of 2–3 mL/s. Scanning begins approximately 40–50 s after the initiation of the injection. Five-mm collimation can be performed with a table speed of 8 mm/s and a reconstruction interval of 5 mm. Images should be obtained from above the thoracic inlet through the liver. In select cases, narrow collimation (i.e., 3 mm) may be used, which is especially useful to assess local tumor spread.

Imaging at deep inspiration with a single breath hold results in better distention of the posterior wall of the trachea. This may be helpful when assessing tracheal invasion by the tumor (1).

Recently, a new barium paste mixture has been described consisting of carboxy-methyl cellulose sodium paste containing barium sulfate (2). This new mixture reportedly improves opacification rates of the esophageal lumen compared with studies using Esoph-o-CAT.

Normal Esophagus

The esophagus is a muscular tube that transports food and liquid from the pharynx to the stomach and prevents the reflux of stomach contents. The esophageal wall comprises five distinct layers: mucosa, muscularis mucosa, submucosa, and the inner and outer muscularis propria. There is no serosal layer. Thus malignant disease can easily spread to adjacent mediastinal structures.

On CT, the esophagus is routinely well visualized because of natural contrast provided by the surrounding lung and mediastinal fat planes. In normal patients the esophagus is typically collapsed, although it may contain a small amount of air on several individual slices (3).

The normal esophageal wall is very thin, usually less than 3 mm when the esophagus is distended (4). Wall thickness greater than 5 mm is definitely abnormal (5). As the esophagus traverses the diaphragmatic hiatus to join the cardia of the stomach, the wall may normally appear thickened. This should not be confused with pathology at the gastroesophageal junction.

Esophageal Cancer

Esophageal carcinoma comprises approximately 1% of all cancers and 6% of the gastrointestinal tract malignancies diagnosed in the United States each year (6). The estimated number of new cases in 1996 was 12,300.

Males are four times more likely to develop esophageal cancer than females, and the risk increases with age. Worldwide, more than 90% of esophageal malignancies are squamous cell carcinomas, most of which are located in the mid-esophagus. Use of tobacco and the consumption of alcohol constitute the two most common risk factors for the development of squamous cell carcinoma of the esophagus. There are also many conditions that predispose to the development of squamous cell carcinoma of the esophagus, including caustic stricture, achalasia, celiac disease, radiation, Plummer-Vinson syndrome, history of oral or pharyngeal cancer, and tylosis palmaris and plantaris.

Adenocarcinoma historically has comprised only a minority of esophageal cancers. However, in the last 20 years, a changing epidemiology has been observed in the United states, where the incidence of adenocarcinoma has risen significantly (7,8). The reason for this trend is not fully understood. Adenocarcinoma almost always arises in Barrett mucosa, a sequela of long-term gastroesophageal reflux. Two-thirds of adenocarcinomas arising in Barrett mucosa are located in the distal esophagus.

Surgery continues to be the most important treatment for patients with either histology who have localized disease. Although advances in surgical techniques have lowered operative mortality and shortened hospital stay, the surgery remains complex, with a reported operative mortality of approximately 30%. Neoadjuvant chemoradiation therapy combined with surgery may help improve survival (9). Recent trends include using chemotherapy and radiation therapy to downstage patients before performing surgery. Initial results with this protocol have been positive, almost doubling the 5-year survival rate compared with surgery alone (9). However, the 5-year survival rate for patients with esophageal cancer continues to be poor, as most patients still present with metastatic or locally advanced stage disease.

TABLE 12-1. *TMN staging of esophageal carcinoma*

Tis	Carcinoma in situ
T1	Invasion of lamina propria or submucosa
T2	Invasion of muscularis propria
T3	Invasion of adventitia
T4	Invasion of adjacent structure
N0	No regional nodes involved
N1	Regional nodes involved
M0	No distant metastasis
M1	Distant metastasis (including nodes outside mediastinum)
Stage 0	Tis, N0, M0
Stage I	T1, N0, M0
Stage IIA	T2/T3, N0, M0
Stage IIB	T1/T2, N1, M0
Stage III	T3, N1, M0 or T4, N0/1, M0
Stage IV	T1-4, N0/1, M1

Staging and Treatment

Adequate preoperative staging of esophageal cancer is essential to determine whether therapy should be directed toward cure or palliation. The TMN system is widely used for the staging of esophageal cancer and is based on information obtained from a variety of sources: endoscopy, biopsy, endoscopic ultrasonography, barium studies, CT, bone scintigraphy, and so on (Table 12-1, Fig. 12-1). In addition, Moss et al. have proposed a staging system that is specific for CT (10) (see Table 12-2).

In patients with limited disease, esophagectomy is the treatment of choice, with or without pre or postoperative chemoradiation therapy. Extraesophageal extension of disease typically precludes curative surgery. Palliative procedures include, surgery, radiotherapy, chemotherapy, esophageal prosthesis, and laser therapy.

Stages I and II

Although the initial diagnosis of esophageal carcinoma is often made at endoscopy or barium esophagography, the primary tumor can often be visualized on CT. The primary tumor can appear as a focal area of wall thickening (>5 mm), circumferential thickening, or a discrete soft-tissue mass (Fig. 12-2). CT is accurate at judging tumor size, and there is a reported association between lesions more than 3.0 cm wide on CT and the presence of periesophageal spread (11). CT estimates of tumor length may not be as

TABLE 12-2. *CT-specific staging of esophageal carcinoma (Moss)*

Stage I	Intraluminal polypoid mass or focal wall thickening of 3–5 mm
Stage II	Focal wall thickening >5 mm
Stage III	Wall thickening and direct invasion of adjacent structures, ± local adenopathy
Stage IV	Distant metastasis

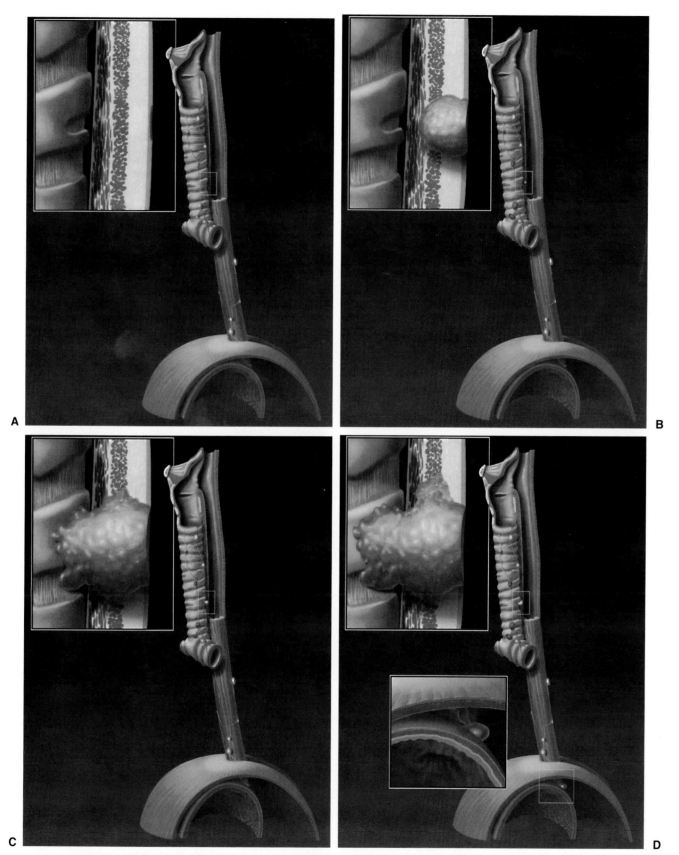

FIG. 12-1. TMN staging system. Schematic diagrams illustrate the TMN staging of esophageal carcinoma. (**A**) Stage O. Carcinoma in situ. (**B**) Stage II (T2, N1, M0). Tumor invasion into muscularis propria with regional nodal involvement. Note that the nodes in red are malignant while those in white are normal. (**C**) Stage III (T4, N1, MO). Tumor extension through the esophageal wall with involvement of the trachea. Regional lymph nodes are also involved. (**D**) Stage IV (T4, N1, M1). Extraesophageal spread of tumor with involvement of regional nodes, trachea, and distant metastases.

213

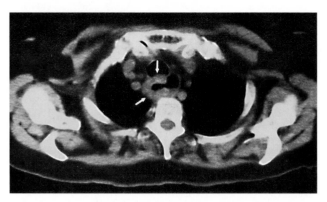

FIG. 12-2. CT stage II esophageal cancer. Seventy-three-year-old female with squamous cell carcinoma of the upper esophagus. CT scan demonstrates tumor involving the right esophageal wall (*arrows*) without evidence of local tumor spread.

accurate, possibly because of surrounding edema or inflammatory changes, especially in patients after chemoradiation therapy (12). Specific areas of difficulty are especially common in tumors of the distal esophagus, where spread into the stomach may be difficult to accurately define.

Complications resulting from the primary tumor can also be detected with CT such as obstruction, perforation, or fistulization (Fig. 12-3).

Stage III

Stage III tumors are characterized by mediastinal extension of tumors with or without local adenopathy. Mediastinal invasion can involve the periesophageal fat, tracheobronchial tree, aorta, pericardium, or diaphragm.

Early periesophageal invasion may appear as increased attention of the fat surrounding the esophagus (13). Tracheobronchial tree involvement is suspected when the posterior wall of the airway is displaced or compressed by the adjacent

tumor mass (14) (Fig. 12-4). Invasion of the aorta is more difficult to assess accurately. The normal esophagus is separated from the aorta by a fat plane. Picus has reported that if 90 degrees or more of the aorta is in contact with the tumor (no discrete fat plane between), this strongly suggests invasion (15) (Fig. 12-5). Similarly, tumor invasion of the pericardium is suspected if the normal surrounding fat plane is obliterated. CT does not appear able to detect diaphragmatic invasion accurately (12), although this typically does not preclude an attempt at surgical resection.

Although fat plane obliteration is a reliable sign of tumor involvement of adjacent structure, the absence of distinct fat planes can occur as a normal variant in cachectic patients, or in patients who have received radiation therapy or surgery (16). In these situations, the fat planes may be absent throughout the mediastinum (4). However, invasion is likely if the fat plane is obliterated at the site of suspected invasion but intact at other nearby levels (14). Overall, the reported sensitivity of CT for detecting mediastinal invasion in patients with esophageal carcinoma ranges from 88% to 100%, with a specificity ranging between 85% and 100% (13–17).

The sensitivity of CT for detection of mediastinal lymphadenopathy is lower, as metastatic involvement of periesophageal nodes may not result in significant enlargement (12). In a study by Picus, almost all the periesophageal nodes containing tumor measured less than 7 mm, indistinguishable on CT from uninvolved nodes (15). Although some studies suggest a decreased postoperative survival in patients with localized nodal spread, at this time metastases to small periesophageal nodes is not considered a contraindication to surgical resection (18–20).

The accuracy of CT for predicting abdominal lymph node involvement ranges between 83% and 87% (1). CT is especially accurate in the detection of metastatic nodes in the celiac and left gastric region, a common site of nodal disease.

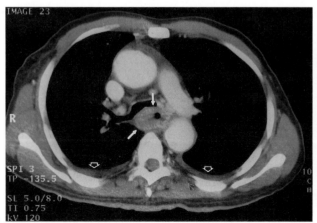
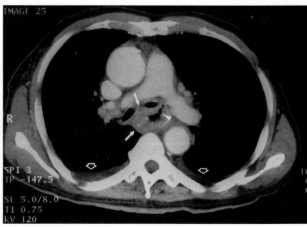

FIG. 12-3. Carcinoma of the esophagus with fistula. **(A)** Spiral CT demonstrates a carcinoma of the mid-esophagus, encasing the airway (*arrows*). **(B)** A fistula is present between the esophagus and left mainstem bronchus (*arrowhead*). Small bilateral pleural effusions are also identified (*open arrows*).

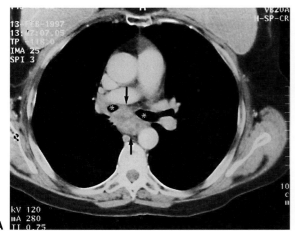
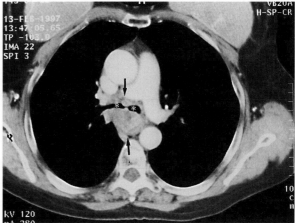

FIG. 12-4. (A,B) CT stage III esophageal cancer with invasion of airway. The spiral CT scan demonstrates a bulky esophageal cancer (*arrows*) with tumor invading both the left and right mainstem bronchi (*asterisks*). Although early invasion of the airway may be difficult to ascertain with CT scanning, with narrow collimation and close interscan intervals (spiral CT) this is easier to document.

Stage IV

Spiral CT is well suited for the detection of metastases to the solid abdominal organs (Fig. 12-6). CT has an established role in the detection of liver metastases in patients with a variety of primary tumors. The detection of liver masses with standard incremental CT varies from series to series but usually ranges from 60% to 75% (21–24). However, the sensitivity of spiral CT for the detection of masses measuring 1 cm or more is around 90% (25). The accuracy of magnetic resonance (MR) and that of CT for evaluation of liver metas-

tases are equivalent (26), but these data were for standard dynamic CT scanning. Currently, spiral CT is the preferred method for liver evaluation.

Spiral scanning with rapid IV contrast injection is considered the preferred technique for liver imaging. With spiral CT the entire liver can be imaged in one breath-hold sequence. Faster scanning eliminates respiratory misregistration and allows imaging during the optimal window for lesion contrast enhancement. A recent study of the detection of hepatic masses using spiral CT demonstrated a better than 90% sensitivity for detecting liver lesions measuring more than 1 cm, and a 56% sensitivity for detecting lesions of less than 1 cm (25). This represents an improvement compared

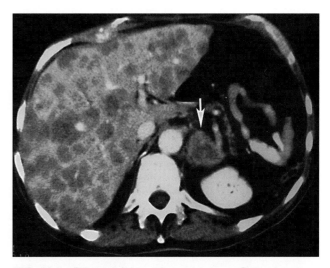

FIG. 12-5. Esophageal carcinoma with aortic involvement. Spiral CT demonstrates diffuse circumferential thickening of the esophageal wall with loss of normal fat planes between the esophagus and aorta, indicating aortic involvement.

FIG. 12-6. CT stage IV esophageal cancer. Sixty-nine-year-old male with squamous cell carcinoma of the esophagus. CT scan demonstrates multiple liver metastases as well as metastases to the left adrenal gland (*arrow*).

with traditional incremental CT scanning. Spiral CT may also promote dual-phase liver imaging (arterial- and portal-phase studies, which can increase the detection rate further (see Chapter 9).

Postoperative Esophagus

The most common surgical procedure performed today for the treatment of malignant disease of the esophagus is the partial esophagogastrectomy. This consists of a transhiatal esophagectomy followed by either a gastric pull-up or colonic interposition. The surgical procedure is complex and can result in a number of postsurgical complications, including anastomotic leak or stricture, mediastinal abscess, chylothorax, or lymphocele. It is important for the radiologist to be familiar with the normal postoperative appearance and to be aware of the potential complications to optimally evaluate these patients in the postoperative period.

Recurrence

Even after curative resection, many patients with esophageal carcinoma experience recurrence (Fig. 12-7). In a recent study by Morita of 187 cases after curative esophagectomy for squamous cell carcinoma, more than 50% of the patients died of recurrence (27). The most common recurrence patterns included lymphatic (48%), hematogenous (24%), mixed lymphatic and hematogenous (23%), and intramural recurrence (4%). The most common organs involved with recurrence are lung, liver, and bone (28). Thus, although endoscopy and endoscopic ultrasound are effective at diagnosis of anastomotic tumor recurrence as well as regional lymph node involvement, CT is important for follow-up to detect distant metastases. The prognosis following recurrence is extremely poor. However, recent advancements with neoadjuvant chemoradiation therapy combined with surgery may help improve survival by decreasing recurrence rates (9).

Benign Diseases

Esophageal Varices

In patients with portal hypertension, increased resistance to portal venous flow in the liver results in the development of portosystemic collaterals. The most common and clinically relevant collaterals involve the paraesophageal venous plexus. Because of the high resistance flow in the liver, blood flows from the portal system retrograde through the left coronary vein or short gastric veins to the esophageal venous plexus and eventually empties into the azygous system.

Spiral CT with intravenous contrast is an excellent modality for the detection and evaluation of portosystemic shunts in patients with portal hypertension (29). The sensitivity of CT for the detection of varices is comparable with that of barium esophogram. However, CT allows better evaluation of the extent and size of varices as well as the ability to detect other portosystemic collaterals (30).

The CT appearance of esophageal varices varies depending on the size and extent of involvement (4). Usually, on unenhanced scans, esophageal varices appear as thickening or nodularity of the esophageal wall. With IV contrast, esophageal varices will appear as enhancing vascular structures within the esophageal wall (31) (Figs. 12-8, 12-9). On noncontrast scans, large varices can simulate adenopathy in the posterior mediastinum, which is a potential pitfall.

CT angiography with volume rendering can also be used to better evaluate portosystemic collaterals. In particular, the CT appearance of esophageal varices is distinctive. Furthermore, the use of 3D reconstruction with volume rendering clearly demonstrates esophageal venous collaterals and their relationship to the portal and systemic venous systems.

Esophagitis

There are many causes of esophagitis, including gastroesophageal reflux, radiation therapy, corrosive ingestions, Crohn disease, and a variety of infections. Immunosup-

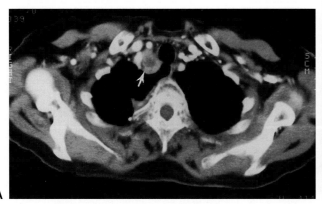
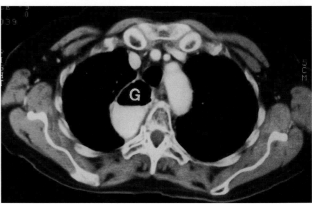

FIG. 12-7. Recurrent esophageal cancer. (**A**) Spiral CT scan demonstrates metastatic involvement of a large mediastinal node (*arrow*) in this patient with a history of esophageal cancer. (**B**) The patient had a history of prior esophagectomy and gastric pull-up (G).

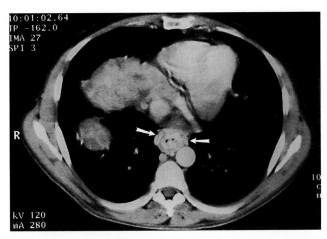

FIG. 12-8. Esophageal varices. Forty-three-year-old male with history of metastatic colon cancer. Spiral CT reveals enhancing vessels within the esophageal wall (*arrows*) compatible with varices. Multiple liver metastases are also present.

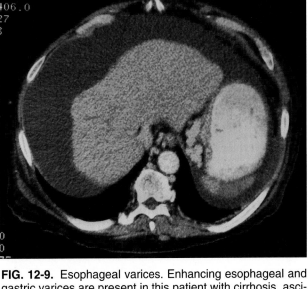

FIG. 12-9. Esophageal varices. Enhancing esophageal and gastric varices are present in this patient with cirrhosis, ascites, and portal hypertension.

pressed patients are particularly prone to certain esophageal infections such as those caused by *Candida,* herpes simplex, cytomegalovirus, and tuberculosis. Candidiasis is the most common cause of infectious esophagitis and results from the spread of the fungus from the oropharynx to the esophagus (4).

Regardless of the etiology, the CT findings of esophagitis usually consist of nonspecific diffuse esophageal wall thickening (Fig. 12-10). Occasionally, deep esophageal ulceration is identified. If ulceration, intramural dissection, and fistula formation are identified, tuberculosis should be considered as the possible etiologic agent (32).

Achalasia

Achalasia is a motor disorder of the esophagus characterized by inadequate relaxation of the lower esophageal sphincter and failure of organized peristalsis in the lower esophagus. Although the condition is usually evaluated with barium studies and endoscopy, CT plays a role.

CT in patients with achalasia demonstrates moderate to marked dilatation of the esophagus, with a mean esophageal diameter of 4.5 cm at the level of the carina (33) (Fig. 12-11). There is often an abrupt transition from the dilated esophagus to normal at the gastroesophageal junction. Air, fluid, or food particles are often present in the lumen (Fig. 12-12). The esophageal wall is usually of normal thickness.

Since achalasia is associated with the development of esophageal carcinoma, CT can detect and demonstrate the extent of esophageal neoplasms occurring in these patients.

STOMACH

Although barium studies and endoscopy have classically been considered the diagnostic modalities of choice for the evaluation of gastric pathology, CT is increasingly used as the first-line imaging study in patients with a variety of symptoms. It is imperative, therefore, that the radiologist be

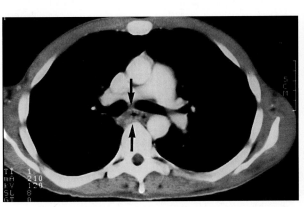

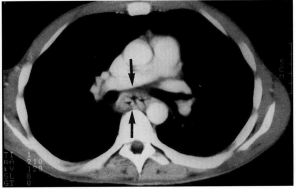

FIG. 12-10. (A,B) Esophagitis. Esophagitis in a patient with a history of AIDS and chest pain. Spiral CT demonstrated definite thickening of the esophagus (*arrows*) with possible ulceration. The patient was subsequently proven to have *Candida* esophagitis. The esophageal wall thickening caused by esophagitis is often impossible to distinguish from carcinoma based simply on the pattern of wall thickening.

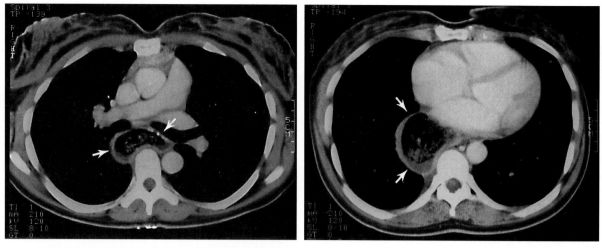

FIG. 12-11. (A,B) Achalasia of the esophagus. CT scan shows a markedly dilated esophagus (*arrows*), with retained food particles. Because of its large size the esophagus is displaced to the right of midline. There is an increased incidence of esophageal cancer; therefore careful follow-up is necessary with these patients.

familiar with the CT appearance of the normal stomach as well as the appearance of a variety of gastric conditions. In addition, CT plays an important role in the staging and follow-up of gastric malignancies, once the diagnosis has been established.

The advent of spiral CT and current interest in the use of water- and air-contrast techniques suggest that the usefulness of CT in evaluating gastric pathology may increase.

Technique

For adequate CT examination of the stomach, careful technique is essential. The key to CT imaging of the stomach

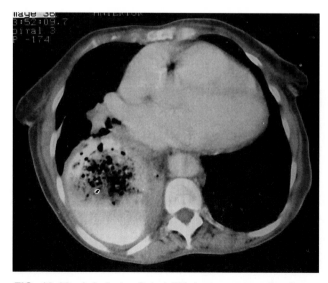

FIG. 12-12. Achalasia. Spiral CT demonstrates classic example of achalasia. The patient presented with mediastinal widening on chest x-ray that was due to the markedly dilated esophagus with food matter within it.

is gastric distention, as wall thickening can be simulated by underdistention. Gastric distention can be accomplished with positive contrast solutions such as Hypaque, with water, or with effervescent gas crystals.

Positive Contrast

Traditionally, for abdominal imaging, positive contrast agents such as Hypaque (Nycomed, Princeton, NJ) have been utilized. Routinely, 500 mL of a 3% oral Hypaque solution is administered 30–60 min before the scan to fill the stomach and small bowel loops. An additional 250 mL of oral contrast is given immediately prior to scanning to ensure maximal distention of the stomach.

Although they are widely used, there is some concern that positive contrast agents may obscure bowel wall pathology when the gastrointestinal wall is simultaneously enhanced with intravenous agents. In addition, there are reports of inadequate mixing of these agents with gastrointestinal contents, sometimes resulting in pseudotumors (34). Finally, the use of positive oral contrast agents interferes with manipulation of the data set in CT angiography. Therefore investigators have explored alternative oral contrast agents for use with abdominal CT.

Water Contrast

Several investigators have advocated the use of water as a neutral contrast agent for imaging the stomach and upper gastrointestinal tract (35–39). Water is safe, well tolerated, and inexpensive. Water may allow better visualization of the enhanced wall of the stomach and small bowel and will not interfere with CT angiography, which positive contrast agents have been said to do. Limitations of the use of water include suboptimal evaluation of the distal small bowel and colon, confusion between water-filled bowel loops and abnormal abdominal fluid collections (abscess), inability to image enteric fistulas, and limited ability to diagnose extravasation of contrast from gastrointestinal perforation (35). If water contrast is desired, 750 mL of water is given 30 min before the exam. An additional 250 mL of water is given to the patient immediately before scanning begins.

Air Contrast

If air contrast is desired, effervescent citrocarbonate granules (4–6 g) can be given with 30 mL of water. Gaseous distention alone, although good for evaluation of stomach pathology, does not provide adequate contrast for the remainder of the bowel. Gas granules can also be administered after the patient has consumed the Hypaque or water for additional air distention of the stomach.

Air is a negative contrast agent and therefore allows better visualization of the bowel wall enhancement without interfering with CT angiography.

IV Contrast

Regardless of the oral contrast agent used, the administration of intravenous contrast is essential for complete evaluation of the stomach. Spiral CT combines rapid scanning and rapid infusion of contrast, resulting in better visualization of bowel loops and the gastric wall (Fig. 12-13). Often subtle changes are well visualized.

Typically, 120 mL of Omnipaque 300 or 100 mL of Omnipaque 350 is injected intravenously, at a rate of 2–3 mL/s. Scanning begins approximately 45 s after the initiation of the contrast injection. Five-millimeter collimation can be performed with a table speed of 5 mm/s and a reconstruction interval of 3 mm though the liver and consecutive 8-mm sections through the remainder of the abdomen and pelvis. Images should be obtained from above the diaphragm through the symphysis pubis.

Occasionally, during the examination, alternate positioning of the patient may be necessary for the best visualization of different regions of the stomach. For example, the prone position is usually optimal for evaluation of pathology at the gastroesophageal junction and greater curvature, whereas supine positioning is appropriate if the lesser curvature or antrum is involved. However, with spiral CT, this is usually unnecessary.

Normal Stomach

The gastric fundus lies in the left upper quadrant of the abdomen. The gastroesophageal junction can be identified as a small soft-tissue mass that indents the medial aspect of the cardia. The body of the stomach obliquely crosses the midline anteriorly and then curves posteriorly to become the antrum. The pylorus can be identified by its narrowed lumen, connecting the antrum to the duodenal bulb (40).

Optimal distention of the stomach results in effacement of the normal folds. The normal gastric wall is very thin, usually measuring 5–7 mm when the stomach is distended (Fig. 12-14). Wall thickness greater than 8–10 mm is definitely abnormal. However, the wall of the fundus and antrum may appear thicker than the remainder of the stomach, because of their orientation within the scanning plane. This should not be confused with pathology at these sites.

The stomach is surrounded by perigastric fat, which should be of uniform density. Increased density in the perigastric fat or loss of fat planes between the stomach and adjacent organs indicates pathology.

Gastric Malignancy

Adenocarcinoma of the Stomach

Adenocarcinoma represents approximately 95% of malignant gastric tumors. The incidence continues to decrease in the United States, with 22,800 new cases expected in the United States in 1996 (6). However, the prevalence of gastric

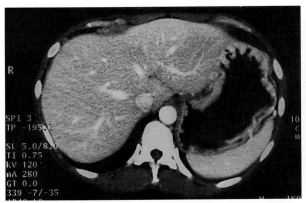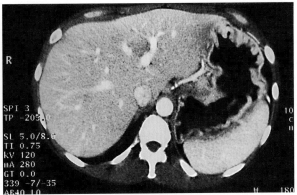

FIG. 12-13. (A,B) Normal gastric folds. CT scan of the stomach with air distention of the stomach demonstrates normal enhancement of the gastric folds. Recent literature suggests that early detection of gastric cancer may be possible by observing changes in the fold enhancement pattern.

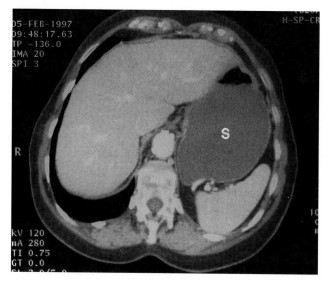

FIG. 12-14. Normal stomach. Spiral CT scan of the abdomen demonstrates adequate gastric distention (s). The wall of the stomach is very thin, measuring only 2–3 mm in this patient.

carcinoma continues to be high in other countries, such as Japan, Chile, and Iceland. The 5-year survival rate is approximately 20%.

Males are affected more commonly than females, with most patients presenting in the sixth decade. Several conditions have been identified that may predispose to the development of adenocarcinoma of the stomach, including pernicious anemia, gastric atrophy, Billroth II, achlorhydria, and hypochlorhydria. In addition, dietary habits, geographic factors, and race are important (41). In the last several years there has been much interest in exploring a possible relationship between *Helicobacter pylori* and gastric cancer (42). Further studies are needed to fully understand *H. pylori*'s role.

Staging and Treatment

CT is the most frequently used imaging modality for staging adenocarcinoma of the stomach. However, its precise role remains controversial. Some surgeons recommend laparotomy in all cases of gastric cancer for either curative resection or palliation, obviating the need for a CT scan. Conversely, many surgeons rely on CT findings to help stage the malignancy, plan patient therapy, and plan the surgical approach. The literature has reported widely varying accuracy for using CT to stage gastric cancer; this has been partly due to differences in scanning techniques during the past two decades. With the advent of spiral CT, combining narrow collimation and close interspace scanning, it is very likely that the accuracy of CT will improve.

Moss proposed a useful CT-based staging system that has been widely accepted (43) (Fig. 12-15) (see color plate 12 following p. 48). The major goal of CT is to determine if there is direct invasion of adjacent organs, enlargement of local nodes, or evidence of distant metastases. Surgical cure

is unlikely in cases representing stage III and IV disease. CT will typically upstage disease from stage II to stage III or IV.

In patients with limited disease (stage I and II), partial gastrectomy is the treatment of choice. The median survival for patients after subtotal gastrectomy is 18 months; after total gastrectomy it is only 12 months. The success of gastrectomy depends on the extent of gastric wall invasion and lymphatic spread. Chemoradiation protocols are being tested in an attempt to improve survival after gastrectomy.

Stages I and II

Common CT appearances of primary gastric carcinoma include discrete soft-tissue mass (Fig. 12-16) with or without ulceration or wall thickening, which may be focal or diffuse (linitis plastica) (44). The average wall thickness in gastric carcinoma is 2 cm, ranging from 6 mm to 4.0 cm. Because of limited spatial resolution, CT is often unable to distinguish the layers within the gastric wall and therefore cannot determine depth of tumor invasion. However, CT can accurately demonstrate wall thickening, which has been shown to correlate directly with probability of transmural extension.

In a recent study by Cho et al. using water contrast, dynamic scanning, rapid intravenous contrast injection, and dual-phase image acquisition, 88% of the primary gastric cancers were detected. This detection rate could improve if spiral scanning were utilized (45).

Stage III

Stage III tumors are characterized by extragastric extension of tumor with or without regional adenopathy (Fig. 12-17). Early perigastric invasion may appear as increased attention of the fat surrounding the stomach or as obliteration of fat planes separating the stomach from adjacent organs (i.e., pancreas) (Fig. 12-18). Although fat plane obliteration is a reliable sign of extragastric tumor invasion, distinct fat planes can be absent as a normal variant in cachectic patients, or in patients with inflammatory conditions such as pancreatitis. The most problematic area for CT in staging gastric neoplasms is in determining pancreatic invasion (46,47). This inability of CT to distinguish between fat plane obliteration due to inflammation from tumor has limited CT's usefulness in staging the primary tumor.

The detection of adenopathy is important in evaluation of gastric carcinomas, as perigastric lymph node involvement decreases median survival by 65% (48). Nodal spread of disease may extend into or around the gastrohepatic ligament. Nodes in this region are considered suspicious for harboring malignancy if they are greater than 8 mm in diameter (49). Although the best indication of lymph node involvement is enlargement, it has been shown that normal-sized nodes may contain tumor, whereas some enlarged nodes do not. Multiple enlarged nodes are more likely to be malignant than a solitary enlarged node (50). Another factor that may

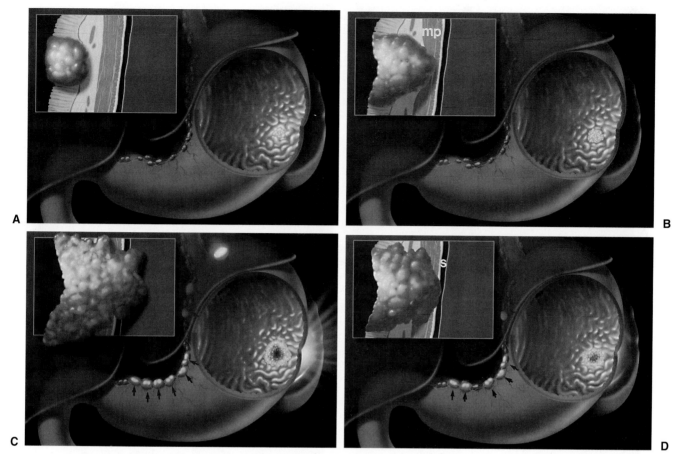

FIG. 12-15. CT staging system (Moss). Schematic diagrams illustrate the CT staging of esophageal carcinoma. (**A**) Stage I. An intraluminal mass is present that invades the mucosa without deeper tumor spread. (**B**) Stage II. There is greater than 1-cm wall thickness that invades through the submucosa into the muscularis propria (mp). There is no evidence of extragastric spread. (**C**) Stage III. The tumor invades through the muscularis propria and serosa (s). Enlarged nodes are seen (*arrows*). (**D**) Stage IV. Tumor has extended through the serosa into the peritoneal cavity. Enlarged nodes and liver metastases are also present.

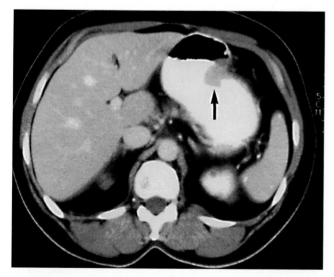

FIG. 12-16. CT stage II adenocarcinoma of the stomach. CT scan shows a polypoid gastric mass (*arrow*) without evidence of extension beyond the stomach. No evidence of metastasis is seen.

help distinguish metastatic from normal nodes is lack of enhancement.

The reported sensitivity of CT for detection of adenopathy in patients with adenocarcinoma of the stomach ranges between 47% and 97% (46,51,52). Although the use of spiral CT may help improve results, the major limitation is CT's inability to detect microscopic involvement of normal-sized nodes.

Stage IV

Spiral CT is excellent for the detection of distant metastases in patients with gastric cancer, as it combines rapid imaging and intravenous contrast injection with three-dimensional imaging display capabilities (Figs. 12-19, 12-20). Common sites for gastric metastatic disease include the liver, adrenal glands, and bone. In addition, gastric cancer can involve the ovaries (Krukenberg tumor) (Fig. 12-21). Gastric cancer may also be associated with carcinomatosis (Fig. 12-22).

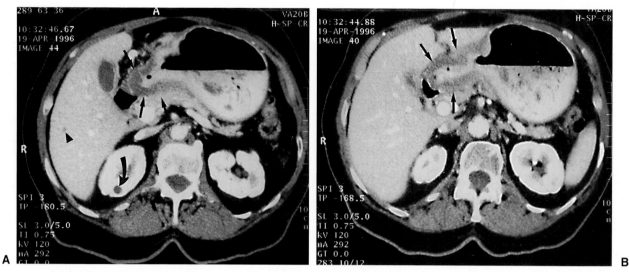

FIG. 12-17. (A,B) CT stage III gastric adenocarcinoma. Spiral CT demonstrates diffuse thickening infiltration of the gastric antrum consistent with gastric adenocarcinoma (*arrows*). Minimal spread into the perigastric soft tissue was seen, but no distal metastasis noted. A small incidental liver cyst (*arrowhead*) and right renal cyst (*curved arrow*) were also seen.

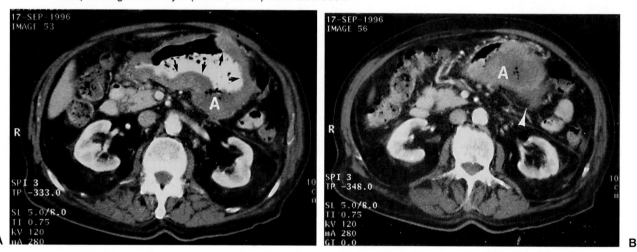

FIG. 12-18. CT stage III gastric adenocarcinoma with spread into the perigastric tissues. Spiral CT demonstrates a large bulky ulcerating gastric mass (*black arrows*). There is a perforation with a walled-off abscess (**A**) in the inferior-posterior aspect of the stomach. Infiltrating of the perigastric tissues can also be identified (*arrowhead* in **B**). This study is a good example that not all bulky tumors represent lymphoma.

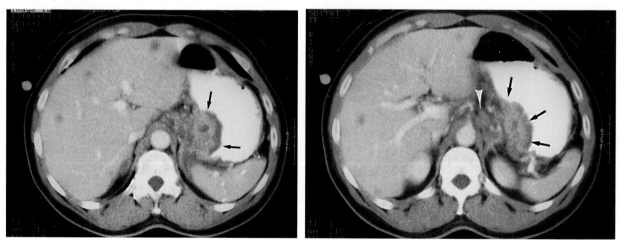

FIG. 12-19. CT stage IV adenocarcinoma of the stomach with liver metastasis. (**A**) Spiral CT demonstrates a bulky tumor in the gastric fundus (*arrows*) with apparent ulceration present. (**B**) There is also evidence of adenopathy in the celiac axis (*arrowheads*). Multiple small liver metastases are seen.

222

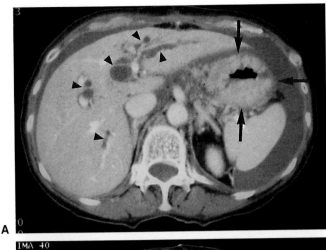

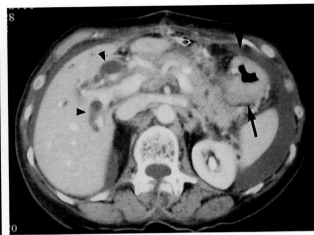

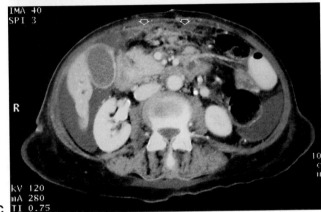

FIG. 12-20. (A–C) Stage IV adenocarcinoma of the stomach. Spiral CT scan demonstrates marked thickening of the gastric fundus (*black arrows*). There are also large, dilated, intrahepatic ducts (*arrowheads*) that are secondary to obstruction of the distal common bile duct by tumor encasement of the porta hepatis. Notice on this examination the encasement of the celiac axis and hepatic and splenic arteries by tumor with collateralization. Tumor implants are also seen on the omentum (*white open arrows*). Para-aortic adenopathy and subcrural nodes are also seen. Ascites is present. These are all pathways of spread of gastric cancer.

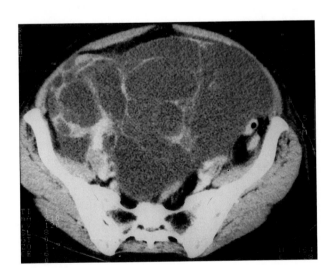

FIG. 12-21. Krukenberg tumor. Patient with metastatic gastric adenocarcinoma to the ovaries. Note the bilateral large cystic pelvic metastases consistent with metastatic Krukenberg tumors.

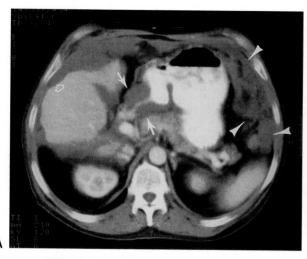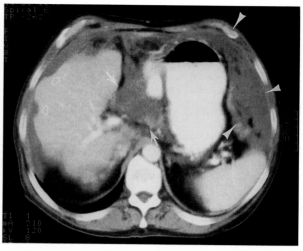

A

B

FIG. 12-22. (A,B) Stage IV adenocarcinoma of the stomach with carcinomatosis. Spiral CT scan demonstrates an infiltrating carcinoma of the gastric antrum (*arrows*). There is widespread carcinomatosis with implants on the mesentery and omentum (*arrowheads*). Scalloped implants on the liver are seen in a pattern suggestive of Pseudomyxoma peritonei (*open arrows*).

Spiral scanning with rapid IV contrast injection is considered the preferred technique for liver imaging. A recent study of the detection of hepatic masses using spiral CT demonstrated a better than 90% sensitivity for detecting lesions of more than 1 cm and a 56% sensitivity for detecting lesions of less than 1 cm (26). This is an improvement compared with traditional CT scanning.

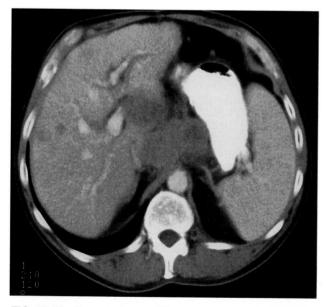

FIG. 12-23. Recurrent stage IV gastric adenocarcinoma. Spiral CT demonstrates tumor recurrence in the celiac axis and porta hepatis with large nodes present. Liver metastases were also seen in this patient following partial gastrectomy.

Postoperative Stomach and Recurrence

In a study by Ha et al. of 36 patients with tumor recurrence following gastrectomy, 69% of recurrences involved nodal spread along the celiac axis or hepatic pedicle (Fig. 12-23), 28% of recurrences involved the anastomotic site or gastric stump, 22% involved the pancreas, and 11% occurred in the anterior abdominal wall (53). A similar study by Mullin of 38 patients with recurrent tumor after gastrectomy for carcinoma also demonstrated that the majority of recurrence involved regional lymph nodes or metastases to organs such as the liver, lung, adrenals, or bone (54). Occasionally, the recurrence can be extensive, involving peritoneal implants and carcinomatosis (Fig. 12-24).

Endoscopic ultrasound, upper endoscopy and barium studies are often capable of detecting recurrence at the anastomosis or in the gastric stump, but they cannot image tumor spread to the abdominal wall or distant organs. In addition, CT is a useful guide for percutaneous biopsy of suspicious lesions.

Lymphoma

Gastric lymphoma comprises approximately 1% to 5% of all gastric malignancies, and represents the most common extranodal site of lymphoma. Most cases are non-Hodgkin's lymphomas, predominantly of the diffuse histiocytic subtype. The CT appearance of gastric lymphoma is variable. Gastric lymphoma may appear as diffuse or segmental wall thickening (Fig. 12-25), with an average wall thickness of 4–5 cm (55,56) (Fig. 12-26). Alternately, gastric lymphoma may present as a localized polypoid mass with or without ulceration (44). Most patients with gastric lymphoma have associated adenopathy, which is often bulky and may extend below the left renal hilum.

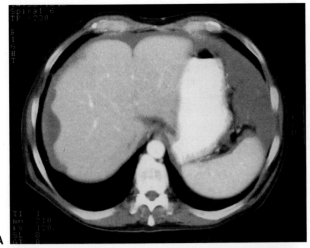

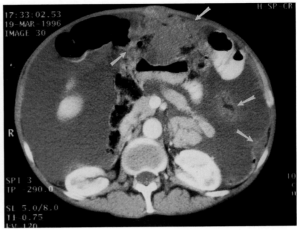

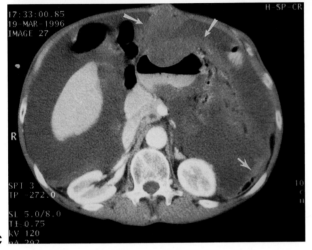

FIG. 12-24. (A–C) Recurrent gastric carcinoma. CT scan of patient with a history of gastric cancer and increasing abdominal distention. Spiral CT demonstrates moderate ascites with extensive tumor implants on omentum and throughout the abdominal cavity (*arrows*).

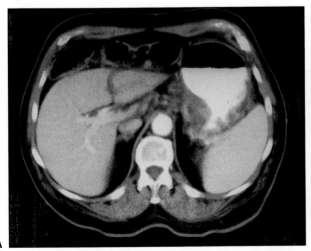

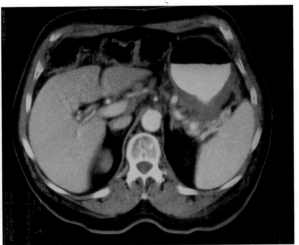

FIG. 12-25. (A,B) Lymphoma of the stomach. CT scan demonstrates thickening of gastric fundal folds. Although the fold thickness was under 3 cm, this was perhaps stable lymphoma. Lymphoma is more likely to give bulky folds than adenocarcinoma, but the differentiation may be possible on select scans.

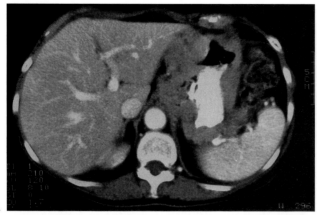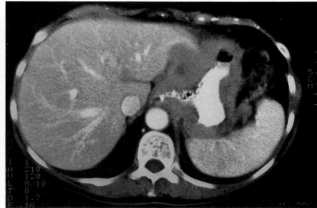

A   B

FIG. 12-26. (A,B) Gastric lymphoma. CT shows marked thickening of gastric folds extending to the gastroesophageal junction. This is the classic CT appearance of gastric lymphoma.

The CT appearance of gastric lymphoma may mimic adenocarcinoma of the stomach. Several key findings have been identified that may help distinguish the two malignancies. First, the gastric wall in lymphoma tends to be thicker (4–5 cm) and more lobular than that in adenocarcinoma (1–3 cm). In addition, although lymphadenopathy may occur in both gastric lymphoma and adenocarcinoma, adenopathy in gastric lymphoma tends to be bulkier and often to extend below the level of the renal hilum. Finally, although gastric lymphomas may appear as large, bulky tumors, they are often pliable and rarely result in gastric outlet obstruction (40).

Spiral CT is valuable for both patients with primary gastric lymphoma and in detecting gastric involvement in patients with more extensive disease. Accurate staging of disease is enhanced with narrower scan collimation and interscan gaps as well as by optimizing organ enhancement and disease detection in the liver, spleen, and kidneys. Solid organ involvement is being detected more commonly, especially in patients whose lymphoma is a result of immunosuppression, whether due to AIDS or to organ transplantation.

With the increased use of CT we are seeing cases of incidental gastric lymphoma. These cases are uncommon, but we are able to identify them, especially if careful attention is paid to scan protocols.

Treatment consists of surgery with postoperative chemoradiation therapy. Radiotherapy alone may be effective in patients with stage I and II disease (57). Chemotherapy is indicated in patients with disseminated disease.

Leiomyosarcoma

Gastric leiomyosarcoma is an uncommon smooth muscle tumor that comprises approximately 1% to 3% of primary gastric malignancies (58,59). Patients typically present with gastric outlet obstruction or bleeding from ulceration.

At CT, leiomyosarcoma appears as a large mass with an average diameter of 12–15 cm (Fig. 12-27). The mass is usually exophytic and often contains areas of decreased attenua-

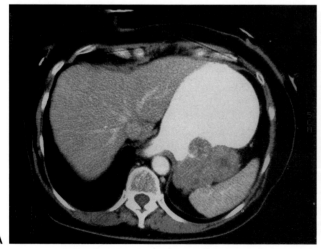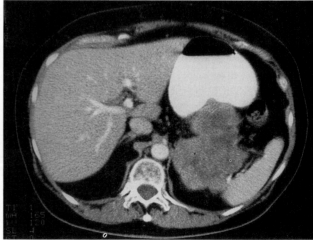

A   B

FIG. 12-27. (A,B) Gastric leiomyosarcoma. CT scan demonstrates a large exophytic ulcerating mass arising near the gastric fundus. The mass has minimal enhancement and its exophytic nature is a common CT appearance for a gastric leiomyosarcoma.

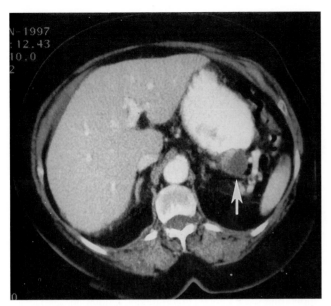

FIG. 12-28. Metastatic melanoma to the stomach. A spiral CT scan was done for staging of this patient with melanoma. Note a 2-cm cystic implant in the fundus of the stomach (*arrow*) consistent with metastatic melanoma.

tion caused by hemorrhage, necrosis, and cystic degeneration. Ulceration is frequent. Calcification is not uncommon.

Leiomyosarcoma can invade adjacent organs such as the pancreas and: Distant metastases may involve liver, lung, or peritoneal surfaces. There is usually no associated perigastric lymphadenopathy, which may help distinguish leiomyosarcoma from gastric adenocarcinoma and lymphoma.

Metastases

Metastases to the stomach occur in approximately 2% of patients who die of cancer each year. Metastases that involve the stomach by hematogenous spread include melanoma (Fig. 12-28), breast and lung, and ovary. Cancers of the esophagus and colon can spread to the stomach by lymphatic invasion. The stomach may also be involved by direct extension of local malignancies originating in the colon, pancreas, or liver (60,61) (Fig. 12-29). Patients can present with a variety of symptoms, including gastrointestinal bleeding, anemia, epigastric pain, and gastric outlet obstruction.

The CT appearance of metastatic disease of the stomach is variable. It can appear as a solitary mass, multiple masses (melanoma), or rigid wall thickening, as in linitis plastica (breast). The appearance of metastatic disease can be indistinguishable from primary gastric malignancies, stressing the importance of clinical information (50). Tumor implants on the stomach are especially common in processes such as ovarian cancer.

Gastric Varices

Gastric varices are tortuous distended collateral vessels fed mainly from the coronary vein that may develop in association with esophageal varices in patients with cirrhosis and portal hypertension. Although intra- or extrahepatic obstruction leads to esophageal and gastric varices, isolated splenic vein occlusion leads to the development of gastric varices, without accompanying esophageal collaterals. Gastric varices may occur in any region of the stomach but are most commonly located in the fundus. Although gastric varices do not bleed as frequently as esophageal varices, hemorrhage from gastric collaterals can be more severe.

The ability of endoscopic and conventional esophograms to diagnose gastric varices is limited, especially if unaccompanied by esophageal varices. In the past, angiography was considered the most reliable method for diagnosis of gastric varices. CT with intravenous contrast was quickly shown to be a sensitive method for the detection of gastric varices

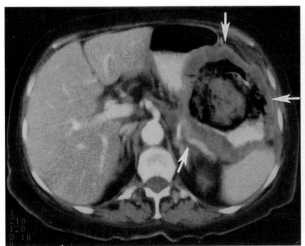

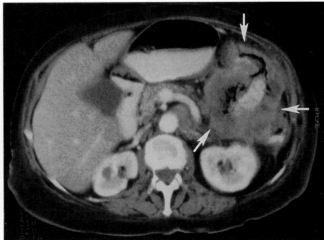

A

B

FIG. 12-29. (A,B) Invasion of the stomach by colon cancer. CT scans reveal a large necrotic mass (*arrows*) in the splenic flexure which invades the stomach.

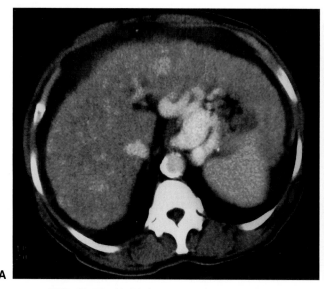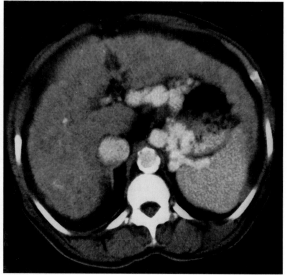

A   **B**

FIG. 12-30. (A,B) Gastric varices. Spiral CT scans demonstrate large varices in the gastric fundus. In this case water was used to distend the stomach, instead of positive contrast, which may obscure the enhancing collateral vessels.

(62). In recent years, spiral CT with intravenous contrast has been shown to provide an accurate means of detecting and evaluating portosystemic shunts in patients with portal hypertension (63).

The CT appearance of gastric varices varies, depending on the size and extent of involvement. Usually, on unenhanced scans, gastric varices appear as a scalloped, lobulated gastric border. With IV contrast, gastric varices appear as enhancing tubular and rounded structures within in the gastric wall (Fig. 12-30). On noncontrast scans, large varices can simulate adenopathy in the posterior mediastinum, which is a potential pitfall (40,44)

CT angiography with volume rendering and 3D image display can also be used to better evaluate gastric varices and their relationship to the portal and systemic venous systems.

Menetrier's Disease

Menetrier's disease (giant hypertrophic gastritis) is an uncommon disorder characterized by giant mucosal hypertrophy in the stomach, excessive mucus production, hypoproteinemia, and hypochlorhydria.

The hallmark of Menetrier's disease on CT is the presence of wall thickening in the proximal stomach and thickening of the rugal folds. Thickened rugal folds are particularly prominent along the greater curvature and fundus (Fig. 12-31). The antrum is typically spared. The CT appearance may

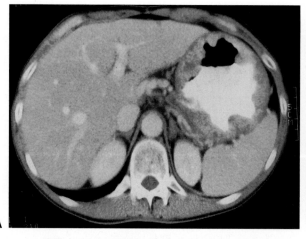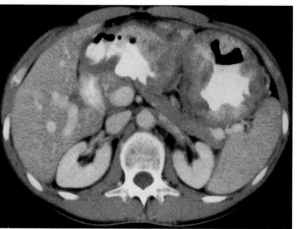

A   **B**

FIG. 12-31. (A,B) Ménétrier's disease. Spiral CT scans demonstrates large, bulky gastric folds. The extent of the fold enlargement is throughout the stomach, and the possibility of an infiltrating tumor such as lymphoma would obviously be considered. At biopsy this proved to be Ménétrier's disease.

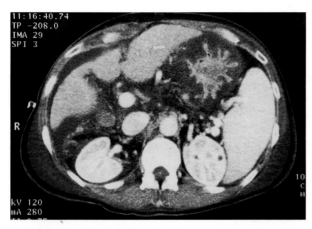

FIG. 12-32. Nonspecific gastritis. CT shows marked gastric wall thickening and edematous gastric folds. Endoscopy revealed nonspecific gastritis.

simulate infiltrating malignancies such as lymphoma. There have been case reports suggesting that patients with Menetrier disease may be predisposed to develop adenocarcinoma (64).

Gastritis

There are many causes of gastritis, including infections (*Helicobacter pylori*, cryptosporidia, cytomegalovirus), inflammatory conditions (Crohn disease, eosinophilic gastroenteritis, Zollinger–Ellison syndrome), radiation, and ingestion of alcohol, corrosive agents, or drugs.

At CT, gastritis usually appears as a gastric fold and wall thickening, regardless of etiology (Fig. 12-32). The thickened wall typically has soft-tissue density. Although if there is significant edema, the wall may have a low density (11). Adequate gastric distention is necessary to avoided confusing wall thickening from gastritis with underdistention. The CT appearances of gastritis and gastric cancer often overlap, requiring biopsy for the definitive diagnosis.

CONCLUSION

Although CT is not the primary imaging modality for gastroesophageal disease, it plays a significant role in the evaluation and staging of esophageal and gastric carcinoma and in the imaging of a variety of benign diseases. With the advent of spiral CT and 3D volume sets, the role of CT in the evaluation of gastroesophageal diseases continues to evolve.

REFERENCES

1. Wolfman NT, Scharling ES, Chen MY. Esophageal squamous carcinoma. *Radiol Clin North Am* 1994;32(6):1183–1201.
2. Noda Y, Ogawa Y, Nishioka A, et al. New barium paste mixture for helical (slip-ring) CT evaluation of the esophagus. *J Comput Assist Tomogr* 1996;20 (5) 773–776.
3. Goldwin RL, Heitzman ER, Proto AV. Computed tomography of the mediastinum. Normal anatomy and indications for the use of CT. *Radiology* 1977;124:235–241.
4. Noh HM, Fishman EK, Forastiere AA, Bliss DF, Calhoun PS. CT of the esophagus: spectrum of disease with emphasis on esophageal carcinoma. *Radiographics* 1995;15:1113–1134.
5. Desai RK, Tagliabue JR, Wegryn SA, Einstein DM. CT evaluation of wall thickening in the alimentary tract. *Radiographics* 1991;11(5): 771–783.
6. Parker SL, Tong T, Bolden S, Wingo PA. Cancer Statistics, 1996. *CA Cancer J Clin* 1996;46:5–27.
7. Heitmiller RF, Sharma RR. Comparison of prevalence and resection rates in patients with esophageal squamous cell carcinoma and adenocarcinoma. *J Thorac Cardiovasc Surg* 1996;112(1)ʷ1–136.
8. Levine MS, Caroline D, Thompson JJ, Kressel HY, Laufer I, Herlinger H. Adenocarcinoma of the esophagus: relationship to Barrett mucosa. *Radiology* 1984;150:305–309.
9. Forastiere AA, Orringer MB, Perez-Tamayo C, Urba SG, Zahurak M. Preoperative chemoradiation followed by transhiatal esophagectomy for carcinoma of the esophagus: final report. *J Clin Oncol* 1993;11: 1118–1123.
10. Moss AA, Schnyder P, Theoni RF, Margulis AR. Esophageal carcinoma: pretherapy staging by computed tomography. *AJR* 1981;136: 1051–1056.
11. Lefor AT, Merino MM, Steinberg SM, et al. Computerized tomographic prediction of extraluminal spread and prognostic implications of lesion width in esophageal cancer. *Cancer* 1988;62:1287–1292.
12. Van Overhagen H, Lameris JS, Berger MY, et al. CT assessment of resectability prior to transhiatal esophagectomy for esophageal/gastroesophageal junction carcinoma. *J Comput Assist Tomogr* 1993;17(3): 367–373.
13. Coulomb M, Lebas JF, Sarrazin R, Geindre M. Computed tomography and esophageal carcinoma (French). *J Radiol* 1981;62:475–487.
14. Thompson WM, Halvorsen RA, Foster WL, Williford ME, Postlethwait RW, Korobkin M. Computed tomography for staging esophageal and gastroesophageal cancer: reevaluation. *AJR* 1983;141:951–958.
15. Picus D, Balfe DM, Koehler RE, Roper CL, Owen JW. Computed tomography in the staging of esophageal carcinoma. *Radiology* 1983; 146:433–438.
16. Daffner RH, Halber MD, Postlethwait RW, Korobkin M, Thompson WM. CT of the esophagus. II. Carcinoma. *AJR* 1979;133:1051–1055.
17. Halvorsen RA Jr, Thompson WM. Computed tomographic staging of gastrointestinal malignancies. I. Esophagus and stomach. *Invest Radiol* 1987;22:2–16.
18. Rosenberg JC, Franklin R, Steiger Z. Squamous cell carcinoma of the thoracic esophagus: an interdisciplinary approach. *Curr Probl Cancer* 1981;5:1–52.
19. Gunnlaugsson GH, Wychulis AR, Roland C, Ellis FH Jr. Analysis of records of 1657 patients with carcinoma of the esophagus and cardia of the stomach. *Surg Gynecol Obstet* 1970;130:997–1005.
20. Parker EF. Carcinoma of the esophagus: is there a role for surgery? The case for surgery. *Am J Dig Dis* 1978;23:730–734.
21. Wernecke K, Rummeny E, Bongartz G, et al. Detection of hepatic masses in patients with carcinoma; comparative sensitivities of sonography, CT, and MR imaging. *AJR* 1991;157:731–739.
22. Miller WJ, Baron RL, Dodd GD 3rd, Federle MP. Malignancies in patients with cirrhosis: CT sensitivity and specificity in 200 consecutive transplant patients. *Radiology* 1994;193:645–650.
23. Matsui O, Takashima T, Kadoya M, et al. Liver metastases from colorectal cancer: detection with CT during arterial portography. *Radiology* 1987;165:65–69.
24. Soyer P, Bluemke DA, Hruban RH, Sitzmann JV, Fishman EK. Hepatic metastases from colorectal cancer: detection and false positive findings with helical CT during arterial portography. *Radiology* 1994;192: 389–392.
25. Zerhouni EA, Rutter C, Hamilton SR, et al. CT and MR imaging in the staging of colorectal carcinoma: report of Radiology Diagnostic Oncology Group II. *Radiology* 1996;200(2):443–445.
26. Kuszyk BS, Bluemke DA, Urban BA, et al. Portal-phase contrast enhanced helical CT for the detection of malignant hepatic tumors: sensitivity based on comparison with intraoperative and pathologic findings. *AJR* 1996;166:91–95.
27. Morita M, Kuwano H, Ohno S, Furusawa M, Sugimachi K. Characteristics and sequence of recurrent patterns after curative esophagectomy for squamous cell carcinoma. *Surgery* 1994;116(1):1–7.
28. Isono K, Onoda S, Okuyama K, Sato H. Recurrence of intrathoracic esophageal cancer. *Jpn J Clin Oncol* 1985;15(1):49–60.

29. Cho KC, Patel YD, Wachsberg RH, Seeff J. Varices in portal hypertension: evaluation with CT. *Radiographics* 1995;15:609–622.

30. Balthazar EJ, Naidich DP, Megibow AJ, Lefleur RS. CT evaluation of esophageal varices. *AJR* 1987;148:131–135.

31. Clark KE, Foley WD, Lawson TL, Berland LL, Maddison FE. CT evaluation of the esophageal and upper abdominal varices. *J Comput Assist Tomogr* 1980;4:510–515.

32. De Silva R, Stoopack PM, Raufman JP. Esophageal fistulas associated with mycobacterial infection in patients at risk for AIDS. *Radiology* 1990;175:449–453.

33. Rabushka LS, Fishman EK, Kuhlman JE. CT evaluation of achalasia. *J Comput Assist Tomogr* 1991;15:434–439.

34. Raptopoulos V, Davis MA, Davidoff A, et al. Fat density oral contrast agent from abdominal CT. *Radiology* 1987;164:653–656.

35. Winter TC, Ager JD, Nghiem HV, et al. Upper gastrointestinal tract abdomen: water as an orally administered contrast agent for helical CT. *Radiology* 1996;201:365–370.

36. Gossios KJ, Tsianos EV, Demou LL, et al. Use of water or air as oral contrast media for computed tomographic study of the gastric wall: comparison of the two techniques. *Gastrointest Radiol* 1991;16:293–297.

37. Baert AL, Roex L, Marchal G, et al. Computed tomography of the stomach with water as an oral contrast agent: technique and preliminary results. *J Comput Assist Tomogr* 1989;13:633–636.

38. Hori S, Tsuda K, Murayama S, Matsushita M, Yukawa K, Kozuka. CT of gastric carcinoma: preliminary results with a new scanning technique. *Radiographics* 1992;12:257–268.

39. Angelelli G, Macarini L, Fratello A. Use of water as oral contrast agent for CT study of the stomach. *AJR* 1987;149:1084.

40. Savader BL, Fishman EK. CT evaluation of the stomach. Contemporary diagnostic. *Radiology* 1992;15(2):1–5.

41. Eisenberg RL. Gastric ulcers. In: RL Eisenberg, ed. Gastrointestinal radiology: a pattern approach. Philadelphia: Lippincott-Raven; 1996: 196–197.

42. NIH consensus conference. *Helicobacter pylori* in peptic ulcer disease. *JAMA* 1994;272:65–69.

43. Moss AA, Margulis AR, Schnyder P, Theoni RF. A uniform, CT based staging system for malignant neoplasms of the alimentary tube. *AJR* 1981;136:1251–1252.

44. Fishman EK, Urban BA, Hruban RH. CT of the stomach: spectrum of disease. *Radiographics* 1996;16:1035–1054.

45. Cho JS, Kim JK, Rho SM, et al. Preoperative assessment of gastric cancer: value of two-phase dynamic CT with mechanical IV injection of contrast material. *AJR* 1994;163:69–75.

46. Sussman SK, Halvorsen RA, Illescas FF, et al. Gastric adenocarcinoma: CT versus surgical staging. *Radiology* 1988;167:335–340.

47. McFee AS, Aust JB. Gastric carcinoma and the CAT scan. *Gastroenterology* 1981;80:196–198.

48. Bedikian AY, Chen TT, Khankhanian N, et al. The natural history of gastric cancer and prognostic factors influencing survival. *J Clin Oncol* 1984;2:305–310.

49. Balfe DM, Mauro MA, Koehler RE, et al. Gastrohepatic ligament: normal and pathologic CT anatomy. *Radiology* 1984;150:485–490.

50. Komaki S. Gastric carcinoma. In: Meyers MA, ed. *Computed tomography of the gastrointestinal tract.* New York: Springer; 1986:23–54.

51. Dehn TC, Reznek RH, Nockler IB, White FE. The preoperative assessment of advanced gastric cancer by computed tomography. *Br J Surg* 1984;71:413–417.

52. Cook AO, Levine BA, Sirinek KR, Gaskill HV III. Evaluation of gastric adenocarcinoma: abdominal computed tomography does not replace celiotomy. *Ach Surg* 1986;121:603–606.

53. Ha HK, Kim HH, Kim HS, Lee MH, Kim KT, Shinn KS. Local recurrence after surgery for gastric carcinoma: CT findings. *AJR* 1993;161:975–977.

54. Mullin D, Shirkhoda A. Computed tomography after gastrectomy in primary gastric carcinoma. *J Comput Assist Tomogr* 1985;90(1):30–33.

55. Megibow AJ, Balthazar EJ, Naidich DP, Bosniak MA. Computed tomography of gastrointestinal lymphoma. *AJR* 1983;141:541–547.

56. Buy JN, Moss AA. Computed tomography of gastric lymphoma. *AJR* 1982;138:859–865.

57. Rao AR, Kagan AR, Potyk D, et al. Management of gastrointestinal lymphoma. *Am J Clin Oncol* 1984;7:213–219.

58. Megibow AJ, Balthazar EJ, Hulnick DH, Naidich DP, Bosniak MA. CT evaluation of gastrointestinal leiomyomas and leiomyosarcomas. *AJR* 1985;144:727–731.

59. Scatarige JC, Fishman EK, Jones B, et al. Gastric leiomyosarcoma: CT observations. *J Comput Assist Tomogr* 1985;9:320–327.

60. Menuck L, Amberg J. Metastatic disease involving the stomach. *Am J Dig Dis* 1975;20:903–913.

61. Radin DR. Halls JM. Cavitary metastases of the stomach and duodenum. *J Comput Assist Tomogr* 1987;11:283–287.

62. Balthazar EJ, Megibow A, Naidich D, LeFleur RS. Computed tomographic recognition of gastric varices. *AJR* 1984;142:1121–1125.

63. Cho KC, Patel YD, Wachsberg RH, Seeff J. Varices in portal hypertension: evaluation with CT. *Radiographics* 1995;15:609–622.

64. Williams SM, Harned RK, Settles RH. Adenocarcinoma of the stomach in association with Menetrier's disease. *Gastrointest Radiol* 1978;3:387–390.

PART 4

Genitourinary Applications

CHAPTER 13

Spiral CT of the Kidney

Elliot K. Fishman and Bruce A. Urban

Spiral computed tomography (CT) provides many advantages in the evaluation of renal pathology. Spiral scanning essentially eliminates data misregistration and allows for visualization of the entire kidney during peak contrast enhancement or in any specific phase of enhancement desired (1–8). The generated data set is free from motion artifact, which improves multiplanar reconstructions and allows accurate three-dimensional (3D) reconstruction of the data sets. These factors are of vital importance for a range of applications, including the evaluation and characterization of small renal tumors (4–7). Spiral CT increases sensitivity in the detection of subtle asymmetries of the cortical nephrogram, which is useful in diagnosing disorders such as renal artery stenosis, renal vein thrombosis, acute pyelonephritis, and renal obstruction. This chapter provides a detailed analysis of the current state of the art of spiral CT evaluation of renal pathology. Such innovative applications as noninvasive renal donor evaluation, renal and ureteral stone detection, and 3D imaging are also addressed.

IMAGING PROTOCOLS

Dynamic CT scanning of the kidneys has long been accepted as the preferred method for evaluation of renal pathology (9–11). Bolus intravenous enhancement aids in the detection and characterization of renal masses and parenchymal disease, allows for assessment of tumor vascularity, and helps to differentiate juxtarenal from intrarenal processes. Dynamic scanning is most sensitive during the early cortical nephrogram phase of renal enhancement, when corticomedullary differentiation is maximal (10). However, conventional scanners are quite limited in obtaining images during this early phase of enhancement. A major advantage of spiral CT is the ability to image the entire length of the kidneys during this ideal period of enhancement, in conjunction with routine dynamic evaluation of the liver and pancreas (8). Newer software for extended spiral capabilities

provides optimal contrast-enhanced images of the kidney during routine evaluation of the entire abdomen.

The protocol for spiral scanning of the kidneys continues to be very controversial, and protocols vary between institutions. Our current protocol for a dedicated kidney study requires a localizing topogram. An initial axial section is then selected in the upper third of the liver. Subsequently, 100–120 mL of nonionic contrast (Omnipaque-350, Nycomed, Inc., Princeton, NJ) is peripherally administered through a power injector, ideally at a rate of 3 mL/s. Following the initiation of contrast injection, spiral scanning begins within 30 s for arterial-phase imaging and within 60 s for the cortical medullary phase. The table incrementation rate is 5 mm/s, with 5-mm collimation at 280 mA and 120 kVp (Siemens Somatom Plus-4). Overlapping reconstruction is usually obtained using 3-mm interscan spacing. Although representative multiplanar and 3D analysis can be performed with these scan parameters in cases where evaluation of vascular anatomy is the focus of the study, such as renal transplant donor evaluation or suspected renal artery stenosis, a different scanning protocol is selected. This protocol often requires imaging during both the arterial and corticomedullary phases of enhancement to obtain key functional data or to image both arterial and venous anatomy. For example, in cases of renal donor evaluation we will obtain 3-mm-thick sections with a table speed of 3–5 mm and reconstruct the data at 1–3-mm increments. In this case dual-phase spiral CT is routinely utilized. In the case of renal artery stenosis we will obtain only arterial-phase images but use 2-mm collimation and reconstruct the data at 1-mm intervals (12–14).

Certain clinical situations require other alterations of the routine renal spiral protocol. Initial precontrast scanning of the entire kidney is performed if renal or ureteral calculi are clinically suspected. In patients presenting with classic signs and symptoms of ureteral colic, recent articles suggest that no additional contrast-enhanced scans are necessary (15–18). In cases of suspected transitional-cell carcinoma, renal infection, or obstruction, delayed scans are obtained

(>4 min after injection) to evaluate the opacified collecting system (19,20). In cases of infection the presence of focal inflammatory changes may only be seen on these delayed images (21). Although a question can be raised about the use of multiphase studies in each patient, we tend to be a bit more pragmatic based on a busy daily clinical workload.

With spiral CT scanning the radiologist has a wider range of capabilities for evaluating the kidney. Noncontrast-enhanced CTs, arterial-phase CT images, corticomedullary-phase CT images, nephrographic-phase images, and excretory-phase CT images are all possible in a single exam. In clinical practice, however, it is unrealistic to get all phases for imaging the kidney in each patient. Therefore optimization of the technique with specific protocols must be designed to maintain realistic patient throughput.

In looking at enhancement patterns of the kidney the classic acquisitions would be considered to be arterial-phase, corticomedullary-phase, nephrographic-phase and delayed-(excretory-) phase imaging. Corticomedullary-phase imaging classically begins at approximately 50 s after initiation of injection. As previously stated, this phase has certain advantages because it provides optimal demarcation between the renal cortex and the medulla. However, several recent articles have focused on some of the potential limitations of early-phase imaging and have focused more on using delayed-phase studies. Szolar et al. (6) reviewed the potential of thin-slice helical CT for detection and characterization of small (<3 cm) renal masses. In this study, images were obtained before and after contrast enhancement, with scans obtained during the corticomedullary and nephrographic phase. The number of masses smaller than 3 cm detected on corticomedullary-phase scans (n = 211) was significantly fewer than that on the nephrographic-phase scans (n = 291). The mean difference in enhancement between the renal cortex and masses was 148 ± 54 HU and 137 ± 44 HU during the corticomedullary and nephrographic phases, respectively. False-positive results occurred only on corticomedullary-phase scans because of the lack of enhancement of the renal medulla. The authors therefore suggested that nephrographic-phase imaging be obtained when looking for small renal masses. Birnbaum et al. (22) similarly addressed the use of thin-section CT during the corticomedullary and nephrographic phases of contrast enhancement in the characterization of renal masses. They found that enhancement of renal neoplasms is time-dependent and that hypervascular tumors may not be evident if analyzed during the early corticomedullary phase and recommended nephrographic-phase evaluation. Similarly, in a study looking at the value of delayed scans, Zeman et al. (23) found that small renal masses could be missed on early-phase images, especially with the less experienced reader.

Cohan et al. (24) reviewed the scans of 33 patients performed during corticomedullary-phase and nephrographic-phase imaging to evaluate suspected renal tumors. In all cases the exam protocols were consecutive 5-mm-thick scans. The authors found a significant difference in tumor detection between the corticomedullary- and nephrographic-phase imaging. The greatest difference was in detection of lesions in the renal medulla, where four times as many lesions were detected in the nephrographic phase than in the corticomedullary phase. The difference in detection was particularly great for smaller lesions (those less than 11 mm), where 6.8 times as many lesions were detected with the nephrographic-phase images. It should be noted, however, that most of these lesions were in fact too small to be characterized and probably represented simple cysts rather than early neoplasm.

Potential reasons for the differential rate of lesion detection are several. A hypervascular carcinoma may enhance to the same extent as a normal renal cortex and so in theory might not be visualized during corticomedullary-phase imaging. False-positive lesions may occur if normal renal medulla that has not yet enhanced to the same degree as renal cortex is misinterpreted as a renal lesion. The authors therefore recommend that a three-phase study be obtained: initial unenhanced spiral CT scans, followed by an enhanced corticomedullary-phase spiral CT images, followed by a series of routine transaxial nephrographic-phase images (beginning 100 s after initiation of contrast injection) (Figs. 13-1–3).

Based on these articles, a focused protocol for patients with suspected renal mass or hematuria can be summarized as follows. Obtain a series of noncontrast spiral scans with 4–5-mm collimation to look for the presence of calcification or renal calculi. Then perform either an arterial-phase study (typically obtained at about 30 s) to optimally visualize the arterial structures or a corticomedullary-phase study (obtained at about 50 s). In both cases, delayed imaging should be obtained at 3–4 min after contrast injection to allow for visualization of an opacified renal pelvis and collecting system as well as to avoid some of the potential pitfalls that Cohan et al. (24) have documented.

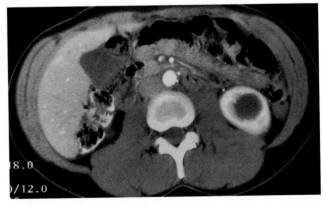

FIG. 13-1. Renal cyst. Spiral CT with early phase imaging clearly demonstrates a well-defined water density lesion with sharp margins in the lower pole of the left kidney consistent with a simple cyst.

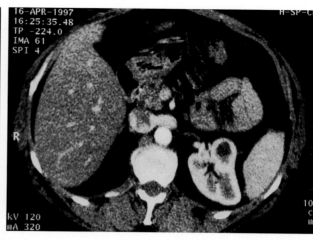

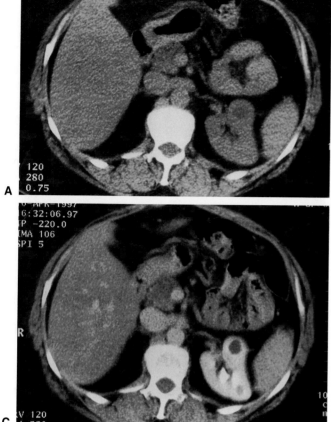

FIG. 13-2. Simple renal cyst. This study was done for evaluation of a questionable abnormality in this patient with hematuria. **(A)** Noncontrast CT demonstrates a low-density region in the superior portion of the left kidney. **(B)** Spiral CT in corticomedullary phase demonstrates the lesion without evidence of enhancement. **(C)** Images in excretory phase demonstrate the sharply defined margins of the lesion consistent with a simple cyst.

THE NORMAL KIDNEY

Following bolus intravenous injection, the renal parenchyma demonstrates four distinct phases of enhancement: the cortical angiogram, the glomerulogram, the cortical nephrogram, and the tubular nephrogram (25). The first two phases occur within a few seconds and are not routinely imaged. Routine spiral CT scanning occurs during the peak of the third phase of renal enhancement, the cortical nephrogram phase. At this time (approximately 40–70 s after injection), contrast fills the cortical capillaries, peritubular spaces, and proximal convoluted tubules, resulting in exquisite corticomedullary differentiation (10,25,26). The density of the cortical nephrogram and the degree of corticomedullary differentiation obtained on the spiral scan depends on the patient's renal function and cardiac output, as well as on the rate and volume of contrast administration. In our experience, bolus injection at 2–3 mL/s usually results in cortical enhancement ranging from 100 to 200 Hounsfield units (HU).

Unlike conventional dynamic scanning, spiral CT is routinely able to image the entire length of the kidneys during this ideal period of enhancement. This can be helpful to discriminate normal cortical variants such as a prominent column of Bertin or dromedary hump from an abnormal renal mass. Spiral CT provides increased sensitivity in the detection of subtle asymmetry of the cortical nephrogram, which reflects abnormal hemodynamics in the setting of either abnormal perfusion or delayed tubular transit (26).

The renal arteries are confidently displayed on spiral CT, and this has an application in the evaluation of renal artery stenosis or thrombosis. Most spiral scans also provide sufficient opacification of the renal veins, although opacification may be delayed in patients with poor renal function. The inferior vena cava is normally nonopacified on early-phase spiral scans. In patients with renal cell carcinoma and suspected vascular invasion, delayed scans may be necessary to better visualize the renal veins and inferior vena cava.

RENAL NEOPLASTIC DISEASE

Renal Cell Carcinoma

CT is widely accepted as the preferred modality for detection and staging of renal cell carcinoma (27–33). The typical carcinoma presents as a bulky, heterogeneous mass that demonstrates inhomogeneous enhancement yet remains relatively hyperdense or hypodense compared with the normally enhancing renal parenchyma (Figs. 13-4, 13-5), depending on the phase of data acquisition, as discussed earlier. Cystic

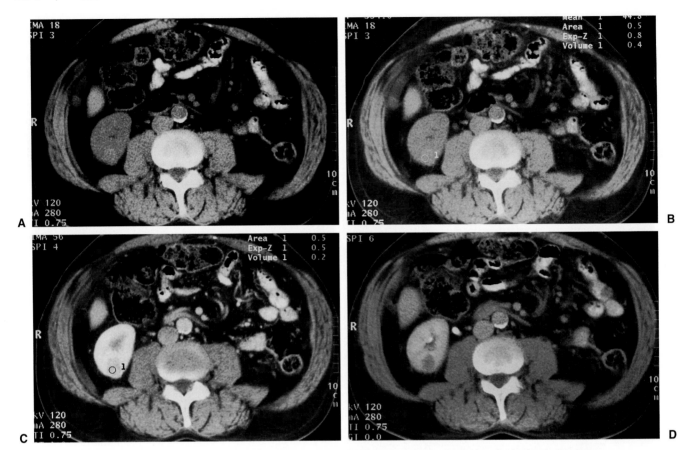

FIG. 13-3. Renal cell carcinoma. **(A,B)** Noncontrast CT demonstrates a high-density lesion in the lower pole of the right kidney measuring 44 HU. **(C)** Images in the corticomedullary phase demonstrate enhancement of the lesion to 126 HU. **(D)** Scans in the excretory phase demonstrate an attenuation of 72 HU. The appearance is consistent with a small hypervascular renal cell carcinoma but could easily be confused with a complicated cyst.

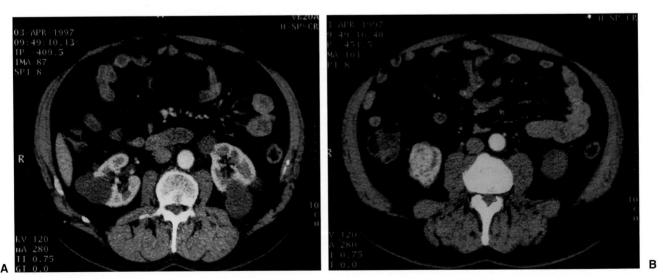

FIG. 13-4. **(A,B)** Hypervascular renal cell carcinoma. The hypervascular nature of the mass in the lower pole of the right kidney (*arrow*) is appreciated because of its vascularity. Compare the tumor with the patient's multiple simple cysts in the midportions of the kidney.

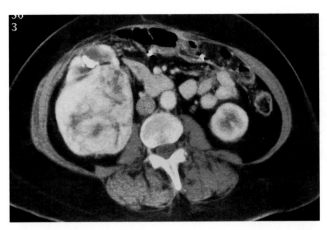

FIG. 13-5. Hypervascular renal cell carcinoma. Spiral CT demonstrates a mass arising off the inferior pole of the right kidney. The mass is hypervascular and consistent with a classic renal cell carcinoma.

renal cell cancers are differentiated from complicated benign cysts by their thick, irregular wall and tumor nodularity (Fig. 13-6). Local spread of renal cell carcinoma typically occurs into the renal vein, para-aortic lymph nodes, or perinephric spaces.

Spiral CT offers many advantages in the evaluation of renal cell carcinoma. The uniform peak vascular opacification that is routinely achieved with spiral scanning improves both detection and characterization of the typically hypervascular renal cell carcinoma. Prognostic significance may also follow, in that tumor size and vascularity may correlate with a renal cell carcinoma's ability to metastasize (34). Optimal vascular opacification also enables the detection of extension of a renal cell carcinoma into the renal vein and inferior vena cava (35) (Figs. 13-7, 13-8). Venous extension of renal cell carcinoma appears to be more common with right-sided tumors, with approximately 10% of renal cell cancers invading the inferior vena cava (36,37). Tumor thrombus presents as a luminal filling defect, and vascular collaterals can occasionally be demonstrated. Delayed scans may improve visualization of the inferior vena cava, which can normally be nonopacified on an early spiral scan.

A particular problem with conventional CT is the precise delineation of the degree of tumor extension into the inferior vena cava. This is particularly true when thrombus approaches the right atrium. Currently, magnetic resonance imaging (MRI) is the most useful modality for tumor thrombus evaluation (38). However, multiplanar reconstruction and 3D imaging obtained from the motion-free spiral data set may prove as effective in the depiction of tumor thrombus extension. Three-dimensional models of the kidneys and their vascular supply can also be helpful in surgical planning for patients eligible for partial nephrectomy (39). In our institution spiral CT with 3D mapping is routinely obtained in all difficult cases of potential partial nephrectomy.

A major advantage of spiral CT over conventional scan-

ning is the increased frequency of detection of small renal cell carcinomas. This advantage results in part from data continuity provided by a single breath-hold acquisition, which eliminates respiratory misregistration and partial volume averaging. This allows for increased visualization of smaller lesions that may otherwise have been missed. Peak contrast enhancement also helps to differentiate small tumors from brightly enhancing normal parenchyma (4,5,40).

Diagnosis of the small renal cell carcinoma also depends, in part, on the detection of "significant" contrast enhancement. On conventional CT, only relatively large increases in attenuation value (>20 HU) indicate true enhancement, in part because smaller increases of attenuation are artificially produced by partial volume averaging. By eliminating this potential source of error, spiral scanning may allow for a decrease in the currently accepted "threshold" level of significant enhancement, thereby increasing our specificity in the characterization of the small renal mass.

Many of these small (<3 cm) renal cell carcinomas are discovered incidentally. Because of disagreement about their clinical course, detection of these lesions poses a problem in clinical management (30). In the past, small tumors were largely felt to represent adenomas with a low potential for metastasis. At present, most pathologists believe these lesions should all be considered carcinomas (28). Because there is no effective cure for advanced renal cell cancer, a potential increase in early detection of small renal cell carcinomas with spiral scanning could provide a valuable role in increasing overall patient survival.

Spiral CT also provides a reliable and reproducible technique for follow-up of patients with small indeterminate renal masses. Spiral CT with breath-hold acquisition ensures accurate size measurements, and even minimal lesion growth can be confidently detected. Such precision greatly improves

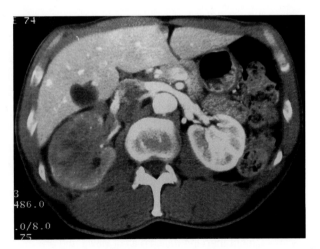

FIG. 13-6. Hypovascular renal cell carcinoma with paracaval adenopathy. Spiral CT demonstrates diffuse infiltration of the right kidney by tumor. The inferior vena cava is displaced forward and retrocaval nodes are present. Note how an infiltrating renal call carcinoma can simulate an advanced stage of transitional cell carcinoma.

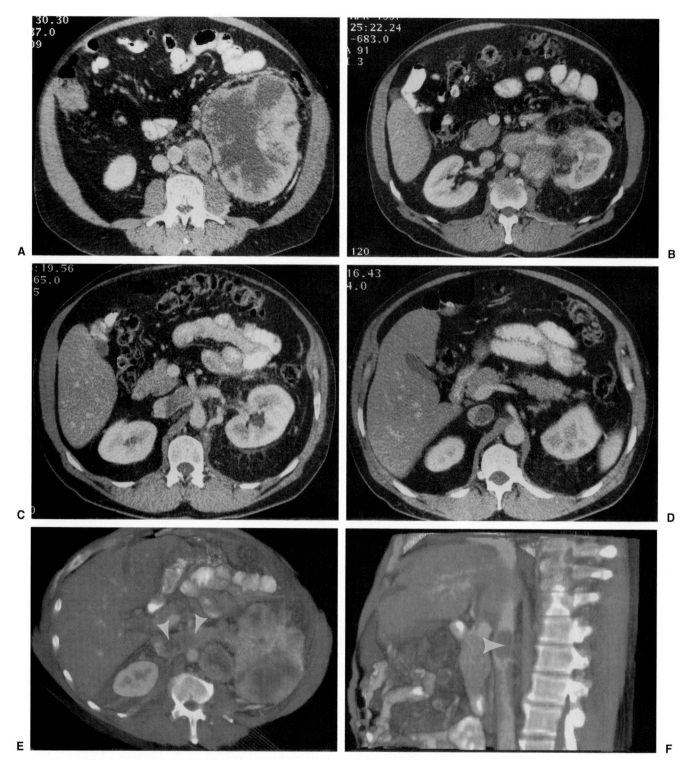

FIG. 13-7. Renal cell carcinoma with renal vein and inferior vena cava extension. (**A**) Spiral CT demonstrates a large hypervascular mass in the inferior portion of the left kidney. Left para-aortic nodes are also seen. (**B–D**) Sequential scans demonstrate the extension of tumor into the renal vein and inferior vena cava (IVC). (**E,F**) Three-dimensional reconstructions better define the renal vein and IVC involvement than the multiple axial views and are more helpful to the surgeon.

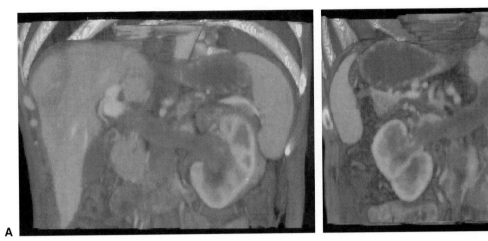

FIG. 13-8. (**A,B**) Renal cell carcinoma with renal vein and inferior vena cava involvement. Three-dimensional reconstructions from anterior and posterior views demonstrate the full extent of vascular involvement.

the management of small renal masses and aids in determining which lesions can be observed and which lesions should undergo resection (7).

Finally, spiral CT provides an excellent means for following the patient after a partial nephrectomy. Thinly collimated slices, with optimal contrast enhancement and absence of artifacts due to partial voluming and motion, permit clear differentiation of postoperative change from small foci of tumor recurrence. Detection of sites of distant metastases, including the lung and liver, is more accurate with spiral CT than with conventional CT scanning (41,42) (Figs. 13-9, 13-10).

Lymphoma

Renal lymphoma invariably results from hematogenous dissemination. Lymphoma can demonstrate multiple appearances on CT (11) (Figs. 13-11, 13-12). Most commonly, the kidneys show diffuse enlargement, with other variations,

including bilateral focal masses, a single dominant mass, or direct invasion by adjacent adenopathy. Lymphomatous masses typically are homogeneous and demonstrate minimal contrast enhancement (10–20 HU). The appearance of focal lymphoma is indistinguishable from that of renal cell carcinoma (Fig. 13-13). Small or subtle lesions are detected on spiral CT with increased frequency, accuracy, and confidence.

Although there are no published results, we feel that corticomedullary-phase imaging is ideal for renal imaging in patients with lymphoma. We do not routinely do multiphase imaging in these patients unless the initial phase of study is indeterminate or primary renal pathology is suspected.

Angiomyolipoma

Angiomyolipomas are focal hamartomas classically seen in middle-aged females or patients with tuberous sclerosis (43). Spiral scanning can help in the detection of subtle foci

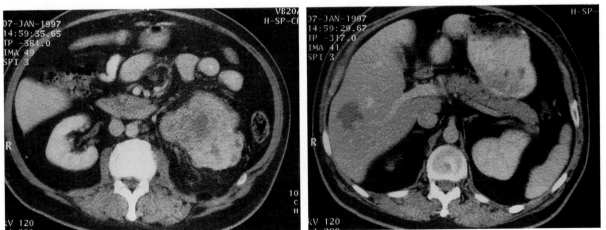

FIG. 13-9. Renal cell carcinoma with liver metastases. (**A**) Spiral CT scan demonstrates a hypervascular left renal tumor that infiltrates and replaces the normal parenchyma. (**B**) A single metastasis was present in the right lobe of the liver.

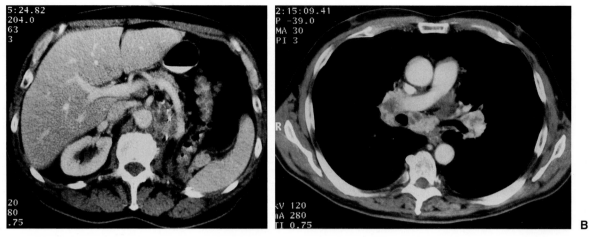

FIG. 13-10. Recurrent renal cell carcinoma. **(A)** Spiral CT demonstrates evidence of prior left nephrectomy with recurrent nodes in the left para-aortic space adjacent to the surgical clips. **(B)** Scans through the chest as part of the follow-up study also demonstrated metastases to hilar and subcarinal nodes.

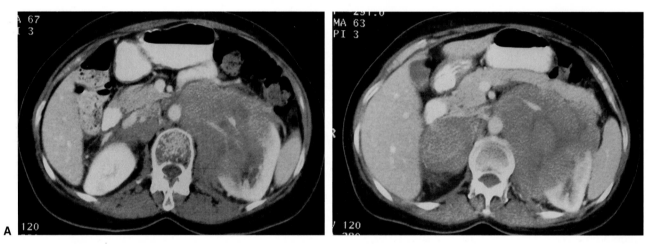

FIG. 13-11. Renal lymphoma. **(A)** Spiral CT demonstrates diffuse infiltration of the left kidney by direct extension secondary to lymphoma. **(B)** The patient also had involvement of both adrenal glands by lymphoma.

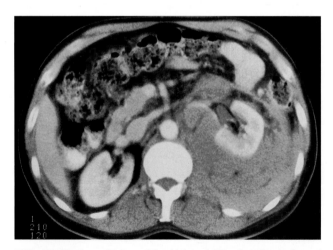

FIG. 13-12. Lymphoma of the kidney infiltrating the peri- and pararenal space. Spiral CT demonstrates diffuse infiltration of the left peri- and pararenal space secondary to tumor. Note delayed excretion of contrast from the left kidney.

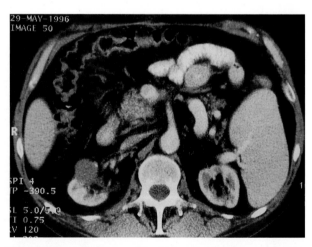

FIG. 13-13. Lymphoma of the kidney presenting as a solitary mass. Spiral CT demonstrates a 3-cm mass in the right kidney that is a biopsy-proven lymphoma. Note how the appearance would be indistinguishable from a primary renal cell carcinoma or metastasis to the kidney.

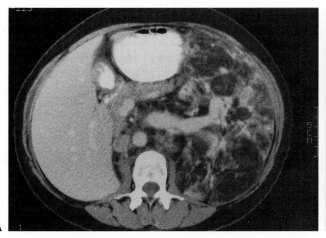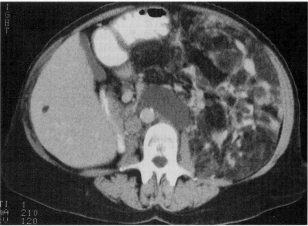

A   B

FIG. 13-14. Renal angiomyololipoma. (A,B) Spiral CT demonstrates near total replacement of the left kidney by a mass with varying amounts of fat with minimal residual normal cortex is seen. Incidental note is also made of a hepatic lipoma. The patient had a prior right nephrectomy for a benign renal tumor that undoubtedly was a angiomyolipoma as well.

of fat within a renal mass. This is considered almost pathognomonic for angiomyolipoma, although reports have described subtle fat deposits in renal cell carcinoma (44,45). Improved lesion characterization provided by the virtual elimination of partial volume averaging can help to differentiate angiomyolipomas from small cysts. Angiomyolipomas can grow quite large and appear almost entirely eccentric to the renal parenchyma. Spiral scanning can help demonstrate that the mass is intrinsic to the kidney, thus ruling out retroperitoneal liposarcoma (Fig. 13-14). Finally, accurate evaluation of larger lesions (greater than 3 or 4 cm) can be helpful for potential presurgical planning.

Transitional Cell Carcinoma

Transitional cell carcinoma accounts for approximately 5% of all renal tumors. Patients frequently present with hematuria. In conjunction with intravenous urography, CT has an important role in the evaluation and staging of transitional cell carcinoma. Several distinct patterns of involvement are described on conventional and spiral CT (46). Urban et al. recently reviewed the CT appearance of transitional cell carcinomas and divided them into early-stage (stages I and II) and late-stage (stages III and IV) disease (19,20). Early-stage disease consists of a central solid mass that expands centrifugally with compression of the renal sinus fat. On noncontrast studies the lesions are in the 5–30-HU range and will only minimally enhance after contrast injection. This enhancement is best seen with spiral CT. Spiral CT cannot reliably distinguish stage I from stage II disease but can distinguish them from more advanced tumors. Delayed scans are very helpful in defining the true extent of tumor, because contrast can pool around the tumor mass on these views.

Renal parenchymal invasion is the key feature in separating early- and late-stage disease. In stage III disease, tumor infiltrates the renal parenchyma or the peripelvic fat. Stage IV disease is defined by local extrarenal extension, lymph node involvement, or distant metastases. Both stage III and stage IV disease can be confused with an infiltrating renal cell carcinoma.

When performing a spiral CT scan of the kidneys, careful attention must be directed to the renal pelvis. Routine spiral scanning does not opacify the renal collecting system. Therefore for patients with any subtle suggestion of intraluminal filling defect, or in studies performed for evaluation of hematuria or known transitional cell carcinoma, delayed scans are necessary for complete evaluation of the renal pelvis and ureter. Although delayed scanning markedly improves detection and conspicuity of transitional cell carcinoma, we have found that most tumors can be suggested even before obtaining the delayed scan (Figs. 13-15–13-17).

Other Tumors

A variety of other neoplasms can commonly involve the kidney. Wilm's tumor is the most common pediatric renal tumor, usually presenting as a large mass that can invade the renal vein and inferior vena cava (Fig. 13-18). Collateral vessels may be demonstrated. Tumor extension is accurately demonstrated using multiplanar reconstruction or 3D images generated by the spiral data set. Oncocytomas usually demonstrate features identical to renal cell carcinoma, although demonstration of a central scar may suggest the diagnosis (Fig. 13-19). Oncocytomas are hypervascular, although this alone is not of significant value in the differentiation from renal cell carcinoma. Most, if not all, patients still require nephrectomy to exclude renal cell carcinoma.

The use of spiral CT for the routine staging of the oncological patient has led to an increase in the number of incidentally discovered renal metastases. Metastases may present as

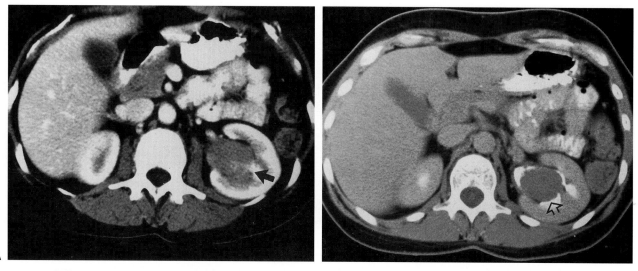

FIG. 13-15. Transitional cell carcinoma. (**A**) Spiral scan reveals mass (*arrow*) distending the left renal pelvis. (**B**) Delayed conventional scan confirms presence of large mass (*arrowhead*).

single or multiple masses, which typically are hypovascular (Fig. 13-20). In many cases the lesions do not distort the renal outline and so can easily be overlooked on noncontrast scans. Some have advocated partial nephrectomy as treatment for small metastases, which are detected with increased frequency on spiral CT scanning.

RENAL CYSTIC DISEASE

The Simple Cyst

Renal cysts are round and usually cortically based. On CT, cysts demonstrate sharp, smooth margins with the nor-

mal renal parenchyma. Attenuation values are near that of water (-10 to 20 HU), with no increase after the administration of contrast. Because of peak contrast enhancement, spiral CT is ideally suited to help define the walls and clearly define the smooth transition with normal, uniformly enhancing renal cortex.

Conventional CT can result in errors in the diagnosis of the simple cyst (47). Errors can result from partial volume averaging of small (<1 cm) cysts or those that are small and completely intrarenal, both of which may falsely elevate the attenuation number. Another common error is the impression of a thick cyst wall that occurs when the parenchymal beak is imaged in cross-section (48). By virtually eliminating

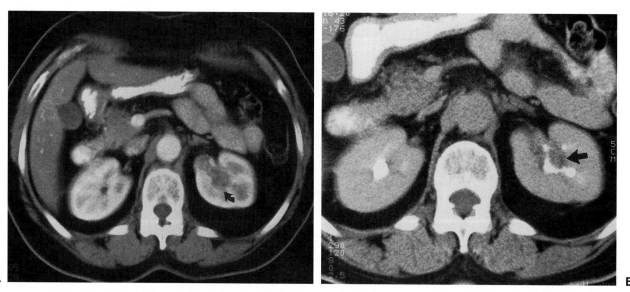

FIG. 13-16. Transitional cell carcinoma. (**A**) Spiral scan suggests possible mass in the renal pelvis (*arrow*). (**B**) Delayed conventional scan definitively confirms presence of renal pelvis filling defect (*arrow*). Delayed scans should routinely supplement the corticomedullary phase spiral CT in patients with hematuria and/or suspected transitional cell carcinoma.

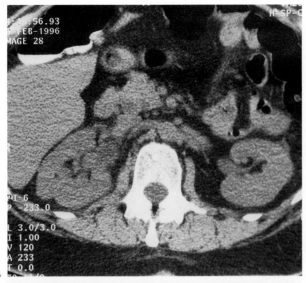

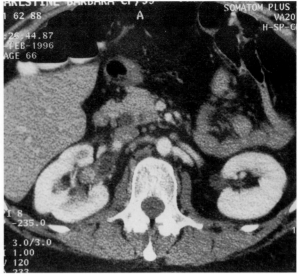

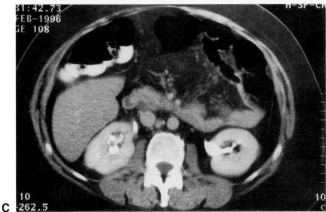

FIG. 13-17. Transitional cell carcinoma of the kidney. **(A)** Noncontrast CT demonstrates an area of increased density (*arrow*) in the right renal pelvis. **(B)** On corticomedullary-phase images the mass minimally enhances relative to its precontrast study. On other sections the tumor appears to extend through the sinus fat representing stage III disease. **(C)** Delayed CT scans in excretory phase demonstrate the calyceal destruction consistent with tumor. Note the variable appearance of the tumor, depending on the phase of enhancement.

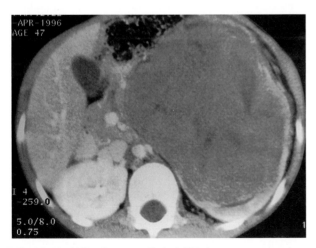

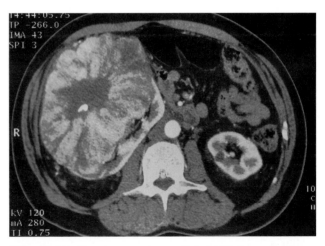

FIG. 13-18. Wilms' tumor. Spiral CT demonstrates a large infiltrating mass of the left kidney. The small residual amount of normal cortex in the posterior portion of the left kidney is seen. This is a classic appearance for Wilms' tumor in a 6-year-old child.

FIG. 13-19. Renal oncocytoma. Spiral CT demonstrates a hypervascular right renal mass. Note the configuration of the mass, with the stellate central scar and central calcification with hypervascularity in the rest of the lesion. This is a classic configuration for an oncocytoma.

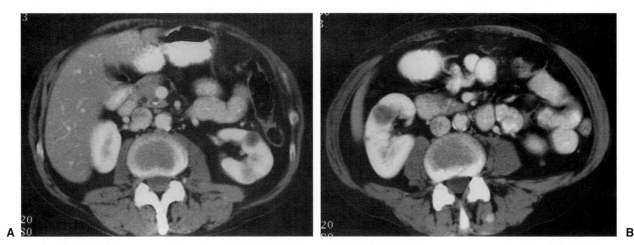

FIG. 13-20. Metastatic melanoma to the kidney. **(A,B)** Spiral CT demonstrates multiple low-density renal masses bilaterally. The cystic nature of the mass is a classic finding in metastatic melanoma.

partial volume averaging, spiral scanning can increase our specificity in the diagnosis of the simple renal cyst, thereby avoiding the erroneous diagnosis of an indeterminate renal mass. Similarly, indeterminate masses found on ultrasound or conventional CT can be confidently characterized on spiral CT. Bosniak and Rofsky (5), in a review of the problems associated with the detection and characterization of small renal masses, felt "that a normal contrast enhanced CT scan of the kidneys with use of 5-mm sections, obtained with a helical scanner, for all practical purposes rules out a clinically significant renal parenchymal neoplasm."

Renal cysts are associated with syndromes such as tuberous sclerosis or von Hippel–Lindau disease. In tuberous sclerosis, the cysts are often small, rarely exceeding 3 cm in diameter (49). Multiple angiomyolipomas are characteristic of tuberous sclerosis. Patients with von Hippel–Lindau disease can also demonstrate multiple renal cysts; however, these cysts may be a precursor to malignancy. Tumors in this setting often present as masses arising from the cyst wall and are frequently bilateral. Careful evaluation is necessary in these patients, as tumors are often small (<2 cm) and very difficult to distinguish from other cysts (50).

The Complicated Cyst

Complicated cysts can be seen in the setting of superimposed infection or hemorrhage. The benign, complicated cyst can be difficult to differentiate from a cystic and septated renal cell carcinoma. In general, if the septae are thin (1 mm or less) and smooth, a benign diagnosis is made with confidence. The septations should not demonstrate enhancement. Minimally complicated cysts may demonstrate calcification in the septations or cyst wall (51). Infected cysts can demonstrate markedly thickened walls that occasionally calcify (52).

If septations measure greater than 1 mm in thickness or are associated with solid or enhancing elements at their attachment to the cyst wall, malignancy must be considered (51). Because of data continuity provided from a single

breath-hold acquisition, spiral CT can visualize the margins of cystic lesions with great precision. This can be helpful in the detection of subtle nodularity or enhancement in the wall of a cystic neoplasm.

Hyperdense renal cysts can be confused with solid masses on CT. Most hyperdense cysts result from hemorrhage or proteinaceous debris, with hemorrhage complicating approximately 6% of simple cysts (48). Two-thirds of patients with polycystic kidney disease have hyperdense cysts (52,53).

Parapelvic Cysts

Parapelvic cysts are likely lymphatic in origin. They can be single or multiple, and commonly present in the perihilar region of the kidney. The CT characteristics are those of the simple cyst. Parapelvic cysts can mimic hydronephrosis or the renal pelvis on dynamic spiral CT evaluation. Delayed scans, which demonstrate characteristic compression of the renal pelvis, are often necessary to establish the proper diagnosis.

Polycystic Kidney Disease

Polycystic kidney disease usually manifests clinically during the third or fourth decade. Patients can present with flank pain, hematuria, hypertension, infection, or a palpable abdominal mass. Some patients are asymptomatic. Spiral CT demonstrates enlarged kidneys with multiple, bilateral cysts of varying size. Cysts can often also be demonstrated in the liver, spleen, and pancreas. The hyperdense cyst (60–90 HU) is a common complication, seen in up to two-thirds of patients. It usually results from prior post-traumatic hemorrhage, followed by clot retraction and protein concentration (54,55). Cyst wall calcification then results in approximately 25% of patients, usually those with more advanced disease. This finding alone is not worrisome for neoplasm unless an associated soft-tissue mass also is present (56).

Flank pain with hematuria is a common clinical dilemma

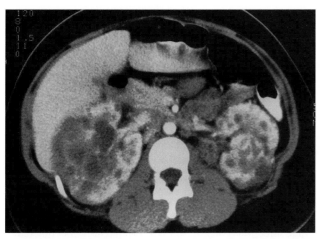

FIG. 13-21. Polycystic kidney disease with secondary infection. Spiral CT demonstrated unsuspected polycystic kidney disease. In the lateral portion of the right kidney the cysts are not well defined and are of increased density. The patient had a positive urine culture for *Escherichia coli* and several of these cysts were secondarily infected. It can be difficult to detect acute polynephritis in a patient with polycystic kidney disease.

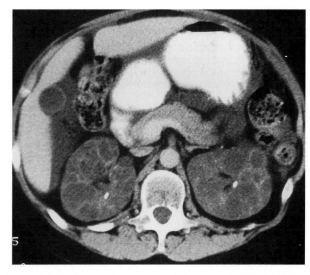

FIG. 13-23. Acquired cystic renal disease. Spiral CT without contrast demonstrates enlarged kidneys with multiple cysts and calcifications. The patient had a history of systemic lupus erythematosus and end-stage renal disease.

in a patient with polycystic kidney disease. This may result from cyst hemorrhage, calculi (found in 20% to 36% of patients), or infection (56). Spiral CT is ideally suited for differentiating these complications. We have found the early dynamic images obtained during spiral CT to be more sensitive than conventional delayed scanning in the detection of secondary pyelonephritis, especially in these patients (Fig. 13-21). Very rarely, neoplasm can complicate polycystic kidney disease (57,58) (Fig. 13-22).

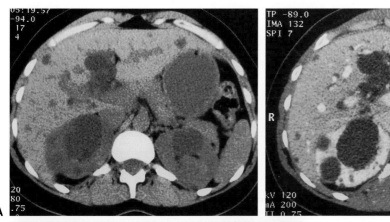

A   B

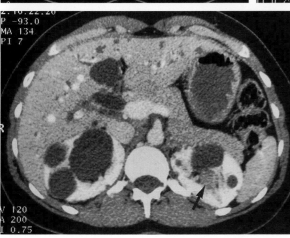

FIG. 13-22. Renal cell carcinoma in a patient with polycystic kidney disease. **(A)** Noncontrast CT demonstrates multiple bilateral renal and hepatic cysts. There is an area in the posterior portion of the left kidney that is of higher CT attenuation, which could represent either a mass or hemorrhage into a cyst. **(B,C)** Spiral CT in cortical medullary phase demonstrates multiple bilateral cysts that meet the classic criteria of simple cysts. There is a mass posteriorly (*arrow*) in the left kidney that corresponds to an area seen on the noncontrast studies. This was biopsied and subsequently removed and was a renal cell carcinoma. Note that with spiral CT these two images are but 4 mm apart.

C

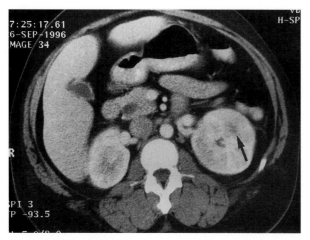

FIG. 13-24. Acute pyelonephritis. Spiral CT demonstrates diffuse enlargement of the left kidney. Note the foci of low density (*arrow*) consistent with the diagnosis of acute pyelonephritis.

Acquired Cystic Disease of Uremia

Although the exact etiology is unclear, cysts can complicate renal failure, typically 3 or more years after the onset of hemodialysis (Fig. 13-23). Uremic cysts can regress after renal transplantation (59). The kidneys in acquired cystic disease of uremia are typically small, and the cysts are commonly intrarenal in location. There is a significant increased incidence of renal carcinomas in these patients. Spiral CT can help differentiate simple uremic cysts from a solid tumor.

RENAL INFLAMMATORY DISEASE

Acute Pyelonephritis

Acute pyelonephritis is usually a clinical diagnosis requiring no diagnostic imaging. Patients may be referred for CT evaluation if there is a poor clinical response and an abscess is suspected or if the diagnosis is in doubt. Ascending retrograde infection typically spreads through the collecting ducts into the renal parenchyma (60). Hematogenous infection may involve the kidney in patients with tuberculosis, fungemia, or staphylococcal sepsis. In pyelonephritis, increased interstitial pressure results in obstruction of the tubules and intense focal vasoconstriction of the blood vessels. Involvement may be focal or diffuse, and the infected kidney is generally enlarged (Fig. 13-24). Enhanced CT scans demonstrate focal areas of striated or wedge-shaped perfusion abnormality, resulting in a characteristic "patchy" nephrogram (21).

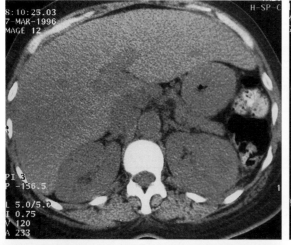

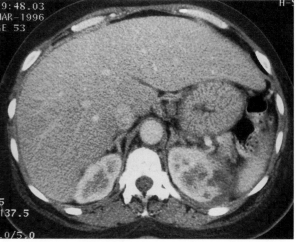

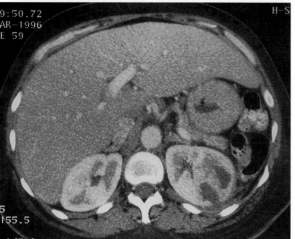

FIG. 13-25. Acute pyelonephritis with perirenal space extension. (**A**) Noncontrast CT demonstrates focal enlargement of the lateral portion of the left kidney with minimal change in attenuation. (**B,C**) Following contrast injection the abnormal enhancement of the left kidney is clearly defined secondary to acute pyelonephritis. In this case the corticomedullary-phase images best demonstrate the extent of disease. Extension into the perirenal space of infection is also seen.

Poorly enhanced areas of focal pyelonephritis can mimic a renal mass on conventional CT. Spiral scanning is probably more specific in differentiating infection from tumor (Fig. 13-25). Spiral CT is also helpful in detecting subtle cases of acute pyelonephritis. Abnormalities only visualized during early dynamic contrast enhancement, such as loss of the normal, sharp corticomedullary differentiation and delayed appearance of the cortical nephrogram, are clues to the diagnosis of underlying infection. Delayed views of the infected kidney may demonstrate a dense nephrogram (Fig. 13-26) or a striated nephrogram.

In the absence of direct visualization of thrombus or vascular collaterals, acute renal vein thrombosis can sometimes mimic conventional CT findings of acute pyelonephritis (61). Both entities can demonstrate renal enlargement and poor renal function. In acute pyelonephritis, low-attenuation wedge-shaped defects extend to the renal cortex, with ill-defined or poorly enhancing parenchymal lesions occasionally seen (62,63). In renal vein thrombosis, focal low-attenuation areas are better defined, representing the renal medulla surrounded by high-attenuation cortex (61). Spiral scanning during peak contrast enhancement can help differentiate these patterns.

In the patient with suspected acute pyelonephritis or other renal infection the sequencing of the spiral CT examination is crucial. Select noncontrast scans are obtained in most cases to exclude the possibility of renal calculi (Fig. 13-27). A spiral CT acquisition in the corticomedullary phase is obtained and may clearly define the presence and extent of infection. Delayed scans are also obtained in the excretory phase, which may in fact define the lesion a bit more specifically, especially if a striated nephrogram is detected. Kawashima (64) has looked into the problem of renal infection with CT and found that there is variability between cases,

and no single set of rules about the optimal image sequence has yet been defined.

Chronic Pyelonephritis

In patients with chronic pyelonephritis, spiral CT demonstrates focal parenchymal scars with underlying calyceal distortion. This is typically most pronounced in the polar regions of the kidney. The kidneys are often small, and renal calculi are frequently seen.

In addition, chronic scarring can produce an irregular, lobulated cortical surface that may mimic a renal mass on sonography or conventional CT. Spiral CT nicely demonstrates the normally enhancing cortex and thus improves detection of focal areas of cortical scarring or thinning. Thus spiral CT helps to distinguish focal scarring from a renal mass. Delayed scans are often helpful to demonstrate the underlying blunted calyces and to confirm the location of renal calculi.

Xanthogranulomatous pyelonephritis is an uncommon form of chronic inflammatory disease, felt to result from obstruction in the presence of infection. CT findings here include a staghorn calculus, an absent or markedly diminished nephrogram, and dilated calyces (62). Extension to the perirenal space and psoas compartment is readily demonstrated by spiral CT.

Renal Abscess

Abscess formation can complicate pyelonephritis or an infected cyst (Figs. 13-28, 13-29). Lesions are low in attenuation, and classically demonstrate an enhancing, thick, and irregular wall, especially when chronic (63). Spiral CT improves lesion characterization because of timed bolus con-

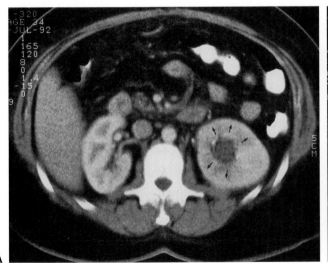
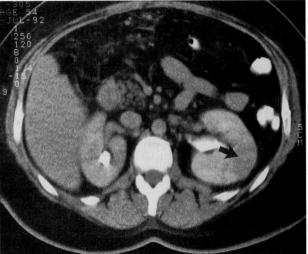

FIG. 13-26. Acute pyelonephritis. **(A)** Spiral CT reveals asymmetrically decreased cortical nephrogram involving focal regions of the left kidney (*arrows*). The kidney is minimally enlarged. **(B)** Delayed conventional scan shows focal regions of pyelonephritis with persistent dense nephrogram. Preserved normal parenchyma is seen laterally (*arrow*).

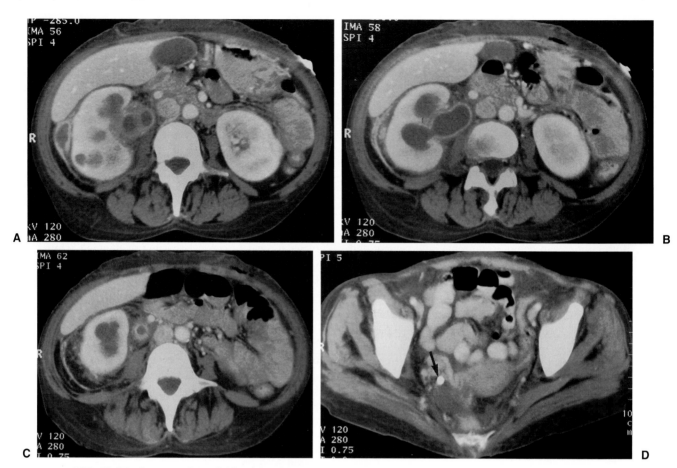

FIG. 13-27. Acute pyelonephritis of the right kidney secondary to ureteral obstruction. **(A–C)** Spiral CT demonstrates a dilated right pelvocalyceal system and ureter. Note that the inflammatory process involves the right pararenal space. **(D)** The obstruction was secondary to stone in distal ureter (*arrow*).

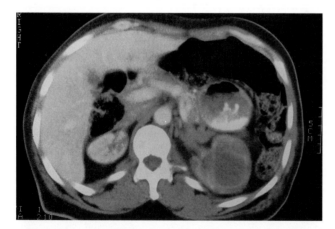

FIG. 13-28. Renal abscess. Spiral CT in this oncological patient demonstrates enlargement of the upper pole of the left kidney with cystic changes and septations seen. The cystic area is of higher attenuation than a simple cyst and has irregular enhancing walls and was newly appearing over several weeks. This was secondary to an *Escherichia coli* abscess.

trast enhancement. Furthermore, the virtual elimination of partial volume averaging provided by spiral scanning can aid in the detection of smaller lesions and in the demonstration of gas bubbles, which are virtually pathognomonic for renal abscess formation. A perinephric abscess can result from extension through the renal capsule. Multiplanar imaging may be helpful in defining the full extent of disease in these patients.

VASCULAR DISEASE

Renal Artery Stenosis

Renal artery stenosis is implicated in approximately 5% of patients with hypertension. With currently available technology, neither color duplex ultrasound nor magnetic resonance angiography has proven adequate in screening patients for significant renal artery stenosis (65–68). Both curved multiplanar and 3D imaging using the spiral CT data set are being shown to provide a reliable, noninvasive screening method for direct visualization of renal artery stenosis. Because imaging occurs during peak arterial opacification, spi-

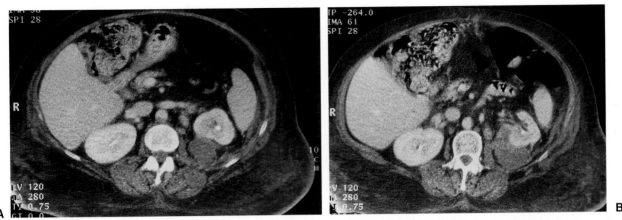

FIG. 13-29. Acute polynephritis with peri- and pararenal space extension. **(A,B)** Spiral CT demonstrates decreased enhancement in posterior portion of the left kidney with extension of the inflammatory process into the left peri- and pararenal space. This was subsequently drained and was an abscess. The patient had presented with a fever of unknown origin with no localizing renal findings.

ral CT clearly defines the location and extent of luminal narrowing (13,69,70).

Brink et al. (71) investigated the optimization of protocols for renal artery evaluation and found that critical renal artery stenosis was best depicted with 2-mm collimation, 2–4-mm table speed (pitch of 1–2), and data reconstruction at 1-mm intervals. Several articles from leading academic institutions have found spiral CT angiography to be equal in accuracy to classic renal angiography (69,70). Because of its noninvasiveness (i.e., freedom from complications) as well as lower cost and speed, spiral CT angiog-

raphy is currently the preferred choice of examination for renal artery evaluation.

On spiral CT the renal artery and any narrowing can be clearly defined and quantified. Other indirect, corroborative evidence of renal artery stenosis is deduced by noting a small and smooth, nonobstructed kidney. Spiral CT may demonstrate an asymmetric delay in the appearance of the cortical nephrogram (Fig. 13-30). The cortical nephrogram is prolonged on delayed images, resulting from decreased glomerular filtration (26). Frequently, other clues to the diagnosis of renal vascular disease are present on the CT scan, such

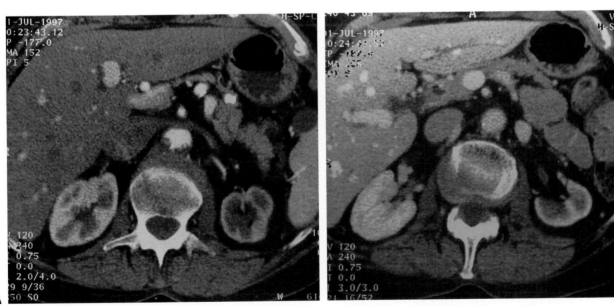

FIG. 13-30. Renal artery stenosis. **(A,B)** Spiral CT demonstrates atrophic left kidney with decreased intensity of enhancement in the cortical medullary phase and persistence of corticomedullary pattern in the delayed phase of enhancement. The cortex is thin in the left kidney compared with the right. Three-dimensional reconstruction demonstrated the patient's renal artery stenosis.

as severe abdominal aortic atherosclerosis or aneurysm formation. The role of spiral CT angiography, including its role in the renal transplant donor, is discussed in more detail in Chapter 20.

Renal Infarction

Renal infarcts are commonly the result of cardiac emboli. The kidney in acute global infarction is rarely enlarged. A characteristic rim of enhancement, representing collateral capsular perfusion, is seen surrounding a hypodense, non-functioning, infarcted kidney (72). The rim usually measures no more than 4 mm in depth (26). Occasionally, vermiform and globular medullary enhancement is demonstrated. Although this finding is of unknown origin, it probably reflects collateral blood flow (73).

Renal infarcts can also be focal, presenting as wedge-shaped defects that extend to the capsular surface. Over time, atrophy occurs in the vascular distribution of the infarction. Segmental infarctions of the anterior or posterior renal arteries demonstrate a characteristic appearance on CT, with the larger ventral branch supplying the anterior lateral portion of the kidney and the smaller dorsal branch supplying the posterior medial aspect (Fig. 13-31). The optimal enhancement of normal renal cortex afforded by spiral technique highlights areas of renal infarction that could be missed on conventional CT.

Renal Vein Thrombosis

The CT diagnosis of renal vein thrombosis is based on direct visualization of an intraluminal filling defect within an enlarged vein. In patients with poor renal function or decreased renal perfusion, care must be taken not to misdiagnose normal delayed filling of the renal veins from thrombus. Delayed scans are often helpful in questionable cases. Indirect signs of renal vein thrombosis include demonstration of collateral vessels, renal enlargement, thickening of Gerota'a fascia, and retroperitoneal hemorrhage. The use of spiral CT with narrow collimation and close interscan reconstruction intervals is ideal for mapping the patency of the renal vein. In our experience, acquisition of data at around 40 s after injection appears to be an ideal protocol.

Spiral CT is sensitive in detection of the asymmetric, abnormally delayed cortical nephrogram seen in patients with renal vein thrombosis. This delay results from diminished glomerular filtration and slowed tubular transit due to compression of the tubules by interstitial edema. Delayed scans may be obtained when the renal veins are opacified to confirm the presence of intraluminal thrombus. Perhaps most importantly, spiral scanning has the potential to be more sensitive than conventional CT in the demonstration of underlying etiologies of renal vein thrombosis, such as renal cell carcinoma.

Small-Vessel Disease

Many diseases can involve the intrarenal vasculature. These include the collagen vascular diseases, radiation nephritis, and hypertension. The spiral CT appearance is nonspecific in these entities, with parenchymal scarring frequently seen. The involved kidneys may be small and poorly functioning, with marked cortical thinning. Areas of hemorrhage may result from rupture of microaneurysms in patients with polyarteritis nodosa, Wegener's granulomatosis, lupus, or intravenous drug abuse. Arterial-phase imaging is ideal

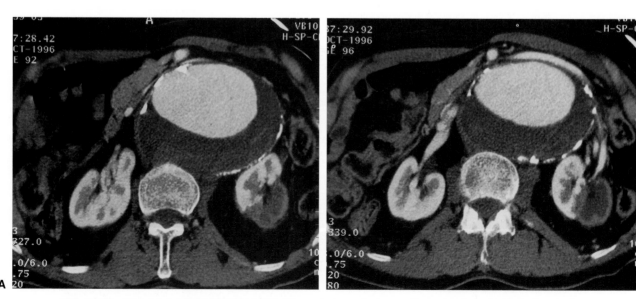

FIG. 13-31. Renal infarct. **(A,B)** Spiral CT demonstrates a large aortic aneurysm with thrombus in its wall. Note the infarcted lateral portion of the left kidney. The study clearly demonstrates lack of enhancement of the lateral portion of the left kidney. The infarct is acute, as the kidney shows no signs of atrophy and a well-defined cortex and medulla.

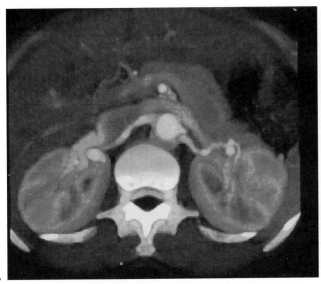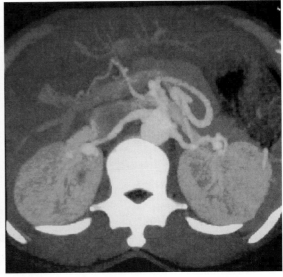

FIG. 13-32. Multiple renal artery aneurysms. Three-dimensional reconstructions with volume-rendering technique (**A**) and MIP (**B**) demonstrate multiple bilateral renal artery aneurysms.

for visualization of these small aneurysms (Fig. 13-32). Radiation nephritis may be acute or chronic, with renal failure ensuing from tubular and glomerular degeneration, as well as vascular fibrinoid necrosis.

Vascular Anomalies

One or more accessory renal arteries are present in up to 40% of normal patients (Fig. 13-33). These usually arise distal to the major artery. Accessory renal branches are best appreciated with spiral CT angiography. Three-dimensional CT angiography with volumetric reconstruction is ideal in these patients and can detect accessory renal arteries with an accuracy equal to classic angiography.

Common venous anomalies include the circumaortic and retroaortic renal vein (74,75). The retroaortic left renal vein is seen in approximately 2% of patients. Demonstration of these vascular anomalies is of vital importance for presurgical planning in patients who are potential renal donors as well as in patients scheduled for resection of renal tumors. Dual-phase spiral CT can define the venous map as well as the arterial map in a single examination (Figs. 13-34, 13-35).

Other Vascular Diseases

Peak contrast enhancement provided by spiral scanning allows for improved detection of congenital and acquired

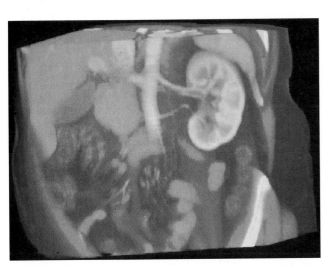

FIG. 13-33. Multiple renal arteries in a potential renal donor. Spiral CT with 3D reconstructions demonstrate the presence of two left renal arteries. The data set was processed with volume rendering.

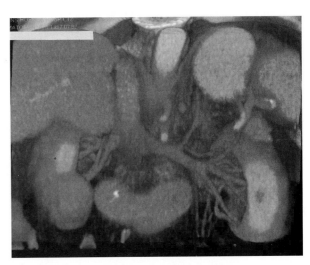

FIG. 13-34. Three-dimensional display of renal venous anatomy. Spiral CT with volume rendering allows generation of highly detailed venous maps as in this case.

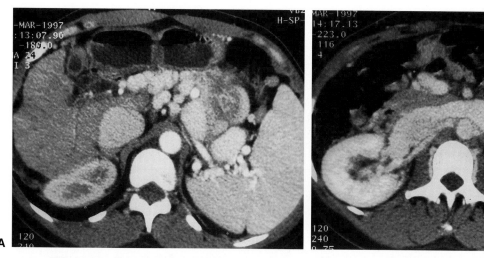

FIG. 13-35. Enlarged left renal vein secondary to splenorenal collateralization due to cirrhosis with portal hypertension. **(A,B)** Spiral CT demonstrates cirrhotic liver with multiple varices. Collateral pathways with splenorenal shunting resulted in large left renal vein.

vascular disease. Renal artery aneurysms can be seen in patients with arteriosclerosis or as a result of septic emboli (76). Congenital arteriovenous malformations are rare. Acquired arteriovenous malformations most commonly result from prior renal biopsy (Fig. 13-36). Dynamic scanning can reveal enlarged feeding vessels and collateral circulation.

RENAL CALCULI

Conventional CT has been shown to be sensitive in the detection of renal calculi (77–79). Theoretically, smaller calculi should be detected with increased frequency and sensitivity on spiral CT. Lack of breathing misregistration ensures continuous coverage of the entire kidney, which improves detection of small stones. Density measurements of small renal calculi are more accurate, as partial volume averaging is virtually eliminated. Olcott et al. (79) found that ''3D spiral CT depicted calculi more sensitively than traditional techniques and provided new information and improved accuracy in the evaluation of nephrolithiasis.''

In performing a spiral CT for suspected stone disease, precontrast scans should be obtained. In most cases no additional scan sequences will be needed. However, even on enhanced studies alone, one is usually able to distinguish renal calculi from potentially obscuring contrast (Fig. 13-37), especially if images are acquired before contrast excretion in the corticomedullary phase. Delayed scans may then be obtained to help localize calculi within a calyx or the renal pelvis.

OBSTRUCTION

Early scanning during the cortical nephrogram phase of enhancement can be useful in the detection of subtle obstruction. Asymmetry in the appearance of the cortical nephro-

gram on spiral CT, manifested by early delay and late persistence, signifies the presence of either abnormal perfusion or tubular transit (26,80). In this setting the finding of a dilated collecting system on delayed scans strongly suggests active obstruction.

However, acute cases of obstruction may demonstrate little or no calyceal dilatation, making spiral CT findings similar to those of renal artery stenosis, renal vein thrombosis, or pyelonephritis. On later images, the nephrogram can appear mottled or striated, and hyperdense (80,81). Delayed images of the collecting system and ureter may help define the cause of obstruction at any point from renal pelvis to the bladder. Suspicious areas can then be rescanned with narrow collimation spiral CT to help characterize the obstructing lesion.

One of the most recently investigated areas of spiral CT applications has been the utility of unenhanced spiral CT for the detection of ureteral calculi and ureteral obstruction in patients presenting with acute flank pain (82–86). Although specific imaging techniques have varied among institutions, most investigators now agree that spiral CT with narrow collimation (3 mm) and close interscan reconstruction (1–3 mm) is the gold standard for calculi detection. Smith et al. found unenhanced CT as effective as intravenous urography (IVU) in determining if ureteral obstruction is present, and more effective than IVU in the identification of stones as the etiology of the obstruction (84–86). This same group evaluated 292 patients with 100 proven ureteral stones and found unenhanced spiral CT to be 97% sensitive, 96% specific, and 97% accurate for the depiction of ureteral calculi.

Other groups, including Sommer et al. (86), have also found noncontrast spiral CT to be a rapid and accurate method for determining the presence of ureteral calculi. Secondary signs—including hydronephrosis, hydroureter, perinephric soft-tissue change, and perinephric edema—can

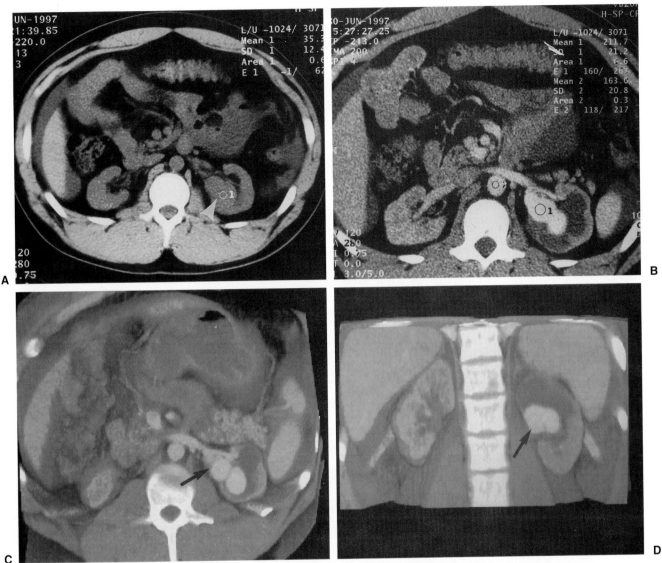

FIG. 13-36. Renal arteriovenous malformation. The patient has a history of progressive renal failure and a biopsy several years earlier. (**A**) Noncontrast CT scans demonstrate an apparent mass (*arrowhead*) in the mid-portion of the left kidney. (**B,C**) Spiral CT with arterial-phase imaging demonstrates that the apparent mass seen on noncontrast CT scans enhanced equal to the aorta consistent with a arteriovenous malformation. On delayed scans there was little difference in enhancement. (**C,D**) Three-dimensional reconstructions clearly define the arteriovenous malformation that caused obstruction of the left upper pole collecting system. Arteriovenous malformations are one of the complications of renal biopsies.

provide supportive evidence for acute obstruction (16–18). Reformatted views using the spiral data set in the curved planar format can produce images similar to those with IVU and can aid in communicating findings with clinicians (86). Most recently, Levine et al. have stressed the limited value of plain-film radiography for the detection of ureteral calculi, instead advocating the immediate use of unenhanced spiral CT in patients presenting with flank pain and symptoms of ureteral calculi. In their study, plain radiographs detected calculi with a sensitivity of only 59% with spiral CT as the standard of reference (82). Without question, spiral CT probably will eventually replace IVU as a rapid screening

technique for evaluating patients with flank pain and suspected ureteral calculi.

RENAL TRAUMA

CT is the imaging modality of choice in the evaluation of renal trauma (87–89) (Figs. 13-38, 13-39). Technical advances in spiral scanning enable ''survey'' coverage of the abdomen during a single breath-hold acquisition. This allows for ideal peak contrast opacification of the entire abdomen. In the kidney, this may be useful in detecting subtle lacerations, contusions, segmental or cortical infarcts, and

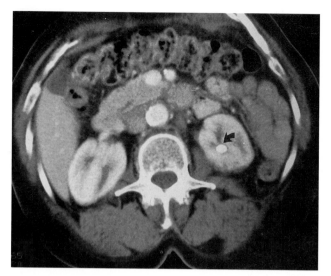

FIG. 13-37. Parenchymal renal calculus. A small stone (*arrow*) is identified in the left kidney. Most stones can be differentiated from enhancing parenchyma on early dynamic spiral scan.

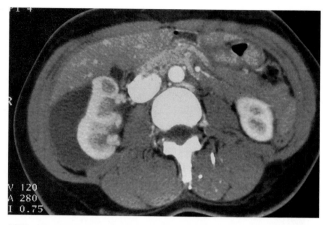

FIG. 13-39. Page kidney. Spiral CT demonstrates increased corticomedullary enhancement of the right kidney secondary to an old subcapsular hematoma. This is the classic appearance of a Page kidney.

subcapsular hematomas. Acute traumatic occlusion or avulsion of the renal artery results in complete absence of renal contrast enhancement shortly after injury. With time, collateral capsular flow is seen, identical to that seen in nontrau-

matic renal infarction. This topic is discussed in more detail in Chapter 18.

CONGENITAL ANOMALIES

Early fusion of the lower poles of the kidneys can result in the horseshoe kidney (Fig. 13-40). This is found in one in 600 people and represents a very common renal fusion

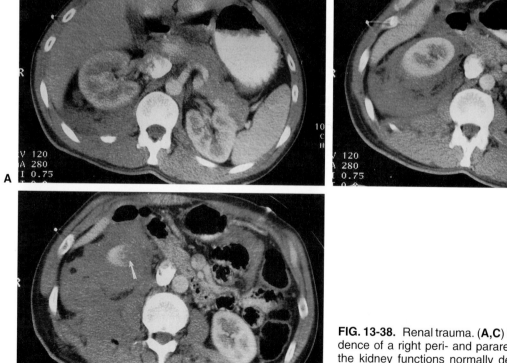

FIG. 13-38. Renal trauma. **(A,C)** Spiral CT demonstrates evidence of a right peri- and pararenal space bleed. Note that the kidney functions normally despite the laceration in the lower pole (*arrow*). Note the dense enhancement of the inferior vena cava, which is secondary to injection through a femoral catheter.

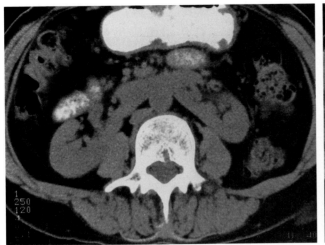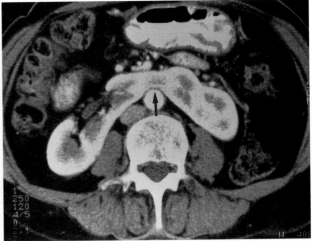

FIG. 13-40. Horseshoe kidney. **(A)** Precontrast and **(B)** postcontrast scans reveal characteristic appearance of horseshoe kidney. Functioning parenchyma is demonstrated in the isthmus (*arrow*).

anomaly (90). The lower poles fuse anterior to the aorta and inferior vena cava via an isthmus of functioning renal tissue or fibrous tissue. Most patients with horseshoe kidney demonstrate multiple, bilateral renal arteries. Other fusion anomalies include crossed fused ectopia and the pancake kidney. Spiral scanning can help define the relationship of the abnormal kidney to the major vessels. Other common congenital anomalies include renal agenesis, renal duplication, and malrotation.

RENAL TRANSPLANTS

Spiral CT has a potential role in the evaluation of the renal transplant patient (91–93). The most important application here may lie in the evaluation of vascular complications, which are a significant cause of graft dysfunction and occur in up to 10% of patients. Common types of vascular complications include arterial and venous stenosis or occlusion, arteriovenous fistulas, and pseudoaneurysms (Fig. 13-41) (see color plate 13 following p. 352). Scanning during peak vascular enhancement increases detection of these potential complications. Other common complications include peritransplant fluid collections and obstruction.

The role of spiral CT for the noninvasive evaluation of potential living, related renal transplant donors is another developing application. At our institution renal transplants are being harvested by a laparoscopic approach rather than with classic open surgery (94). Patients have fewer postprocedure complications and return to work after 3.9 ± 1.8 weeks versus 6.4 ± 3.1 weeks, with full activity at an earlier

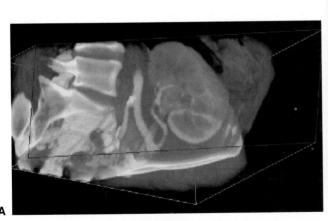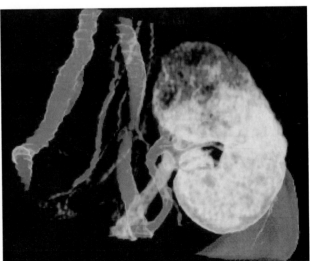

FIG. 13-41. Patent renal artery in a transplanted kidney. **(A,B)** Spiral CT with 3D reconstruction demonstrates the patent renal artery anastomosis. Color enhancement can be helpful in select cases. Vessel patency could not be defined on the basis of axial images only.

date. Dual-phase 3D spiral CT has proved to be a viable alternative to angiography and has become the study of choice at our institution. The use of volumetric 3D rendering has been critical to our success in these patients.

SUMMARY

Spiral CT represents an exciting advance in evaluation of renal disease, offering several technical advantages in evaluation of the kidney. Scans can be obtained during specific phases of renal contrast enhancement, densitometry measurements are accurate, and minimal respiratory artifact results in less potential errors in diagnosis. As a result of the newer techniques, smaller cancers are detected with increased frequency, which will likely impact upon overall patient survival. Subtle asymmetries of the cortical nephrogram can be readily detected, increasing sensitivity and often specificity in the diagnosis of renal obstruction, renal artery stenosis, or pyelonephritis. Findings from partial volume averaging of benign lesions with normal parenchyma are minimized. Finally, improved lesion characterization should decrease the incidence of the diagnostically frustrating indeterminate renal mass. Newer vascular applications as well as 3D imaging suggest that the role of spiral CT in evaluation of the kidneys will only increase in the near future.

REFERENCES

1. Kalender WA, Seissler W, Klotz E, Vock P. Spiral volumetric CT with single-breath-hold technique, continuous transport, and continuous scanner rotation. *Radiology* 1990;176:181–183.
2. Kalender WA, Polacin A. Physical performance characteristics of spiral CT scanning. *Med Phys* 1991;18:910–915.
3. Heiken JP, Brink JA, Vannier MW. Spiral (helical) CT. *Radiology* 1993;189:647–656.
4. Bosniak MA. The small (≤3.0 cm) renal parenchymal tumor: detection, diagnosis, and controversies. *Radiology* 1991;179:307–317.
5. Bosniak MA, Rofsky NM. Problems in the detection and characterization of small renal masses. *Radiology* 1996;198(3):638–641.
6. Szolar DH, Kammerhuber F, Altziebler S, et al. Multiphasic helical CT of the kidney: increased conspicuity for detection and characterization of small (<3-cm) renal masses. *Radiology* 1997;202(1):211–217.
7. Urban BA. The small renal mass: what is the role of multiphasic helical scanning? *Radiology* 1997;202(1):22–23.
8. Zeman RK, Fox SH, Silverman PM, et al. Helical (spiral) CT of the abdomen. *AJR* 1993;160:719–725.
9. Burgener FA, Hamlin DJ. Contrast enhancement in abdominal CT: bolus vs. infusion. *AJR* 1981;137:351–358.
10. Ishakawa I, Onouchi Z, Saito Y, et al. Renal cortex visualization and analysis of dynamic CT curves of the kidney. *J Comput Assist Tomogr* 1981;5:695–701.
11. Lee JKT, Sagel SS, Stanley RJ. *Computed body tomography with MRI correlation*. New York: Raven Press, 1989;627–639.
12. Cochran ST, Krasny RM, Danovitch GM, et al. Helical CT angiography for examination of living renal donors. *AJR* 1997;168:1569–1574.
13. Brink JA. Spiral CT angiography of the abdomen and pelvis: interventional applications. *Abdom Imag* 1997;22:365–372.
14. Beregi JP, Elkohen M, Deklunder G, et al. Helical CT angiography compared with arteriography in the detection of renal artery stenosis. *AJR* 1996;167:495–501.
15. Fielding JR, Fox LA, Heller H, et al. Spiral CT in the evaluation of flank pain: overall accuracy and feature analysis. *J Comput Assist Tomogr* 1997;21(4):635–638.
16. Heneghan JP, Dalrymple NC, Verga M, Rosenfield AT, Smith RC. Soft-tissue "rim" sign in the diagnosis of ureteral calculi with use of unenhanced helical CT. *Radiology* 1997;202(3):709–711.
17. Katz DS, Lane MJ, Sommer FG. Unenhanced helical CT of ureteral stones: incidence of associated urinary tract findings. *AJR* 1996;166:1319–1322.
18. Kawashima A, Sandler CM, Boridy IC, Takahashi N, Benson GS, Goldman SM. Unenhanced helical CT of ureterolithiasis: value of the tissue rim sign. *AJR* 1996;168:997–1000.
19. Urban BA, Buckley J, Soyer P, Scherrer A, Fishman EK. CT appearance of transitional cell carcinoma of the renal pelvis: part 1. early-stage disease. *AJR* 1997;169:157–161.
20. Urban BA, Buckley J, Soyer P, Scherrer A, Fishman EK. CT appearance of transitional cell carcinoma of the renal pelvis: part 2. advanced-stage disease. *AJR* 1997;169:163–168.
21. Soulen MC, Fishman EK, Goldman SM, Gatewood OMB. Bacterial renal infection: role of CT. *Radiology* 1989;171:703–707.
22. Birnbaum BA, Jacobs JE, Ramchandani P. Multiphasic renal CT: comparison of renal mass enhancement during the corticomedullary and nephrographic phases. *Radiology* 1996;200(3):753–758.
23. Zeman RK, Zeiberg A, Hayes WS, Silverman PM, Cooper C, Garra BS. Helical CT of renal masses: the value of delayed scans. *AJR* 1996;167:771–776.
24. Cohan RH, Sherman LS, Korobkin M, Bass JC, Francis IR. Renal masses: assessment of corticomedullary-phase and nephrographic-phase CT scans. *Radiology* 1995;196(2):445–451.
25. Boijsen E. Anatomic and physiologic considerations In: Abrams HL et al., eds. Abrams Angiography, Boston: Little, Brown and Company, 1983;1118–1119.
26. Birnbaum BA, Bosniak MA, Megibow AJ. Asymmetry of the renal nephrogram of CT: significance of the unilateral prolonged cortical nephrogram. *Urol Radiol* 1991;12:173–177.
27. Zimmer WD, Williamson Jr B, Hartman GW, Hattery RR, O'Brien PC. Changing patterns in the evaluation of renal masses: economic implications. *AJR* 1984;143:285–289.
28. Curry NS, Schabel SI, Betsill WL. Small renal neoplasms: diagnostic imaging, pathologic features, and clinical course. *Radiology* 1986;158:113–117.
29. Balfe DM, McClennan BL, Stanley RJ, Weyman PJ, Sagel SS. Evaluation of renal masses considered indeterminate on computed tomography. *Radiology* 1982;142:421–428.
30. Levine E, Huntrakoon M, Wetzel LH. Small renal neoplasms: clinical, pathologic, and imaging features. *AJR* 1989;153:69–73.
31. Smith SJ, Bosniak MA, Megibow AJ, Hulnick DH, Horii SC, Raghavendra BN. Renal cell carcinoma: earlier discovery and increased detection. *Radiology* 1989;170:699–703.
32. Dunnick NR. Renal lesions: great strides in imaging. *Radiology* 1992;182:305–306.
33. Chernoff DM, Silverman SG, Kikinis R, et al. Three-dimensional imaging and display of renal tumors using spiral CT: a potential aid to partial nephrectomy. *Urology* 1994;43:125–129.
34. McClennan BL. Computed tomography in the diagnosis and staging of renal cell carcinoma. *Semin Urol* 1985;3:111–131.
35. Silverman SG, Lee BY, Seltzer SE, Bloom DA, Corless CL, Adams DF. Small (≤3 cm) renal masses: correlation of spiral CT features and pathologic findings. *AJR* 1994;163:597–605.
36. Goncharendo V, Gerlock Jr AJ, Kadir S, Turner B. Incidence and distribution of venous extension in 70 hypernephromas. *AJR* 1979;133:263–265.
37. Madayag MA, Ambos MA, Lefleur RS, Bosniak MA. Involvement of the inferior vena cava in patients with renal cell carcinoma. *Radiology* 1979;133:321–326.
38. Roubidoux MA, Dunnick NR, Sostman HD, Leder RA. Renal carcinoma: detection of venous extension with gradient-echo MR imaging. *Radiology* 1992;182:269–272.
39. Smith PA, Marshall FF, Urban BA, Heath DG, Fishman EK. Three-dimensional CT stereoscopic visualization of renal masses: impact on diagnosis and patient management. *AJR* 1997;169:1331–1334.
40. Foster WL, Roberts L, Halvorsen RA, Dunnick NR. Sonography of small renal masses with indeterminate density characteristics on computed tomography. *Urol Radiol* 1988;10:59–67.
41. Buckley JA, Scott Jr WW, Siegelman SS, et al. Pulmonary nodules: effect of increased data sampling on detection with spiral CT and confidence in diagnosis. *Radiology* 1995;196:395–400.

42. Kuszyk BS, Bluemke DA, Urban BA, et al. Portal-phase contrast-enhanced helical CT for the detection of malignant hepatic tumors: sensitivity based on comparison with intraoperative and pathologic findings. *AJR* 1996;166:91–95.

43. Bret PM, Bretagnolle M, Gaillard D, et al. Small, asymptomatic angiomyolipomas of the kidney. *Radiology* 1985;154:7–10.

44. Strotzer M, Lehner KB, Becker K. Detection of fat in a renal cell carcinoma mimicking angiomyolipoma. *Radiology* 1993;188:427–428.

45. Helenon O, Chretien Y, Paraf F, Melki P, Denys A, Moreau JF. Renal cell carcinoma containing fat: demonstration with CT. *Radiology* 1993;188:429–430.

46. Baron RL, McClennan BL, Lee JKT, Lawson T. Transitional cell carcinoma of the pelvis and ureter: CT evaluation. *Radiology* 1982;144:125–130.

47. Hartman DS. Cysts and cystic neoplasms. *Urol Radiol* 1990;12:7–10.

48. Segal AJ, Spitzer RM. Pseudothick-walled renal cyst by CT. *AJR* 1979;132:827–828.

49. Mitnick JS, Bosniak MA, Hilton S, Raghavendra BH, Subramanyam BR, Genieser NB. Cystic renal disease in tuberous sclerosis. *Radiology* 1983;147:85–87.

50. Levine E, Collins DL, Horton WA, Schimke RN. CT screening of the abdomen in von Hippel–Lindau disease. *AJR* 1982;139:505–510.

51. Bosniak MA. The current radiological approach to renal cysts. *Radiology* 1986;158:1–10.

52. Levine E, Grantham JJ. High-density renal cysts in autosomal dominant polycystic kidney disease demonstrated by CT. *Radiology* 1985;154:477–482.

53. Meziane MA, Fishman EK, Goldman SM, Friedman AC, Seigelman SS. Computed tomography of high density renal cysts in adult polycystic kidney disease. *J Comput Assist Tomogr* 1986;10:767–770.

54. Sussman S, Cochran ST, Pagani JJ, et al. Hyperdense renal masses: a CT manifestation of hemorrhagic renal cysts. *Radiology* 1984;150:207–211.

55. Fishman MC, Pollack HM, Argre PH, Banner MP. Case report. High protein content: another cause of CT hyperdense benign renal cyst. *J Comput Assist Tomogr* 1983;5:104–111.

56. Levine E, Grantham JJ. Calcified renal stones and cyst calcifications in autosomal dominant polycystic kidney disease: clinical and CT study in 84 patients. *AJR* 1992;159:77–81.

57. Gabow PA. Autosomal dominant kidney disease: more than a renal disease. *Am J Kidney Dis* 1985;5:104–111.

58. Gregoire JR, Torres VE, Holley KE, Farrow GM. Renal epithelial hyperplasia and neoplastic proliferation in autosomal dominant polycystic kidney disease. *Am J Kidney Dis* 1987;9:27–38.

59. Levine E, Grantham JJ, Slucher SL, Greathouse JL, Krohn BP. CT of acquired cystic kidney disease and renal tumors in long-term dialysis patients. *AJR* 1984;142:125–131.

60. Roberts JA. Pyelonephritis, cortical abscess, and perinephric abscess. *Urol Clin North Am* 1986;13:637–645.

61. Glazer GM, Francis IR, Gross BH, Amendola MA. Computed tomography of renal vein thrombosis. *J Comput Assist Tomogr* 1984;8:288–293.

62. Goldman SM, Hartman DS, Fishman EK, Finizio JP, Gatewood OMB, Siegelman SS. CT of xanthogranulomatous pyelonephritis: radiologic-pathologic correlation. *AJR* 1984;142:963–969.

63. Dunnick NR, McCallum RW, Sandler CM. *Textbook of uroradiology.* Baltimore: Williams and Wilkins, 1991.

64. Kawashima A, Sandler CM, Goldman SM, Ravel BK, Fishman EK. CT of renal inflammatory disease. *Radiographics* 1997;17:851–866.

65. Desberg AL, Paushter DM, Lammert GK, et al. Renal artery stenosis: evaluation with color Doppler flow imaging. *Radiology* 1990;177:749–753.

66. Middleton WD. Doppler evaluation of renal artery stenosis: past, present and future. *Radiology* 1992;184:307–308.

67. Berland LL, Koslin DB, Routh WD, Kellar FS. Renal artery stenosis: prospective evaluation of diagnosis with color duplex US compared with angiography. *Radiology* 1990;174:421–423.

68. Kim D, Edelman RR, Kent KC, Porter DH, Skillman JJ. Abdominal

69. aorta and renal artery stenosis: evaluation with MR angiography. *Radiology* 1990;174:727–731.

69. Galanski M, Prokop M, Chavan A, Schaefer CM, Jandeleit K, Nischelsky JE. Renal arterial stenoses: spiral CT angiography. *Radiology* 1993;189(1):185–192.

70. Halpern EJ, Wechsler RJ, DiCampli D. Threshold selection for CT angiography shaded surface display of the renal arteries. *J Digit Imag* 1995;8(3):142–147.

71. Brink JA, Lim JT, Wang G, Heiken JP, Deyoe LA, Vannier MW. Technical optimization of spiral CT for depiction of renal artery stenosis: in vitro analysis. *Radiology* 1995;194(1):157–163.

72. Glazer GM, London SS. CT appearance of global renal infarction. *J Comput Assist Tomogr* 1981;5:847–850.

73. Malmed AS, Love L, Jeffrey RB. Medullary CT enhancement in acute renal artery occlusion. *J Comput Assist Tomogr* 1992;16:107–109.

74. Beckmann CF, Abrams HL. Circumaortic venous ring: incidence and significance. *AJR* 1979;132:561–565.

75. Reed MD, Friedman AC, Nealey P. Anomalies of the left renal vein: analysis of 433 CT scans. *J Comput Assist Tomogr* 1982;6:1124–1126.

76. DuBrow RA, Patel SK. Mycotic aneurysm of the renal artery. *Radiology* 1981;138:577–582.

77. Segal AJ, Spataro RF, Linke CA, Frank IN, Rabinowitz R. Diagnosis of nonopaque calculi by computed tomography. *Radiology* 1978;129:447–450.

78. Federle MP, McAninch JW, Kaiser JA, Goodman PC, Roberts J, Mall JC. Computed tomography of urinary calculi. *AJR* 1980;136:255–258.

79. Olcott EW, Sommer FG, Napel S, et al. Accuracy of detection and measurement of renal calculi: in vitro comparison of three-dimensional spiral CT, radiography, and nephrotomography. *Radiology* 1997;204(1):19–25.

80. Samin A, Becker JA. CT nephrogram in acute obstructive uropathy. *Urol Radiol* 1991;12:178–180.

81. Bigongiari LR, Davis RM, Novak WG, Wicks JD, Kass E, Thornbury JR. Visualization of the medullary rays on excretory urography in experimental ureteric obstruction. *AJR* 1977;129:89–93.

82. Levine JA, Neitlich J, Verga M, Dalrymple N, Smith RC. Ureteral calculi in patients with flank pain: correlation of plain radiography with unenhanced helical CT. *Radiology* 1997;204(1):27–31.

83. Smith RC, Verga M, McCarthy S, Rosenfield AT. Diagnosis of acute flank pain: value of unenhanced helical CT. *AJR* 1995;166:97–101.

84. Smith RG, Rosenfield AT, Choe KA. Acute flank pain: comparison of noncontrast enhanced CT and intravenous urography. *Radiology* 1995;194:789–794.

85. Smith RC, Verga M, Dalrymple N, McCarthy S, Rosenfield AT. Acute ureteral obstruction: value of secondary signs on helical unenhanced CT. *AJR* 1996;167:1109–1113.

86. Sommer FG, Jeffrey Jr RB, Rubin GD, et al. Detection of ureteral calculi in patients with suspected renal colic: value of reformatted noncontrast helical CT. *AJR* 1995;165:509–513.

87. Federle MP, Kaiser JA, McAninch JW, Jeffrey RB, Mall JC. The role of computed tomography in renal trauma. *Radiology* 1981;141:455–460.

88. Sandler CM, Toombs BD. Computed tomographic evaluation of blunt renal injuries. *Radiology* 1981;141:461–466.

89. Bretan PN, McAninch JW, Federle MP, Jeffrey RB. Computerized tomographic staging of renal trauma: 85 consecutive cases. *J Urol* 1986;136:561–565.

90. Moore KL. *The developing human: clinically oriented embryology.* Philadelphia: WB Saunders, 1988.

91. Alfrey EJ, Rubin GD, Kuo PC, et al. The use of spiral computed tomography in the evaluation of living donors for kidney transplantation. *Transplantation* 1995;59(4):643–645.

92. Dodd III GD, Tublin ME, Shah A, Zajko AB. Imaging of vascular complications associated with renal transplants. *AJR* 1991;157:449–459.

93. Rubin GD, Alfrey EJ, Dake MD, et al. Assessment of living renal donors with spiral CT. *Radiology* 1995;195(2):457–462.

94. Ratner LE, Kavoussi LR, Schulam PG, Bender JS, Magnuson TH, Montgomery R. Comparison of laparoscopic live donor nephrectomy versus the standard open approach. *Clin Imag* 1997;96:138–139.

CHAPTER 14

Spiral CT Evaluation of the Pelvis

Bruce A. Urban and Elliot K. Fishman

Computed tomography has a well-established role in evaluating the pelvis (1–3). The utility of conventional CT has focused on the demonstration of pathology in the female pelvis, providing accurate staging of cervical, ovarian, and uterine cancer. Spiral CT provides an opportunity for improved evaluation of the pelvis (4,5). Data misregistration is essentially eliminated as the patient is advanced through the gantry at a constant rate during continuous data acquisition (6). Scans are obtained during optimal vascular opacification following bolus contrast administration. Together these advantages allow for potentially improved accuracy in the detection and staging of pelvic pathology, better definition of pelvic anatomy, and improved multiplanar and three-dimensional images. In our experience, spiral CT represents the state-of-the-art technique for CT evaluation of the pelvis (4,5). Most of this chapter focuses on the usefulness of spiral CT in the evaluation of the female pelvis.

TECHNIQUE

Because most older-generation spiral units have a specific length limitation, dedicated spiral CT scanning of the pelvis is usually performed using caudal-to-cranial data acquisition. This ensures coverage of the pelvic organs during peak vascular opacification (4,5). Spiral scanning begins at the level of the symphysis pubis following the administration of nonionic iodinated contrast at a rate of 1.5–2.0 mL/s. Scanning is initiated 90–120 s after the onset of contrast injection. This scanning delay—longer than the typical delay for spiral scanning in the upper abdomen—is necessary to optimize venous opacification and is critical for differentiating iliac blood vessels from lymph nodes (Fig. 14-1). Bolus contrast enhancement also delineates the endometrial cavity from the brightly enhancing myometrium and can help to differentiate tumor from the normal enhancing uterus (Fig. 14-2). When arterial anatomy is of major interest, scanning should begin earlier (50–70 s) following contrast injection at

a faster rate (2.0–3.0 mL/s). ''Pseudothrombosis,'' or partial opacification, of the femoral and iliac veins is a potential pitfall seen with early arterial-phase spiral scanning, or in patients with stagnant venous flow (Fig. 14-3). Care must be taken not to mistake partial venous opacification for deep venous thrombosis: ''pseudothrombosis'' is always bilateral and symmetric, and the veins are of normal caliber; clots are often unilateral and acutely increase the venous diameter.

Typical scanning parameters are 5–8-mm collimation, 5–8-mm table speed, with 4–5-mm reconstruction incrementation. Thinner collimation (3–5 mm) is helpful in the evaluation of known masses or tumors, when accurate staging and lesion characterization are important. Delayed images should be obtained in cases with complicated or confusing pathology. This is especially important in the evaluation of large ovarian masses or fluid collections, which can be difficult to differentiate from the unopacified bladder (Figs. 14-4, 14-5). Delayed images are usually obtained 5–8 min following contrast injection, allowing adequate time for contrast to reach the bladder.

Newer-generation spiral CT scanners have certainly increased protocol options in the pelvis. Most new machines now allow for multiple repeat scans with a negligible interscan delay. Furthermore, with the advent of subsecond scanning, improved reconstruction algorithms, and high-performance tubes, newer spiral scanners can routinely provide quality thin-collimation images of the entire chest, abdomen, and pelvis in one or two long breath-hold scans. Therefore with newer machines, pelvic spiral scans can be obtained utilizing the conventional superior-to-inferior acquisition, as adequate coverage of the pelvic organs is ensured. Usually, images of the chest and abdomen are obtained prior to pelvic scanning to optimize contrast dynamics in the mediastinum, liver, pancreas, and kidneys. Images of the pelvis are then obtained during the ideal phase of pelvic enhancement, 90–110 s following the start of contrast administration.

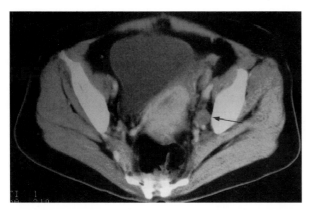

FIG. 14-1. Spiral CT technique. Optimal vascular opacification with spiral CT allows for confident display of the pelvic arteries and veins, and enables differentiation of abnormal lymph nodes from vessels, as in this patient with metastatic cervical cancer. Cancerous node is demonstrated in the left obturator chain (*arrow*). (Used with permission from Urban BA, Fishman EK. Spiral CT of the female pelvis: clinical applications. *Abdom Imaging* 1995;20:9–14.)

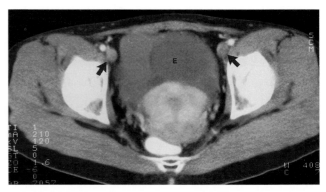

FIG. 14-3. Spiral CT technique. The veins of the lower extremities and pelvis are often partially opacified on spiral CT, and care must be taken not to misdiagnose normal veins (*arrows*) for thrombosed veins, as in this patient with a cystic endometrioma (E). (Used with permission from Urban BA, Fishman EK. Spiral CT of the female pelvis: clinical applications. *Abdom Imaging* 1995;20:9–14.)

NORMAL ANATOMY

Spiral scanning optimizes enhancement of the pelvic organs and improves definition of pelvic vascular anatomy. In the female pelvis spiral CT is very helpful for delineating the relationships between the uterus, cervix, and ovaries (7). Following bolus contrast administration, marked enhancement of the normal myometrium is seen, reflecting the rich uterine vascular supply (4,7). At times, in our experience, the normal myometrium can enhance inhomogeneously. This is particularly true in younger patients. In the normal uterus, delayed scans reveal a homogeneous myometrium (Fig. 14-6). The lower-attenuation secretions of the centrally located endome-

trial cavity are routinely demonstrated on spiral CT (4). The cervix often demonstrates enhancement, particularly in a peripheral distribution. The vaginal mucosa can also demonstrate prominent enhancement. The normal ovarian relationships to the broad ligaments are nicely demonstrated on spiral CT (Fig. 14-7). The normal ovaries do not enhance appreciably, even following rapid contrast injection.

Vascular opacification of the major pelvic arteries and veins is essential in differentiating vessels from lymph nodes. This is especially true of the pelvic veins, which typically do not reach peak opacification until 2–4 min following contrast injection. In the female pelvis, paired branches from the internal iliac arteries—the uterine arteries—provide the majority of blood flow to the uterus. The uterine veins parallel the arterial supply via a prominent plexus of vessels embedded within the parametrium. Adequate vascular opacification is crucial in differentiating these vessels from abnor-

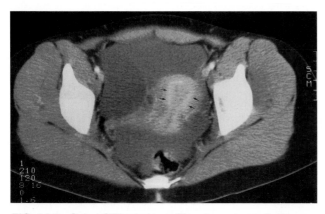

FIG. 14-2. Spiral CT technique. The uterus normally demonstrates marked myometrial enhancement on spiral CT (*arrows*), as in this patient with a cystic pelvic mass. The normal endometrium is seen as a central region of decreased attenuation within the uterus. (Used with permission from Urban BA, Fishman EK. Spiral CT of the female pelvis: clinical applications. *Abdom Imaging* 1995;20:9–14.)

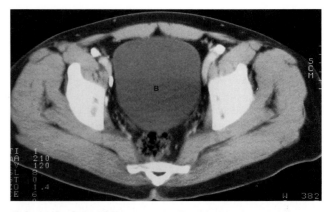

FIG. 14-4. Spiral CT technique. The bladder is normally unopacified on spiral CT. Delayed views following bladder opacification are unnecessary in most patients, as the bladder is easily identified (B).

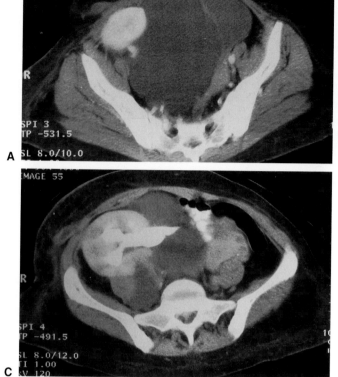

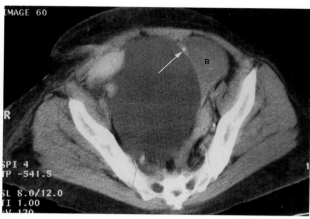

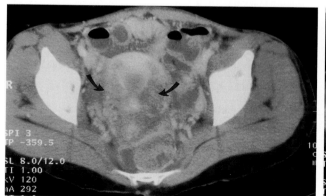

FIG. 14-5. Spiral CT technique. Delayed views are essential in cases with cystic pelvic masses, as in this patient with a large fluid collection following renal transplant. (**A**) Spiral CT identifies two fluid collections adjacent to the renal transplant. The bladder cannot be confidently localized. (**B,C**) Conventional delayed images obtained 5 min after contrast injection confidently identify the bladder (B), now partially opacified, displaced laterally by the large fluid collection. The ureter is compressed (*arrow*), resulting in hydronephrosis of the transplant kidney.

mal parametrial soft-tissue stranding, especially in patients with cervical cancer referred for staging CT scan.

CERVICAL CARCINOMA

Cervical carcinoma is a common gynecological malignancy (1,8). More than 90% of these carcinomas are squamous cell carcinomas arising in the external surface of the cervix; the remainder are adenocarcinomas arising from the endocervix. Although the overall accuracy of MRI is slightly superior to CT in the staging of cervical carcinoma, CT remains an important ancillary modality (8–12). Older-generation CT scanners have demonstrated an overall staging accuracy of between 58% and 88%. Spiral scanning may improve accuracy by differentiating normal parametrial vessels and ligaments from adenopathy and tumor extension.

Accurate staging defines the optimal therapy for patients with cervical carcinoma (8,9,11,12). A stage I tumor is con-

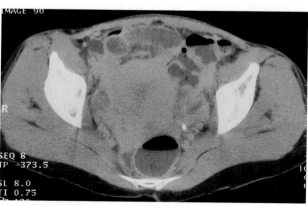

FIG. 14-6. Normal uterus. (**A**) The normal uterus (*arrows*) can demonstrate striking enhancement on spiral CT. Occasionally, as in this case, the enhancement is heterogeneous and presents a confusing appearance. (**B**) Delayed scans are helpful to confirm the normal appearance of the uterus.

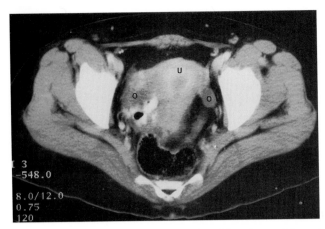

FIG. 14-7. Normal uterus and ovaries. The uterus (U) and ovaries (O) are confidently displayed in most patients following spiral CT.

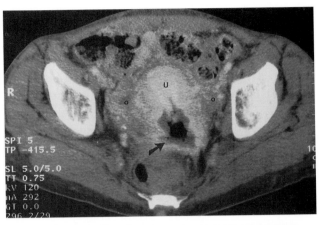

FIG. 14-9. Necrotic cervical cancer. Larger cervical tumors can present as necrotic masses. In this patient, spiral technique allows for differentiation of the mass (arrow) from the normal uterus (U) and ovaries (O).

fined to the cervix. The tumor appears as a hypodense mass against the enhancing cervical stroma, with intact peripheral margins in the absence of parametrial stranding (13) (Fig. 14-8). In our experience, we have been able to confidently detect tumors as small as 2 cm using spiral technique. Larger tumors, often measuring 4 cm or larger in diameter, can demonstrate areas of central necrosis (1) (Fig. 14-9). Retained endometrial secretions from obstruction of the endocervical canal provide a helpful secondary diagnostic sign of cervical cancer (14) (Fig. 14-10). A stage II neoplasm extends beyond the cervix with obvious parametrial involvement and does not involve the pelvic side wall. Parametrial invasion is demonstrated on spiral CT by the presence of parametrial stranding or an eccentric parametrial mass (13). Recent instrumentation or inflammation can result in a false-positive diagnosis of tumor extension (1).

Advanced-stage cervical cancers are nicely demonstrated on spiral CT (4). A typical stage III carcinoma demonstrates extension into the lower third of the vagina, pelvic sidewall

extension, lymph node enlargement, or ureteral obstruction (Figs. 14-11, 14-12) (8). Pelvic sidewall extension by confluent tumor spread can invade the piriformis and/or the obturator internus muscles. Pelvic lymph nodes greater than 1.5 cm in diameter should be considered abnormal (11,15). Abnormal lymph nodes can also demonstrate peripheral or heterogeneous enhancement following bolus contrast enhancement. Stage IV tumors invade the adjacent bladder or rectum, or spread outside the true pelvis (8,12). Retroperitoneal lymph nodes larger than 1.0 cm in diameter suggest metastasic involvement (1). The lungs are also a common site of distant metastasis.

OVARIAN CANCER

The primary ovarian malignancies include adenocarcinoma and serous or mucinous cystadenocarcinoma. Ultrasound remains the study of choice in the characterization of most ovarian masses and is routinely performed for lesion detection and characterization. Ovarian cancers typically appear as large, complex solid and cystic masses. Conventional CT confidently demonstrates most larger masses (1,16). Spiral CT can provide useful information regarding internal architecture of ovarian masses (4,5). Features that suggest malignancy include papillary projections, enhancing solid elements, and a thick wall or septations (Figs. 14-13, 14-14). Spiral CT, in combination with bolus contrast enhancement, accentuates the vascular solid component of ovarian masses, and in many cases can differentiate tumors from benign cysts (4,5). Despite optimal imaging, however, many cystic masses remain indeterminate on spiral CT, and definitive diagnosis can be established only at surgery (Fig. 14-15).

Many ovarian tumors present at an advanced stage. Tumor spread often involves the intestine, ureters, mesentery, and omentum. Accurate staging of ovarian cancer is crucial for determining which patients may benefit from aggressive cy-

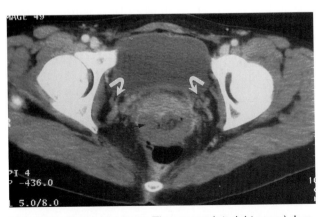

FIG. 14-8. Cervical cancer. The cancer (straight arrow) demonstrates relatively decreased enhancement following bolus contrast injection. Note the opacified parametrial vessels (curved arrows). There is no evidence for adenopathy.

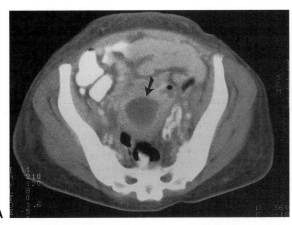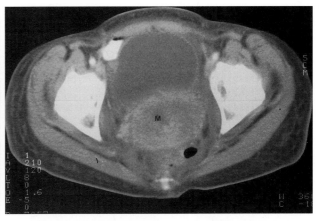

FIG. 14-10. Cervical cancer with retained secretions. Secretions within the endometrial cavity can be secondary to outlet obstruction from a cervical stenosis or mass. **(A)** In this patient, moderate fluid is seen with the endometrial cavity (*arrow*). **(B)** Inferiorly, the obstructing mass (M) is identified arising from the cervix.

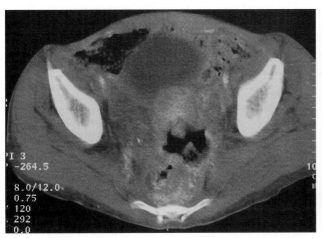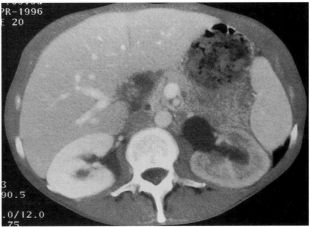

FIG. 14-11. Cervical cancer with hydronephrosis. **(A)** A large, necrotic tumor is seen arising from the cervix. **(B)** The left kidney demonstrates hydronephrosis. Ureteral obstruction by cervical cancer constitutes a more advanced stage III tumor.

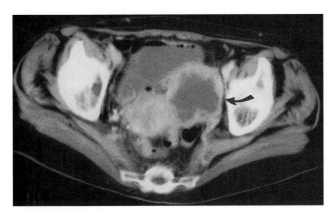

FIG. 14-12. Cervical cancer with pelvic sidewall extension. Direct left parametrial extension of the necrotic tumor is demonstrated (*arrow*). (Used with permission from Urban BA, Fishman EK. Spiral CT of the female pelvis: clinical applications. *Abdom Imaging* 1995;20:9–14.)

toreductive surgery (17–19). Past studies utilizing conventional CT have demonstrated a sensitivity range of 58% to 92% and a specificity range of 79% to 100% for the staging of ovarian carcinoma (18,19). Spiral scanning, with improved imaging characteristics, may increase detection of small omental and peritoneal implants and may therefore provide improved staging accuracy. Spiral technique also provides a confident and reliable imaging modality for follow-up management of the postoperative patient.

Smaller ovarian cysts are often incidentally discovered on CT (20) (Fig. 14-16). On spiral scanning, simple ovarian cysts appear as smooth-walled masses with a central attenuation close to that of water. Thin-collimation spiral scanning helps confirm the ovarian origin of cysts by demonstrating a rim of ovarian tissue near the cyst (4,5). Often cysts are demonstrated in younger women and represent prominent follicles or functional cysts. We often suggest clinical corre-

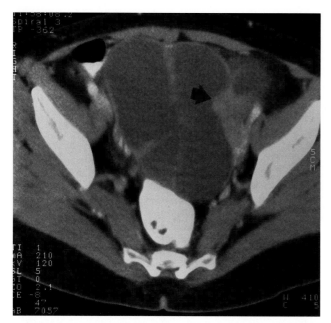

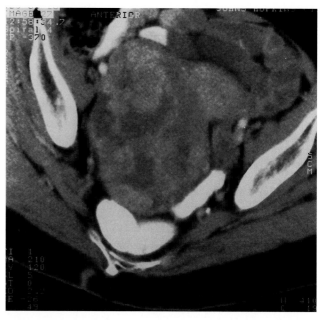

FIG. 14-13. Ovarian cystadenocarcinoma. The predominately cystic mass demonstrates thick, enhancing septations. A solid nodule (*arrow*) is seen within the lateral aspect of the mass. Spiral technique following bolus contrast administration optimizes the detection of subtle enhancing septations and nodules. (Used with permission from Urban BA, Fishman EK. Spiral CT of the female pelvis: clinical applications. *Abdom Imaging* 1995;20:9–14.)

FIG. 14-14. Ovarian cystadenocarcinoma. Heterogeneous enhancing solid and cystic components are characteristic features of an ovarian malignancy.

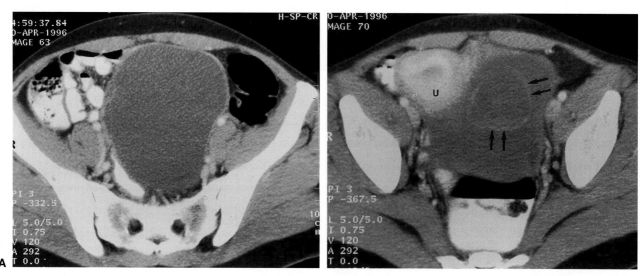

FIG. 14-15. Ovarian cystadenoma. (**A**) A large cystic mass is seen in the pelvis. (**B**) Very fine, minimally enhancing septations are demonstrated within the inferior portion of the cyst (*arrows*), an indeterminate finding for malignancy. Surgery revealed a benign serous cystadenoma. Note the brightly enhancing uterus (U).

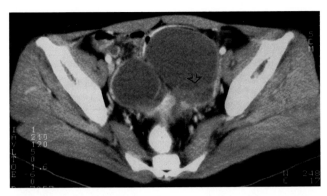

FIG. 14-16. Indeterminate ovarian cysts on spiral CT. There are bilateral, predominantly cystic adnexal masses. The larger left adnexal cyst demonstrates increased attenuation or enhancement posteriorly (*arrow*). In this case, spiral CT cannot accurately differentiate a benign from malignant etiology. At surgery, the right adnexal mass revealed endometrioma; the left adnexal mass revealed a benign teratoma with coexistent endometrioma. (Used with permission from Urban BA, Fishman EK. Spiral CT of the female pelvis. *Radiol Clin of North Am* 1995;33:933–948.)

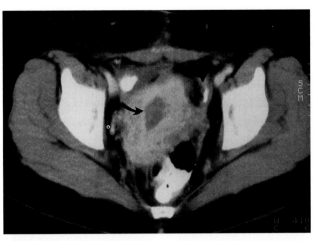

FIG. 14-17. Endometrial carcinoma. The centrally located carcinoma (*arrow*) is easily appreciated against the enhanced myometrium.

lation from the referring physician and rarely advise further work-up. In the post- or perimenopausal patient, however, we always advise further work-up of any detectable ovarian cysts and recommend evaluation with sonography in the vast majority of cases. Sonography remains more sensitive for the depiction of septations, nodules, and other indicators of malignancy.

OTHER TUMORS OF THE FEMALE PELVIS

Endometrial carcinoma is the most frequently invasive gynecological malignancy (21–23). Endometrial carcinoma commonly presents with postmenopausal bleeding. Most patients with endometrial cancer present with localized stage I or II disease. Spiral CT depicts endometrial tumors as central hypodense uterine masses against the brightly enhancing myometrium (Fig. 14-17) (23,24). Invasion of the myometrium is suggested by interruption of this enhancement (Fig. 14-18). Occasionally, tumor involvement of the cervical canal (stage II) results in a bulky mass that can mimic a cervical carcinoma (21). Stage III disease is present when tumor extension involves the parametrium or pelvic sidewall. Stage IV disease involves the bladder or rectum, or demonstrates distant metastases (21–24).

Teratomas account for 10% to 15% of all ovarian tumors (2). The great majority of ovarian teratomas are benign (25–27). Imaging findings vary, depending on the components present in the mass (2). Calcifications are frequently seen. Fat is commonly present in a mass containing a mixture of fluid, hair, and debris. Cystic teratomas can demonstrate a solid element (the dermoid plug) arising from the wall. CT remains the most sensitive and specific imaging modality to confirm the fatty nature of this tumor (26,27). Volumetric

data acquisition with spiral scanning ensures accurate lesion characterization (4,5) (Fig. 14-19).

Gestational trophoblastic disease ("molar pregnancy") encompasses a spectrum of disorders from the benign hydatidiform mole to malignant choriocarcinoma, and results from proliferation of trophoblastic elements of the blastocyst with resultant invasive tendencies (28–30). The uterus is often enlarged and can demonstrate areas of decreased attenuation centrally. Interruption of the brightly enhancing myometrium suggests the diagnosis of an invasive mole or choriocarcinoma (28–30). Other portions of the tumor can demonstrate striking hypervascularity, the presence of which is nicely appreciated using spiral CT technique. The ovaries in gestational trophoblastic disease often demonstrate characteristic theca lutein cysts.

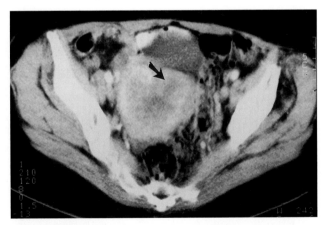

FIG. 14-18. Invasive endometrial carcinoma. Low-density material fills the endometrial cavity. Disruption of the normally enhancing myometrium is demonstrated laterally (*arrow*). (Used with permission from Urban BA, Fishman EK. Spiral CT of the female pelvis: clinical applications. *Abdom Imaging* 1995;20:9–14.)

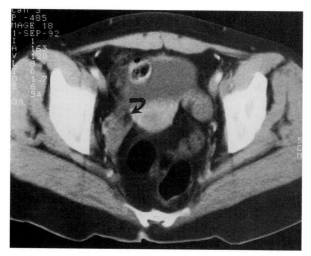

FIG. 14-19. Small right ovarian dermoid. The patient was referred following sonographic depiction of a small echogenic lesion in the right adnexa. Spiral CT scan reveals a small focus of fat (*arrow*) within right ovary, establishing the correct diagnosis (Used with permission from Urban BA, Fishman EK. Spiral CT of the female pelvis: clinical applications. *Abdom Imaging* 1995;20:9–14.)

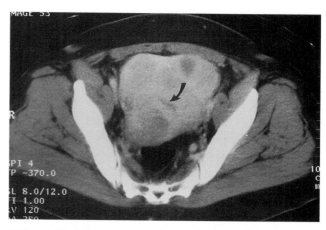

FIG. 14-20. Fibroid uterus. Spiral CT scan depicts an enlarged, lobulated uterus containing multiple hypodense leiomyomas. Dynamic contrast enhancement of the myometrium enables depiction of the endometrium (*arrow*).

Uterine leiomyomas (fibroids) are common benign neoplasms resulting from smooth muscle proliferation. CT typically demonstrates a lobulated uterine surface contour, deformity of the endometrial cavity, or focal uterine masses with or without calcification (Fig. 14-20) (2,31,32). Cystic degeneration is seen following infarction or hemorrhage into a leiomyoma. The complicated uterine leiomyoma should be included in the differential of most pelvic masses involving the uterus (33). The often hypervascular nature of many uterine leiomyomata can be appreciated on spiral scanning, at times suggesting sarcomatous degeneration (4,5). This potential pitfall can by clarified on delayed scans obtained several minutes following the spiral acquisition: delayed images will demonstrate the more familiar homogeneous appearance of the fibroid uterus (Fig. 14-21).

PELVIC INFLAMMATORY DISEASE

Typical CT findings in patients with pelvic inflammatory disease include unilateral or bilateral adnexal masses, hydrosalpinx, and pelvic ascites (2). Spiral CT can accurately localize the ovaries and demonstrate the tubular nature of the hydrosalpinx (Fig. 14-22). Tubo-ovarian abscess can complicate pelvic inflammatory disease and present as thick-walled, complex masses with septations and irregular walls (2,34). Spiral technique helps demonstrate characteristic peripheral enhancement of the abscess capsule (Fig. 14-23). Occasionally, air is present within the mass, and a diagnosis

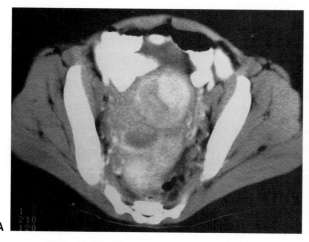

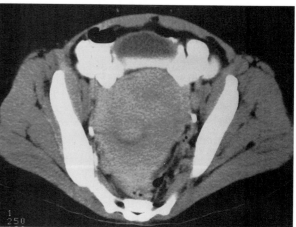

FIG. 14-21. Hypervascular fibroid uterus. (**A**) Spiral CT scan demonstrates a bulky, enlarged uterus with markedly enhancing uterine fibroids. (**B**) Fibroid enhancement is not appreciated on the delayed CT scan. (Used with permission from Urban BA, Fishman EK. Spiral CT of the female pelvis: clinical applications. *Abdom Imaging* 1995;20:9–14.)

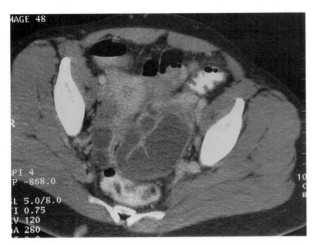

FIG. 14-22. Pelvic inflammatory disease. The tubular nature of the pyosalpinx is appreciated. Spiral technique with bolus contrast enhancement helps demonstrate subtle enhancement of the fallopian tube wall.

of abscess is made with certainty. Tubo-ovarian abscesses can be difficult to differentiate from ovarian neoplasms, or abscesses secondary to other etiologies such as inflammatory bowel disease or appendicitis. Spiral scanning, by providing excellent opacification of the nearby vascular structures, is also very helpful in planning the approach of potential percutaneous drainage.

THE POSTPARTUM UTERUS

CT scanning is occasionally used for evaluation of the postpartum patient (5). The normal postpartum uterus demonstrates a moderately thickened wall and a central low-attenuation fluid cavity (Fig. 14-24). Air can be seen within the endometrial canal immediately following delivery; it should disappear within several days. The continued presence of air and fluid within the endometrial cavity suggests

retained products and/or infection. Following caesarean section, the transverse uterine incision site is often appreciated as a normal finding (35). A variety of postpartum complications—including abscesses, retained products, and deep venous thrombosis—can be confidently and efficiently evaluated with a single spiral CT scan (36,37). Fluid collections near the site of surgery are not uncommon.

FLUID COLLECTIONS

Abnormal fluid collections in the pelvis can result from ascites, prior surgery, hemorrhage, infection, or tumors. Ascites is the most frequently encountered pelvic fluid collection and has a CT density close to that of water. Thickening or nodularity with enhancement of the periphery of the collection suggests the presence of malignant ascites. Spiral CT following bolus contrast enhancement accentuates these features. Ancillary findings of malignant ascites include matted bowel loops, lymphadenopathy, and peritoneal implants.

Pelvic abscesses represent localized infected fluid collections. They are most frequently related to prior surgery, appendicitis, inflammatory bowel disease, colonic perforation, or pelvic inflammatory disease (2). Pelvic abscesses usually demonstrate a characteristic enhancing, irregular outer rim (Fig. 14-25). Spiral CT is helpful in demonstrating small foci of air within infected fluid collections. In the absence of internal gas, noninfected inflammatory masses or cystic or necrotic tumors cannot always be excluded.

THE POSTOPERATIVE PATIENT

Spiral CT is very useful for monitoring the postoperative patient (2,5). It is the modality of choice for the long-term follow-up of patients with cervical, endometrial, or ovarian

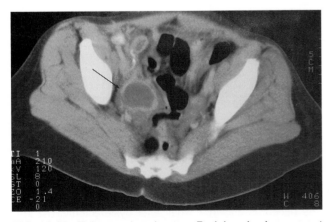

FIG. 14-23. Tubo-ovarian abscess. Peripheral enhancement (*arrow*) of the low-density lesion in the right adnexa raises the suspicion for abscess. (Used with permission from Urban BA, Fishman EK. Spiral CT of the female pelvis: clinical applications. *Abdom Imaging* 1995;20:9–14.)

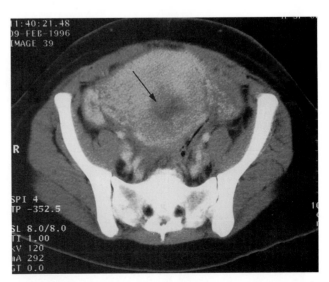

FIG. 14-24. Normal postpartum uterus, day 1. The uterus is enlarged and demonstrates minimal retained fluid within the endometrial cavity (*arrow*). The deep veins are normal.

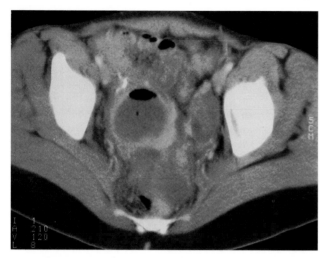

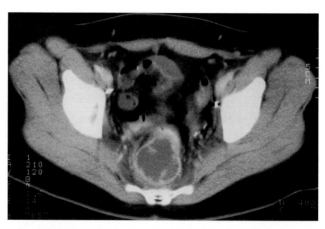

FIG. 14-25. Postoperative abscess. The patient is shown several months after vaginal hysterectomy. A well-defined abscess cavity with air is seen in the region of the vaginal cuff. (Used with permission from Urban BA, Fishman EK. Spiral CT of the female pelvis: clinical applications. *Abdom Imaging* 1995;20:9–14.)

FIG. 14-26. Recurrent cervical cancer. An enhancing soft-tissue mass is identified in the surgical bed of the pelvis. The mass demonstrates imaging characteristics similar to the primary cervical tumor.

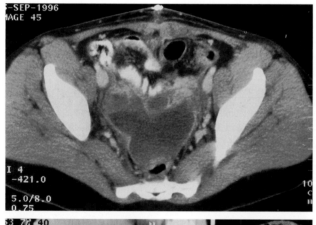

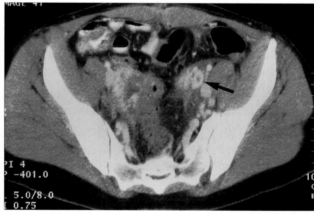

FIG. 14-27. Gonadal vein thrombosis and pelvic abscess. The patient is shown 1 week after hysterectomy. (**A**) The pelvic abscess demonstrates characteristic rim enhancement. (**B**) Superiorly, the left gonadal vein demonstrates a central filling defect (*arrow*) compatible with thrombosis. (**C**) Coronal reconstruction nicely demonstrates the full extent of the gonadal vein thrombosis (*arrows*).

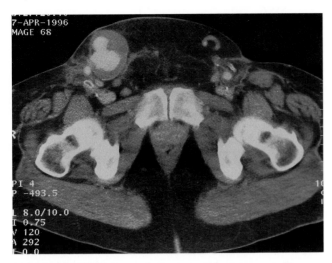

FIG. 14-28. Right femoral artery pseudoaneurysm. The patient demonstrates a large pseudoaneurysm near the anastomosis of a fem-fem bypass graft. Spiral CT following bolus contrast enhancement defines the aneurysm and the extent of thrombus.

contrast enhancement, essentially free from motion artifact. Postprocessing of the spiral data set using maximum-intensity projection or shaded-surface display techniques can provide an exquisite display of the normal anatomy, as well as help create angiographic road maps for preoperative planning for repair of aneurysms, pseudoaneurysms, and so on (38–40) (Fig. 14-28). As in the chest and abdomen, spiral CT angiography in the pelvis offers an exciting, less invasive imaging technique for the evaluation of vascular anatomy.

cancer. Tumor recurrence often presents as focal masses or implants that demonstrate CT characteristics similar to the primary cancer (Fig. 14-26). Spiral CT is also helpful in the perioperative period for the detection of postoperative fluid collections and abscesses. Other common postoperative complications include hematomas and venous thrombosis. Hematomas initially present as high-density masses, which become increasingly cystic over time. Occasionally, hematomas can be mistaken for cystic tumors or abscesses (2). Deep venous thrombosis appears as a central luminal filling defect. Vessels which are difficult to examine with conventional sonography, particularly the deep veins of the pelvis, are well visualized using spiral CT (4,5) (Fig. 14-27).

RADIATION THERAPY TREATMENT PLANNING

Spiral CT scanning provides an improved technique for radiation therapy planning. This is very useful for pelvic malignancies such as prostate cancer and cervical cancer. Spiral CT provides reliable and reproducible depiction of tumor volume, and is very helpful in localizing radiation portals. Sagittal reconstruction is especially valuable for side ports and in decreasing the radiation exposure of the rectum and sigmoid colon.

Reformatted images, free from motion artifact, can be made easily available on an independent workstation. When therapy planning is done, it is important to use a flat board placed on the CT scanner to more accurately simulate radiation delivery. Spiral CT with multiplanar display is also useful in simulating the implant zone for radium implants.

VASCULAR APPLICATIONS

An important advantage of spiral scanning is the ability to consistently demonstrate vascular anatomy during uniform

REFERENCES

1. Walsh JW. Computed tomography of gynecologic neoplasms. *Radiol Clin North Am* 1992;30:817–830.
2. Langer JE, Dinsmore BJ. Computed tomographic evaluation of benign and inflammatory disorders of the female pelvis. *Radiol Clin North Am* 1992;30:831–842.
3. Gross BH, Moss AA, Mihara K, et al. Computed tomography of gynecologic diseases. *AJR* 1983;141:765.
4. Urban BA, Fishman EK. Spiral CT of the female pelvis: clinical applications. *Abdom Imaging* 1995;20:9–14.
5. Urban BA, Fishman EK. Spiral CT of the female pelvis. *Radiol Clin of North Am* 1995;33:933–948.
6. Heiken JP, Brink JA, Vannier MW. Spiral (helical) CT. *Radiology* 1993;189:647.
7. Foshager MC, Walsh JW. CT anatomy of the female pelvis: a second look. *Radiographics* 1994;14:51.
8. Walsh JW, Goplerud DR. Prospective comparison between clinical and CT staging in primary cervical carcinoma. *AJR* 1981;137:997.
9. Kim SH, Choi BI, Lee HP, et al. Uterine cervical carcinoma: comparison of CT and MR findings. *Radiology* 1990;175:45.
10. Klein L, Pollack HM. Computed tomography and magnetic resonance imaging of the female lower urinary tract. *Radiol Clin North Am* 1992;30:843–860.
11. Grumbine FC, Rosenshein NB, Zerhouni EA, et al. Abdominopelvic computed tomography in the preoperative evaluation of early cervical cancer. *Gynecol Oncol* 1981;286:12.
12. Kilcheski TS, Arger PH, Mulhern CB Jr, et al. Role of computed tomography in the presurgical evaluation of carcinoma of the cervix. *J Comput Assist Tomogr* 1981;5:378.
13. Vick CW, Walsh JW, Wheelock JB, et al. CT of the normal and abnormal parametria in cervical cancer. *AJR* 1984;143:597.
14. Scott WW Jr, Rosenshein NB, Siegelman SS, et al. The obstructed uterus. *Radiology* 1981;141:767.
15. Teefey SA, Baron RL, Schulte SJ, Shuman WP. Differentiating pelvic and enlarged lymph nodes: optimal CT technique. *Radiology* 1990;175:683–685.
16. Fukuda T, Ikeuchi M, Hashimoto H, et al. Computed tomography of ovarian masses. *J Comput Assist Tomogr* 1986;10:990.
17. Megibow AJ, Bosniak MA, Ho AG, et al. Accuracy of CT in detection of persistent or recurrent ovarian carcinoma: correlation with second-look laparotomy. *Radiology* 1988;166:341.
18. Meyer JI, Kennedy AW, Friedman R, et al. Ovarian carcinoma: value of CT in predicting success of debulking surgery. *AJR* 1995;165:875.
19. Nelson BE, Rosenfield AT, Scwartz PE. Preoperative abdominopelvic computed tomographic prediction of optimal cytoreduction in epithelial ovarian carcinoma. *J Clin Oncol* 1993;11:166.
20. Sawyer RW, Vick CW, Walsh JR, et al. Computed tomography of benign ovarian masses. *J Comput Assist Tomogr* 1985;9:784.
21. Balfe DM, Van Dyke J, Lee JKT, et al. Computed tomography in malignant endometrial neoplasms. *J Comput Assist Tomogr* 1983;7:677.
22. Dore R, Moro G, D'Andrea F, et al. CT evaluation of myometrium invasion in endometrial carcinoma. *J Comput Assist Tomogr* 1987:11:282.
23. Walsh JW, Goplerud DR. Computed tomography of primary, persistent, and recurrent endometrial malignancy. *AJR* 1982;139:1149.
24. Hamlin DJ, Burgener FA, Belcham JB. CT of intramural endometrial carcinoma. Contrast enhancement is essential. *AJR* 1981;137:551.

25. Brammer HM III, Buck JL, Hayes WS, et al. Malignant germ cell tumors of the ovary: radiologic-pathologic correlation. *Radiographics* 1990;10:715.

26. Buy J, Ghossain MA, Moss AA, et al. Cystic teratoma of the ovary: CT detection. *Radiology* 1989;171:697.

27. Friedman AC, Pyatt RS, Hartman DS. CT of benign cystic teratomas. *AJR* 1982;138:659.

28. Sanders C, Rubin E. Malignant gestational trophoblastic disease: CT findings. *AJR* 1987;148:165.

29. Miyasaka M, Hachiya J, Furuya A, et al. CT evaluation of invasive trophoblastic disease. *J Comput Assist Tomogr* 1985;9:459.

30. Davis WK, McCarthy S, Moss AA, et al. Computed tomography of gestational trophoblastic disease. *J Comput Assist Tomogr* 1984; 8–1136.

31. Sawyer RW, Walsh JW. CT in gynecologic pelvic diseases. *Semin Ultrasound CT MR* 1988;9:122–142.

32. Casillas J, Joseph RC, Guerra JJ Jr. CT appearance of uterine leiomyomas. *Radiographics* 1990;10:999.

33. Togashi K, Nishimura K, Nakano Y, et al. Cystic pedunculated leiomy-omas of the uterus with unusual CT manifestations. *J Comput Assist Tomogr* 1986;10:642.

34. Wilbur A. Computed tomography of tuboovarian abscesses. *J Comput Assist Tomogr* 1990;4:625.

35. Twickler DM, Setiawan AT, Harrell RS, Brown CEL. CT appearance of the pelvis after cesarean section. *AJR* 1991;156:523–526.

36. Sgaffer PB, Johnson JC, Bryan D, et al. Diagnosis of ovarian vein thrombophlebitis by computed tomography. *J Comput Assist Tomogr* 1981;5:436.

37. Savader SJ, Otero RR, Savader BL. Puerperal ovarian vein thrombosis: evaluation with CT, US, and MR imaging. *Radiology* 1988;167:637.

38. Zeman RK, Silverman PM, Berman PM, Weltman DI, Davros WJ, Gomes MN. Abdominal aortic aneurysms: findings on three-dimensional display of helical CT data. *AJR* 1995;164:917–922.

39. Bluemke DA, Chambers TP. Spiral CT angiography: an alternative to conventional angiography. *Radiology* 1995;195:317–319.

40. Zeman RK, Silverman PM, Berman PM, Weltman DI, Davros WJ, Gomes MN. Abdominal aortic aneurysms: evaluation with variable-collimation helical CT and overlapping reconstruction. *Radiology* 1994;193:555–560.

PART 5

Other Applications

CHAPTER 15

Spiral CT of the Musculoskeletal System

Elliot K. Fishman

Despite the widespread belief that magnetic resonance imaging (MRI) is the modality of choice for imaging the musculoskeletal system, computed tomography (CT) remains extremely effective for a wide range of clinical applications. Spiral CT provides definite advantages over standard dynamic CT in nearly all of these applications and in clinical practice is almost universally the technique of choice (1–4). The specific advantages of spiral CT enable us to define its role in musculoskeletal imaging. Spiral CT is particularly well suited in the following clinical applications.

1. Examinations where even minimal intrascan or interscan motion may compromise the study. Typical problem areas have been the shoulder, sternum, and wrist. Lack of interscan motion is especially important in any study of these regions when multiplanar or three-dimensional imaging (3D) is planned.

2. Smaller anatomic regions of interest like the foot or wrist benefit from a spiral acquisition of a volume data set combining narrow collimation (2–4 mm) and a pitch of 1 with small reconstruction increments (1–2 mm) (Fig. 15-1).

3. CT studies for suspected infection in muscle or soft tissue, or a suspected soft-tissue or muscle mass require iodinated intravenous contrast to optimize detection of the presence and extent of disease (4–6). Spiral CT allows data to be acquired during the phase of maximum contrast enhancement, thereby optimizing lesion detection. The enhancement patterns may also prove useful in the differential diagnosis of a lesion. Optimization of vascular enhancement is also valuable for definition of vascular anatomy. Three-dimensional images using maximum-intensity projection (MIP) or volume-rendering techniques require optimal contrast administration (7–9) if vascular maps are to be generated (Fig. 15-2).

4. Spiral CT may be valuable in specific studies like CT arthrotomography of the shoulder. In these cases, high-resolution images can be acquired in a volume of data that rivals, and in many cases is superior to, MRI. How-

ever, no clinical series has yet been published on the advantages of this technique for this application (10) (Fig. 15-3).

EXAMINATION TECHNIQUE AND SCANNING PROTOCOLS

Specific spiral CT scanning techniques will depend on the clinical problem to be evaluated. Scanning parameters that must be selected include slice thickness or collimation, table speed, and interscan spacing. These decisions typically are

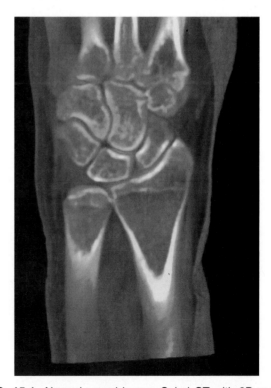

FIG. 15-1. Normal carpal bones. Spiral CT with 3D reconstruction was done to rule out a carpal fracture or dislocation. Note detail of carpal bones on these cutaway views.

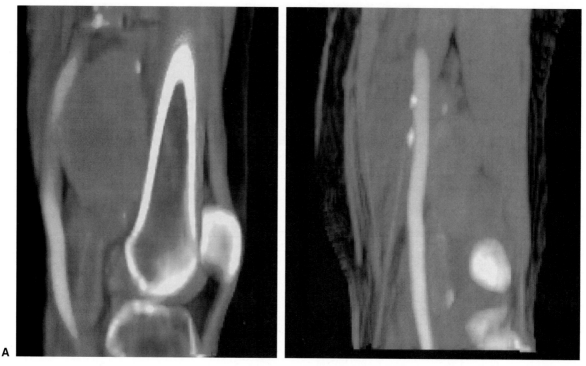

FIG. 15-2. Aneurysm of a thrombosed femoral artery with patent graft. The patient had a history of multiple aneurysms and palpated a mass behind the knee and worried about a sarcoma. **(A,B)** Three-dimensional vascular display defines a patent femoral popliteal graft and an aneurysm of the thrombosed native vessel.

based on the distance of the area to be scanned and whether multiplanar reconstruction and/or 3D imaging is to be obtained following the routine CT scan. Use of intravenous contrast material will be variable, but a good rule of thumb is that if soft tissue or muscle is to be evaluated, then contrast is always helpful. This is true whether one is looking at tumor or inflammatory disease.

Several specific scanning protocols are commonly used

and can be modified to meet the specific scan parameters available on any commercially available spiral scanner. The parameters listed here should therefore only be used as a guide and may need to be modified. Please consult your CT scanner's manual or contact your applications specialist for specific recommendations.

If the study is primarily to evaluate isolated musculoskeletal trauma, for example, following a motor vehicle injury to

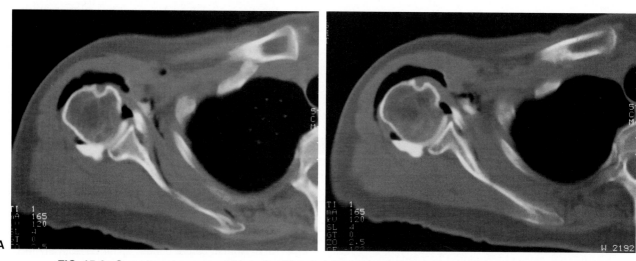

FIG. 15-3. Seventy-seven-year-old female with spiral CT arthrogram to rule out labral tear. **(A,B)** Spiral CT scan demonstrates normal anatomy of the rotator cuff. The labrum was also normal.

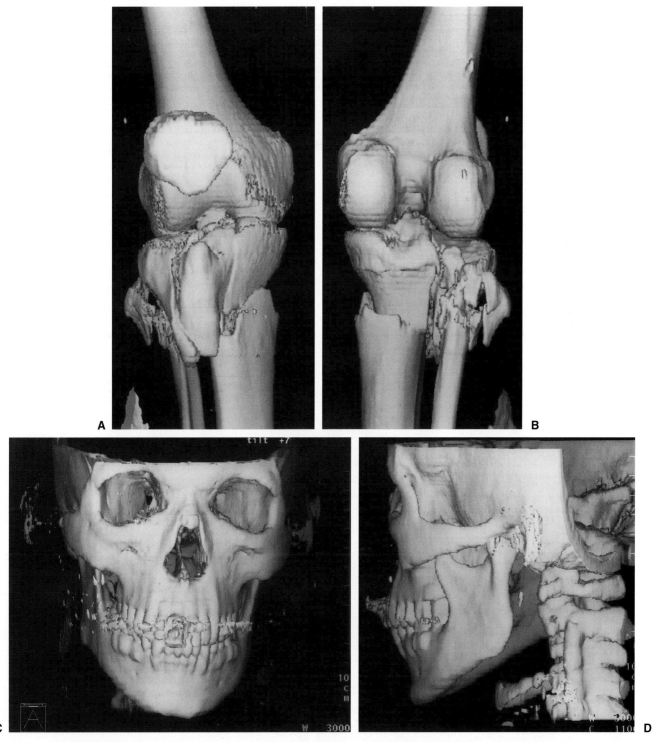

FIG. 15-4. Shaded-surface technique for 3D reconstruction. **(A,B)** Select views of a comminuted fracture of the proximal tibia and fibula demonstrate some of the problem with thresholding-based techniques for small fragments. **(C,D)** Three-dimensional images of the skull do provide a good representation but are lacking the fine detail of the transaxial CT, such as the sinuses and the different densities of various bony structures.

the bony pelvis or shoulder, we would typically not use any intravenous contrast material. Depending on the area to be scanned, the spiral length will vary from 32 to 40 s and will generally use a pitch of 1. Depending on the scanner used, a pitch of up to 2 will also be satisfactory in most cases. Slice thickness is usually 3 mm with a table speed of 3–6 mm/s. Our reconstruction interval would be 2 or 3 mm. The kilovolt peak (kVp) is 120 with 280 milliamperes (mA) on a Siemens Somatom-Plus-4 scanner. If the area of interest is a smaller anatomic area, such as the sternoclavicular joint or possibly the carpal bones, then spiral CT can be done with thinner sections (1–2 mm) and a pitch of 1–2. Data reconstruction will be in 1-mm increments. In reconstructing the data in skeletal trauma cases we typically use the high or ultrahigh reconstruction mode. This tends to make the images sharper, which is of critical importance when generating images to detect subtle fractures. In terms of the quality of the 3D reconstruction, we have generally found little problem with using a high or ultra-high filter. Occasionally, the ultra-high filter introduces too much noise and the 3D images may be suboptimal. If 3D rendering is required following reconstruction data, a second set of reconstructions can be done with a standard algorithm. Depending on the scanner, this may or may not require saving the raw data from the spiral CT acquisition.

Although a detailed analysis of the principles and techniques of 3D imaging is beyond the scope of this chapter, several important concepts should be reinforced. In musculoskeletal 3D imaging, the principal techniques used are shaded-surface rendering (Fig. 15-4) and volume rendering (Fig. 15-5) (11–16). Although both techniques have their advocates, numerous articles have stressed the advantages of volume rendering. Kuszyk et al. (17) evaluated both techniques by comparing 3D images generated with both rendering techniques. He concluded that

> surface renderings show gross 3D relationships most effectively, but suffer from more stair step artifacts and fail to effectively display lesions hidden behind overlying bone or located beneath the bone cortex. Volume rendering algorithms effectively show subcortical lesions, minimally displaced fractures, and hidden areas of interest with few artifacts. Volume algorithms show 3D relationships with varying degrees of success depending on the degree of surface shading and opacity. While surface rendering creates three-dimensionally realistic imaging of the bone surface, it may be of limited clinical utility due to numerous artifacts and the inability to show subcortical pathology. Volume rendering is a flexible 3D technique that effectively displays a variety of skeletal pathology with few artifacts.

Current systems now allow volume rendering to be done in "real time" with no preediting of the data set required. This is our technique of choice for all applications.

Another common clinical problem is the case where the primary area of interest is soft tissue or muscle. In these cases we are usually trying to rule out the presence of infection or a mass or to define its extent. Once again the table speed and slice thickness will vary based on the anatomic area that needs to be covered. As stated previously, in cases where muscle or soft tissue need to be evaluated, contrast material is mandatory to optimize the differential enhancement between normal and abnormal tissue. We usually use a scan delay of approximately 50 s from initiation of contrast injection. If images of the lower extremity are to be obtained, a delay of up to 70 s may be warranted. The key to timing the acquisition of CT data after contrast administration is an

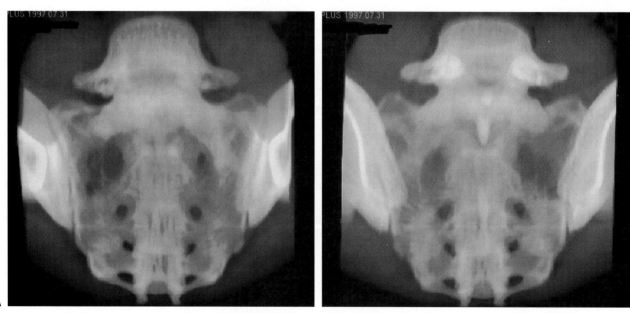

A   B

FIG. 15-5. Volume rendering of the sacrum. **(A-B)** Three-dimensional reconstruction defines the extent of the lytic nature of the tumor that involves the foramen at S-1. Note the fine detail of bone, including definition of the individual sacral elements.

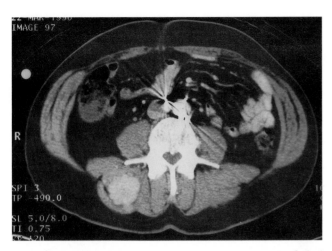

FIG. 15-6. Renal cell carcinoma metastatic to muscle. Spiral CT was performed in this patient status post left nephrectomy as a routine follow-up. Note the enhancing metastasis in the right paraspinal muscles.

understanding of iodinated contrast and its distribution in muscle. Regardless of the pathological process, in most cases normal muscle will enhance more than either inflammatory disease or neoplastic disease. Two exceptions might be desmoid tumors and occasional metastatic tumors to muscle, which are typically hyperdense or hypervascular (5,18) (Fig. 15-6).

For most muscle or soft-tissue evaluations, a typical spiral CT study would be 24–40 s with a pitch of 1–2. Slice thickness would be 5 or 8 mm, depending on the length of the area to be scanned, and the table speed would correspond to 5 or 16 mm/s. The reconstruction interval will vary but typically ranges from 5 to 8 mm. The kVp is 120 with 280 mA. When soft tissues or muscles are evaluated, the standard reconstruction algorithm (or soft-tissue algorithm) is used. Using a high or ultrahigh algorithm tends to create too much noise and detracts from the quality of the CT image. In select cases, images may need to be reconstructed using both the standard and high-resolution/ultra-high-resolution algorithm.

Occasionally, we have found that delayed scans following the spiral CT may be helpful in better understanding a pathological process involving muscle. Tumors such as desmoid tumors will show persistent intense delayed enhancement. Also on occasion, abscesses will become more obvious on delayed studies done 10–15 min after contrast injection. In these cases, a dense enhancing rim may be seen.

CLINICAL APPLICATIONS

The number of potential applications of spiral CT in musculoskeletal imaging cannot be covered in detail in a single chapter. Therefore some representative applications are presented that suggest the unique capabilities of this technique.

Sternum and Sternoclavicular Joint

Evaluation of the sternum and sternoclavicular (S/C) joint is most often requested to rule out fracture or fracture/dislocation, to define the extent of a fracture or dislocation, to evaluate suspected inflammation or abscess, and occasionally to clarify indeterminant or confusing findings on plain film or bone scan. The sternoclavicular joint is especially difficult to evaluate with plain radiographs, and several articles have stressed the value of CT. The use of transaxial CT, supplemented by multiplanar imaging in select obliquities, is especially valuable when looking at the sternoclavicular joint (5,19–21).

Sternal or sternoclavicular injury is most often a direct result of closed-chest trauma following a motor vehicle accident (Fig. 15-7). Although often an isolated injury, involvement of the shoulder or ribs is not uncommon. Injuries associated with S/C joint dislocation, especially posterior dislocation, include injury to the aorta and great vessels. In these cases, intravenous contrast should always be used to exclude vascular injury. Spiral CT is invaluable in these cases by providing both an excellent vascular study and an excellent study of the skeletal structures involved.

In the patient with S/C joint injury, we routinely do multiplanar and 3D imaging. The coronal views and oblique coronal images are most helpful in defining any involvement of the sternum, including displacement due to fracture. A z-axis 3D study is optimal for looking at the orientation of S/C joint dislocations and in helping to determine the mechanism of injury. These reconstructions can be done with either a surface-rendering or volumetric technique. We have found that these 3D images are most useful after associated bony structures have been edited.

Because chest trauma is often complex, it is important to carefully evaluate the entire shoulder joint complex and not

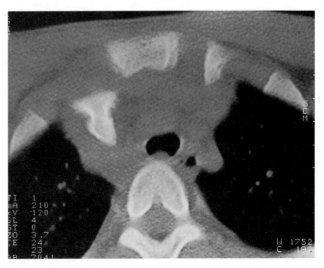

FIG. 15-7. Posterior dislocation of the clavicle. Spiral CT demonstrates a posterior sternoclavicular fracture. This dislocation is often associated with vascular injury. A CT angiogram should be performed.

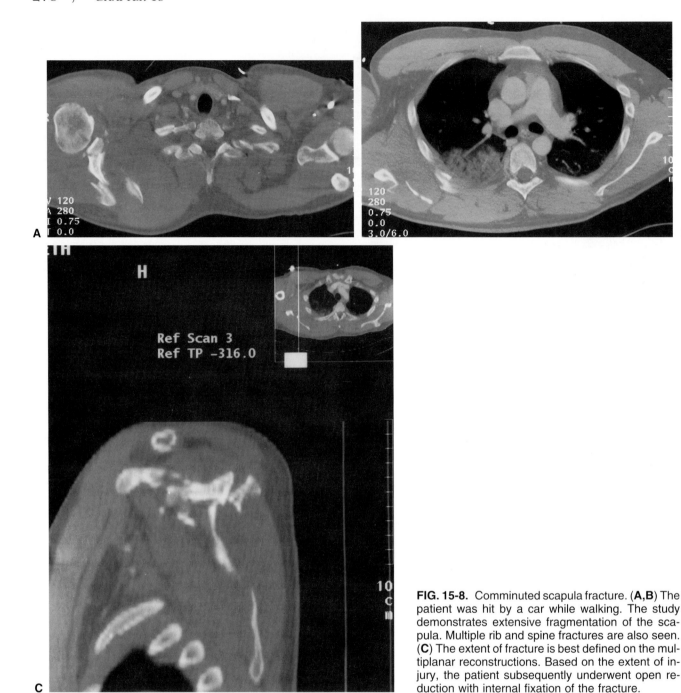

FIG. 15-8. Comminuted scapula fracture. **(A,B)** The patient was hit by a car while walking. The study demonstrates extensive fragmentation of the scapula. Multiple rib and spine fractures are also seen. **(C)** The extent of fracture is best defined on the multiplanar reconstructions. Based on the extent of injury, the patient subsequently underwent open reduction with internal fixation of the fracture.

overlook fractures in other structures, including the scapula (22) (Fig. 15-8). Scapular injuries are often overlooked in over 40% of cases on plain radiographs. CT excels at detecting the full extent of injuries and is especially valuable at evaluating pathology involving the scapula.

Infection of the sternoclavicular joint is more common in the patient with a history of either drug abuse, steroid use, or prior surgery to the head and neck region. It is especially common in the HIV-positive or AIDS patient, although we have recently seen several cases in patients without any known risk factors. Spiral CT excels at defining both the

soft-tissue and muscle component of disease as well as associated bony involvement (Fig. 15-9). Extension into adjacent muscle (pectoralis major, pectoralis minor, or sternocleidomastoid muscle) and retrosternal soft tissues is not uncommon. In rare cases, untreated mediastinitis may, in fact, develop (Figs. 15-10, 15-11). Spiral CT can be used to both plan therapeutic intervention and monitor response to therapy whether surgical and/or medical. In cases of suspected infection contrast enhancement is particularly useful. We recently reviewed a series of seven patients with infection of the sternoclavicular joint and found spiral CT to be invalu-

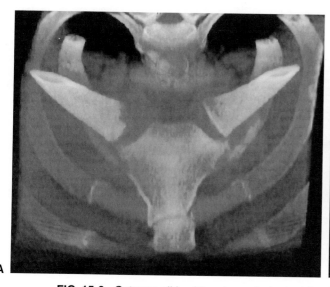
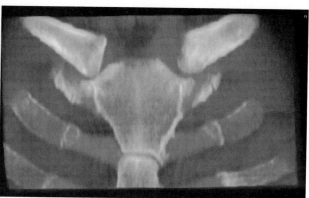

FIG. 15-9. Osteomyelitis of the sternoclavicular joint. **(A)** Three-dimensional display defines the destruction of the right clavicular head and early involvement of the right side of the manubrium. **(B)** A view of the sternum from a posterior orientation.

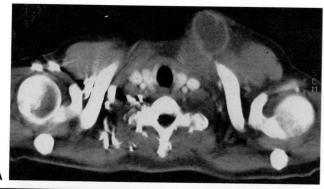
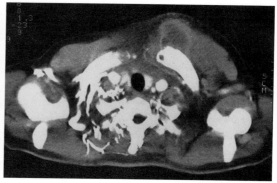

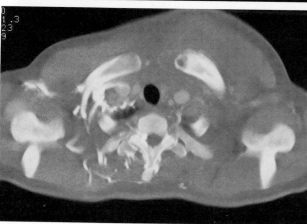

FIG. 15-10. Staphylococcus abscess of the chest wall with clavicular destruction. **(A,B)** Spiral CT scan demonstrates abscess involving the left pectoralis major and minor muscle. The abscess appears to extend toward the left sternoclavicular joint. Notice the wall enhancement of the abscess. **(C)** CT scan at bone settings demonstrates destruction of the medial portion of clavicle with periosteal reaction.

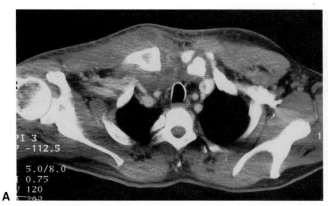
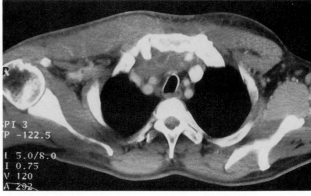

A   B

FIG. 15-11. Osteomyelitis of the right sternoclavicular joint with abscess and retrosternal extension. **(A,B)** Spiral CT demonstrates the inflammatory process involving the anterior chest wall with extension retrosternally to involve the anterior mediastinum. Images with bone windows demonstrate early destruction of the right clavicular head. In our experience involvement of the anterior mediastinum is not unusual with chest wall infections.

able at arriving at a correct diagnosis and in guiding management (15). When evaluating the sternoclavicular joint we have found the use of a high spatial filter to be valuable in accentuating subtle details, including early bone erosions or periosteal reaction (Fig. 15-12).

Spiral CT is also of value for the detection of bone fragments or foreign matter in the shoulder joint. The combination of narrow slice collimation with closely spaced sections (1–2 mm) and targeted images is invaluable for the detection of small intra-articular fragments. Multiplanar reformations or 3D reconstructions (Figs. 15-13–15-15) can help localize the lesion in three planes and/or perspectives. Similarly, complex humeral injuries can be mapped with spiral CT scanning.

Shoulder CT Arthrograms

The optimal radiological evaluation of suspected shoulder pathology is constantly undergoing change. A recent state-of-the-art article in *Radiology* by Stiles and Otte (22) carefully analyzed various imaging modalities, including Arthrography, CT Arthrography, MRI, and ultrasound. Their conclusions were that although each of these techniques does have merit in certain situations, there is no clear-cut "best study." In reviewing the relative values of each imaging modality, the authors note that Wilson et al. (23) showed that CT Arthrotomography provides accurate evaluation of labral disorders with a sensitivity of 100% and a specificity of 97%. Similarly, complete rotator cuff tears were also well

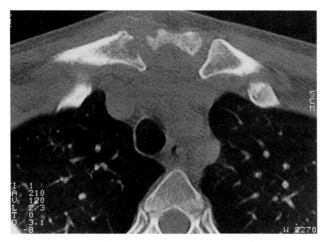

FIG. 15-12. Osteomyelitis of the right sternoclavicular joint. Spiral CT demonstrates the destructive process involving the right clavicular head and medial portion of the sternum. An associated soft-tissue mass is seen. Evaluation in this case was done with high-resolution kernel, which limits detail of soft-tissue involvement.

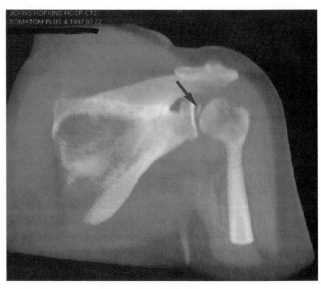

FIG. 15-13. Intra-articular fragment in shoulder joint. The 3D views define the presence and location of the fragment (*arrow*) which was not seen on plain radiographs.

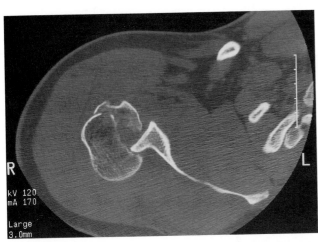

FIG. 15-14. Humeral head fracture with dislocation. High-resolution spiral CT images demonstrate an impacted fracture and dislocation of the humeral head. No associated glenoid fracture was seen.

demonstrated with this technique. CT Arthrography is also useful for detecting intra-articular fragments and for looking at the position and status of the biceps tendon. Spiral CT may increase the value of these studies by providing narrow interscan spacing (2 mm) and a volumetric data set. The volumetric data set with reconstructions into oblique and coronal planes can be most helpful in defining the presence or extent of labral injuries. A combination of spiral CT and arthrotomography may be most helpful in the future in the evaluation of the unstable shoulder (Fig. 15-16).

Spiral CT scanning with narrow collimation is also valuable in the evaluation of the acromion either pre- or postoperatively (Fig. 15-17). This may prove useful in patients with shoulder instability or in those with an impingement syndrome. When evaluating the shoulder for spiral CT Arthrography or standard spiral CT, a protocol might be 3-mm slice thickness, 3-mm/s table speed with reconstructions at 1–2-mm intervals. One technical point that we should mention is that in cases of CT Arthrography only about 3 mL of

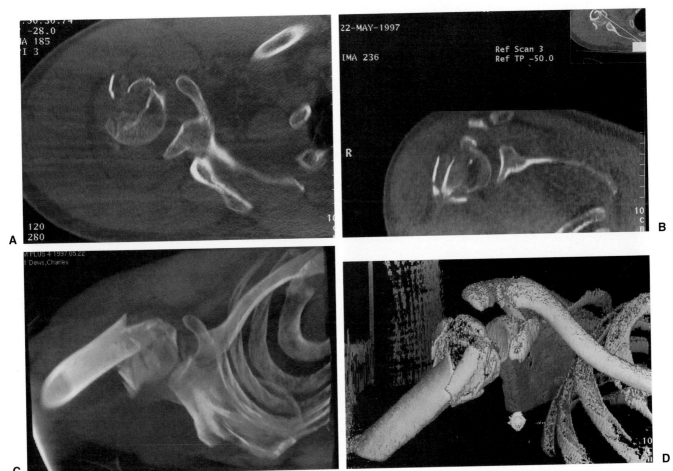

FIG. 15-15. Comminuted fracture of the humeral head. (**A**) Spiral CT demonstrates a comminuted fracture of the right humeral head. (**B**) Multiplanar reconstruction in oblique mode demonstrates orientation of the humeral head to the joint space as well as proximal humerus. Three-dimensional reconstructions with volume (**C**) and shaded-surface techniques (**D**) clearly show the advantages of volume rendering in these cases.

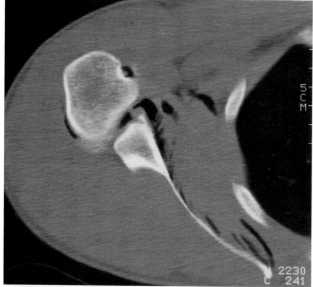

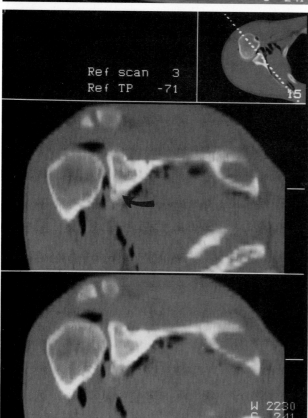

FIG. 15-16. Glenoid fracture with labral tear. **(A)** Transaxial CT arthrogram demonstrates prior fracture of glenoid as well as tear of labrum. **(B)** Oblique axis reconstruction demonstrates the extent of injury (arrow).

positive contrast media is injected into the joint space prior to the CT scan. It is important not to overdistend the joint space.

Skeletal Trauma

Possibly the most obvious ideal application for spiral CT is in the evaluation of musculoskeletal trauma. Because closely spaced scans can be obtained in a short scanning cycle, there is likely to be less chance for intrascan or interscan motion. Once a volumetric data set is generated, the images can be used for multiplanar and 3D reconstruction. The value of rapid acquisition is particularly apparent in trauma patients when the trauma involves areas where patients may have difficulty remaining still, such as the shoulder, sterno-clavicular joint, elbow, or wrist. Because arbitrary interscan spacing can be chosen following data acquisition, it is possible to obtain very closely spaced scans as needed for image postprocessing. Prior work has shown that the quality of multiplanar reconstruction and 3D images from helical or spiral CT is equal to that of conventional CT (24). In an article by Ney (24) to test whether spiral CT scans are equal to or superior to those of standard dynamic CT, two objects were used to study the effects of spiral CT: an angled cylindrical bone phantom and a human cadaver femur specimen with a simulated 1-mm fracture. Both objects were scanned in a water bath, and a series of spiral and standard CT scans was obtained with various parameters. Volumetric rendering was then done with the resultant data sets to create 3D images. Three radiologists reviewed the images to rate fidelity, accuracy, and diagnostic usefulness. The results showed that for similar parameters (slice thickness, interscan spacing) spiral and dynamic CT data resulted in images similar in quality. However, because spiral CT is approximately five times faster than dynamic CT, it is possible to use thinner collimation and obtain more sectional data with spiral CT.

Several other studies have shown similar results. McEnery et al. (25) studied the capabilities of spiral CT versus conventional CT to represent minimal fracture displacement on multiplanar reconstruction images and found with correctly selected scan parameters that "spiral CT derived reconstructions demonstrate similar edge profile resolution to reconstructions obtained from conventional CT." Link et al. (26) studied artificial spine fractures with spiral and conventional CT and found that "helical CT requires thinner collimation for fracture detection comparable with that of conventional CT."

Several authors have recently questioned the value of conventional CT versus spiral CT for musculoskeletal image reconstruction and 3D imaging (27). However, these studies have been in phantom experiments where real-life problems such as patient cooperation and potential interscan or intrascan movement as well as time to complete study are not considered. It is our experience that in the clinical environment, spiral CT is the technique of choice in the trauma patient.

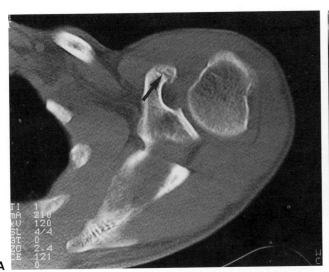
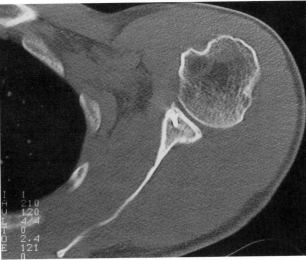

FIG. 15-17. Acromion fracture. **(A-B)** Spiral CT scan of the left shoulder demonstrates subtle fracture of acromion with attempt at healing at fracture line (*arrow*). Pin placed in glenoid from repair of prior fracture/dislocation is noted in **(B)**.

Although this chapter cannot review in detail all the specific applications for CT imaging of trauma, several of the more common applications should be noted. These anatomic zones include the pelvis and acetabulum, the knee (including the tibial plateau), the ankle joint, the wrist, and the spine. Even in the prespiral CT era it became clear that transaxial CT supplemented by multiplanar reconstruction (MPR) and 3D imaging could have a major impact on both diagnosis and patient management. Although precise numbers vary by clinical application, we found a consistent 20% to 30% rate of altered management by using MPR and 3D imaging versus transaxial CT alone. These changes in management were of predominantly two types: tentative surgery scheduled because of a situation worse than anticipated and acute surgery deferred in favor of later definitive arthrodesis or arthroplasty, again usually when the images revealed a clinical picture worse than anticipated.

In acetabular and pelvic trauma, spiral CT data sets coupled with a real-time 3D volume-rendering program allow visualization of the entire pelvis through any plane or perspective (28). The interactive nature of an imaging display was previously shown to be of value in creating arbitrary 360-degree rotation into any inlet or tangential view desired. Editing of the data set is of particular value in isolating the fracture, and in select cases disarticulating the femur from the acetabulum may be useful. By scanning and creating 3D maps of the entire pelvis we can easily detect any associated sacral or sacroiliac injuries (Figs. 15-18, 15-19).

Finally, in a single examination we can also use intravenous contrast to create vascular maps of the iliac and femoral vessels to rule out any associated vascular injuries (Fig. 15-20). Vascular injuries are critical components of complex pelvic fractures and in the past were studied exclusively with catheter angiography. With spiral CT angiography, classic angiographic studies may often be replaced.

CT is especially useful in lower-extremity trauma involving either the knee joint or the ankle. In the patient with a tibial plateau fracture, spiral CT with sagittal and coronal reformatting of data is an important study in defining whether or not a patient needs surgical intervention. The use of these displays coupled with 3D images is ideal for defining plateau depression and quantifying it (Fig. 15-21). In cases of proximal tibiofibular dislocation the 3D images are especially valuable. McEnery et al. (29) did an analysis to determine the value of spiral CT for detecting displacement of fractures of the tibial plateau. The authors found that "spiral CT can detect clinically important inferior depressions of tibial plateau fractures." The authors felt that to achieve optimal results the scan protocol should be 2-mm section collimation and 2-mm/s table speed, with image reconstruc-

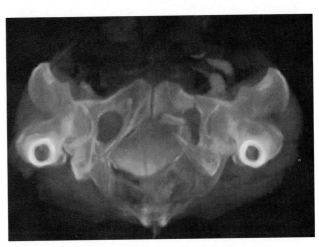

FIG. 15-18. *Fracture of the symphysis pubis.* Three-dimensional views clearly define both the extent of the superior and inferior pubic rami fractures as well as the degree of angulation.

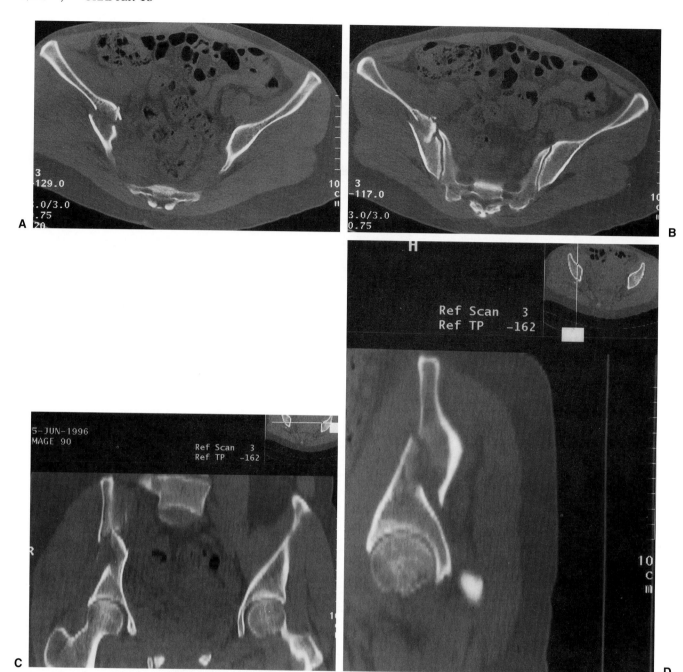

FIG. 15-19. Iliac wing fracture. **(A,B)** The transaxial views demonstrate the iliac fracture with extension to the right sacroiliac joint. **(C,D)** The extent of fracture is well demonstrated in multiplanar views, particularly on the sagittal reconstruction. *(continued)*

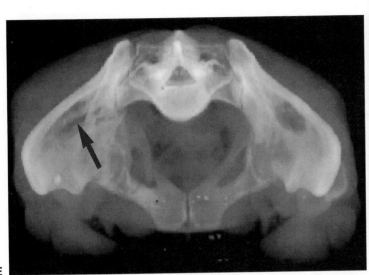
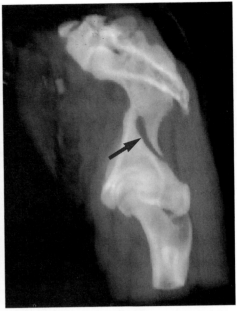

E   F

FIG. 15-19. *Continued.* **(E,F)** Three-dimensional reconstructions are useful because of their display of the entire injury from any perspective, as in this case.

tion at 1-mm intervals. Trauma to the distal femur can also benefit from spiral 3D studies in select cases (Fig. 15-22).

Severe ankle trauma also illustrates the role of multiplanar and 3D imaging in finalizing assessment and surgical planning (30) (Figs. 15-23, 15-24). Pilon fractures, with severe impaction and destruction of the articular plafond, may be triaged into those patients needing immediate surgery and those who will be treated later with arthroplasty. Injuries to the talus, calcaneus, or tarsal bones are well imaged with spiral CT protocols. Follow-up of patients, whether managed by surgery or more conservatively, is easily done with spiral CT. MPR and 3D images are often successful even in the face of metal pins and plates (Fig. 15-25).

Spiral CT with direct coronal reconstructions is an excellent approach to the traumatized wrist (31). This technique combines 2-mm collimation, 2–3-mm/s table speed, and reconstruction of data at 1-mm intervals. The technique is successful in evaluating occult or complex fractures, and the postsurgical wrist to determine healing. High-resolution al-

gorithms are helpful in these cases, as are targeting image reconstructions to achieve the best details in the data set (Figs. 15-26, 15-27)

Trauma to the spine can be routinely visualized successfully with a combination of transaxial CT, MPR images, and 3D studies. Nunez et al. (32) analyzed the standard radiographs and spiral scan in 88 patients and found that in 32 patients (*n* = 50) fractures were either missed or incompletely defined on conventional studies and defined on CT. In fact, the authors felt strongly enough to recommend routine screening with spiral CT in polytrauma victims.

Similar success has also been noted in the rest of the spine. In the thoracic and lumbar spine, CT coupled with sagittal reconstruction and 3D images helps define the presence and extent of injury. Specific applications include, in addition to fracture detection, detecting subluxations and locked facets, as well as localizing foreign matter, such as bullets. Sacral fractures, which can be overlooked on plain radiographs, are easily detected with spiral CT (Figs. 15-28, 15-29).

Soft-Tissue or Muscle Evaluation

The evaluation of soft-tissue or muscle infection and/or tumor is another clinical application for spiral CT. With the use of iodinated contrast material, we can scan through an area of suspected musculoskeletal abnormality during peak levels of contrast enhancement. It has been previously documented that contrast enhancement allows for better detection of intramuscular pathology, whether inflammatory or neoplastic (33,34). With spiral CT we can get an excellent idea of the vascularity of the lesion, and its detectability is en-

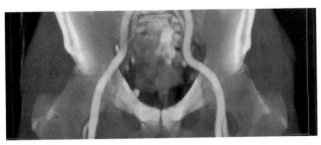

FIG. 15-20. Pelvic trauma without vascular injury. A spiral CT angiogram demonstrates normal arterial system without vascular injury.

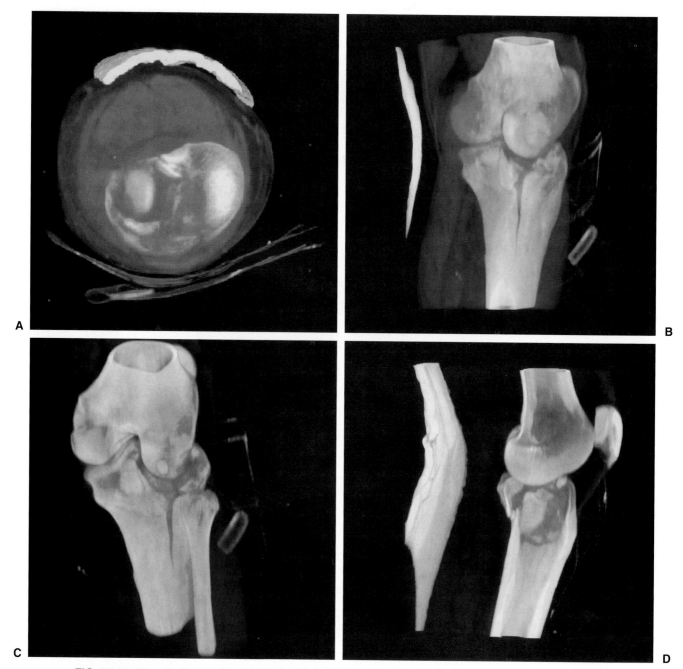

FIG. 15-21. Tibial plateau fracture. **(A-D)** Sequence of 3D views provides the surgeon with a comprehensive analysis of the fracture extent.

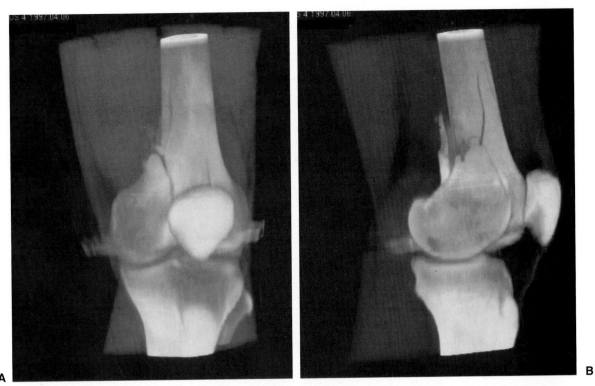

A B

FIG. 15-22. Comminuted fracture of the distal femur. (**A,B**) The fracture was secondary to a gunshot wound. Note that artifact related to the high-attenuation bullet is present but does not detract from the image quality.

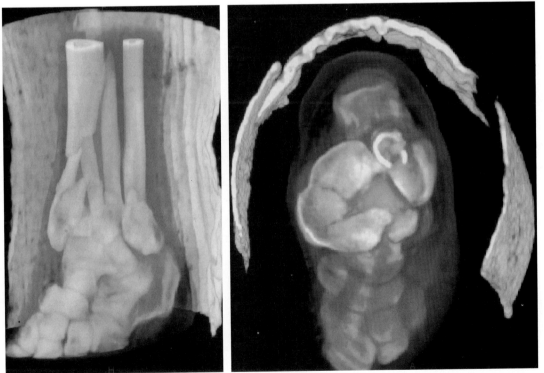

A B

FIG. 15-23. Comminuted fracture/dislocation of the distal tibia and fibula. (**A,B**) These views define the fracture extent as well as the disruption at the ankle mortise and tibiofibular ligament.

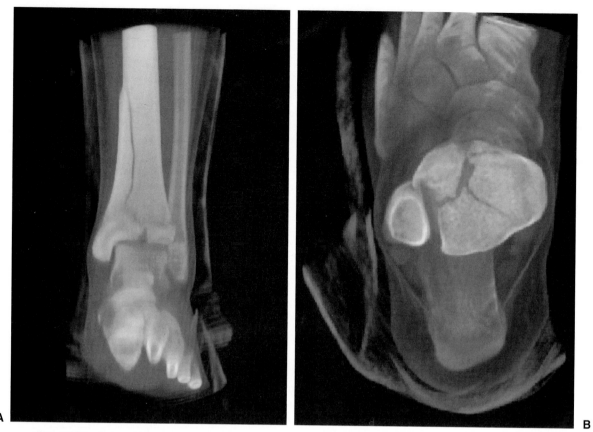

A

B

FIG. 15-24. Salter IV fracture of the distal tibia. (**A,B**) Select 3D views defines the fracture extent as well as the intact tibiofibular ligament.

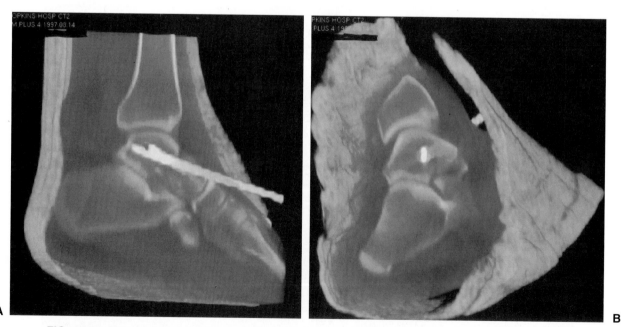

A

B

FIG. 15-25. Postoperative assessment of a talus fracture. (**A,B**) Multiple views define the location of the surgical pins to the fractures as well as the resultant repair. Note the study quality despite metal pins in place.

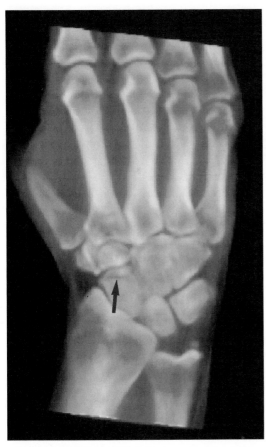

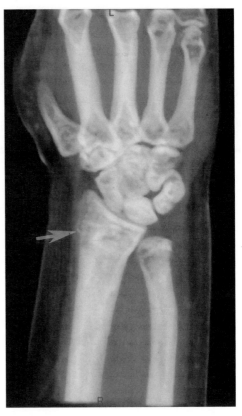

FIG. 15-26. Navicular fracture. Three-dimensional rendering defines a minimally displaced navicular fracture. Note how the fracture line is best defined with interactive editing and display of the data volume.

FIG. 15-27. Impacted fracture of the distal radius. Three-dimensional reconstruction of a spiral CT data set defines the subtle fracture line and impaction site (*arrow*).

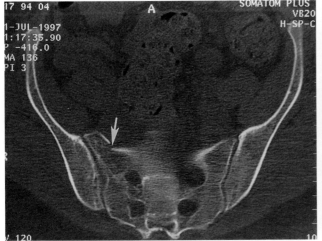

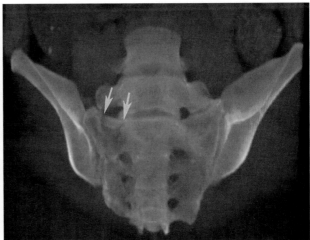

FIG. 15-28. Sacral fracture. (**A,B**) Plain radiographs were negative but transaxial CT detected a subtle fracture on the right side of the sacrum. The full extent of the fracture is best defined on the 3D views (**B**).

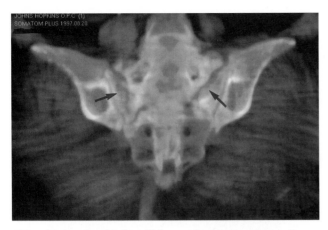

FIG. 15-29. Sacral insufficiency fractures. Three-dimensional representation of fractures through both the right and left sacral foramina (*arrows*). The right fracture extended to the sacroiliac joint.

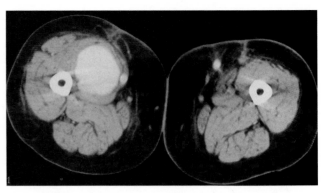

FIG. 15-30. Pseudoaneurysm. The patient had a history of a vascular graft and an enlarging thigh mass. The enhancement on the spiral CT is consistent with a pseudoaneurysm.

hanced by optimizing normal muscle enhancement. The local vascular supply is also optimally visualized, which can be valuable in patients with tumors where resection is being considered. Vascular thrombosis, aneurysms, or pseudoaneurysms are also easily detected with these techniques (Fig. 15-30). The timing of spiral image acquisition after contrast injection is critical. We have found that a delay of about 50–60 s is ideal in most clinical situations. In cases where an arteriovenous malformation or another arterial process is suspected, images at 25–30 s are preferred. In cases of vascular processes, surface or volumetric 3D reconstruction or MIP images may be helpful.

One patient population where we have found spiral CT of the muscle to be especially helpful is in the AIDS patient. This population appears to have an increased incidence of muscle infections and abscesses, although in many cases the presentation is best occult or subtle. Contrast-enhanced spiral CT optimizes detection of lesions during the preequi-

librium phase, even in patients with poor tissue planes (Figs. 15-31–15-35). The extent of involvement is well demonstrated on multiplanar reconstruction of the spiral CT data set. Multiplanar imaging is particularly useful in surgical planning, especially when the inflammatory process is extensive (Fig. 15-36). In many of these cases, delayed scans may also be helpful in defining the full extent of pathology.

Spiral CT is also useful in distinguishing vascular masses from hematoma, abscess, or tumor. In the postoperative vascular patient, aneurysms or pseudoaneurysms may present as a palpable mass. Although in many cases the diagnosis can be made clinically or with Doppler ultrasound, in other cases spiral CT with 3D rendering is most valuable. As more experience is gained with spiral CT angiography, its role continues to expand in vascular imaging across a wide range of applications.

One interesting finding related to spiral CT is the frequency of detection of musculoskeletal metastasis as inci-

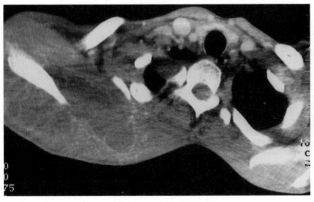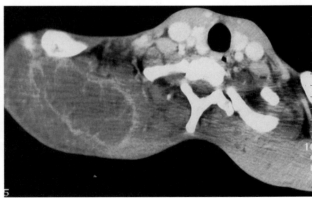

FIG. 15-31. Intramuscular abscess involving the posterior deltoid, suprascapular and subscapular musculature. (**A,B**) Spiral CT demonstrates multiple low-density areas with enhancing rims in muscle consistent with abscess. The patient had a history of intravenous drug abuse. The use of spiral CT with iodinated contrast optimizes detection of these abscesses.

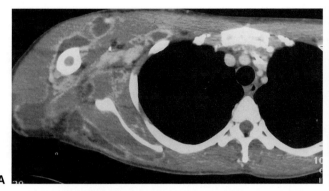
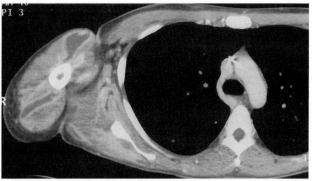

A B

FIG. 15-32. Multiple intramuscular abscesses involving the chest wall and upper extremity. (**A,B**) Spiral CT demonstrates multiple low-density lesions with peripheral enhancement consistent with multiple abscesses. The patient had a history of lupus, renal failure, and intravenous drug use. The CT appearance also suggested some degree of myositis. Culture of the abscesses grew group A strep.

dental findings. We have seen many cases of metastasis to muscle presenting as hypervascular lesions ranging in size from 5 mm to 5 cm. In most cases the patients have not been symptomatic as a result of these lesions. The common tumors where we have found this to occur have been lung cancer, breast cancer, and lymphoma.

Skeletal Tumors

Spiral CT is helpful in defining the full extent of primary or metastatic bone tumors. This information can be used for either image analysis or therapy planning, whether surgical, radiation therapy, or chemotherapy. Multiplanar and/or 3D reconstruction may be of special value in this group of patients. Spiral CT is especially valuable in areas such as the ribs, spine, sternum, and shoulder when other examinations are equivocal for tumor infiltration (Figs. 15-37–15-39). The combination of thin-section CT (2–4 mm) with narrow interscan spacing (1–3 mm) can be useful for the detection of subtle tumor infiltration. For example, in Fig. 15-40, we

evaluated a patient with a known pelvic mass prior to biopsy and prior to final management decision making. Spiral CT was done from the upper thigh in a cranial direction to optimize definition of tumor extent as well as vascular involvement. In this case, both vascular encasement and bony involvement were detected and defined. This information was helpful in the eventual resection of this tumor.

In bony metastases or primary tumors, spiral CT can help define the presence and extent of disease. Although bone scans are an excellent screening study for metastases, CT is more valuable when symptoms are localized to a specific zone or anatomic region. In these cases, targeted examinations are the ideal screening study. Multiplanar and 3D studies are often critical in these cases for defining the true extent of lesions for the referring orthopedic surgeon or oncologist

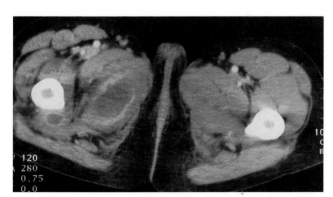

FIG. 15-33. Intramuscular thigh abscess. The patient developed fever several days subsequent to a gunshot wound to the pelvis and thigh. CT scan demonstrates two enhancing lesions. The largest one involved the adductor magnus muscle. This was an intramuscular abscess with classic peripheral enhancement.

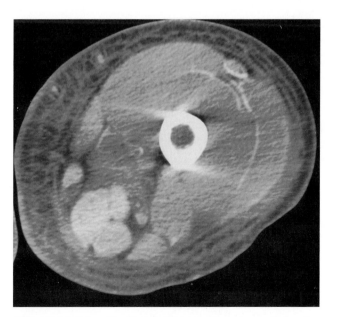

FIG. 15-34. Myositis. Spiral CT scanning demonstrates the decreased attenuation of the muscles of the left upper thigh. This was secondary to myositis in this intravenous drug abuse patient.

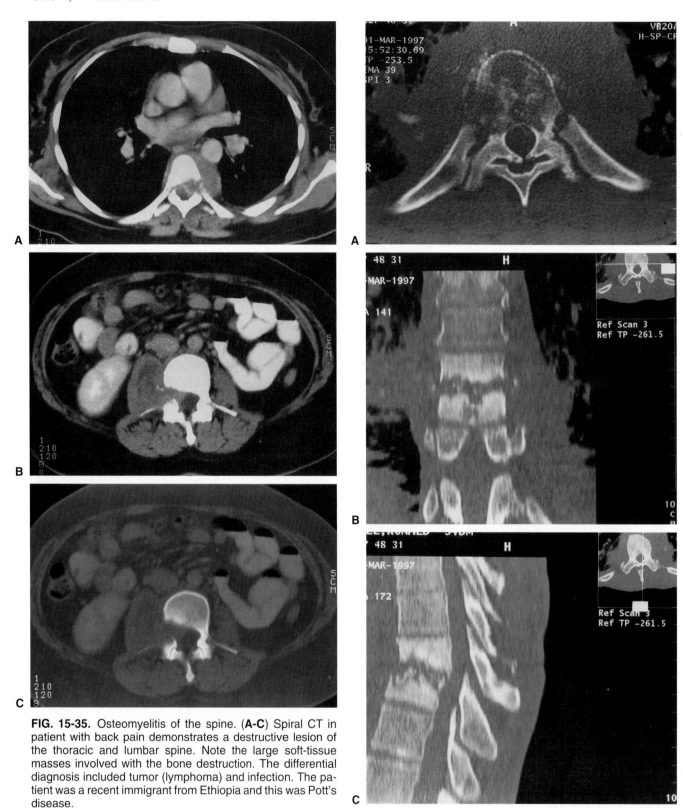

FIG. 15-35. Osteomyelitis of the spine. **(A-C)** Spiral CT in patient with back pain demonstrates a destructive lesion of the thoracic and lumbar spine. Note the large soft-tissue masses involved with the bone destruction. The differential diagnosis included tumor (lymphoma) and infection. The patient was a recent immigrant from Ethiopia and this was Pott's disease.

FIG. 15-36. Tuberculous osteomyelitis of the thoracic spine. **(A-C)** Spiral CT demonstrates evidence of osteomyelitis of the lower spine with bony destruction seen and associated paraspinal abscess.

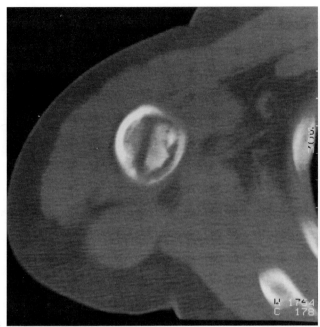

A

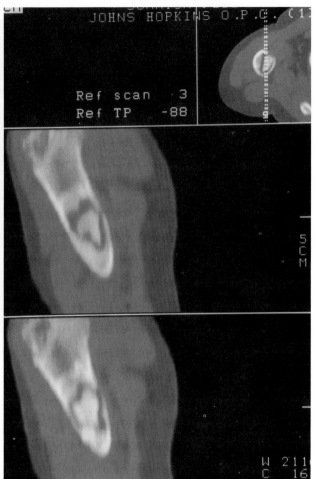

B

FIG. 15-37. Fibrous dysplasia of right humerus. **(A)** Spiral demonstrates a lesion involving both cortex and medulla of right humerus with fallen fragment sign seen. This was consistent with the diagnosis of fibrous dysplasia. **(B)** Sagittal reconstruction of the lesion demonstrates its full extent.

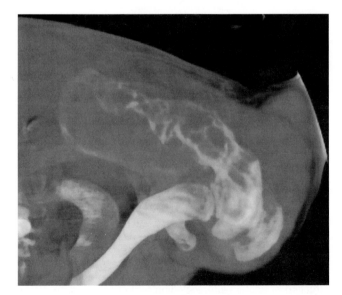

FIG. 15-38. Multiple myeloma. Three-dimensional representation of a large expansile lytic lesion of the scapula that was due to multiple myeloma.

(Fig. 15-41). The recognition that image display is important for the referring physician is often overlooked in a busy radiological practice.

CT is also worthwhile in patients with benign tumors such as suspected osteoid osteoma (Fig. 15-42). The use of narrow collimation (2 mm) and small interscan spacing (1 mm) allows for detection of the nidus even in the most difficult of cases. This information can be used for percutaneous CT-guided removal of the nidus or for standard surgical planning (35).

Oncological applications for musculoskeletal spiral CT, including its role in radiation therapy planning, are discussed in more detail in Chapter 17.

Problem-Solving Studies

The initial role of CT scanning in the musculoskeletal system was as a problem-solving tool. CT often became the final arbiter in cases in which radiological studies, clinical presentation, and/or physical examination were in conflict (Fig. 15-43). Spiral CT helps increase the value of CT in this clinical situation. Spiral CT scanning provides a volume data set that can allow for multiple sections through an area

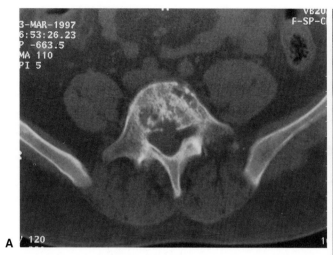

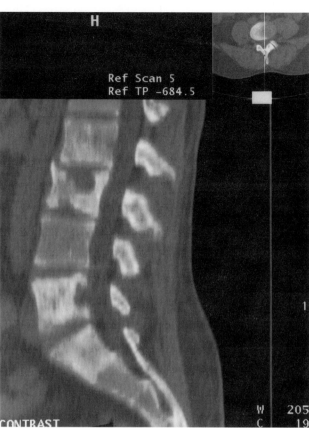

FIG. 15-39. Lymphoma of the lumbar spine and sacrum. (**A, B**) Transaxial CT supplemented by sagittal multiplanar reconstruction demonstrates multiple abnormal vertebral bodies. The lesions could be described as mixed lytic and sclerotic and were biopsy-proven lymphoma.

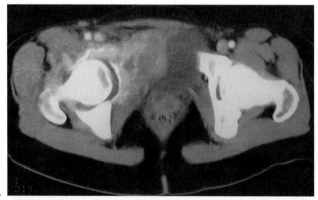

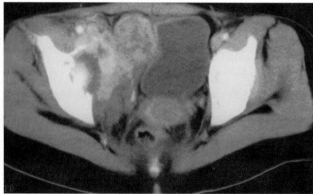

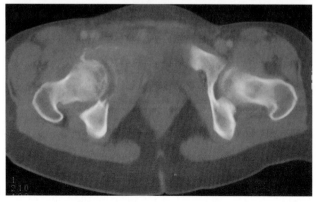

FIG. 15-40. Aggressive aneurysmal bone cyst. (**A,B**) Spiral CT scan demonstrates hypervascular mass destroying right anterior medial wall of acetabulum with large soft-tissue mass extending into pelvis, compressing and possibly invading the bladder. Note the hypervascular nature of this mass seen on spiral CT scan with data acquired in a caudal-to-cranial direction. (**C**) Corresponding bone image demonstrates destruction of acetabulum, including roof of acetabulum.

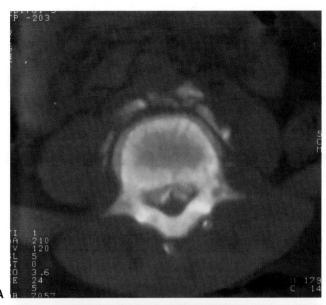

A

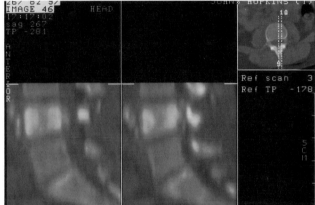

B   C

FIG. 15-41. Osteosarcoma involving the L4 and S1 vertebral bodies. (A) Transaxial CT demonstrates osteoblastic component of tumor with extension both anterior and posterior to the vertebral body. (B,C) Coronal and sagittal reconstructions demonstrate the full extent of the lesion, including extension of tumor into spiral canal on sagittal view.

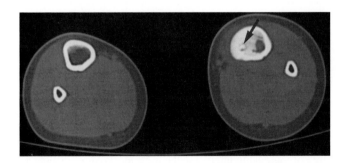

FIG. 15-42. Osteoid osteoma. Spiral CT with sections reconstructed at 2 mm demonstrates a small central nidus within the cortex of the left mid tibia (*arrow*). Notice the remodeling of the tibia with endosteal reaction.

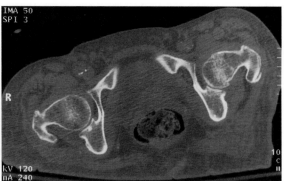

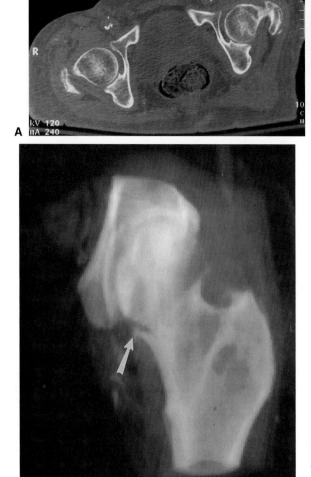

FIG. 15-43. Impacted femoral neck fracture. **(A,B)** The plain radiographs were negative and the transaxial CT subtle. **(C)** The 3D rendering with editing and optimal plane projection clearly defines the fracture extent and impaction (*arrow*).

of suspicious pathology. Spiral CT is excellent in detecting the presence of subtle lesions with even minimal destruction or resorption. In most cases when bone involvement is evaluated, intravenous contrast material is not used. It may be helpful, however, in demonstrating soft-tissue extension of tumor and vascular invasion. It is therefore important to understand the clinical questions to be answered prior to performing the spiral CT examination.

CONCLUSION

Spiral CT combined with multiplanar reconstruction and 3D imaging has replaced conventional tomography in a wide range of applications. The role of spiral CT musculoskeletal imaging undoubtedly will increase with more clinical experience as well as with the advancement of spiral CT technique and the refinement of reconstruction algorithms to improve image quality.

In the first edition of this book, we listed several specific limitations of musculoskeletal spiral CT scanning at its current state. The key limitations included a relatively low mA value on some systems for the basic 24–32-s spiral as well as bone reconstruction algorithms that did not seem to create high-resolution images that are as sharp as those generated from nonspiral CT data. Additionally, the length of the spiral CT scan (32 s) was often not long enough when a larger area was to be imaged for multiplanar or 3D reconstruction. However, these problems have been solved on most systems and the potential roadblocks to imaging have been removed.

Although most of the original excitement of spiral CT centered around applications in the chest and abdomen, an area of increasing interest is the musculoskeletal system. As illustrated in this chapter, the potential applications in a wide range of problems are exciting and have only recently begun to be addressed. The current trend by major CT manufacturers toward workstations will increase the routine use of multiplanar and 3D imaging, two applications for which spiral CT is particularly well suited. Other applications—including surgical planning, custom hip design, and joint reconstruction—will all benefit from the use of spiral CT, and we look forward with cautious optimism to its continued growth (Figs. 15-44, 15-45).

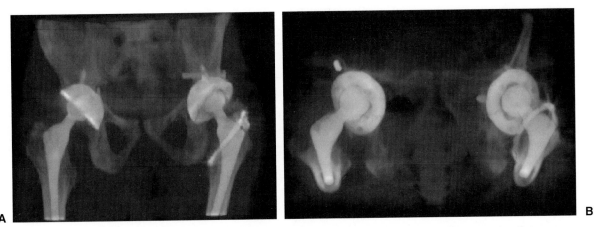

FIG. 15-44. Failed left total hip replacement. (**A,B**) Despite hip implants the 3D reconstruction are detailed with minimum of artifact. The left prosthesis cup has rotated superior and posteriorly. Note that the screw holes can be seen clearly on (**B**).

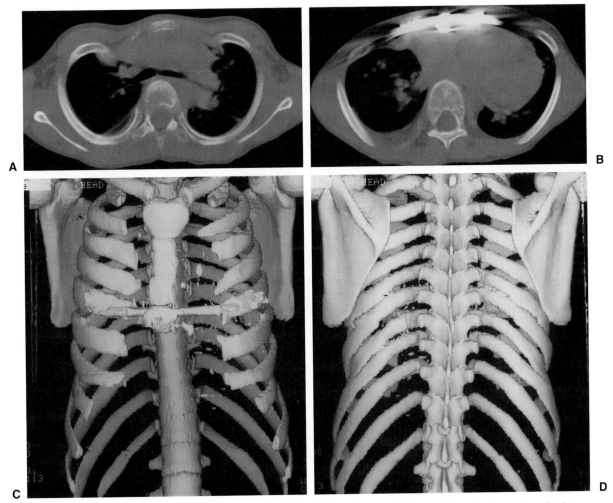

FIG. 15-45. Acquired Jeunes syndrome. (**A**) Transaxial views demonstrate deformity of anterior ribs in relationship to sternum. (**B**) The sternum was elevated with surgical repair. Three-dimensional reconstruction views (**C,D**) demonstrate the reconstruction of the thoracic cage.

REFERENCES

1. Fishman EK, Wyatt SH, Bluemke DA, Urban BA. Spiral CT of musculoskeletal pathology: preliminary observations. *Skeletal Radiol* 1993; 22:253–256.
2. Heiken JP, Brink JA, Vannier MW. Spiral (helical) CT. *Radiology* 1993;189:647–656.
3. Fishman EK. Spiral CT evaluation of the musculoskeletal system In: Fishman EK, Jeffrey RB, eds. *Spiral CT: principles, techniques and clinical applications.* New York: Raven Press; 1995.
4. Pretorius ES, Fishman EK. Helical (spiral) CT of the musculoskeletal system. *Radiol Clin North Am* 1995;33(5):949–978.
5. Tecce PM, Fishman EK. Spiral CT with multiplanar reconstruction in the diagnosis of sternoclavicular osteomyelitis. *Skeletal Radiol* 1995; 24:275–281.
6. Scott WW Jr, Fishman EK. Soft tissue masses. In: Scott WW Jr, Magid D, Fishman EK, eds. *Computed tomography of the musculoskeletal system.* New York: Churchill Livingstone; 1987;8:1–27.
7. Dillon EH, van Leenwen MS, Fernandez MA, Mali WPTM. Spiral CT angiography. *AJR* 1993;160:1273–1278.
8. Costello P, Gaa J. Spiral CT angiography of the abdominal aorta and its branches. *Eur Radiol* 1993;3:359–365.
9. Rubin GD, Dake MD, Napel S, et al. Spiral CT of renal artery stenosis: comparison of three-dimensional rendering techniques *Radiology* 1994;190:181–189.
10. Scott WW Jr, Fishman EK. Spiral CT arthrography of the shoulder. (*Work in progress.*)
11. Fishman EK, Magid D, Ney DR, et al. Three-dimensional Imaging. *Radiology* 1991;181:321–337.
12. Magid D, Fishman EK, Sponseller PD, Griffin PP. 2D and 3D computed tomography of the pediatric hip. *Radiographics* 1988;8:901–934.
13. Magid D, Fishman EK. Imaging of musculoskeletal trauma in three dimensions. *Radiol Clin North Am* 1989;27:945–956.
14. Ney DR, Drebin RA, Fishman EK, Magid D. Volumetric rendering of computed tomographic data: principles and techniques. *IEEE Comput Graph Applic* 1990;10:24–32.
15. Drebin RA Carpenter L, Hanrahan P. Volume rendering. *Comput Graph* 1988;22:65–74.
16. Drebin RA, Magid D, Robertson DD, Fishman EK. Fidelity of three-dimensional CT imaging for detecting fracture gaps. *J Comput Assist Tomogr* 1989;13:487–489.
17. Kuszyk BS Heath DG, Bliss DF, Fishman EK. Skeletal 3-D CT: advantages of volume rendering over surface rendering. *Skeletal Radiol* 1996; 25:207–214.
18. Olson PN Everson LI, Griffiths HJ. Staging of musculoskeletal tumors. *Radiol Clin North Am* 1994;32:151–162.
19. Pretorius ES, Scott WW Jr, Fishman EK. Acute trauma to the shoulder: role of spiral computed tomographic imaging. *Emerg Radiol* 1995;2(1): 13–17.
20. Kuhlman JE, Fishman EK, Ney DR, Magid D. Complex shoulder trauma: three-dimensional CT imaging. *Orthopedics* 1988;11: 1561–1563.
21. Kuhlman JE, Fishman EK, Scott WW Jr, Magid D, Siegelman SS. Two-dimensional and three-dimensional evaluation of the painful shoulder. *Orthop Rev* 1989;18:1201–1208.
22. Stiles RG, Otte MT. Imaging of the shoulder. *Radiology* 1993;188: 603–613.
23. Wilson A, Totty WG, Murphy WA, et al. Shoulder joint: arthrography CT and long-term follow-up with surgical correlation. *Radiology* 1989; 173:329–333.
24. Ney DR, Fishman EK, Kawashima A, Robertson Jr DD, Scott WW Jr. Comparison of helical and serial CT with regard to three-dimensional imaging of musculoskeletal anatomy. *Radiology* 1992;185(3): 865–869.
25. McEnery KE, Wilson AJ, Murphy Jr WA. Comparison of spiral computed tomography versus conventional computed tomography multiplanar reconstructions of a fracture displacement phantom. *Invest Radiol* 1994;29(7):665–670.
26. Link TM, Meier N, Rummeny EJ, et al. Artificial spine fractures: detection with helical and conventional CT. *Radiology* 1996;198(2): 515–519.
27. Kasales CJ, Mauger DT, Sefczek RJ, et al. Multiplanar image reconstruction and 3D imaging using a musculoskeletal phantom: conventional versus helical CT. *J Comput Assist Tomogr* 1997;21(1):162–169.
28. Scott WW Jr, Fishman EK, Magid D. Optimal imaging of acetabular fractures. *Radiology* 1987;11:1017–1020.
29. McEnery KW, Wilson AJ, Pilgram TK, Murphy Jr WA, Marushack MM. Fractures of the tibial plateau: value of spiral CT coronal plane reconstructions for detecting displacement in vitro. *AJR* 1994;163: 1177–1181.
30. Magid D, Michelson JD, Ney DR, Fishman EK. Adult ankle fractures: comparison of plain films and interactive two- and three-dimensional CT scans. *AJR* 1990;154:1017–1023.
31. Kuszyk BS, Fishman EK. Direct coronal CT of the wrist: helical acquisition with simplified patient positioning. *AJR* 1996;166:419–420.
32. Nunez DB Jr, Zuluaga A, Fuentes-Bernardo DA, Rivas LA, Becerra JL. Cervical spine trauma: how much more do we learn by routinely using helical CT? *Radiographics* 1996;16(6):1307–1318.
33. Magid D, Fishman EK. Musculoskeletal infections in patients with AIDS: CT findings. *AJR* 1992;158:603–607.
34. Beauchamp NJ, Scott WW Jr, Gottlieb LM, Fishman EK. CT evaluation of soft tissue muscle infection and inflammation: a systematic compartmental approach. *Skeletal Radiol* 1995;24(5):317–324.
35. Ayala A, Murray JA, Erling MA. Osteoid osteoma: intraoperative tetracycline-fluorescence demonstration of the nidus. *J Bone Joint Surg (Am)* 1988;68:747–751.

CHAPTER 16

Spiral CT: Pediatric Applications

George A. Taylor

Computed tomographic (CT) imaging in children is associated with a unique set of problems that make obtaining diagnostic images in children a challenge: Rapid respiratory rate and voluntary movement can cause significant artifacts; there is typically little fat surrounding and therefore highlighting normal structures in children; the patients are small; and radiation dose to the patient must be very seriously taken into account (1).

Spiral CT offers potential solutions to several of these problems. In this chapter we will discuss techniques and applications of spiral CT in the pediatric population and how this technique can be maximized for solving imaging problems in children.

GENERAL TECHNIQUE

The following approach represents what has worked well in our own clinical practice with children. However, it is important to recognize that there are a variety of approaches to scanning the pediatric patient. Differences in local preference and institutional practices are such that no single regimen is used universally.

Sedation

One of the most striking benefits of spiral CT in children is the significantly reduced time necessary for image acquisition. Our current scanner can cover up to a 120-cm volume in 60 s using 20-mm/s table increments and a 5-mm beam collimation. This has resulted in the possibility of reduced sedation in younger children. In a recent study, White showed an 8% reduction in sedation rate in children undergoing abdominal or chest CT with the advent of helical scanning (2). We have also observed that sedation can be reduced or completely avoided in many young children by using spiral techniques. Immobilization can be achieved in children less than 6 months of age without sedation by swaddling, or with the use of Velcro straps or adhesive tape. Children

as young as 2 years have undergone abdominal CT scans using only a parent's physical presence and reassurance. A variety of sedation regimens can be used in children who cannot cooperate for the necessary time (3). Intravenous pentobarbital at a dose of 2–6 mg/kg has been used quite safely and successfully in children (4).

The advantages of intravenous (IV) sedation are rapid onset, predictable effect, and the ability to titrate to desired effect. Children under 18 months of age can also be well sedated with oral chloral hydrate (50–80 mg/kg).

All sedated children should be monitored both visually by medical and nursing personnel, and mechanically. Pulse oximetry with respiratory monitoring and electrocardiogram are the safest tools for monitoring the pediatric patient (5).

Breathing Techniques

Cooperative older children can almost always be taught to hold their breath without great difficulty. However, reliable breath-holding is usually impossible in children younger than 10 years of age. In these patients, spiral CT examinations (including the lung and mediastinum) can be adequately performed during quiet respiration without significant motion artifacts (6).

Intravenous Contrast

Although extensive noncontrast scanning in children is usually unnecessary, it can be useful when the detection of calcification or hemorrhage is important. In the initial evaluation of abdominal masses we recommend obtaining two or three sequential CT images of the region of interest before administration of IV contrast.

As in conventional CT, IV contrast during spiral CT can be quite helpful in children because of the relatively little amount of fat and inherent tissue contrast in these patients. However, administration of IV contrast with spiral CT dif-

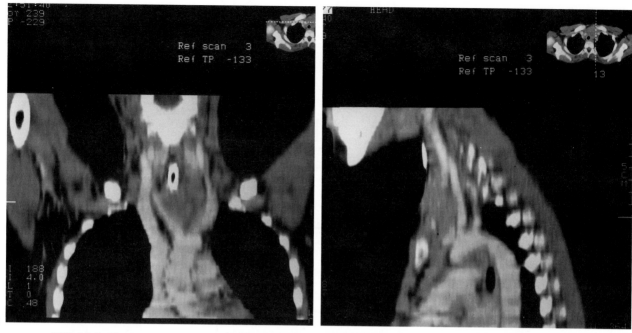

A

B

FIG. 16-1. Fourteen-year-old boy with laryngeal papillomatosis and metallic tracheostomy tube, unsuitable for magnetic resonance imaging. Sagittal (**A**) and coronal (**B**) reconstructions of a spiral CT of the neck and chest after injection of 1.5 mL/kg iohexal show posterior and lateral displacement of common carotid arteries by mass surrounding trachea. Note excellent opacification of the great vessels of the mediastinum with reduced dose of intravenous contrast.

fers from that used with conventional CT in two important ways: volume of contrast required and method of administration. Because of the very short scanning times, the total volume of contrast used for spiral CT can be reduced when compared with that needed for conventional CT. In adult patients, the volume of contrast may be reduced by 25% to 50% without sacrificing vascular and tissue opacification (7). Similar reductions can be achieved in pediatric patients. Excellent opacification can be routinely obtained using nonionic, iso-osmolar contrast 300–320 mg/mL (1.5–2 mL/kg) by rapid bolus injection (Fig. 16-1). This is especially helpful when the amount of contrast needs to be limited because of diminished cardiac or renal function, or because of tenuous venous access.

Time delay after contrast administration is also an important variable in optimizing contrast enhancement. This poses a special challenge because injection rates can vary widely in children. Contributing factors include differences in heart rate, and cardiac output, and use of hand injections for contrast administration (8). Nonetheless, most pediatric sites use hand injection to avoid the potential risk of contrast extravasation. Optimization of contrast enhancement can be achieved in a number of ways, including bolus timing and monitoring techniques (9). At this time, most pediatric injection protocols are empirically based and not standardized to specific time delays (10). At our institution, we set the delay relative to the end of injection, so that scanning begins approximately 10–15 s after completion of injection when ex-

amining the chest, and after a 20–30-s delay for abdominal applications. This approach has resulted in excellent parenchymal opacification of the liver and is consistent with recommendations by other pediatric specialists (9,10).

A dose of 2 mL/kg is suggested for the combined chest and abdomen study. Rather than delivering half of the total dose at the start of the mediastinum and the remainder at the level of the diaphragm by separate bolus infusion, a single rapid bolus of contrast can be administered at the beginning of the scan.

When an abnormality is suspected in the pelvis, one-third of the contrast dose can be reserved and given at the level of the pelvic inlet for better evaluation of the regional anatomy.

GI Contrast

Normal fat distribution in children is different than that in adults. Even overweight children tend to accumulate fat almost exclusively in the subcutaneous tissues and not within the peritoneal cavity. Without the intrinsic contrast of intraperitoneal fat, distinguishing bowel loops from adenopathy, abscess, or tumor can be quite difficult. This is why we recommend the use of oral contrast with spiral CT for most examinations of the abdomen.

When opacifying the GI tract from the stomach to the terminal ileum, a single dose of oral contrast given 60–90 min before scanning is usually sufficient. In examinations involving the pelvis, a dose of contrast may be given 2–4

TABLE 16-1. *Suggested schedule of oral contrast administration*

Age	60 min prior to study (in ounces)	15 min prior to study (in ounces)
<1 month	2–3	1–1.5
1 month to 1 year	4–8	2–4
1–5 years	8–12	4–6
6–12 years	12–16	6–8
13–15 years	16–20	8–10
>15 years	20	11

hours before scanning followed by a second dose 30 min prior to scanning. Either a dilute (1% to 2%) barium solution or water-soluble, iodine-based contrast may be used. Contrast may be mixed with fruit juice or Kool-Aid to disguise the taste and may be given per nasogastric tube if the child refuses to drink. Amount and timing of contrast administration are based on the age of the patient (11). In the past, 4–6-hour schedules have been used with excellent results. However, more streamlined protocols are in use at most children's hospitals that allow scanning without inordinate delay and during normal working hours. Below is a suggested schedule of oral contrast administration (Table 16-1).

For children who have difficulty tolerating large amounts of contrast (e.g., oncology patients on chemotherapy or patients with partial bowel obstruction), time can be increased to 4 hours or overnight, particularly if the patient is an outpatient to be scanned the following day.

The following are circumstances in which oral contrast is not routinely used in pediatrics:

Acute abdominal trauma;

Follow-up for known splenic/hepatic laceration;

Suspected fungal abscesses in immunocompromised patients.

Under the preceding circumstances, patients may be scanned without oral contrast administration.

Contraindications for use of oral contrast include patients without a gag or cough reflex and intubated patients with an uncuffed endotracheal tube.

When contrast is given rectally, opacification of the distal colon and rectum can be achieved with 1.5% Hypaque solutions. This can be performed by slow administration through a small-caliber catheter. Suggested volumes for rectal administration are 50 mL for infants, 100 mL for young children, and 250 mL for older children.

Spiral Technique

For each spiral CT scan the radiologist must specify several scanning and reconstruction parameters, including the collimation, table speed, total scan time, and image reconstruction, all the while keeping in mind the goals for the particular study and the relative radiation dose to the child.

As with standard CT, the choice of collimation depends on the particular imaging task and age of the patient. Routine thoracic and abdominal spiral scanning in children is generally performed using the following slice thickness:

Age (years)	Slice Thickness (mm)
<2	3–5
2–10	5–7
>10	8–10

Another important consideration in scanning pediatric patients is pitch, or table speed relative to slice thickness. To balance radiation dose considerations against significant loss of anatomic detail, we recommend a pitch of 1.5:1 for most pediatric body CT applications, except for abdominal trauma examinations, in which we often use a pitch of 2:1 for faster or extended anatomic coverage. When three-dimensional (3D) or multiplanar reconstructions are necessary, we use approximately 50% overlapped reconstructions.

Detailed examination of specific areas, such as the tracheobronchial tree or complex fractures may require 1–2-mm collimation and a pitch of 1:1 to achieve greater delineation of anatomic detail.

Relative radiation dose is a key consideration in pediatric CT imaging. In general, total dose for a spiral CT examination using a pitch of 1:1 is equivalent to that of contiguous conventional CT images obtained with the same collimation and milliamperage (mA) (12). It is important to note that the resolution along the longitudinal axis of spiral CT can be increased to approximately half the original collimation thickness without any additional increase in radiation dose (13). In addition, increasing the pitch to 1.5:1 or 2:1 will result in theoretical total dose reductions of approximately 33% and 50%, respectively. As with conventional CT, the most important radiation dose savings are achieved by limiting the use of spiral CT to specific high-yield clinical indications and by limiting the scans to well-defined areas of interest.

SPIRAL CT APPLICATIONS IN CHILDREN

For many of the reasons outlined earlier, most CT examinations of the chest and abdomen in young children at our institution are currently performed with spiral technique. In this section, we will cover common indications for spiral CT in children, as well as some specific circumstances in which conventional CT techniques are preferable.

Applications in the Chest

Tumors involving the mediastinum are an excellent indication for spiral CT (14). In these patients, the primary goal of preoperative imaging is accurate definition of the location and extent of the lesion. Spiral CT with multiplanar reformatting can be very useful in the identification of encasement or compression of vital structures, or intraspinal extension; information necessary to determine resectability; and

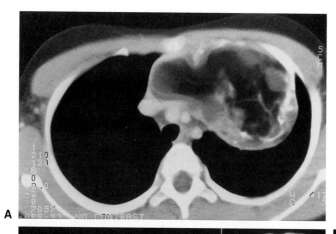

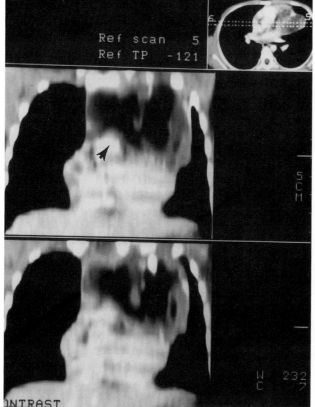

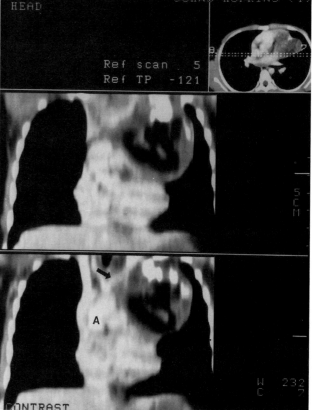

FIG. 16-2. Nine-year-old boy with mediastinal mass. Axial spiral CT obtained during quiet breathing using 8-mm collimation and 8-mm/s table speed. Four-millimeter axial reconstruction (**A**) shows heterogeneous mass containing fat, intermediate soft-tissue density, and calcification typical of teratoma. Coronal reconstructions (**B,C**) show intimate relationship between mass and main pulmonary artery (*arrowhead*), ascending aorta (A), and left subclavian vessels (*arrow*).

need for neurosurgical consultation (Fig. 16-2). Although possible in many cases, precise preoperative histological diagnosis of a solitary mass is not essential for surgical planning. The major exceptions to this are inflammatory masses that might be treated by antibiotics and/or percutaneous drainage, and lymphoma, the prognosis of which is not altered by resection.

As with tumors of the mediastinum, spiral CT can be very useful in the evaluation of masses involving the chest wall. Although uncommon in children, tumors of the chest wall proper are frequently malignant and may aggressively invade the pleural space, lung, spinal canal, or mediastinal vessels. Preoperative imaging evaluation should focus on assessment of size and extent of the primary tumor, bony

invasion, and involvement of the chest wall musculature (Fig. 16-3).

Spiral CT can also be used to evaluate the pulmonary parenchyma in children. The technique can be especially useful in infants or young children in whom rapid respiratory rate can cause significant artifacts on conventional CT. In congenital cystic lesions of the lung such as cystic adenomatoid malformation or sequestration, imaging is important in establishing accurate anatomic location, and extent of disease, prior to attempted resection (Fig. 16-4). Preoperative spiral CT may be very useful in confirming the diagnosis and establishing precise anatomic relationships even in the tachypneic infant.

Tumor involvement of the lungs in children is most often

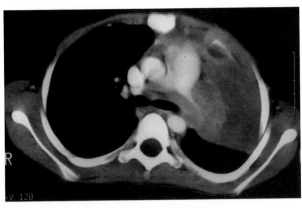

FIG. 16-3. Eleven-year-old boy with rhabdomyosarcoma of the chest wall. Enhanced 10-mm axial scan shows tumor involvement of the left anterior chest wall and encasement of the left main pulmonary artery.

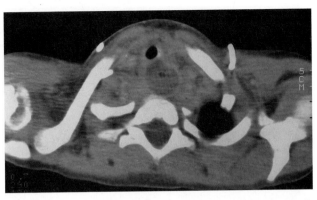

FIG. 16-5. Seven-year-old boy with lymphoma and aspergillus infection of the cervical esophagus. Contrast-enhanced 4-mm axial scan obtained with spiral technique during quiet respiration shows 3-cm hypodense mass surrounding gas-containing esophagus.

the result of metastatic disease. Survival of children with pulmonary metastases may be significantly influenced by resection of isolated lesions, especially with osteosarcoma (15). In adults, spiral CT during suspended respiration appears to have an advantage in eliminating misregistration from respiratory motion (16). Its utility in children has not been systematically explored.

In addition, spiral CT can be helpful in imaging difficult anatomic areas such as cervicothoracic junction or diaphragm (Fig. 16-5). In patients with focal tracheal narrowing, spiral CT can define the causes of extrinsic compression, associated vascular anomalies, and length and site of narrowing (Fig. 16-6). Evaluation of associated vascular anomalies can also be easily achieved using spiral technique.

Applications in the Abdomen

Aside from the evaluation of traumatized children, CT of the abdomen is most commonly used in the evaluation of children with blunt trauma, neoplasms, adenopathy, abscesses, complex fluid collections, and extent and complications of inflammatory bowel disease. CT should not be the first imaging study performed in the assessment of the newborn and young infant. Ultrasound often contributes far more information in this age group, and CT should be reserved for specific problems not resolved by ultrasound. A clearly defined role for spiral CT of the pediatric abdomen at this time is in the evaluation of neoplasms (17). The most commonly occurring tumors of the abdomen in children are neuroblastoma (Fig. 16-7) and Wilms' tumor of the kidney (Fig. 16-8), followed by rhabdomyosarcoma, hepatoblastoma, and hepatocellular carcinoma. On occasion, undifferentiated tumors of uncertain primary origin can be seen in the liver, peritoneal cavity, or retroperitoneum. Rapid scan times and multiplanar capability may provide significant anatomic in-

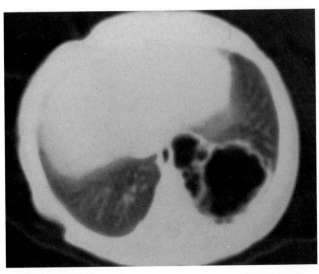

FIG. 16-4. Newborn with cystic adenomatoid malformation. Unenhanced 4-mm axial scan obtained with spiral technique during quiet respiration clearly shows well-defined, thin-walled cystic lesion in left lower lobe.

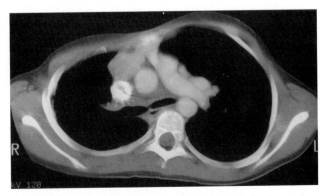

FIG. 16-6. Twelve-year-old boy with asymmetric chest size. Enhanced 10-mm axial spiral CT image shows absent right pulmonary artery.

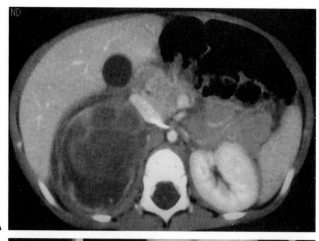

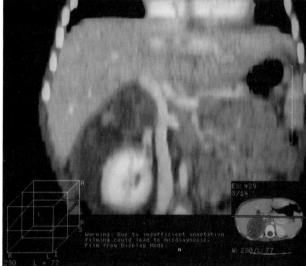

FIG. 16-7. Eighteen-month-old with adrenal neuroblastoma. Enhanced 5-mm axial (**A**), coronal (**B**), and sagittal (**C**) reconstructions show a right suprarenal mass inferiorly displacing the right kidney and anteriorly displacing the inferior vena cava.

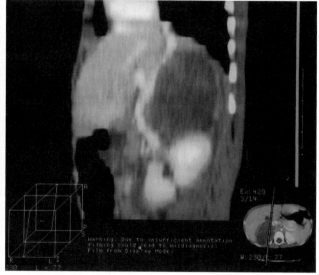

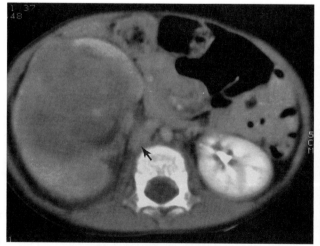

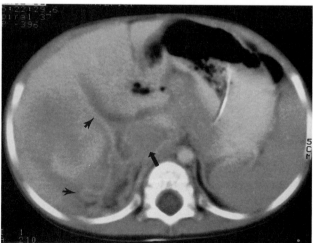

FIG. 16-8. Two-year-old with Wilms' tumor. Contrast-enhanced axial CT using spiral technique at level of kidneys (**A**) shows a large, hypodense mass arising from midportion of right kidney. Note inferior vena cava (IVC, *arrowhead*) is normal in size and patent at this level. Axial scan at higher level (**B**) shows enlarged, thrombus-filled IVC (*arrow*) and tortuous collateral retroperitoneal vessel entering porta hepatis (*arrowheads*). *(continued)*

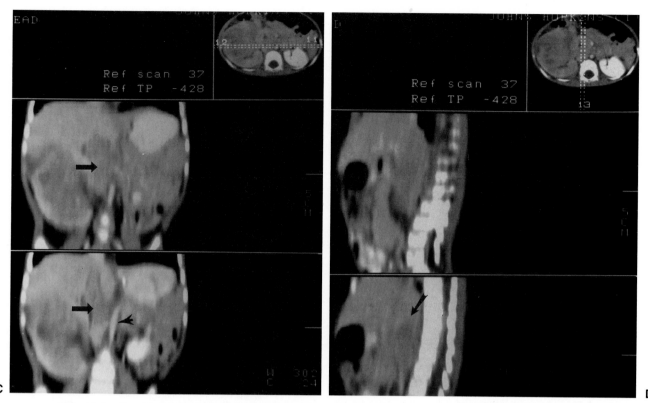

FIG. 16-8. *Continued.* Coronal reconstruction (**C**) shows thrombus-filled IVC (*arrow*) and contrast-enhanced, dilated azygous vein (*arrowhead*). Sagittal reconstruction to right of spine (**D**) shows superior extent of tumor thrombus at level of intrahepatic IVC (*arrow*).

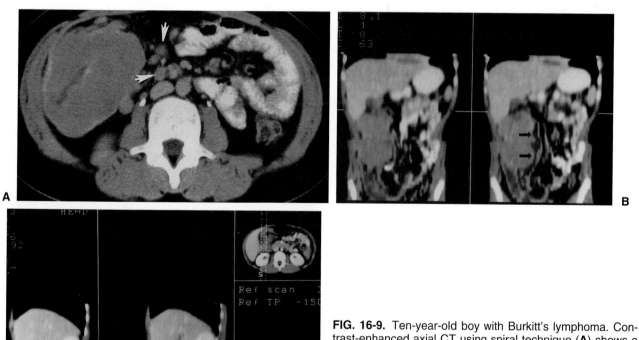

FIG. 16-9. Ten-year-old boy with Burkitt's lymphoma. Contrast-enhanced axial CT using spiral technique (**A**) shows a homogeneous mass in right lower quadrant containing a small amount of fat within (*black arrowheads*). Adenopathy at base of mesentery is also present (*white arrowheads*). Coronal (**B**) reconstruction of two separate volume acquisitions shows soft-tissue mass arising from and medially displacing ascending colon (*arrows*). Sagittal reconstruction (**C**) shows mass is separate from liver and right kidney.

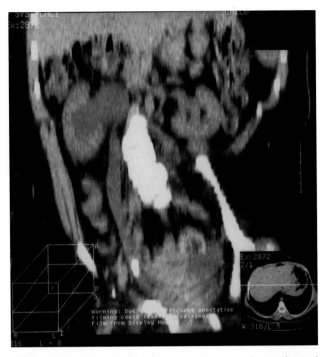

FIG. 16-10. Sixteen-year-old girl with lipomeningocele and new onset of hematuria. Coronal reconstructions from a non-enhanced spiral CT obtained using 10-mm collimation and pitch of 1.5:1 show a calculus in the distal right ureter causing right hydroureteronephrosis.

formation, especially in determining resectability of hepatic tumors, evaluation of large tumors in which determination of organ of origin can be difficult (Fig. 16-9), and tumors in which vascular or spinal invasion is common, such as Wilms' tumor or neuroblastoma.

Spiral CT can be very helpful in the evaluation of children with suspected renal calculi, particularly older children with spinal dysraphism in whom evaluation of the kidneys with sonography can be difficult due to body habitus. Non–contrast-enhanced CT with curved reconstructions can be used to identify the location of ureteral calculi and to depict the presence of associated hydronephrosis (Fig. 16-10).

Another area in which spiral CT may play a significant role is in the acute evaluation of children with blunt abdominal trauma. Rapid scanning may allow for quicker disposition of a traumatized child, especially critically ill children with multiple injuries.

LIMITATIONS OF SPIRAL CT IN CHILDREN

The most important limitations of spiral CT in children are increased image noise, decreased longitudinal resolution (12), and sensitivity to high-amplitude motion. The resulting loss of spatial resolution limits the use of spiral CT in the evaluation of small or complex structures in children. We currently prefer conventional to spiral technique for high-resolution CT of the lung, for the evaluation of complex

fractures involving the growth plate or small bones of the wrist, and for evaluation of tarsal coalitions. Finally, in children who are combative and unable to be restrained appropriately, incremental CT scanning using short scan times often results in less motion artifacts than spiral CT.

CONCLUSIONS

Spiral CT is rapidly evolving as an important new tool for imaging children. It has immediate applications, particularly for the rapid evaluation of children in whom prolonged sedation is contraindicated and in critically ill children in whom rapid throughput is essential. In addition, it provides a viable alternative to magnetic resonance imaging for patients with difficult airway management or monitoring requirements.

REFERENCES

1. Kaufman RA. Expert advice: technical aspects of abdominal CT in infants and children. *AJR* 1989;153:549–553.
2. White KS. Reduced need for sedation in patients undergoing helical CT of the chest and abdomen. *Pediatr Radiol* 1995;25:344–346.
3. Thompson JR, Schneider S, Ashwal S, Holden BS, Hinshaw DB Jr, Hasso AN. The choice of sedation for computed tomography in children: a prospective evaluation. *Radiology* 1982;143:475–479.
4. Strain JD, Campbell JB, Harvey LA, Foley LC. IV Nembutal: safe sedation for children undergoing CT. *AJR* 1988;151:975–979.
5. Pruitt AW, Anyan WR, Kaufman RE, et al. American Academy of Pediatrics Committee on Drugs, Section on Anesthesiology: guidelines for monitoring and management of pediatric patients during and after sedation for diagnostic and therapeutic procedures. *Pediatrics* 1992; 89:1110–1115.
6. Cox TD, White KS, Weinberger E, Effman EL. Comparison of helical and conventional chest CT in the uncooperative pediatric patient. *Pediatr Radiol* 1995;25:347–349.
7. Costello P, Dupuy DE, Ecker CP, Tello R. Spiral CT of the thorax with reduced volume of contrast material: a comparative study. *Radiology* 1992;183:663–666.
8. White KS. Helical/spiral CT scanning: a pediatric radiology perspective. *Pediatr Radiol* 1996;26:5–14.
9. Silverman PM, Brown B, Wray H, et al. Optimal contrast enhancement of the liver using helical (spiral) CT: value of SmartPrep. *AJR* 1995; 164:1169–1171.
10. Luker GD, Siegel MJ, Bradley DA, Baty JD. Hepatic spiral CT in children: scan delay time-enhancement analysis. *Pediatr Radiol* 1996; 26:337–340.
11. Kirks DR, Hedlund GL, Gelfand. Techniques. In: Kirks DR, ed. *Practical pediatric imaging,* 2nd ed. Boston: Little, Brown; 1991:2–55.
12. Heiken JP, Brink JA, Vannier MW. Spiral (helical) CT. *Radiology* 1993;189:647–656.
13. Kartakura T, Kimura K, Midorikawa S, et al. Improvement in resolution along the patient axis in helical-volume CT. *Radiology* 1990;177:188.
14. Mooney DP, Sargent SK, Pluta D, Mazurek P. Spiral CT: use in the evaluation of chest masses in the critically ill neonate. *Pediatr Radiol* 1996;26:15–18.
15. Di Lorenzo M, Collin P-P. Pulmonary metastases in children: results of surgical treatment. *J Pediatr Surg* 1988;23:762–765.
16. Remy-Jardin M, Remy J, Giraud F, Marquette CH. Pulmonary nodules: detection with thick-section spiral CT versus conventional CT. *Radiology* 1993;187:513–520.
17. Plumley DA, Grosfeld JL, Kopecky KK, Buckwalter KA, Vaughan WG. The role of spiral (helical) computerized tomography with three-dimensional reconstruction in pediatric solid tumors. *J Pediatr Surg* 1995;30:317–321.

CHAPTER 17

Oncological Applications of Spiral CT

Elliot K. Fishman

Over the past 5 years numerous articles have addressed the advantages of spiral CT over standard dynamic CT for a wide range of oncological applications (1–6). In these reports, spiral CT has been shown to be more accurate in detecting disease as well as in staging the extent of the disease process. The advances of spiral CT, including the technological developments that allowed dual-phase CT, have proven especially valuable in detecting disease in the liver, pancreas, and kidney. Other chapters in this book discuss the importance of technique and technical optimization of studies for the evaluation of a wide range of clinical problems. In addition, many new and exciting applications are being developed. For example, the combination of advanced spiral CT imaging combined with three-dimensional (3D) reconstructions has provided a new paradigm in patient care and treatment (7,8).

We believe that the true excitement of spiral CT in oncological patients is far more than simply increased detection of disease. Although we can surely detect more lung metastasis or liver metastasis with spiral CT than with conventional CT, other important applications would be impossible with dynamic CT scanning. These examinations are closely tied to postprocessing of the CT data, whether with multiplanar or 3D reconstruction. In addition, radiologists move from the more passive role of film interpretation to an active role of image rendering and study optimization, which places them in the core function of patient care. As continued improvements in CT technology and computer hardware and software evolve, many new and exciting applications will be developed. In this chapter, we look at some of these new and exciting applications and look forward to the changes that they will bring to radiological imaging and patient evaluation.

LIVER VOLUMETRICS FOR LIVING DONOR TRANSPLANT

Liver transplantation is currently used for a wide range of problems, including biliary cirrhosis, chronic active hepa-titis, and primary hepatic neoplasms. The indications for pediatric liver transplantation include biliary atresia, metabolic diseases, rare cholestatic syndromes (including tyrosinemia), and malignant hepatic tumors (9,10). Biliary atresia is by far the most common indication in the pediatric patients and comprises approximately 60% of all cases. Unfortunately, the number of patients awaiting transplant far exceeds the number of available donor livers. A procedure now done in several institutions where the recipient is a child is the living-donor transplant (11,12). That is, a portion of the left lobe of the liver from a parent is removed and placed in a child with hepatic failure. In these cases most patients are very young and the donor liver must ''fit'' in the liver fossa (Figs. 17-1, 17-2). To make sure this is possible, we obtain spiral CT scans of both the donor and recipient liver and then do volumetrics of the recipient liver and the donor left lobe. Depending on size, we may calculate the volume of either the entire left lobe or just the lateral segment. This allows the surgeon to minimize the amount of liver resected from the donor and optimize the transplant process. Future work will include actual simulation of the surgical procedure and optimization of liver transplant placement using 3D reconstruction. The role of virtual reality may loom large in these types of simulations.

TUMOR VOLUMES

One of the important applications of CT scanning in the oncological patient is the ability to obtain objective measurements of response to therapeutic intervention. CT scanning has been shown to be an accurate method for defining changes in tumor size and has been the mainstay for measuring tumor volumes in the oncological patient (13). Spiral CT, with its single breath-hold study and volume data sets, should prove ideal for accurate and reproducible measurement of tumor volumes. Van Hoe et al. (14) recently assessed the reproducibility of one-, two-, and three-dimensional measurements of the size of liver metastasis by measuring

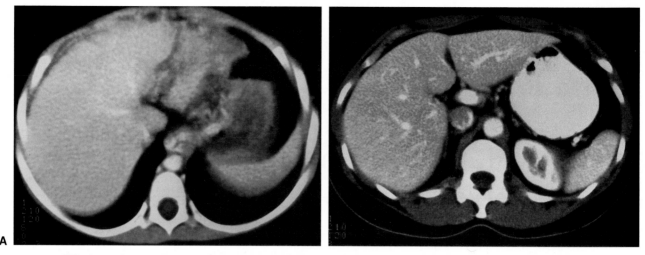

FIG. 17-1. Spiral CT scans done for preoperative planning of living donor liver transplant. **(A)** Three-year-old female with a history of primary biliary cirrhosis prior to transplantation. The spiral CT scan demonstrates the nodularity of the liver as well as varices near the esophagus. **(B)** Forty-year-old female who is mother of the child in scan **(A)**. The spiral CT demonstrates the key anatomic and vascular landmarks. Based on the volume of the child's liver, the segment of the liver lateral to the falciform ligament was removed at surgery and transplanted.

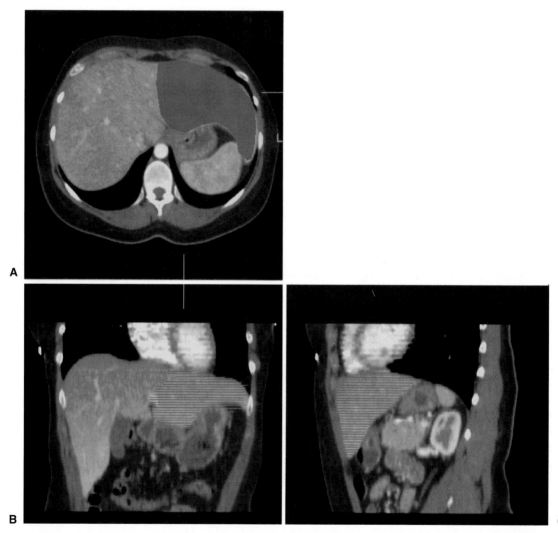

FIG. 17-2. Liver volumes in potential living related liver donor. **(A–C)** Image demonstrates a multiplanar profile of the lateral portion of the left lobe of the liver in potential donor. The volume of the liver was 362 mL. The child's liver volume (not shown) was 460 mL, making this a potentially perfect fit. *(continued)*

308

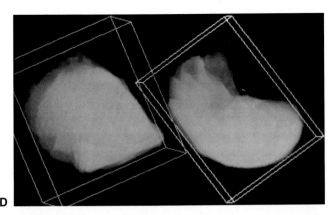

D

FIG. 17-2. *Continued.* (**D**) Display defining the child's liver and the donor's lateral segment. Computer simulations such as this are helpful in preoperative planning.

the sizes of liver metastases using 10 observers with multiple measurement techniques. These measurement techniques include the maximum diameter, product of diameters, area, volume, and product of three diameters. The authors had the observers do these measurements several times in separate sessions. The conclusion was that 3D measurements proved to be as reproducible as one- and two-dimensional measurements and could be used in place of them.

The importance of the use of accurate measurements is underscored by the definition of response to therapy by the World Health Organization (WHO). According to the WHO, a measurable lesion is defined as a mass that can be measured in two perpendicular axes and followed by imaging (15,16). With this criterion a partial response is greater than 50% reduction in two-dimensional size, and progression is a 25% increase in size of preexisting disease or the occurrence of new disease.

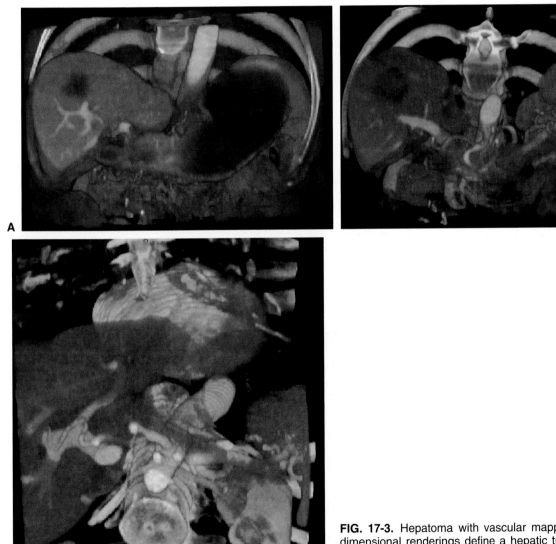

A

B

C

FIG. 17-3. Hepatoma with vascular mapping. (**A-C**) Three-dimensional renderings define a hepatic tumor with arterial and venous mapping. This technique provides a noninvasive method for preoperative planning.

PREOPERATIVE SURGICAL PLANNING AND SURGICAL SIMULATION

Spiral CT data sets acquired either from peripheral arterial or venous injection provides both excellent detail of the hepatic venous anatomy and lesion definition. This allows for the creation of 3D maps of the liver and affords the potential for true surgical planning (17,18). Using faster workstations like the Silicon Graphics Infinite Reality provides the potential for nearly real-time 3D display of data. Development of new algorithms for more automated segmentation promises to move this plan from the drawing board to the clinical arena over a short period of time. In addition to liver resection, the data created from the 3D imaging of the kidney may prove important in helping determine candidates for partial nephrectomy (19).

Although we initially used the data from SCTAP (spiral computed tomographic arterial portography) to create our 3D images, there was little doubt from our initial experience that similar studies could be done using peripheral injection (20) (Figs. 17-3–17-5). With peripheral injection, high rates of contrast injection (3–5 mL/s) are needed, as are larger volumes of contrast (probably 150 mL vs. 100–125 mL with standard spiral techniques). The one question that has not yet been answered is whether or not spiral CT with peripheral injection will prove to be as accurate as intra-arterial injection with the computed tomographic during arterial portography (CTAP) technique. Future studies will have to determine the advantages of this technique.

One of the major advantages of spiral CT noted in nearly every published article is its ability to define vascular anatomy. This is especially important in the region of the porta hepatis and pancreatic head. Currently, standard angiography is routinely obtained presurgically in patients to define the vascular anatomy prior to Whipple procedure for pancreatic tumors. It would be a significant improvement if spiral CT with peripheral injection could provide similar information without need for a ''classic'' angiogram. Our initial

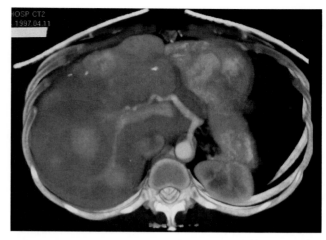

FIG. 17-5. Metastatic islet cell tumor of the pancreas. Three-dimensional view defines the extent of the vascular metastases as well as a vascular map of the celiac and hepatic artery. This image was generated with volume rendering.

experience is that key structures like the hepatic artery can be identified from their origin regardless of their takeoff. The accuracy for defining these structures will have to be assessed in a combined angiographic/spiral CT study before routine clinical use is accepted.

VIRTUAL ENDOSCOPY

Another area of great interest that may have a significant impact on oncological imaging is the development of virtual endoscopy (21–23). This technique is a direct result of advances in CT data acquisition, 3D imaging processing, computer graphics, and computer hardware. Unlike classic 3D imaging, which presents an object as if one were holding it in one's hand, the endoscopic technique tries to place one inside an organ, as if you were in an endoscope and ''looking around.''

This technique has been applied to imaging the colon (vir-

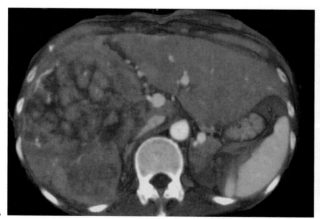
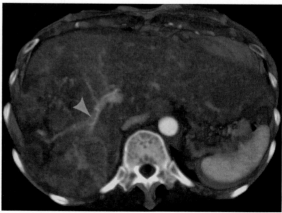

A   B

FIG. 17-4. Hepatoma with vascular invasion. **(A,B)** The 3D maps demonstrate a large vascular mass involving both lobes of the liver. Vascular invasion is also seen (*arrowhead*).

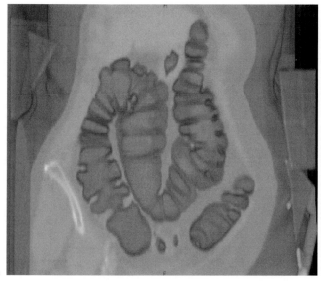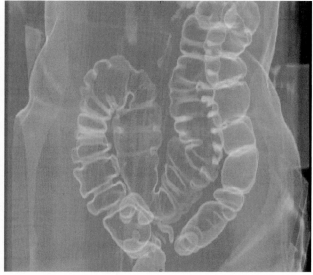

A   B

FIG. 17-6. Three-dimensional reconstruction of the colon. (**A,B**) Manipulation of rendering parameters allows a detailed view of the colon similar to the prospective provided by a double-contrast barium study.

tual colonoscopy) (Figs. 17-6–17-10), the stomach (virtual endoscopy), and the airways (virtual bronchoscopy) (Figs. 17-8–17-10). Some of the results have been promising, although in most cases the sample sizes are too small to make definitive conclusions.

Although much progress has been made with this technique there are still many technical obstacles to overcome before it can become mainstream and replace more intense or invasive examinations. Among the problems to be overcome is the design of a computer interface that is easy to

use and yet meets the needs of viewing the data set in a user-controlled fashion.

When reviewing a volume data set for virtual colonoscopy or virtual imaging, it is imperative that an easy-to-use navigation scheme be developed. For the airways the ability to maintain control and follow a set travel or flight path tends to be a bit simpler than in the colon, because the colon is particularly variable in terms of its configuration (i.e., redundancy). Therefore it is significantly more challenging to image the colon in a coordinated fashion

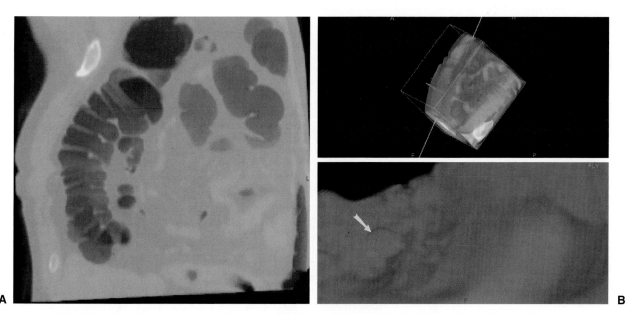

A   B

FIG. 17-7. Virtual colonoscopy with polyp. (**A**) Three-dimensional view of the right colon and its well-defined haustral markings. (**B**) Virtual colonoscopic views detected an 8-mm polyp (*arrow*). Guidance of the flight of travel is critical in this application.

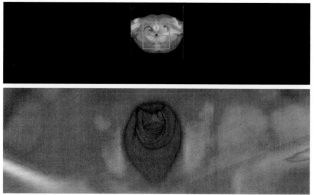

FIG. 17-8. Virtual endoscopy of the trachea. Three-dimensional display of the trachea looking down to the bifurcation with guidance system.

and to make sure a successful examination is completed.

Why is a flight plan needed and what specific obstacles does it face? There are several reasons for its use, including the following:

1. To guarantee a review of the entire data set. (That is, if we examine the colon we would like to make sure we evaluate the entire colon.)
2. To localize an abnormality as seen on a 3D data set and have it registered on the 2D data set. (If we see a polyp we need to know exactly where that polyp is, so that the endoscopist can biopsy it.)
3. To perform the study quickly, without user frustration or confusion.

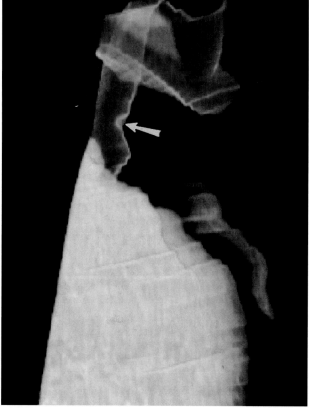

FIG. 17-9. Tracheal papilloma. **(A)** Transaxial CT demonstrates a 3-mm intraluminal lesion (*arrow*) **(B)** Three-dimensional reconstruction defines the true lesion extent (*arrow*) on this edited view.

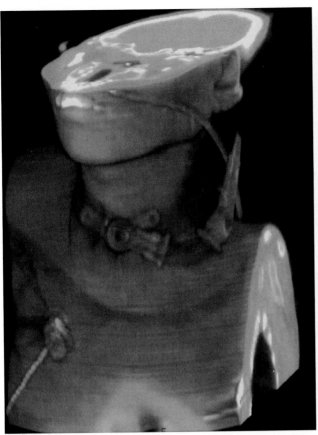 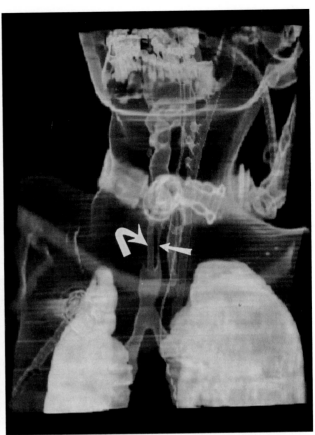

FIG. 17-10. Tracheal stenosis. The flexibility of volume rendering is well documented in this case. Image (**A**) is with the skin opaque and shows the tracheostomy site and connections. Image (**B**) shows the airway stenosis (*arrows*) and the endotracheal tube (*curved arrow*).

In thinking about potential display techniques for this task we could have the user design a flight path on a series of multiplanar images (coronal, sagittal, transaxial). Another technique might have the user mark the beginning and end of the flight and have the computer generate the flight path by staying within the center of the colon or airway based on boundary detection. McFarland et al. addressed this problem, and noted that, regardless of what flight planning is used, that a technique be developed that allows the user to have registration of the flight path and the data set (24).

THREE-DIMENSIONAL ANGIOGRAPHIC APPLICATIONS IN THE ONCOLOGICAL PATIENT

The ability to acquire true volume data sets in a single breath-hold provides several important capabilities across a wide range of oncological applications (25,26). The common denominator in these applications relates to the role of CT angiography and its ability to combine thin-section CT with optimally timed intravenous contrast administration and data acquisition. This is then combined with the real-time interactive 3D capabilities becoming available to provide the radiologist with unprecedented noninvasive imaging capabilities.

Many oncological applications have been discussed in detail in other chapters of this book. These range from the detection and staging of renal cancer to the detection and staging of hepatic tumors and the detection and staging of lung cancer (Fig. 17-11). The advantages of spiral CT compared with dynamic CT were defined, and in many cases the use of CT angiography was noted. Rather than repeat these discussions, several salient points germane to all these applications are noted. They are the following:

1. The key to accurate detection and staging of tumor is differentiation between normal and abnormal tissue. Iodinated contrast material delivered at the "right" time optimizes this detection. This is especially critical for smaller tumors and for specific organs like the liver.
2. Volume data sets, which are a feature of spiral CT, are ideal when subsecond scanning eliminates any cause of intrascan or interscan motion by scanning the area in question in one-third less time than required with one second spiral CT (Fig. 17-12).
3. Generation of 3D images consisting of vascular maps increases both the understanding of extent of disease and the accuracy of staging. For example, tumor encasement of vessels like the superior mesenteric artery or

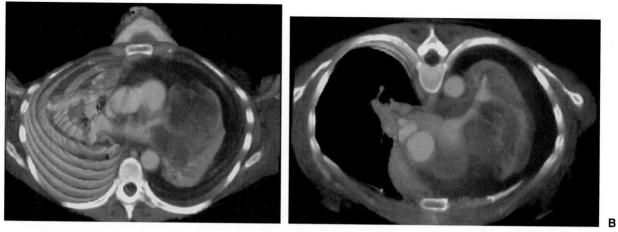

FIG. 17-11. Lung cancer invades heart. (**A,B**) Three-dimensional renderings from inferior and superior projection demonstrates tumor invading the left atrium and pulmonary artery.

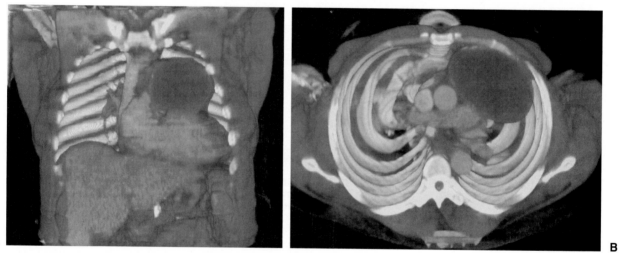

FIG. 17-12. Cystic thymoma. (**A,B**) Large anterior mediastinal mass that is cystic with faint peripheral calcification. No evidence of vascular invasion was seen.

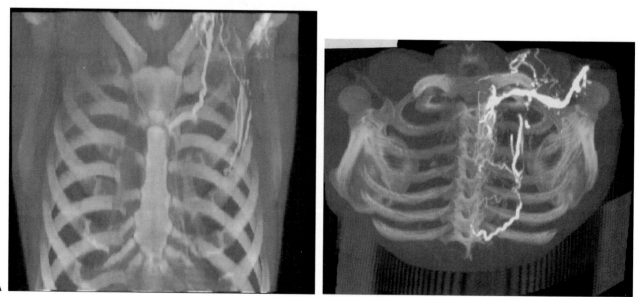

FIG. 17-13. SVC syndrome with collateral pathways. Three-dimensional renderings define obstruction of the left innominate vein as it joins the SVC. Note the collaterals anteriorly (**A**) through the internal mammary veins and posteriorly (**B**) through the paravertebral vessels.

celiac artery is often best defined in planes other than the axial one.

4. Three-dimensional vascular maps are critical for determining tumor encasement in areas such as the mediastinum and can define processes such as superior vena cava syndrome (Fig. 17-13) or pulmonary artery encasement. The value of these displays and the effect on therapy planning is in many cases first being systematically analyzed. Outcome studies as well as cost–benefit analysis of these techniques will be critical.

5. CT-angiographic displays meet the needs of the referring physician who has been trained in reviewing classic angiography. The ability to create displays that are familiar with CT angiography is one of the reasons for its rapid acceptance by referring physicians (27) (Fig. 17-14).

RADIATION THERAPY TREATMENT PLANNING

CT scanning has always been used as a guide for radiation therapy treatment planning. This has been especially true in pelvic malignancies such as prostate cancer and cervical cancer. The use of spiral CT coupled with multiplanar reconstruction is especially valuable in therapy planning because it is a superior diagnostic study (i.e., stage disease by looking at nodal disease) and it provides a 3D approach to therapy planning. Spiral CT with multiplanar reconstruction is also useful when intrauterine devices are placed to simulate the

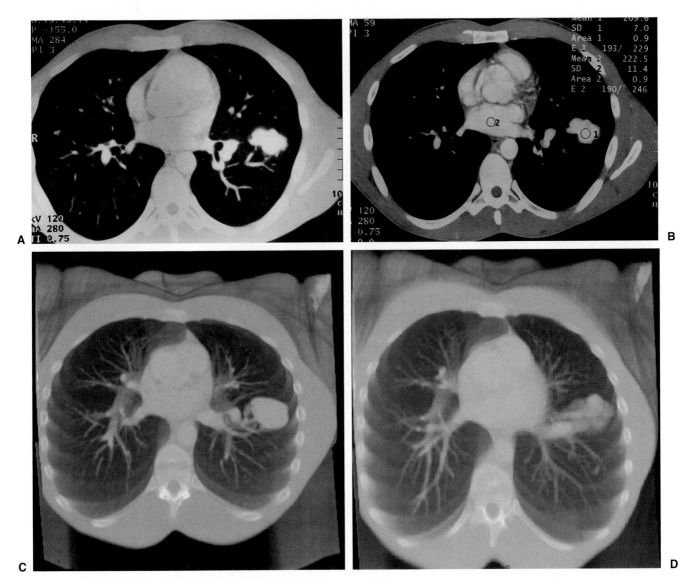

FIG. 17-14. Pulmonary arteriovenous malformation. (**A,B**) Axial CT demonstrates a left mid-lung mass that enhances equal to the cardiac chambers consistent with an arteriovenous malformation (AVM). (**C,D**) The 3D reconstructions provide clear definition of the arterial supply and venous drainage of the aneurysm. Several other tiny AVMs are seen.

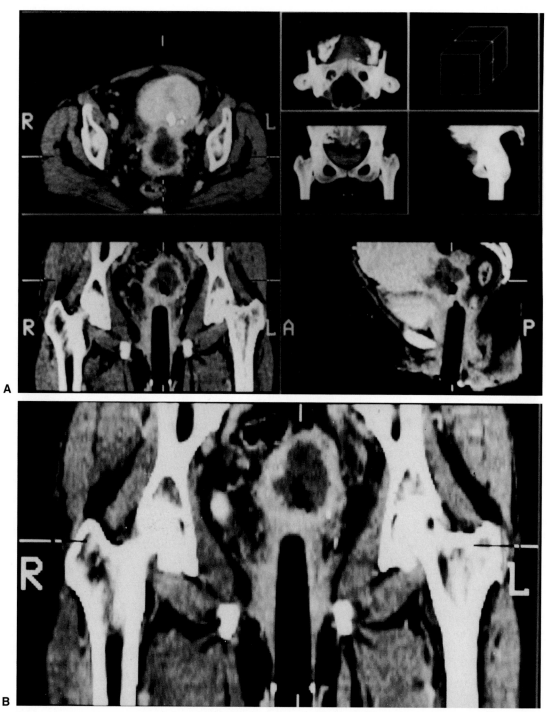

FIG. 17-15. Cervical cancer for radiation therapy planning. (**A**) Spiral CT in multiplanar display demonstrates necrotic lesion in the cervical canal. The data were acquired with 4-mm-thick sections at 4-mm intervals. A cylinder simulating the therapy implants was placed in the patient's vagina. The coronal and sagittal reconstructed views clearly demonstrate the location of the tumor in relationship to the implant. (**B**) The coronal view defines therapy simulator and relationship to tumor.

implant zone for radium implants (Fig. 17-15). A typical spiral CT scan protocol for pelvic tumors would be a 4–5-mm slice thickness, 4–5-mm/s table speed, and 3–4-mm reconstruction interval. In cases of pelvic pathology we typically begin scanning at the level just beneath the symphysis and scan cranially. Our initial experience suggests a delay of 60–70 s from start of contrast infusion (2–3 mL/s) to the beginning of scanning. We currently use a pitch of 1 to scan these patients, although a pitch of up to 1.5 can be used without much loss of detail and will provide near total coverage of the abdomen. In the past, the only disadvantage of spiral CT of the pelvis was the relatively low milliamperage values in an area where patient bulk may be greatest. Upgrades in system capabilities (300 mA) make this a nonissue. When therapy planning is done it is important to use a flat board placed on the CT scanner rather than the standard curved CT couch to simulate more accurately the actual therapy delivery.

In cases of pelvic malignancies like prostate or cervical cancer when we scan the patient from a caudal-to-cranial direction, delayed scans will often be done if bladder opacification is needed. Delayed scans may also prove useful if a fistula is suspected. In the male pelvis, spiral CT can be used for treatment planning for radiation therapy of prostate cancer. In this case the radiation oncologist wants to ensure that the entire prostate is within the designated therapy ports and that no nodes are present that are not covered by these ports. The use of sagittal reconstruction is especially valuable for the side ports and in decreasing the radiation exposure of the rectum and sigmoid colon.

PARTIAL NEPHRECTOMY FOR RENAL CANCER

Partial nephrectomy is an important surgical alternative for patients with a prior contralateral nephrectomy, decreased renal function, or bilateral renal masses. One of the primary radiological criteria for successful partial nephrectomy is a clear margin between tumor and renal pelvic fat and a clear margin around the major renal vessels. Spiral CT can be done with narrow collimation and can be supplemented by multiplanar reformations to provide a surgical road map. Three-dimensional reconstructions of the kidney are also proving useful in this clinical situation and are being explored at several institutions (Figs. 17-16, 17-17).

The typical scanning protocol in the patient being consid-

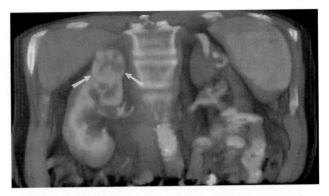

FIG. 17-17. Renal carcinoma with partial nephrectomy planning. The tumor arises off the upper pole of the right kidney (*arrows*), making the patient an ideal candidate for nephron-sparing surgery.

ered for a partial nephrectomy would include a 120-mL injection of Omnipaque-300 at the rate of 3 mL/s, and a dual spiral CT acquisition, including arterial-phase imaging. In cases where the patient has had a prior nephrectomy or partial nephrectomy or in the patient with decreased renal function, less contrast material can be used, and between 70 and 90 mL of contrast typically will suffice.

EVALUATION OF SUSPECTED BONE METASTASES

CT has always been used to help detect the presence of bone metastases when there was discordance between radiographic studies (plain films and bone scans) or when there is discordance between radiographic studies and clinical examination. In other cases, spiral CT may be valuable in detecting the presence or in confirming the absence of skeletal pathology. Spiral CT scanning is especially valuable in areas

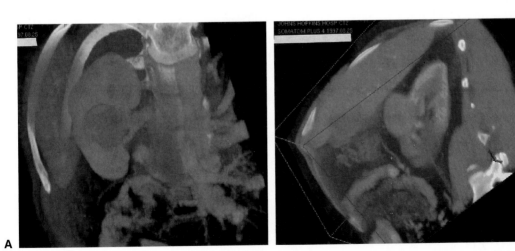

FIG. 17-16. Renal carcinoma with partial nephrectomy planning. (**A,B**) The 3D displays define the tumor arising off the kidney. On the cutaway view, extension of tumor into the renal pelvis would not make the patient an ideal candidate for nephron-sparing surgery.

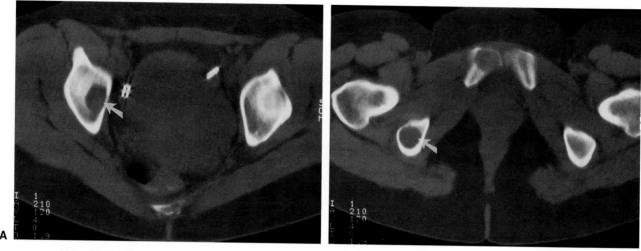

FIG. 17-18. Breast cancer and right hip pain but negative plain films. **(A,B)** Spiral CT demonstrates a 2 × 1-cm lytic lesion in the dome of the right acetabulum consistent with metastatic breast cancer (*arrow*). Other metastases were noted in the symphysis and ischium (*arrow*).

where patient compliance is often difficult such as the shoulder, sternum, and ribs. Standard CT scans are supplemented by multiplanar and 3D imaging. Although imaging protocols will vary, we combine thin collimation, narrow interscan spacing, and a high spatial frequency algorithm (Figs. 17-18–17-20).

A typical scanning protocol in these patients might be a spiral scan of 32 s using 2–4-mm slice thickness and 2–4-mm/s table speed. Reconstruction intervals are at 2–3 mm, depending on the clinical situation. The choice of slice thickness and the table speed will have to be adjusted to the length of area that needs to be scanned. One technical point that we have found important is that in cases where bone involvement is to be evaluated, reconstructions using the high-resolution algorithm on the scanner are important. We are aware that different scanners will have different names for this algorithm. However, we find that using the high-resolution edge enhancement algorithm, the computer-generated edge blur with spiral CT tends to be less noticeable (28,29).

In cases where a soft-tissue mass or extension of a bone tumor into the soft tissues is suspected, we use iodinated contrast (120 mL of Omnipaque-350 injected at 3 mL/s)

material. The contrast is injected approximately 40 s before scanning begins. This allows for excellent detection of intramuscular pathology (Fig. 17-21).

THE POST-WHIPPLE'S PATIENT

The Whipple's procedure is commonly used for resection of pancreatic or ampullary carcinomas. The procedure typically involves resection of the pancreatic head, distal common duct, and duodenum with or without antrectomy. Once a tumor has been resected, it is now common for radiation therapy to be given to the tumor bed, even in cases without tumor spread and negative surgical margins. This dose, which is in the range of 4,000 rad, will often result in radiation gastritis and radiation enteritis. CT is used to monitor any recurrence or to determine response to therapy (30). This is often difficult in the face of complex postoperative anatomy, but with spiral CT the combination of vascular opacification and multiple sampling of the data volume seems to provide excellent results (Fig. 17-22). Vascular involvement, including vascular encasement, and venous thrombosis are well seen with this protocol (Fig. 17-23). Small liver metastases can also be detected. The spiral CT

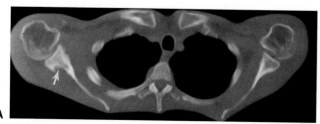

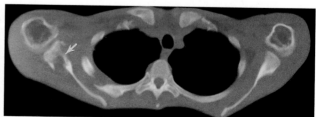

FIG. 17-19. Adenocarcinoma of the lung with right shoulder pain. **(A,B)** Spiral CT scan demonstrates a lytic lesion involving the right scapula (*arrows*) with destruction in the region of the inferior glenoid. Periosteal reaction and associated soft-tissue mass are noted.

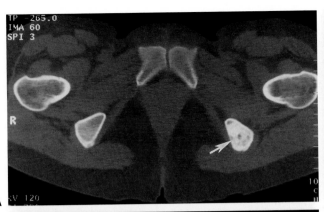

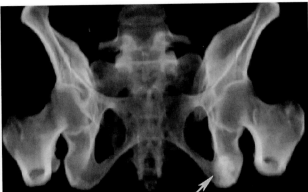

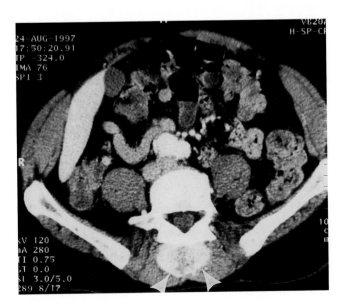

FIG. 17-20. Metastatic breast cancer. **(A-C)** The patient had pelvic pain but bone scans and plain radiographs were inconclusive. CT clearly demonstrates blastic metastases to the ischium (*arrows*).

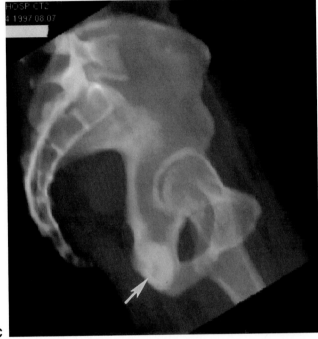

FIG. 17-21. Metastatic poorly differentiated carcinoma metastatic to muscle. The patient presented with abdominal pain and a 3-cm enhancing mass posterior to the L-5 vertebral body (*arrowheads*) was incidently discovered. This was biopsied and consistent with metastases from a lung primary.

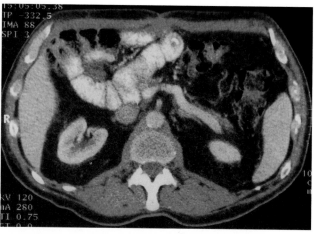

FIG. 17-22. Normal post-Whipple's procedure spiral CT. (**A,B**) Sequential images clearly define the surgical bed with no evidence of tumor recurrence. The opacified bowel anastomoses are well-defined on this study.

scans are also commonly used to design radiation therapy portals in these patients.

ADRENAL GLAND

CT remains the primary imaging modality for the evaluation of known or suspected adrenal disease (31–38). Numerous articles have stressed the importance of proper CT technique, which combines narrow collimation (3–4 mm) with narrow interscan incrementation (2–4 mm). Several articles have also addressed the problem of differentiating benign from malignant adrenal disease based solely on CT criteria. Berland et al. found that CT features of a benign lesion included homogeneous low attenuation (possibly with punctate contrast enhancement), an enlarged gland with configuration maintained, a thin or absent rim, and discrete sharp margins. Malignant lesions typically had a thick enhancing rim, invasion of adjacent structures, irregular or poorly defined margins, and inhomogeneous attenuation (Fig. 17-24).

The positive predictive value for a series of 37 patients with 44 lesions was 100% for a benign diagnosis and between 62% and 82% for a malignant diagnosis. Lee et al. found that mean CT attenuation on noncontrast scans was −2.2 HU ± 16 for benign adrenal masses and 28.9 HU ± 10.6 for malignant lesions (Fig. 17-25). Korobkin et al. (36–38) further analyzed adrenal adenomas and found that the presence and amount of lipid accounts for the low attenuation of these lesions. They also found that lesion attenuation on noncontrast scans allowed for an accurate discrimination of benign and malignant lesions.

Spiral CT has proven to have some excellent applications in the evaluation of the adrenal gland. By using a combination of single breath-hold volume acquisition, narrow collimation (3–4 mm), and interscan spacing (every 3 mm), excellent data sets without respiratory motion are routinely obtainable. Hounsfield unit measurements tend not to be

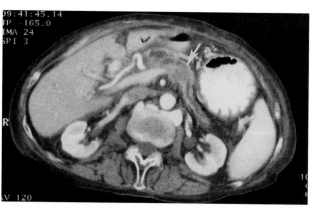

FIG. 17-23. Recurrent pancreatic cancer following a Whipple's procedure. Spiral scan demonstrates a mass (*arrow*) at the site of prior resection. Encasement of portal vein is also seen.

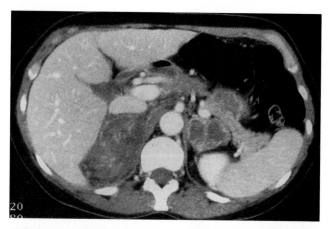

FIG. 17-24. Adrenal metastases with hemorrhage. Spiral CT demonstrates bilateral adrenal metastases with hemorrhage involving the right adrenal gland. The patient presented with severe abdominal pain, and subsequent work-up detected a primary lung cancer as the source of the metastases.

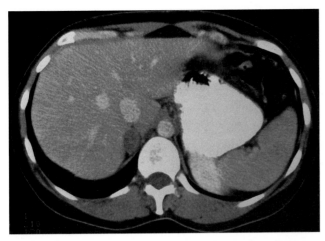

FIG. 17-25. Incidental adrenal adenoma. CT scan obtained for evaluation of abdominal pain to exclude a malignancy. Spiral CT demonstrates 2-cm right adrenal lesion of low CT attenuation consistent with an incidental adrenal adenoma.

limited by partial averaging, as has been shown by Seltzer et al., and are accurate for measuring density values.

Spiral CT is also valuable for the staging of adrenal carcinoma (Fig. 17-26). The use of multiple thin sections and a volume data set may provide increased accuracy in terms of vascular invasion and local extension. The presence of liver metastases can also be defined on the spiral study. Multiplanar reformatting in the coronal and/or sagittal plane may be helpful in defining adjacent organ extension and/or invasion. The information provided by the multiplanar views may be valuable in surgical planning especially in cases of larger tumors.

Spiral CT can also be useful for the evaluation of the patient following resection for adrenal carcinoma. The early detection of tumor recurrence as well as its extent may be optimized on these studies. Since metastases from adrenal cancer may be vascular in nature, the use of spiral CT with

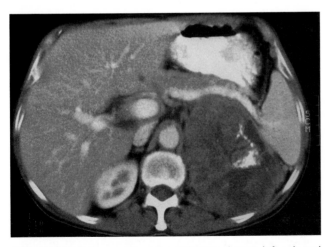

FIG. 17-26. Primary adrenal carcinoma. Large left adrenal mass with foci of calcification is a classic appearance for primary adrenal carcinoma.

the rapid infusion of iodinated contrast may help detect early recurrence, especially in or near the tumor bed.

Although in most cases it is easy to determine if a mass is or is not of adrenal origin, in others this may be more difficult, especially if a mass is very large (i.e., adrenal mass versus retroperitoneal sarcoma versus splenic mass versus liver mass). This may be especially important in the pediatric patient, where differentiating a neuroblastoma from a Wilms' tumor may be difficult. In these cases the information provided by vascular opacification and supplemented by multiplanar reconstruction will usually allow the clinician to make the correct diagnosis. The use of sagittal reconstruction of the CT data is especially valuable.

Spiral CT is also valuable in the patient with an incidentally discovered adrenal mass where conservative management is warranted. Spiral CT can be used as a technique to allow for interscan reproducibility over time, which can help determine whether interval growth has occurred.

INTERVENTIONAL PROCEDURES WITH SPIRAL CT

The biopsy of a suspected primary tumor or metastatic lesion is an everyday procedure in a busy radiological department. With experience, biopsy success rates in the 90% to 100% range have been documented for the liver, pancreas, and adrenal glands. Recent articles have evaluated the use of spiral CT to perform these procedures optimally by decreasing the length of study time while increasing their success rate.

Silverman et al. reviewed a series of 40 patients with abdominal masses to compare the efficacy of spiral CT needle localizations with that of conventional CT (39). The mean time for biopsy for spiral CT was 35 s compared with 105 s for conventional CT ($p < .001$). The advantages were especially apparent in biopsies in the upper abdomen, which included the liver, pancreas, kidney, and adrenal glands. The authors thought that this improvement was mainly related to elimination of respiratory misregistration with spiral CT as compared with conventional CT. Spiral CT was especially valuable for lesions that were smaller or more difficult to localize and biopsy.

Another potential interventional direction with spiral CT is what is commonly called CT fluoroscopy. The continuous-rotation scanners can be designed to reconstruct and display images in real time. Scanners such as those from Toshiba and Siemens Medical Systems can obtain up to six images per second. Several reports have shown that CT fluoroscopy can reduce the time needed for a cutaneous needle biopsy. A recent article by White et al. (40) also suggests that CT fluoroscopy can be used as a guide for transbronchial needle aspiration for sampling nodes in the hilum, subcarinal regions, or mediastinum. The authors felt that CT fluoroscopic guidance of transbronchial needle aspiration would be particularly valuable for bronchoscopists who have only minimal experience or in cases where nodal size was less than 2.5 cm and the success rate might be limited. There appears to be great potential for the role of CT in difficult-to-biopsy situations.

The potential of CT fluoroscopy (41) for biopsy must be considered not merely in light of the current status of biopsy techniques but in a more forward-looking fashion, to the time when therapy may be individually designed based on the patient's tumor cell sampling. In these cases the radiologist may be called upon to sample ever smaller lesions to get material that can be used to develop either vaccines or tumor gene models for patients. The role of the radiologist would therefore expand in this important clinical situation.

CONCLUSION

The role of spiral CT continues to evolve, with new and exciting applications. In the oncological arena, spiral CT has the promise to increase our sensitivity for the detection of disease with hopefully increased specificity as well.

Spiral CT may be especially applicable in those oncological studies where standard CT has had relatively low sensitivity and/or specificity. Whether or not spiral will help to more accurately stage oncological patients remains to be seen, but initial published results have been very encouraging. The clinical applications of spiral CT will continue to evolve with advances in scanner technology, as well as postprocessing applications on free-standing workstations. The radiologist must also be aware of the needs of our referring physicians and tailor specific applications to meet these needs. As we move toward the millennium, oncological applications for CT will be a driving force in medical imaging.

REFERENCES

1. Zeman RK, Fox SH, Silverman PM, et al. Helical (spiral) CT of the abdomen. *AJR* 1993;160:719–725.
2. Bluemke DA, Fishman EK. Spiral CT of the abdomen: clinical applications. *Crit Rev Diagn Imaging* 1993;34(3):103–158.
3. Heiken JP, Brink JA, Vannier MW. Spiral (helical) CT. *Radiology* 1993;189:647–656.
4. Lu DSK, Reber HA, Krasny RM, Kadell BM, Sayre J. Local staging of pancreatic cancer: criteria for unresectability of major vessels as revealed by pancreatic-phase, thin section helical CT. *AJR* 1997;168:1439–1443.
5. Bluemke DA, Cameron JL, Hruban RH, et al. Potentially resectable pancreatic adenocarcinoma: spiral CT assessment with surgical and pathologic correlation. *Radiology* 1995;197:381–385.
6. Yuh BI, Cohan RH. Helical CT for detection and characterization of renal masses. *Semin Ultrasound CT MR* 1997;18(2):82–90.
7. Chernoff DM, Silverman SG, Kikinis R, et al. Three-dimensional imaging and display of renal tumors using spiral CT: a potential aid to partial nephrectomy. *Urology* 1994;43(1):125–129.
8. Heath DG, Soyer PA, Kuszyk BS, et al. Three-dimensional spiral CT during arterial portography: comparison of three rendering techniques. *Radiographics* 1995;15:1001–1011.
9. Todo S, Fung JJ, Tsakis A, et al. One hundred and ten consecutive primary orthotopic liver transplants under FK 506 in adults. *Transplant Proc* 1991;23:1397–1402.
10. Otte JB, Yandza T, de Ville de Goyet J, et al. Pediatric liver transplantation: report on 52 patients with a 2-year survival of 86%. *J Pediatr Surg* 1988;23:250–253.
11. Broelsch CE, Lloyd DM. Living related donors for liver transplants. In: Cameron JL, ed. *Advances in surgery.* St. Louis: Mosby-Year Book; 1993;25:209–231.
12. Busuttil RW, Sev P, Millis JM, et al. Liver transplantation in children. *Ann Surg* 1991;213:48–57.
13. Yang NC, Leichner PK, Fishman EK, et al. CT volumetrics of primary liver cancers. *J Comput Assist Tomogr* 1986;10:621–628.
14. Van Hoe L, Van Cutsem E, Vergote I, Baert AL, Bellon E, Dupont P, Marchal G. Size quantification of liver metastases in patients undergoing cancer treatment: reproducibility of one-, two- and three-dimensional measurements determined with spiral CT. *Radiology* 1997;212(3):671–675.
15. Miller AB, Hoogstraten B, Staquet M, Winkler A. Reporting results of cancer treatment. *Cancer* 1981;47:207–214.
16. Breiman RS, Beck JW, Korobkin M, et al. Volume determinations using computed tomography. *AJR* 1982;138:329–333.
17. Ney DR, Fishman EK, Niederhuber JE. Three-dimensional display of hepatic venous anatomy generated from spiral computed tomography data: preliminary results. *J Digit Imaging* 1992;5(4):242–245.
18. Woodhouse CE, Ney DR, Sitzmann JV, Fishman EK. Spiral computed tomography arterial portography with three-dimensional volumetric rendering for oncologic surgery planning: a retrospective analysis. *Invest Radiol* 1994;29(12):1031–1037.
20. Bluemke DA, Fishman EK. Spiral CT arterial portography of the liver. *Radiology* 1993;186:576–579.
21. Vining DJ. Virtual endoscopy: is it reality? *Radiology* 1996;200:30–31.
22. Lee HL, Young TK. Gastric lesions: evaluation with three-dimensional images. *AJR* 1997;169:787–789.
23. Hara AK, Johnson CD, Reed JE, et al. Colorectal polyp detection with CT colonography: two- versus three-dimensional techniques: work in progress. *Radiology* 1996;200:49–54.
24. McFarland EG, Wang G, Brink JA, Balfe DM, Heiken JP, Vannier MW. Spiral computed tomographic colonography: determination of the central axis and digital unraveling of the colon. *Acad Radiol* 1997;4:367–373.
25. Frush DP, Siegel MJ, Bissett GS III. From the RSNA refresher courses. *Radiographics* 1997;17:939–959.
26. Zeman RK, Cooper C, Zeiberg AS, et al. TNM staging of pancreatic carcinoma using helical CT. *AJR* 1997;169:459–464.
27. Chambers TP, Fishman EK, Bluemke DA, Urban B, Venbrux AC. Identification of the aberrant hepatic artery with axial spiral CT. *J Vasc Interv Radiol* 1995;6(6):959–964
28. Kalender WA, Seissler W, Klotz E, Vock P. Spiral volumetric CT with single-breath-hold technique, continuous transport, and continuous scanner rotation. *Radiology* 1990;176:181–183.
29. Kalender WA, Polacin A. Physical performance characteristics of spiral CT scanning. *Med Phys* 1991;18:910–915.
30. Bluemke DA, Fishman EK, Kuhlman JE. CT evaluation following Whipple procedure: potential pitfalls in interpretation. *J Comput Assist Tomogr* 1992;16(5):704–708.
31. Berland L, Koslin D, Kenney P, Stanley R, Lee J. Differentiation between small benign and malignant adrenal masses with dynamic incremented CT. *AJR* 1988;151:95–101.
32. Herrera M, Grant C, van Heerden J, Sheedy P II, Ilstrup D. Incidentally discovered adrenal tumors: an institutional perspective. *Surgery* 1991;110:1014–1021.
33. Francis I, Gross M, Shapiro B, Korobkin M, Quint L. Integrated imaging of adrenal disease. *Radiology* 1992;184:1–13.
34. Schultz C. T and MR of the adrenal glands. *Semin Ultrasound CT MR* 1986;7(3):219–233.
35. Lee M, Hahn P, Papanicolaou N, et al. Benign and malignant adrenal masses: CT distinction with attenuation coefficients, size, and observer analysis. *Radiology* 1991;179:415–418.
36. Korobkin M, Giordano TJ, Brodeur FJ, et al. Adrenal adenomas: relationship between histologic lipid and CT and MR findings. *Radiology* 1996;200:743–747.
37. Korobkin M, Brodeur FJ, Francis IR, Quint LE, Dunnick NR, Goodsitt M. Delayed enhanced CT for differentiation of benign from malignant adrenal masses. *Radiology* 1996;200:737–742.
38. Korobkin M, Francis IR. Adrenal imaging. *Semin Ultrasound CT MR* 1995;16(4):317–330.
39. Silverman SG, Bloom DA, Seltzer SE, Tempany CMC, Adams DF. Needle-tip localization during CT-guided abdominal biopsy: comparison of conventional and spiral CT. *AJR* 1992;159:1095–1097.
40. White CS, Templeton PA, Hasday JD. CT-assisted transbronchial needle aspiration: usefulness of CT fluoroscopy. *AJR* 1997;169:393–394.
41. Katada K, Kato R, Anno H, et al. Guidance with real-time CT-fluoroscopy: early clinical experience. *Radiology* 1996;200:851–885.

CHAPTER 18

Spiral CT in Blunt Thoracoabdominal Trauma

R. Brooke Jeffrey, Jr.

Over the past 15 years dynamic incremental contrast-enhanced computed tomography (CT) has gained widespread clinical acceptance in the evaluation of hemodynamically stable patients with blunt abdominal trauma. Accurate diagnosis with CT has played a key role in the increasing trend toward nonoperative management of many visceral injuries (1,2).The technological advances with spiral CT further enhance this diagnostic capability. The vast majority of clinically significant visceral injuries can be readily detected by CT, thus facilitating rapid diagnosis and patient management. When positive, CT provides an accurate assessment of the extent of abdominal injuries and associated hemorrhage. In conjunction with clinical parameters of hemodynamic stability, the information provided by CT is crucial in determining the need for surgery. When negative, CT provides a reliable means of excluding serious intra-abdominal injury. A very small percentage of patients, however, may have occult visceral injuries. These are typically due to lacerations of the luminal gastrointestinal tract or pancreas (3). Therefore a negative CT scan for trauma does not entirely exclude the possibility of visceral injury.

Current state-of-the-art spiral CT represents a significant technical advance in the evaluation of blunt trauma patients. It affords a number of important imaging advantages when compared with dynamic contrast-enhanced CT, including significantly faster scanning acquisition, improved contrast enhancement to more clearly demonstrate both visceral injuries and active arterial extravasation, and more accurate multiplanar reconstructions.

TECHNIQUE

Intravenous contrast enhancement is essential for accurate diagnosis of visceral injuries and to assess renal perfusion and excretion. Parenchymal lacerations result in avascular hematomas that do not appreciably enhance with intravenous contrast. Thus visceral injuries are identified on CT as low-attenuation areas compared with normally enhancing parenchyma (Fig. 18-1). Noncontrast CT scans may occasionally be helpful in identifying very small parenchymal hematomas such as a rare occult splenic laceration. However, the diagnostic yield does not justify the time, expense, and additional radiation required for routine use of noncontrast spiral CT scans in trauma.

Breath-held spiral imaging of the upper abdomen (requiring 25–30 s) is performed whenever feasible. Alternatively, in tachypneic patients, clusters of 10–15-s breath-held spiral scans may be obtained. A significant number of severely traumatized patients, however, are unresponsive or in such pain that even relatively short breath-held spiral acquisitions are impossible. In these patients, motion and respiratory artifacts still occur with spiral scanning and can significantly degrade image quality. In a select number of patients, limited repeat scans may be required for accurate diagnosis. For contrast injection, 150 mL of 60% iodinated contrast is administered as a uniphasic bolus at a rate of 3 mL/s. Scanning of the abdomen is initiated 70 s after the start of the intravenous contrast bolus injection. Whenever possible, the patient is hyperventilated during the injection delay so that a single spiral acquisition may be obtained of the upper abdomen. Quiet breathing is then initiated as scans proceed from the lower abdomen to the pelvis in a second spiral acquisition. Slice collimation is generally 7–8 mm using a pitch of at least 1.5 to 1. The data set is then reconstructed at the slice collimation to ensure optimal registration of images.

Following an initial digital scout radiograph of the lower chest and abdomen, scans are performed from several centimeters above the diaphragm to the symphysis pubis. In addition to soft-tissue windows, both bone and lung windows are routinely viewed in trauma patients. Lung windows should first be scrutinized to exclude an unsuspected pneumothorax. Bone windows, similarly, are essential for diagnosis of subtle vertebral and pelvic fractures. These can be viewed rapidly by ''paging through'' multiple images at the console with a track ball. It is essential to view images of the chest and abdomen with very wide windows (preferably

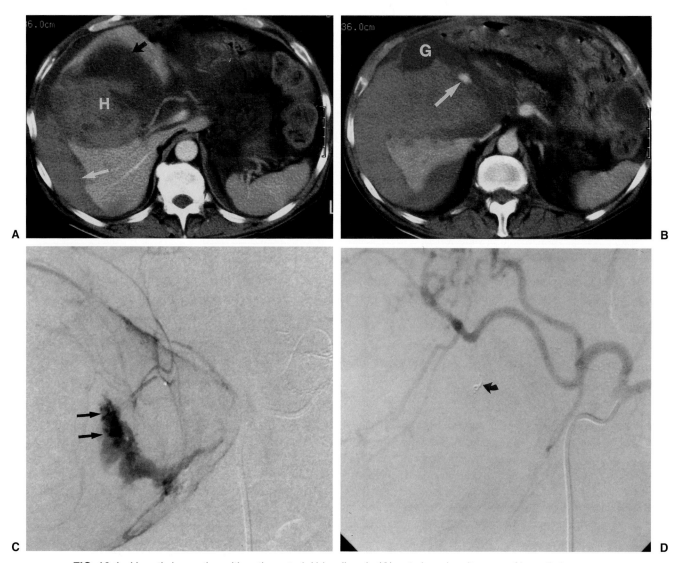

FIG. 18-1. Hepatic laceration with active arterial bleeding. In (**A**) note low-density area of hepatic lacera-tion (*black arrow*). Higher-attenuation hematoma (H) representing clotted blood is also noted. Large amount of surrounding perihepatic hemoperitoneum is demonstrated (*curved arrow*). In (**B**) note focus of active arterial extravasation (*arrow*) adjacent to gallbladder (G). Elective hepatic arteriography (**C**) demonstrates active arterial extravasation (*arrows*). Following embolization with a steel coil (*arrow*, **D**) no further arterial extravasation is evident.

800–1,000) to detect subtle areas of pneumoperitoneum (Fig. 18-2). Delayed scans obtained at 3–5 min after contrast injection are essential to evaluate renal excretion in patients with flank trauma to exclude disruption of the collecting system.

In addition to intravenous contrast, oral contrast is essen-tial for diagnosis of pancreatic, duodenal, and proximal small bowel injuries (Fig. 18-3). Concern about possible tracheo-bronchial aspiration of orally administered contrast has proved to be unfounded. The collective experience of 15 years of orally administered contrast agents from multiple trauma centers has clearly demonstrated its usefulness in evaluating bowel and pancreatic injuries and the virtual ab-sence of any complications. In a recent study of 506 trauma

patients receiving oral contrast, only one patient experienced tracheobronchial aspiration (4). This was due to inadvertent placement of a nasogastric tube into the right mainstem bron-chus (4). When administering oral contrast, no attempt should be made to delay the CT study to opacify the distal gastrointestinal tract. It is sufficient to opacify the stomach, duodenum, and proximal jejunum. Approximately 450 mL of 1% to 2.5% water-soluble contrast is administered via nasogastric tube placed during the patient's resuscitation in the emergency room. Whenever possible, conscious patients may ingest the oral contrast. Prior to scanning, the nasogas-tric tube is withdrawn to the distal esophagus to minimize streak artifacts. In patients going to surgery, all remaining oral contrast in the stomach is withdrawn by simply reinsert-

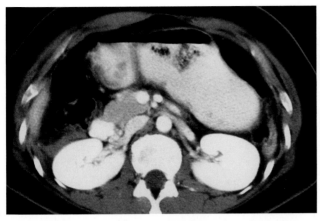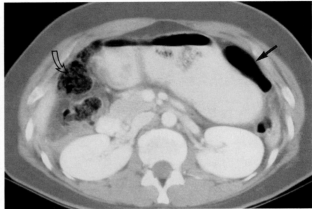

A

B

FIG. 18-2. Value of wide windows to demonstrate pneumoperitoneum. **(A)** This image is obtained at windows of 400 and the area of pneumoperitoneum is not evident. **(B)** This image is obtained using a window of 800, the pneumoperitoneum (*black arrow*) is clearly identified adjacent to the stomach. The stool containing right colon (*curved arrow*) is readily identified as a loop of bowel.

ing the nasogastric tube into the stomach and aspirating the gastric contents with a syringe.

USEFUL SIGNS IN THE CT EVALUATION OF BLUNT ABDOMINAL TRAUMA

Sentinel Clot Sign

Because of its hemoglobin content, blood is typically higher in attenuation value than other serous fluid collections such as urine, ascites, bile, or lymph (5). In patients without anemia, free lysed blood in the peritoneal cavity is generally greater than 30 Hounsfield units (HU) (5). In a small number of patients, however, blood may be less than 20 HU (6).

This is particularly true of hepatic lacerations that may be associated with bilomas of near water attenuation. Clotted blood is typically higher in attenuation than free lysed blood and is generally on the order of 45–70 HU. Active arterial extravasation may result in extremely high attenuation areas with blood mixed with iodinated contrast (often more than 100 HU). The "sentinel clot sign" refers to the observation that blood is highest in attenuation in close proximity to the site of visceral injury (7; Fig. 18-4). This observation may be helpful in patients with subtle visceral injuries that are not apparent on initial inspection of the solid viscera.

Active Arterial Extravasation

One of the main values of spiral CT in trauma is identifying areas of acute hemorrhage with active arterial extravasa-

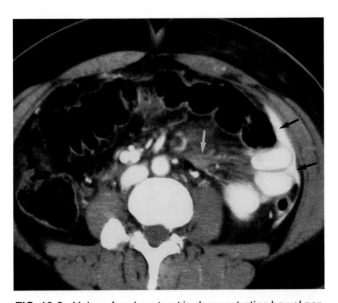

FIG. 18-3. Value of oral contrast in demonstrating bowel perforation. Note extravasated oral contrast in left paracolic gutter (*black arrows*) in a patient with jejunal laceration. No hemoperitoneum was evident. Note triangular high attenuation hematoma in the mesentery (*white arrow*).

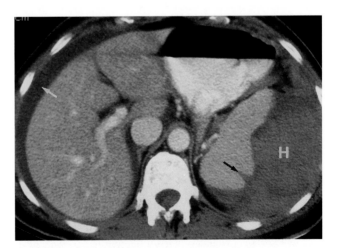

FIG. 18-4. Perisplenic sentinel clot sign from splenic laceration. Note high-density perisplenic hematoma (H). The perisplenic hematoma is higher in attenuation than the perihepatic hemoperitoneum (*white arrow*). Note the small splenic laceration (*black arrow*).

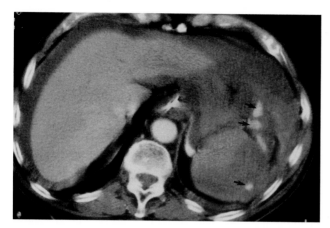

FIG. 18-5. Active arterial extravasation from splenic artery laceration. Ruptured subcapsular hematoma of the spleen demonstrates high-attenuation foci (*arrows*) adjacent to the spleen consistent with active arterial extravasation. Note similar attenuation to the aorta.

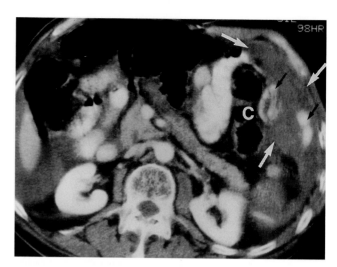

FIG. 18-7. Active arterial extravasation from splenic laceration mimics extravasation of oral contrast. Note high-attenuation foci in left pericolic gutter (*black arrows*) adjacent to the descending colon (C). Note large surrounding hematoma (*white arrows*).

tion. The rapid acquisition of spiral CT facilitates scanning during peak opacification of the contrast bolus. Areas of active arterial extravasation appear on CT as foci of high-attenuation fluid similar in attenuation to adjacent major arterial structures (8,9; Figs. 18-5–18-8). Surrounding an area of active arterial extravasation is invariably a large hematoma. At times the high-attenuation fluid may be so dense as to mimic extravasated oral contrast (see Fig. 18-7). However, the identification of the large adjacent hematoma is a key differentiating feature. The accurate CT diagnosis of active arterial extravasation is of major clinical significance

for patient management. It indicates the need for either urgent surgery or angiographic embolization. A trial of nonoperative management is generally unwarranted because of the potential hazard of ongoing blood loss. Accurately identifying the anatomic site of the bleeding is also critical in directing therapy. In patients with extraperitoneal foci of active extravasation (such as from a laceration of a lumbar artery), angiographic embolization is the treatment of choice. In patients with intraperitoneal active arterial extravasation, ur-

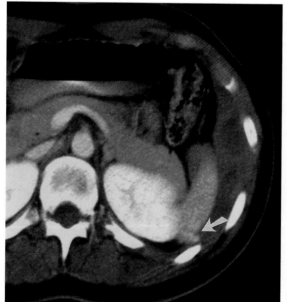

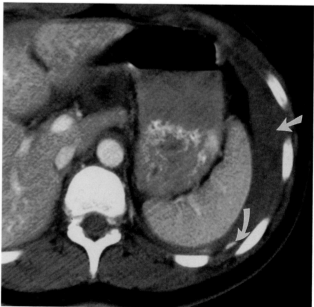

A   **B**

FIG. 18-6. Active arterial extravasation from subtle splenic laceration. In (**A**) note subtle defect in the outer margin of the splenic contour consistent with laceration (*arrow*). In (**B**) high-attenuation focus is identified (*curved arrow*) consistent with active arterial extravasation. Note surrounding perisplenic hemoperitoneum (*arrow*).

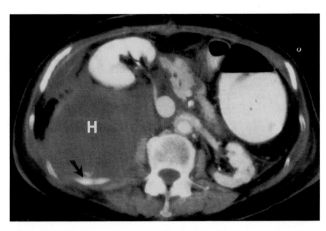

FIG. 18-8. Extraperitoneal active arterial extravasation from lumbar artery bleed. Note large extraperitoneal hematoma (H) and high-attenuation focus (*arrow*) from active arterial extravasation from the lumbar artery.

gent laparotomy is generally undertaken because of associated multiple injuries.

CT Signs of Shock and Hypovolemia

CT is generally performed only in trauma patients who are hemodynamically stable. Hypotensive patients are generally sent directly to surgery after rapid resuscitation. Rarely, some patients who are initially stable after resuscitation become hypotensive during CT scanning. Thus frequent patient monitoring of vital signs is mandatory. There are several CT signs that indicate systemic hypovolemia and/or hypotension. Persistent flattening of the intrahepatic inferior vena cava is reliable evidence of decreased central venous return and should prompt immediate fluid resuscitation and central venous pressure monitoring (9; Fig. 18-9). Hypovolemic but

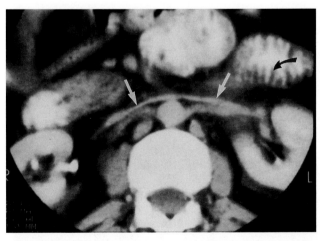

FIG. 18-9. The collapsed cava sign of hypovolemia. Note marked flattening of the inferior vena cava of the renal veins (*white arrows*) from central hypovolemia. Small bowel fold thickening is also noted, and that is a finding consistent with "shock bowel."

normotensive patients, however, may demonstrate renal excretion of contrast. In patients with hypovolemic shock, however, uniformly dense nephrograms will be noted without evidence of renal excretion on delayed images. This mimics the appearance of the kidneys after an allergic reaction to contrast.

In patients with prior shock the aorta and mesenteric vessels may undergo intense vasoconstriction and appear small in caliber. Vasoconstriction of mesenteric vessels may result in submucosal edema of the bowel that causes thickening of small bowel folds (10; Fig. 18-9). This is distinct from the diffuse mural thickening of the small bowel wall caused by an intramural hematoma. There may also be intense enhancement of the small bowel wall because of prolonged mural transit time (10). Vasoconstriction of the splenic artery is a common physiological response to shock and results in a small hypodense spleen. Recognition of any of the preceding findings indicating hypovolemia or shock should lead to immediate termination of the CT and transfer of the patient to the emergency room or intensive care unit for stabilization or surgery.

ANALYSIS OF INTRAPERITONEAL FLUID

Intraperitoneal fluid following blunt trauma may be due to blood, small bowel contents, bile, urine, or lymphatic fluid. Attenuation values greater than 30 HU are consistent with blood. Negative attenuation values may be noted with lymphatic fluid due to the lipid content of chylomicrons (11). The anatomic location of the intraperitoneal fluid may be an important clue to its origin. Intraloop fluid between the reflections of the mesentery strongly suggests a bowel or mesenteric injury.

In a small number of patients, intraperitoneal fluid may be the only abnormal finding on abdominal CT. Close clinical observation is generally all that is required in these patients, because they typically do well with conservative therapy (12). Surgery is generally indicated in patients with large amounts of fluid to exclude bowel or mesenteric injury (12).

SPECIFIC ORGAN INJURIES

Hepatic Trauma

The liver is the second most frequently injured abdominal organ after the spleen. The right lobe is injured much more frequently than the left in patients sustaining blunt trauma. Associated with right hepatic lobe lacerations are right lung contusion and pneumothorax, right rib fractures, right renal lacerations, and right adrenal hemorrhage (13). Injuries to the left lobe are associated with pancreatic, duodenal, and transverse colon lacerations.

In patients who are hemodynamically stable, the vast majority of blunt hepatic lesions can be treated nonoperatively (1,14). This includes even extensive parenchymal lacerations. Identification of active arterial extravasation within

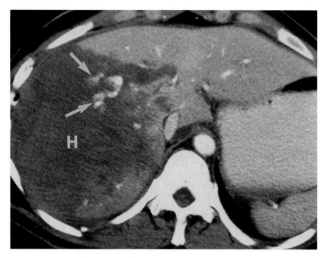

FIG. 18-10. Hepatic laceration with active arterial extravasation. Note large right lobe hepatic low-attenuating hematoma (H). Foci of high attenuation are noted (*arrows*), indicating active arterial extravasation.

the liver, however, indicates the need for immediate surgical intervention or embolization (Figs. 18-10, 18-11). CT findings that indicate patients at high risk for complications include complex perihilar injuries and lacerations involving major hepatic veins (13). Transection of the hepatic veins is a life-threatening injury and is a challenging surgical problem. The surgeon in many cases must devascularize the liver by clamping the portal vein and hepatic artery. In some instances an atrial-caval bypass is performed.

In patients treated conservatively for blunt hepatic trauma, follow-up CT may be useful to document healing and to exclude post-traumatic complications such as bilomas or hepatic abscesses. In patients who are asymptomatic, however, the value of follow-up CT is questionable. Most of the symptomatic post-traumatic complications of hepatic trauma may be treated with percutaneous techniques.

Splenic Trauma

Splenic injuries occur in approximately one-fourth of all patients sustaining major blunt abdominal trauma. CT has a sensitivity of approximately 95% for diagnosing splenic injury (15; see Figs. 18-4–18-7). A small percentage of injuries are occult and can only be suggested by identification of a perisplenic "sentinel clot sign" (7). The spleen is the most common abdominal site of active arterial extravasation. This finding necessitates either urgent splenectomy or embolization. As previously mentioned, in patients with hypovolemic shock, vasoconstriction of the splenic artery may result in a small, diffusely hypoattenuating spleen (16). This should not be misinterpreted as splenic infarction or rupture.

Delayed rupture of the spleen has been a feared complication following blunt abdominal trauma. More recent information suggests that, in fact, delayed hemorrhage is often "delayed diagnosis" of an ongoing splenic injury with either

intermittent hemorrhage or slow, continuous bleeding (17). In a very small percentage of patients, the initial CT will be normal or demonstrate a superficial laceration (18). Days later there may be life-threatening hemorrhage from the splenic injury. Attempts to classify splenic injuries on the basis of CT severity scores have largely been disappointing (19–21). This is due to the capricious nature of splenic injuries. Relatively superficial lacerations can unpredictably go on to massive and near exsanguinating hemorrhage days or hours later. Conversely, patients (particularly pediatric patients) with extensive splenic fractures who are hemodynamically stable may go on to near complete resolution without significant hemorrhage.

Renal Trauma

Contrast-enhanced spiral CT is an extremely accurate technique for evaluating renal trauma. Renal injuries are quite common in patients with blunt abdominal trauma. As with hepatic injuries, the majority can be treated conservatively without surgery. Although most parenchymal injuries can be clearly diagnosed on the initial scans of the upper abdomen obtained with a spiral acquisition starting at 60–70 s, delayed images performed 3–5 min after the initial contrast injection should be performed to assess renal excretion and diagnose rupture of the collecting system (Fig. 18-12). Delayed images may also be of value in determining if there is ongoing hemorrhage from the kidney (Fig. 18-13).

Complete absence of renal perfusion and excretion is diagnostic of traumatic renal artery occlusion (22,23). The CT appearance is so characteristic that angiography should be deferred and immediate surgical reconstruction of the thrombosed renal artery should be undertaken without delay (Fig. 18-14). Renal fractures typically occur in an axial plane, as there is dissociation of the upper and lower poles via a

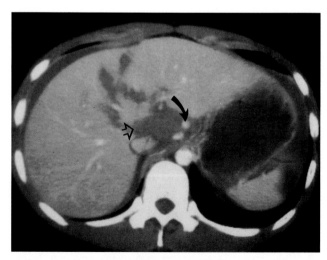

FIG. 18-11. Hepatic laceration with active arterial extravasation. Notice low-density hepatic laceration (*open arrow*) and foci of active arterial extravasation (*curved arrow*). Patient required urgent surgery for control of hemorrhage.

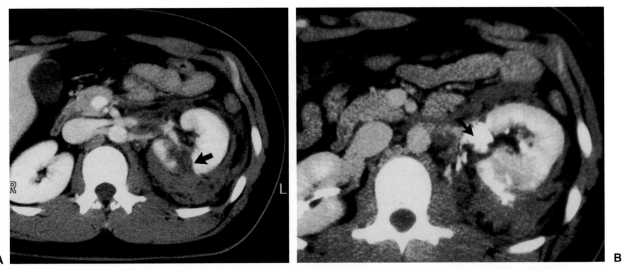

FIG. 18-12. Value of delayed scans in documenting perforation of the renal pelvis. In (**A**) note the deep laceration to the left kidney with surrounding perirenal hemorrhage (*arrow*). Delayed images demonstrate extensive contrast extravasation consistent with rupture of the collecting system.

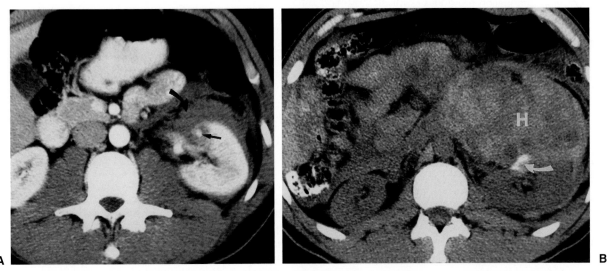

FIG. 18-13. Value of delayed scans in demonstrating ongoing hemorrhage from the kidney. In (**A**) note high-attenuation focus involving the left anteromedial aspect of the renal cortex (*straight arrow*). There is a small surrounding perirenal hematoma (*curved arrow*). Follow-up delayed images (**B**) demonstrates marked interval progression of perirenal hematoma (H) and high-attenuation focus (*curved arrow*) consistent with active arterial extravasation from ongoing hemorrhage.

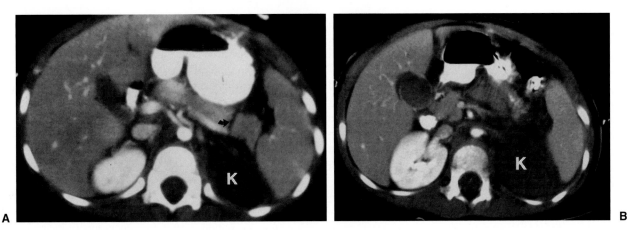

FIG. 18-14. Traumatic renal artery occlusion. Note in both (**A**) and (**B**) complete absence of enhancement of left kidney (K) consistent with traumatic renal artery occlusion. In addition, in (**A**) note a fracture of the tail of the pancreas (*curved arrow*).

329

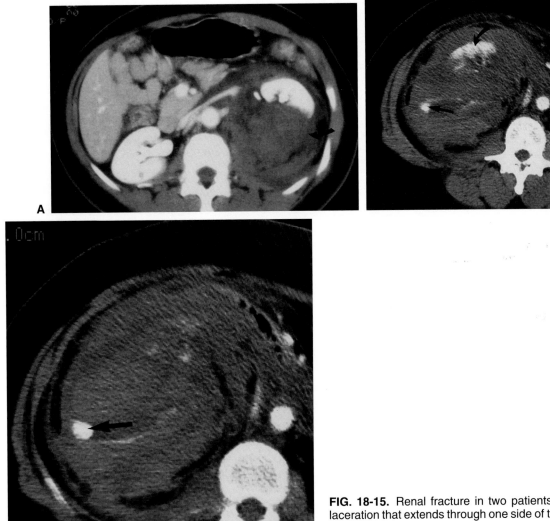

FIG. 18-15. Renal fracture in two patients. In (**A**) note the laceration that extends through one side of the cortex through the collecting system and out the other side of the cortex. There is a large surrounding perirenal hematoma (*curved arrow*). In another patient (**B,C**) with a renal fracture, note small segment of perfused kidney anteriorly (*curved arrow* in [**B**]) and active arterial extravasation (*arrow* in [**C**]).

through-and-through laceration that extends from the collecting system through the renal hilum (Fig. 18-15). Although the vast majority of renal fractures are treated surgically, in a small percentage of patients who are hemodynamically stable even extensive renal fractures may heal with conservative management. Most superficial lacerations that do not extend into the collecting system can be treated nonoperatively. However, lacerations that do extend deep into the renal hilum may be associated with injuries to large segmental vessels and may require surgical intervention for ongoing hemorrhage.

Gastrointestinal Tract

Most patients with gastrointestinal lacerations have multiorgan trauma and do not undergo CT because of hemody-

namic instability. Isolated injuries to the bowel and mesentery, however, may be diagnosed with CT by identification of pneumoperitoneum, interloop fluid, mesenteric hematomas, and intramural hematomas (3,24,25). A small percentage of gastrointestinal lesions, however, are "occult" and may have a deceptively normal initial CT. Patients may present 4–6 weeks later with either localized abscesses from bowel perforation or small bowel obstruction from inflammatory adhesions.

The luminal gastrointestinal tract is most often injured near points of relative anatomic fixation. The proximal jejunum just beyond the ligament of Treitz is a frequent site of bowel injury. Often this segment of the bowel does not contain gas within it; therefore pneumoperitoneum is an infrequent finding with jejunal laceration. An important observation indicating bowel injury, however, is water density

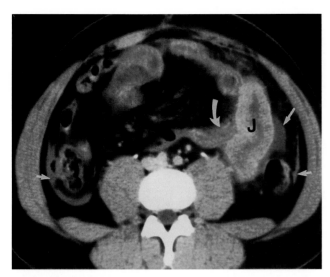

FIG. 18-16. Water density fluid as a sign of bowel perforation. Note marked mural thickening of the jejunum with increased enhancement of the bowel wall (J). High-density hematoma is seen in the adjacent mesentery (*curved arrow*). Water density fluid is seen along the lateral aspect of the jejunal loop consistent with bowel perforation. Note that there is no pneumoperitoneum. A small amount of hemoperitoneum is noted in both paracolic gutters (*short white arrows*).

fluid (small bowel contents) between the leaves of the mesentery. The "interloop fluid sign" is a characteristic hallmark of bowel or mesentery injury and should raise a very strong suspicion for this entity (3; Figs. 18-16, 18-17). Interloop hemorrhage may also occur if there is extension of lacerations into the mesenteric vessels. Most patients with hepatic and splenic injuries do not have blood collecting within the interloop compartment of the abdomen. Hemoperitoneum from hepatic or splenic lacerations extends from the upper abdominal peritoneal cavity to the pelvis via the lateral paracolic gutters (Fig. 18-18).

Hemorrhage into the bowel wall typically results in focal

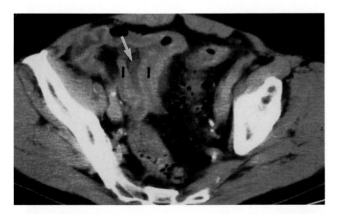

FIG. 18-17. Interloop fluid as the sign of bowel perforation. A small amount of water density fluid (*arrow*) is noted adjacent to the terminal ileum (I). Perforation of the terminal ileum was noted at surgery.

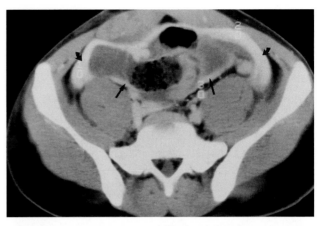

FIG. 18-18. Active arterial extravasation from mesenteric arterial laceration. Note high-attenuation fluid within interloop compartments (*long arrows*). High-attenuation fluid is also seen in the paracolic gutters (*curved arrows*). At surgery mesenteric arterial laceration was noted with active arterial extravasation.

mural thickening. This is often best assessed with oral contrast which facilitates diagnosing bowel injuries. In the absence of pneumoperitoneum or other signs of perforation, focal hematomas of the bowel wall may be cautiously observed. This is particularly true in pediatric patients with duodenal hematomas. A low threshold for operative intervention exists, however, because of the potential for increased morbidity associated with unrecognized peritonitis.

Pancreatic Trauma

Pancreatic injuries are relatively uncommon. It is estimated that they represent no more than 3% to 12% of all intra-abdominal injuries (26–28). However, the morbidity and mortality of pancreatic lacerations are substantial. Mortality rates of 20% have been reported with complete pancreatic transection (26–28). In most instances pancreatic injury occurs in the setting of multiorgan trauma, but on rare occasion isolated pancreatic injuries may occur. One of the major factors contributing to the high morbidity and mortality of pancreatic injuries is delay in diagnosis. The clinical signs of pancreatic injury may be challenging and fraught with difficulty. A classic surgical dictum states that pancreatic trauma results in pain out of proportion to the physical findings. Peritoneal signs are often inconspicuous in these patients.

The surgical classification of pancreatic injury largely depends on whether there is disruption of the duct of Wirsung and an associated duodenal injury (29). Category I injuries typically result in pancreatic contusions and superficial hematomas. Category II injuries involve complete transection of the duct of Wirsung generally in the body or tail of the pancreas. Category III injuries are related to pancreatic ductal disruption in the head of the pancreas. Category IV lesions involve both head of pancreas and duodenal or common bile duct injury.

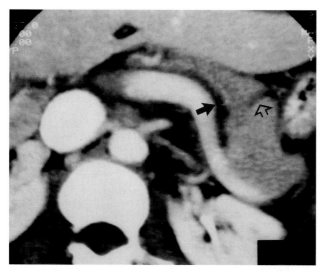

FIG. 18-19. Retropancreatic fluid as a major sign of pancreatic trauma. Note laceration of the pancreatic parenchyma (*open arrow*). A large amount of retropancreatic fluid is seen adjacent to the splenic vein, indicating transection of the pancreatic duct and extensive pancreatic injury (*arrow*).

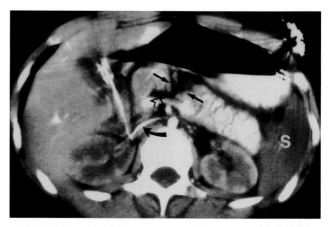

FIG. 18-21. Pancreatic laceration and CT signs of shock. Note the small hypodense spleen (as consistent with shock). Other signs of hypovolemia include the collapsed inferior vena cava (*curved arrow*). Note pancreatic fracture in the midbody (*arrows*). Retropancreatic fluid is seen adjacent to the splenic vein (*open arrow*).

It may be extremely difficult to diagnose subtle pancreatic injuries soon after blunt abdominal trauma. Therefore the initial CT scan may be negative, and if there is a high clinical suspicion of pancreatic injury, a repeat CT scan may be of significant value in clarifying the diagnosis. Post-traumatic pancreatitis may be the predominant CT finding with soft-tissue infiltration along the anterior reflection of Gerota's fascia. Another finding recently noted on spiral CT is the presence of fluid dissecting between the splenic vein and the posterior body of the pancreas (Fig. 18-19). Active arterial extravasation can be identified in a small percentage of patients. In other patients, low-attenuation lacerations can be identified adjacent to normally enhancing parenchyma (Figs. 18-20, 18-21).

One of the main advantages of spiral CT is that the intense enhancement of the normal pancreatic parenchyma can be obtained with a uniphasic bolus of contrast. In addition, thin cuts (3–5 mm) can be obtained through the pancreas with spiral technique, which further facilitates the diagnosis of subtle pancreatic abnormalities.

It is not uncommon for the diagnosis to be missed clinically and for patients to present days to weeks later with peripancreatic fluid collections. In some instances patients develop well-defined pseudocysts at sites of prior pancreatic injury. Spiral CT may be of considerable value in diagnosing complications of pancreatic trauma, including abscess, hematoma, and pseudoaneurysm formation.

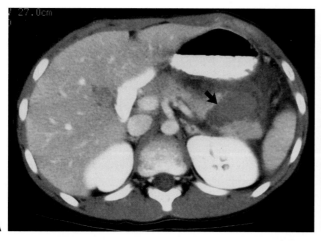

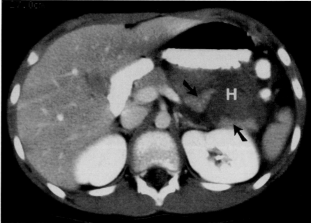

FIG. 18-20. Fracture of the pancreatic tail. In (**A**) note laceration traversing the tail of the gland. In (**B**) note the separation of normally perfused segments of the pancreatic parenchyma (*arrows*) with large hematoma extending into the lesser sac (H).

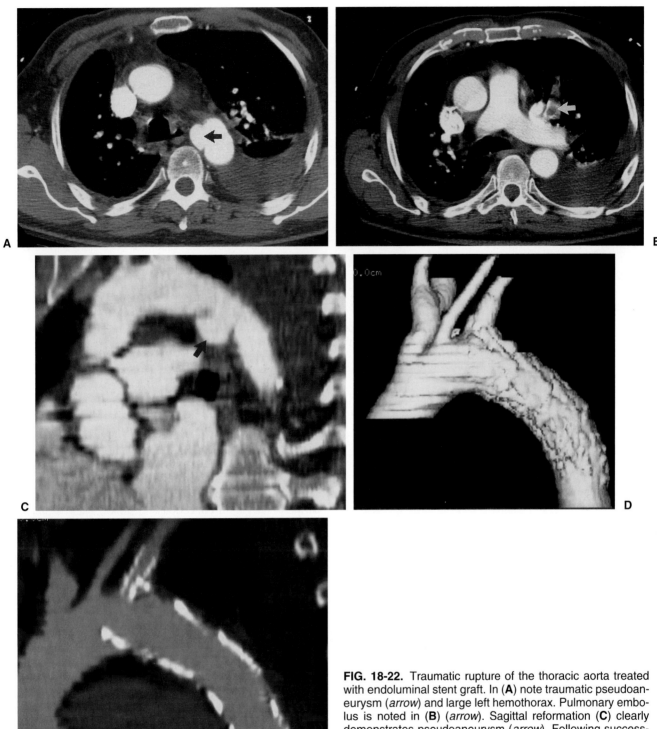

FIG. 18-22. Traumatic rupture of the thoracic aorta treated with endoluminal stent graft. In (**A**) note traumatic pseudoaneurysm (*arrow*) and large left hemothorax. Pulmonary embolus is noted in (**B**) (*arrow*). Sagittal reformation (**C**) clearly demonstrates pseudoaneurysm (*arrow*). Following successful endoluminal stent graft placement, shaded-surface display (**D**) and curved planar reformation (**E**) demonstrate occlusion of pseudoaneurysm.

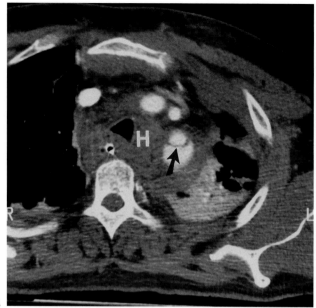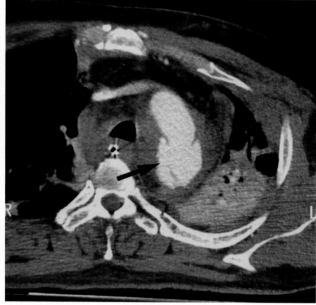

A B

FIG. 18-23. Traumatic rupture of the thoracic aorta. In (**A**) note mediastinal hematoma (H) and intimal flaps (*arrow*) at top of aortic arch. Pseudoaneurysm is noted in (**B**) (*arrow*).

THORACIC AORTIC INJURY

Thoracic rupture following blunt trauma is a highly lethal injury (30). In the small percentage of patients who survive the initial injury, establishing the diagnosis may be exceedingly difficult, based on history, physical examination, and chest radiographs. Thoracic aortography has been widely used to diagnose this potentially life-threatening injury. However, up to 80% of studies are negative.

CT may play an important role in triaging patients for angiography (Fig. 18-22). In a large retrospective study, mediastinal hemorrhage was shown to be 87% specific for aortic injury (31). It is likely that with better contrast enhancement and speed of acquisition with spiral CT, the direct visualization of the aortic pseudoaneurysm is improved (Fig. 18-23).

REFERENCES

1. Goff CD, Gilbert CM. Nonoperative management of blunt hepatic trauma. *Am Surg* 1995;61:66–68.
2. Roberts JL, Dalen K, Bosanko CM, Jafir SZ. CT in abdominal and pelvic trauma. *Radiographics* 1993;13:735–752.
3. Nghiem HV, Jeffrey RB Jr, Mindelzun RE. CT of blunt trauma to the bowel and mesentery. *AJR* 1993;160:53–58.
4. Federle M. Should patients who undergo CT scanning of the abdomen for blunt trauma always have a CT scan of the pelvis as well, regardless of the severity and location of the trauma? *AJR* 1995;164:762.
5. Federle MP, Jeffrey RB Jr. Hemoperitoneum studied by computed tomography. *Radiology* 1983;148:187–192.
6. Levine CD, Patel UJ, Silverman PM, Wachsberg RH. Low attenuation of acute traumatic hemoperitoneum on CT scans. *AJR* 1996;166: 1089–1093.
7. Orwig D, Federle MP. Localized clotted blood as evidence of visceral trauma on CT: the sentinel clot sign. *AJR* 1989;153:747–749.
8. Jeffrey RB Jr, Cardoza JD, Olcott EW. Detection of active intraabdomi-

nal arterial hemorrhage: value of dynamic contrast-enhanced CT. *AJR* 1991;156:725–729.
9. Jeffrey RB Jr, Federle MP. The collapsed inferior vena cava: CT evidence of hypovolemia. *AJR* 1988;150:431–432.
10. Mirvis SE, Shanmuganathan K, Erb R. Diffuse small-bowel ischemia in hypotensive adults after blunt trauma (shock bowel): CT findings and clinical significance. *AJR* 1994;163:1375–1379.
11. Watanabe AT, Jeffrey RB Jr. CT diagnosis of traumatic rupture of the cisterna chyli. *J Comput Assist Tomogr* 1987;11:175–176.
12. Levine CD, Patel UJ, Wachsberg RH, Simmons MZ, Baker SR, Cho KC. CT in patients with blunt abdominal trauma: clinical significance of intraperitoneal fluid detected on a scan with otherwise normal findings. *AJR* 1995;164:1381–1385.
13. Jeffrey RB Jr, Olcott EW. Imaging of blunt hepatic trauma. *Radiol Clin North Am* 1991;29:1299–1310.
14. Knudson MM, Lim RC Jr, Oakes DD, Jeffrey RB Jr. Nonoperative management of blunt liver injuries in adults: the need for continued surveillance. *J Trauma* 1990;30:1494–1500.
15. Federle MP, Griffiths B, Minagi H, Jeffrey RB Jr. Splenic trauma: evaluation with CT. *Radiology* 1987; 162:69–71.
16. Berland LL, VanDyke JA. Decreased splenic enhancement on CT in traumatized hypotensive patients. *Radiology* 1985;156:469–471.
17. Olsen WR, Polley TJ. A second look at delayed splenic rupture. *Arch Surg* 1977;112:422–425.
18. Taylor CR, Rosenfield AT. Limitations of computed tomography in the recognition of delayed splenic rupture. *J Comput Assist Tomogr* 1984;8:1205–1207.
19. Becker CD, Spring P, Glattli A, Schweizer W. Blunt splenic trauma in adults: can CT findings be used to determine the need for surgery? *AJR* 1994;162:343–347.
20. Jeffrey RB Jr. CT diagnosis of blunt hepatic and splenic injuries: a look to the future [editorial]. *Radiology* 1989;171:17–18.
21. Scatamacchia SA, Raptopoulos V, Fink MP, Silva WE. Splenic trauma in adults: impact of CT grading on management. *Radiology* 1989;171: 725–729.
22. Steinberg DL, Jeffrey RB, Federle MP, McAninch JW. The computerized tomography appearance of renal pedicle injury. *J Urol* 1984;132: 1163–1164.
23. Malmed AS, Love L, Jeffrey RB. Medullary CT enhancement in acute renal artery occlusion. *J Comput Assist Tomogr* 1992;16:107–109.
24. Mirvis SE, Gens DR, Shanmuganathan K. Rupture of the bowel after blunt abdominal trauma: diagnosis with CT. *AJR* 1992;159:1217–1221.

25. Cox TD, Kuhn JP. CT scan of bowel trauma in the pediatric patient. *Radiol Clin North Am* 1996;34:807–818.

26. Jurkovich GJ, Carrico CJ. Pancreatic trauma. *Surg Clin North Am* 1990; 70:575–593.

27. Frey C. Trauma to the pancreas and duodenum. In: Blaisell FW, Trunkey DD, eds. *Abdominal trauma.* New York: Thieme-Stratton; 1982: 87–122.

28. Bach RD, Frey CF. Diagnosis and treatment of pancreatic trauma. *Am J Surg* 1971;121:20–29.

29. Lucas CE. Diagnosis and treatment of pancreatic and duodenal injury. *Surg Clin North Am* 1977;57:49–65.

30. Kirsh MM, Behrendt DM, Orringer MB, et al. The treatment of acute traumatic rupture of the aorta: a 10-year experience. *Ann Surg* 1976; 184:308–316.

31. Mirvis SE, Shanmuganathan K, Miller BH, White CS, Turney SZ. Traumatic aortic injury: diagnosis with contrast-enhanced thoracic CT—five-year experience at a major trauma center. *Radiology* 1996; 200:413–422.

PART 6

Spiral CT Angiography

CHAPTER 19

Principles and Techniques of 3D Spiral CT Angiography

Sandy Napel

CT angiography (CTA) is a new and important application of spiral CT that permits the imaging of vascular structures in three dimensions (3D) using an intravenous (IV) injection of iodinated contrast agent. In general, CTA consists of the following three steps:

1. The choice of three parameters describing the design of an IV bolus of contrast: (a) injection rate (mL/s), (b) injection duration (s), and (c) delay between injection initiation and the start of the scan sequence (s).
2. The choice of three parameters describing a spiral CT acquisition timed to occur while the target vasculature is maximally opacified: (a) scan duration (s), (b) collimation (mm), and (c) table speed (s).
3. Creation of an ''angiogram-like'' image display from the reconstructed transaxial CT sections.

This chapter describes these steps in detail as a prelude to the chapters that discuss clinical applications of CTA in various parts of the body. Before getting into technical details, however, we begin by setting the historical context within which CTA has arisen and by discussing conventional angiography (the ''gold standard'' for vascular imaging) in comparison to CTA.

CTA is neither the first nor the only method of vascular imaging. The first images of the vascular system in a living human were obtained in 1926 by Egas Moniz, who imaged the intracranial arteries (1). Shortly thereafter, in 1928, Raynaldo Dos Santos developed translumbar aortography (2). Both techniques, though highly invasive, were the mainstays of vascular imaging until the Seldinger technique was developed in 1953 (3). Since then, a number of other vascular imaging techniques have become available, including ultrasound, magnetic resonance angiography (MRA), and now CTA.

It is perhaps worth noting that although the medical application of CT began a decade before that of magnetic resonance (MR) imaging, the development of MRA preceded that of CTA. The reason for this is that the imaging of blood vessels using x-rays requires the introduction of a contrast agent (typically an iodinated compound) that is toxic and may only be used in small doses. Using an intravenous injection, the concentration of the iodine required to opacify the arterial vasculature sufficiently is such that the permitted dose of iodine must be administered as a bolus. To capture the first pass of a bolus through the target vasculature requires the rapid acquisition speed afforded by continuous scanning technology. Early MR images of blood vessels, however, did not require the use of a contrast agent, relying instead on the motion of molecules in magnetic field gradients (4,5) or between radiofrequency excitations (6) to provide the vascular signal. Thus the development of MRA was not delayed by its relatively long acquisition times. (Note, however, that the use of MR contrast agents has increased [7] and is now often used for MRA [8–12].)

This historical juxtaposition is not only interesting but important. For when spiral CT enabled the development of CTA, many techniques for producing 3D angiograms from the acquired CT data had already been developed and aggressively utilized for MRA. The reader is referred to ref. 13 for a comprehensive discussion and extensive list of references on the creation and presentation of MR angiograms.

CONVENTIONAL ANGIOGRAPHY VS. CTA

It is not our intent to review and compare all vascular imaging techniques. For an in-depth treatment, see the review article by Mistretta (14). However, a brief review of conventional angiography, the still reigning ''gold standard'' for vascular imaging, is important to put into context the strengths and weaknesses of CTA.

Conventional angiography utilizes a catheter inserted directly into the arterial system to inject a contrast agent. An x-ray exposure of the target artery is made simultaneously with the contrast injection (15). A projection of the target imaging volume is acquired either by analog (e.g., film–screen combinations) or by digital means. With digital techniques, detected x-rays are converted to digital format and stored in a computer without the use of film. The high acquisition speed of the digital techniques permit a preinjection image to be subtracted from subsequent images that have contrast material present, resulting in real-time images of the contrast column alone (digital subtraction angiography, or DSA) (16). (Hereafter the term *conventional angiography* will imply intra-arterial injection and will include both analog and digital recording techniques.)

The spatial and temporal resolution of these conventional angiographic techniques is currently unsurpassed. Film–screen combinations have spatial resolution on the order of five or six line pairs per millimeter. Newer DSA units with 1,024 × 1,024 matrix arrays also approach this spatial resolution. Conventional film–screen combinations permit exposures as short as 0.25 s/frame, and approximately

10–12 frames are exposed per injection. DSA allows for more rapid imaging, with up to 25–30 frames per second used in cardiac imaging. With both of these techniques, the additional attribute of high contrast-to-noise ratio obtained using intra-arterial injections makes conventional angiography the definitive diagnostic examination for assessing vascular disease and/or abnormalities.

Unlike conventional angiography, CTA is a 3D imaging technique. Within any plane of section, the CT reconstruction process itself separates structures that are superimposed in the projection direction. The reconstruction of individual cross-sections of the acquired volume further separates structures that overlay each other in the longitudinal direction. Once the entire volume is reconstructed, viewing directions can be chosen arbitrarily (e.g., try obtaining a direct craniocaudal projection through the chest with conventional angiography) and retrospectively. Also unlike conventional angiography, CTA utilizes an IV injection, which significantly reduces the risk of complications compared with arterial injections. Table 19-1 further describes these and other

TABLE 19-1. *Advantages of CT versus conventional angiography*

Conventional angiography	CT angiography
Selection of View Angles	
Biplane systems can acquire at most two view angles of a given vascular structure per contrast injection. Alternate views and examination of additional structures require added x-ray exposure and contrast media.	CTA acquires an entire volume of 3D data using a single injection of contrast agent. Thus, arbitrary views can be retrospectively targeted and reconstructed without the need for additional iodine or x-ray exposure.
Patient Recovery	
Because an arterial puncture is made, patients must recover from the procedure with close nursing observation and strict bedrest for a minimum of 6–8 hours. An overnight hospital stay may also be required. Thus, recovery time adds significantly to the cost of the examination.	Peripheral intravenous injections permit a true outpatient examination with minimal postprocedure observation required.
Potential Complications	
Serious complications from angiography can include reactions to contrast media, and thromboembolic complications from catheterization of arteries that can lead to infarctions, strokes, arterial dissections, pseudo-aneurysms, and arterial bleeding. Using cerebral angiography as an example, the risk of a neurological complication such as a transient ischemic attack or stroke is about 4% and the risk of developing a permanent neurological deficit from a disabling stroke is about 1% (81–83).	Though the contrast agent is the same, peripheral IV injections significantly reduce the risk of thromboembolic complications.
Interpretation	
Conventional angiography is a projection imaging technique that produces 2D images of 3D structures. Therefore blood vessels and other structures that overlap in the direction of the projection may obscure the site of interest.	CTA is a 3D examination. Overlying structures may be eliminated by postprocessing.
Soft-Tissue Imaging	
Conventional angiography is an intraluminal technique and as such does not display mural abnormalities or true mural dimensions, making percent stenosis and aneurysm size measurements difficult.	CT is a cross-sectional imaging modality that exhibits excellent soft-tissue discrimination. As such, it has utility for depicting mural thrombus, calcifications, and true mural dimensions.

potential advantages of CTA. Because conventional intra-arterial angiography is still superior in terms of spatial, temporal, and contrast resolution, there is no clear overall winner. However, early studies of CTA compared with conventional angiography are showing that in selected applications, CTA provides equivalent diagnostic and pretherapeutic information at significantly less cost and risk (17–27). Of course, further studies are required to validate these capabilities and discover new ones.

The following section describes the technical aspects of CTA data acquisition, with emphasis on bolus timing and protocol selection.

CT ANGIOGRAPHY DATA ACQUISITION STRATEGY

By nature of its rapid coverage of anatomy in the z direction, spiral CT is readily applicable to vascular imaging of all parts of the body (except the heart, where the temporal resolution is thus far inadequate to suppress motion blurring and artifacts). By initiating a spiral scan subsequent to starting a bolus of intravenous contrast agent, opacification of the desired vascular anatomy can be obtained.

Bolus Timing

CT angiography with IV injections require choosing the duration of the bolus and an appropriate delay time between the initiation of the injection and the start of the spiral sequence. An ideal choice would result in scanning while the target vascular structures are opacified and without opacification of surrounding structures. This perfect situation, however, is seldom achieved because the scanning rate in the z direction is much slower than the speed of the bolus. This is illustrated in Fig. 19-1, which shows the location of an ideal contrast bolus at several points in time as it travels at an average rate of v_b mm/s through a target vessel. (Note that in practice, the first-pass arterial phase of an IV bolus will not be the ideal "slug" depicted in Fig. 19-1. Rapid mixing in the right side of the heart and passage through the lungs dilute the bolus and stretch it out in length and duration. However, we use the ideal bolus as shown to represent the region of maximal opacification.)

If the bolus was injected over T_b seconds, then its length l is given by

$$l = v_b T_b. \tag{1}$$

Suppose we begin scanning at the proximal aspect immediately upon the arrival of the bolus and that we scan distally at a rate of v_s for T_s seconds covering $v_s T_s$ mm. Then the distance d that the scan location falls behind the leading edge of the bolus in T_s seconds is

$$d = (v_b - v_s)T_s. \tag{2}$$

Thus, to ensure opacification of the target vessels during

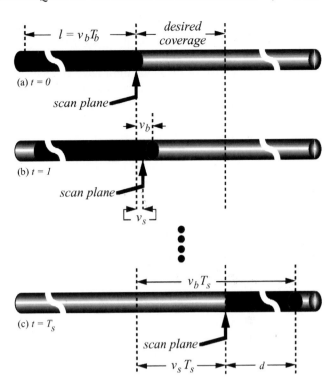

FIG. 19-1. Bolus length calculation. (**A**) Ideal bolus (*black*) as it first enters the target portion of the vessel. The length of the bolus l along the vessel is the product of the velocity of the blood, v_b, and the time T_b, over which the bolus was injected. The initial scan plane is as shown. (**B**) After 1 s, the leading edge of the bolus has traveled v_b mm but, assuming the blood travels faster than the patient can be translated, the scan plane has advanced only v_s mm. (**C**) After scanning for T_s seconds, the leading edge of the bolus and the scan plane have advanced to the positions shown. Note that the distance that the scan plane has fallen behind by the end of the scan (given by $d = v_b T_s - v_s T_s$) is equivalent to the length l of the bolus. Thus the time duration of the bolus can be computed as given by Eq. (4).

the entire scan, we must choose the length l of the bolus, such that $l \geq d$, or

$$l \geq (v_b - v_s) \div v_b. \tag{3}$$

By substituting Eq. (1) into Eq. (3) we see that the duration of the bolus T_b must satisfy the relationship

$$T_b \geq T_s(v_b - v_s) \div v_b. \tag{4}$$

If we could keep up with the bolus (i.e., if $v_s = v_b$), then we would require only that $T_b \geq 0$ (i.e., we could use a very short bolus). However, in practice $v_b \gg v_s$, resulting in the requirement that $T_b \geq T_s$ (i.e., the bolus duration must be at least as long as the scan time).

Given that the bolus duration should be as long as the scan time, we have to worry about the possibility that surrounding venous structures and perfused tissue will enhance before the scan is complete. Note, for example, the enhancement of the jugular vein during the last two-thirds of a spiral CT scan shown in Fig. 19-8. Assuming that scanning began at the inferior aspect simultaneous with the arrival of iodine and proceeded superiorly at a fixed rate, we see that after 12 s the leading edge of the bolus must have crossed the capillary bed in the brain and started to collect in the draining veins. This time will vary among different patients and may be much shorter in pathological instances such as arteriovenous malformations.

Reducing parenchymal and venous enhancement of course argues for short scan times, which in turn require faster patient translation. But with a fixed gantry rotation period, faster translation reduces the spatial resolution in the z direction. Also, without simultaneously increasing the photon flux, faster translation reduces the exposure to the volume, which in turn correlates the noise in the z direction. Therefore unwanted enhancement is always a concern. The best that we can do, then, is to make the scan time and bolus duration as short as possible to cover the target region, and to ensure that the spiral scan sequence begins immediately upon entry into the target region. (Note that recent advancements, such as multidetector ring scanners [28] and faster gantry rotations, permit faster translation without increasing pitch; that is, without reducing spatial resolution in the z direction. We might speculate that continued advancement in these directions will reduce the magnitude of unwanted enhancement sometime in the future.)

Because circulation time varies considerably from patient to patient and even within a given patient at different times, ensuring proper timing is nontrivial (29). However, a test injection may be used to determine the transit time from the venous injection site to target vasculature. Typically, the test injection rate is the same as the rate intended to be used for the actual study (e.g., 5 mL/s), but the duration is significantly shorter (e.g., 4 s). Figures 20-2 and 21-1 give examples of using this technique for scanning the abdominal aorta and carotid arteries, respectively. Eight seconds after the initiation of the test injection, 1-s scans of the proximal section of the volume were repeatedly scanned at a rate of one scan every 2 s. The figures show plots of enhancement in the target vessels as a function of time. The rising edge of these plots is typical of what we expect from the actual injection to be used for the CT angiogram. Thus we can use the plots to deduce the time of onset of maximal enhancement, and use this time as the delay time for the actual study. Use of a test injection has proven to be quite reliable; however, it does result in increased dose to the proximal aspect and in a small, but not insignificant, increase in iodine burden.

Scan Duration, Collimation, and Pitch

Many aspects of the intended goals of a CTA study must be taken into account to determine an appropriate protocol. A very important tradeoff, which has to be made, is the amount of coverage versus the spatial resolution in the z direction. High spatial resolution in this direction requires narrow collimation and relatively slow patient translation.

However, slow table feeds limit the amount of coverage that can be obtained in a fixed time interval. Therefore with present-day scanners it is important to target a study to the smallest possible volume that will reveal the required information. For example, the major vessels of the circle of Willis can be covered in a 3-cm slab and can usually be localized with a noncontrast scan. Thus 1-mm collimation and table feed of 1 mm/s (pitch = 1) can be used to cover this territory in a scan time of 30 s at the highest possible spatial resolution. In contrast, a study of the abdominal aorta requires coverage of approximately 18 cm. A maximum 30-s breath-holding scanning interval therefore requires a table feed of 6 mm/s. At this speed, choices of pitch between 1.0 and 2.0 require collimator settings of 6 mm (pitch = 1.0), 5 mm (pitch = 1.2), 4 mm (pitch = 1.5), and 3 mm (pitch = 2.0). (Note that not all collimation settings are available from every manufacturer). Narrower collimation results in higher spatial resolution and reduced dose. For some applications, the increase in noise may result in decreased low-contrast lesion conspicuity (30). For CT angiography, however, the literature has supported the use of the smallest collimation possible that permits coverage of the desired volume with pitch of 2.0 or less (31,32). (Note, however, that higher pitch can result in increased artifactual content; see, for example, Chapter 1, Fig. 1-9.) Example protocols and results for applications in the abdomen and brain are given in Chapters 20 and 21.

ANGIOGRAM GENERATION

Three-dimensional vascular anatomy is difficult to discern in transaxial slice format, and direct comparison with conventional angiography, which provides projection images, is impossible. The CT data are inherently 3D and provide the opportunity to generate views from many directions and to restrict the volume to the structures of interest. However, all conventional image-viewing techniques are two-dimensional (2D); that is, images will be viewed either on film or on a computer monitor. Thus the 3D data must be processed and displayed in 2D. In the remaining sections, we discuss algorithms and techniques for creating and presenting angiogram-like depictions of the CT data. Because there are some excellent treatments of this subject with respect to MR imaging (see, for example, ref. 13), we will place particular emphasis on the unique challenges presented by the CT data.

Many available 3D display techniques result in images that are more directly comparable to angiograms (33–35). These methods include volume rendering (VR) (36–39) and shaded-surface display (SSD) (40–44). All 3D rendering methods produce 2D images, which portray the 3D anatomy from an arbitrary view angle along with 3D cues such as surface shading, depth shading, or rotational motion from frame to frame in a movie loop. Thus orientations can be chosen that are comparable to conventional angiograms; indeed, orientations can also be chosen that would be impossible to obtain by projection imaging. In addition, internal perspectives can be computed and displayed to simulate angioscopy (45–48). The following sections describe the theory and practical application of these techniques to exploration and display of CT angiographic images.

Volume Rendering

Volume-rendering techniques build up a 2D image by casting mathematical rays in some desired viewing direction through a stack of reconstructed slices (Fig. 19-2.) The rendering can be done using divergent rays (see the section entitled "Use of Perspective"), giving perspective to the final image or, as is most common, using parallel rays. The simplest form of VR is the average projection, in which the intensity of each pixel in the resulting image is the average of the intensities encountered along each ray connecting the

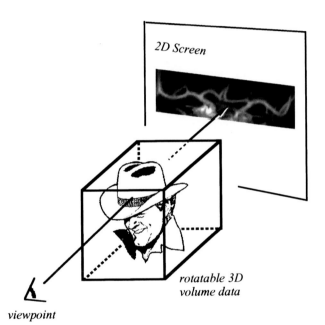

FIG. 19-2. Three-dimensional reconstruction by volume rendering. The 3D volume data may be composed of a stack of acquired and reconstructed 2D CT images. The first step is to set the viewing orientation with respect to the observer's viewpoint and a hypothetical 2D screen. The coronal projection direction is shown, but other orientations (e.g., sagittal, axial, left anterior oblique, etc.) may be chosen. Next, the computer casts mathematical rays from the observer's viewpoint through the reoriented volume data to each pixel on the 2D screen. (The figure shows a single such ray.) The shade of gray (or color) assigned to each pixel is a function of the voxel data encountered by the associated ray. For example, with MIP, the shade of gray chosen is the brightest encountered along the ray. Note that in general, rays do not pass through the centers of acquired voxels. Thus some form of interpolation is required to estimate samples of each ray as it traverses the volume. The most commonly used interpolation methods are "nearest neighbor interpolation," which chooses the value of the voxel closest to the desired sample point, and "tri-linear interpolation," which computes an inverse-distance weighted average of the eight nearest voxels to the desired sample point.

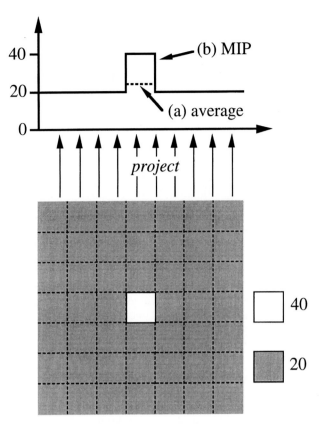

FIG. 19-3. Two-dimensional example of (**A**) average projection and (**B**) MIP in the left-to-right direction. Suppose the white square represents a blood vessel perpendicular to the plane shown and that it has twice the intensity of the surrounding pixels illustrated by the gray squares. Note that the vessel-to-background ratio for the average projection is 8 : 7 (1.14 : 1) whereas the same ratio for MIP is 2 : 1. Also note that as the number of pixels traversed by each ray gets larger (i.e., the volume size increases), the vessel-to-background ratio for the average projection decreases, whereas for MIP it remains at 2 : 1.

pixel to the observer's viewpoint as it traverses the volume. However, the average projection suffers from the same low-contrast resolution as conventional x-ray imaging, and for the same reasons. Figure 19-3 illustrates this effect and also compares the average projection with another form of VR known as maximum-intensity projection (MIP), to be discussed in the section of the same name, and shows MIP to have superior contrast for blood vessel imaging.

A more general case of VR permits the specification of a relationship between pixel intensity and ray transmission characteristics such as opacity and color, as shown by Fig. 19-4 (see color plate 14 following p. 352). Such a mapping can be thought of as an attempt to divide the density (measured in Hounsfield units [HU]) range up into distinct subranges for individual tissue types. The VR algorithm uses these tables to classify every sample point along each ray and looks up the sample's opacity and color. The algorithm then accumulates the opacity and blends the color with results obtained so far for the ray. When the opacity reaches

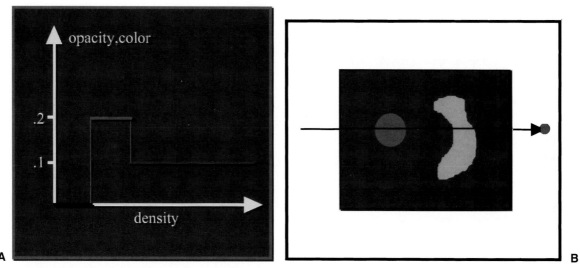

FIG. 19-4. Generalized volume rendering. (**A**) Look-up tables map density to opacity and color; for example, in this case low-density voxels have zero opacity (i.e., are transparent), mid-density voxels have opacity of 0.2 per unit length and map to red, and higher-density voxels have opacity of 0.1 per unit length and map to blue. (**B**) Example of a ray passing through a single plane of voxels. Brighter shades of gray map to higher densities. According to look-up table (**A**), when the ray traverses the circle it accumulates twice the "amount" of red per voxel compared with the "amount" of blue it accumulates per voxel as it traverses the higher-density irregular shape. Other (low-density) tissue maps to zero opacity and therefore does not contribute to the exiting color and saturation. Assuming a ray does not saturate, the exit color is a mixture of red and blue. If the path length through the circle were large enough, the ray could saturate before entering the irregular shape, resulting in an exit color of red. Note that look-up tables may be adjusted during rendering to alter the relative visibilities of tissues with different densities.

1.0, the ray saturates and the current color is assigned to the output pixel. Note that discrete ranges, such as those shown by Fig. 19-4, are not required; in general, every intensity value can have its own opacity and color. Smooth curves, instead of piece-wise continuous functions as shown, can be used to lessen the impact of pixel misclassification, which can happen as a result of noise and partial volume effects, and can also reduce aliasing caused by inadequate sampling of sharp edges (49).

The principal advantage of generalized VR is that all the image data remain available to contribute to the display of each rendered image. The opacity and color tables may be altered to increase or decrease the contribution of a given density range to the rendered image, and the results of the change are viewable in the time it takes to render a single frame. Also noteworthy is that spatial gradients can be computed from the image data and used to compute the simulated reflection of light from surfaces within the volume. Figure 19-5 illustrates the use of opacity tables and lighting (see color plate 15 following p. 352).

Although VR is not a new idea, its use has been limited for medical imaging because of its high computational complexity and the size of radiological data sets. Shaded-surface display and MIP, both computationally simpler approaches (see the following two sections), have had much more widespread use for CTA applications. However, in the previous 2 years, the price/performance ratio of computer

workstations and the cost of computer memory chips have dropped drastically, to the point that VR is possible at nearly interactive rates for the price of a $20,000 workstation. Accordingly, the use of VR is increasing and may in the future be the dominant method for visualization of CT angiograms (45,50). Shaded-surface displays are still popular, however, and are discussed next.

Shaded-Surface Display

The SSD technique is an alternative to VR and MIP for generating CT angiograms (Fig. 19-6). This method first computes a mathematical model of a surface that connects all pixels with CT intensities above a preset threshold. Although many algorithms exist for constructing the model, they all result in the coordinates of points (or small regions) on the surface together with their respective surface normal vectors describing the orientation of the surface at each coordinate (40,41). This computation is done once for a given threshold and generally reduces the volume data considerably. Next, for a given view direction, an image is created that shades or colors the surface in proportion to the amount of light it would reflect from a simulated light source back to the observer, and may darken the reflections in proportion to distance. These computations are fairly simple and, because of the reduced number of points to consider, can be performed about 10–50 times faster than generalized VR on equivalent hardware.

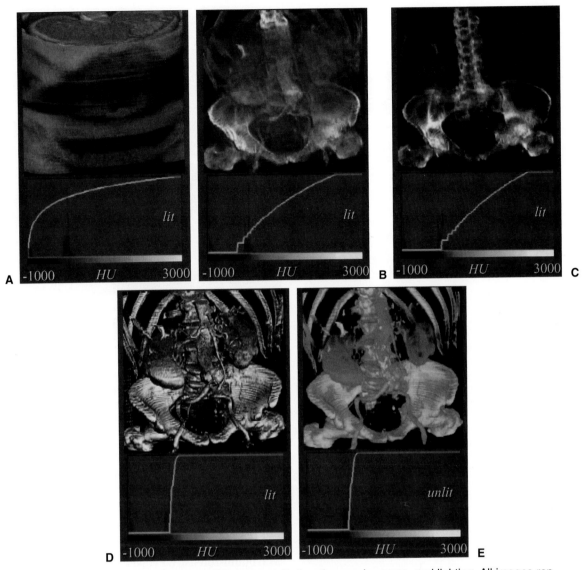

FIG. 19-5. Volume rendering with different opacity functions, color maps, and lighting. All images rendered at the same orientation in orthographic mode. Each subfigure consists of a rendered image, voxel density histogram with superimposed opacity function, and color map, from top to bottom, respectively. First peak in histogram is air voxels, second is soft tissue, third is iodine/bone. In (**A–D**) the lighting is on; in (**E**) it is off. (**A**) Opacity map adjusted to saturate rays as soon as they enter soft tissue, thereby rendering skin surface. (**B**) Opacity map shifted to right makes soft tissue translucent and bone opaque. (**C**) Opacity map shifted further to right makes soft tissue transparent and bone/iodine translucent. (**D**) Steep opacity function near iodine peak renders iodine/bone/opaque. (**E**) Same as (**D**) but with lighting turned off.

In many cases SSDs result in clear and even dramatic depiction of vascular anatomy; however, the threshold must be carefully picked, based on the intensity of the contrast material in the anatomy of interest. This is not always straightforward, because imperfect bolus timing, reduced flow distal to stenoses, noise and partial volume effects may result in nonuniform lumen intensity. As shown by Fig. 19-7, the choice of threshold strongly affects the depiction of stenosis degree. Also, choosing too low a threshold may cause noise and higher-density soft tissue to obscure the target vasculature; choosing too high a threshold may result in small vessels disappearing and/or stenoses falsely implied.

Another problem with SSD is that SSDs do not preserve CT gray-scale levels; that is, the reduction of the CT volume data to isodense surfaces eliminates the wide range of density values inherent in the CT data. Therefore displayed intensity in SSDs of blood vessels do not allow one to distinguish between calcified plaques and the contrast column. Further, dark regions, which might be mistaken for stenoses, can be produced because of the angle of the surface with respect

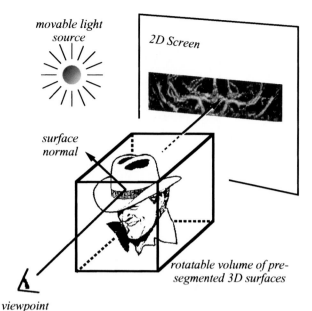

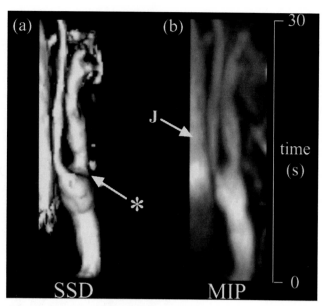

FIG. 19-8. Comparison of (**a**) SSD and (**b**) MIP in the extracranial carotid artery. Both images were computed from the same inferior-to-superior 30-s CTA acquisition. Note that both the SSD and the MIP show jugular enhancement (J) approximately 12 s into the acquisition. The apparent disruption of the external carotid artery (*) shown by SSD is not confirmed by MIP. This effect is most likely caused by reduced surface reflection due to the angle of the carotid bulb at this location with respect to the simulated light source.

FIG. 19-6. Three-dimensional reconstruction by shaded-surface display. The first step is to segment the volume, usually by using some type of thresholding, into mathematical descriptions of surfaces. Next, the user sets the viewing orientation and the location of one or many simulated lighting sources. As with volume rendering (see Fig. 19-2), the algorithm then casts rays along the viewing direction onto a hypothetical 2D screen. However, as soon as the ray intersects a surface, a lighting model based on the surface normal at the intersection and the location of the light source(s) is computed. The shade of gray (or color) assigned to each pixel depends on the lighting model. For example, a Lambertian lighting model results in reflections whose brightness depends only on the angle between rays from the light source to the surface location and the surface normal (84).

to the simulated light source (Fig. 19-8). However, because of the loss of depth-dependent information with MIP, there are some instances where SSDs depict anatomic relationships better then MIPs.

Maximum-Intensity Projection

Maximum-intensity projection, a simple form of VR, is widely used in MRA because of its improved contrast resolution compared with the average projection (6,51). A MIP image is easy to compute: the intensity of each pixel in a MIP image is the maximum intensity encountered along each projected ray (as shown in Fig. 19-3). Another advantage of MIP is that pixel values are represented quantitatively in Hounsfield units (HU). (For example, bone and calcified structures are bright and distinguishable from the iodinated contrast, soft tissue, and air by familiar brightness relationships.) Many examples of MIPs of CTA data appear in Chapters 20 and 21.

Pitfalls of MIP

Although MIP is simple to compute, is easy to understand, and has become very popular for rendering vascular structures from CT of MR data, it has several drawbacks. Many of these are nicely described in ref. 13 in the context of MRA. Although for CTA the concepts are similar, we present them

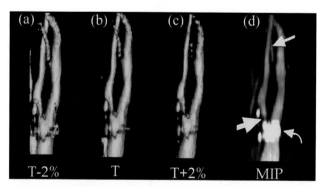

FIG. 19-7. Illustration of the sensitivity of SSD (**a–c**) to small changes in the chosen surface threshold compared with MIP (**d**). The threshold T was varied by 2% about that used in image B. The broad *arrow* shows a tight stenosis at the origin of the internal carotid artery superior to a heavily calcified carotid bulb (*curved arrow*). Note the varying degrees of stenosis depicted by SSD as a function of threshold and the loss of CT density information. Also note the change in depiction of a branch of the external carotid artery (*smaller straight arrow*) from continuous (**a**) through barely visible (**c**).

here with particular emphasis on the implications of using CT data.

Obscuration

Because MIP always projects the brightest pixel encountered along each ray, bone either in front of or behind a vascular structure will obscure it. Calcifications in the arterial wall, particularly when they are circumferential, can present a difficult problem, often obscuring the view of the vessel lumen. This is because the use of IV injections does not result in higher densities within arteries compared with bone and other calcified structures. Thus the use of MIP for CTA often requires preprocessing of the volume data to eliminate bone and other undesirable bright structures. Preprocessing is also useful for SSD and generalized VR, and will be discussed under "Other Variants of MIP."

Ambiguous Projection Direction

Because MIP causes a given structure to occlude another based on relative brightness alone (i.e., independent of relative spatial position), MIP does not provide a constant spatial perspective to the observer (52). First, MIP images are always ambiguous with respect to the antiparallel viewing directions (e.g., an anteroposterior [AP] MIP is simply the mirror image of a PA MIP). Second, MIP images display only the brightest features in the projection direction. These effects, combined with obscuration, may cause an apparent sudden reversal of rotation direction during viewing of a cine-loop. Even in a static MIP image, one must also remember that the bright structures are not the closest structures and may not be the most important or clinically relevant.

Data Loss

Consider for a moment that MIP is performed on a 512- × 512- × 100-voxel volume and produces a 512- × 512-pixel image. Because MIP projects only the maximum values found along rays drawn from the observer to the output image grid, the values selected by MIP for the output image are a very small subset of the input data. For example, if nearest-neighbor interpolation in the volume is used, the ratio of the number of voxels used to the number of voxels in the volume is less than or equal to 1%. Even if trilinear interpolation is used during the volume-sampling process, the ratio rises at most to 8%. The effects of this loss of data are several and depend on the voxel data. One effect is an increase in noise compared with, for example, an average projection, which uses all the voxel data. However, it is generally accepted that the increase in noise is more than compensated for by an increase in the contrast-to-noise ratio for the MIP image (53). Nonetheless, this severe reduction in data has been a major impetus to attempting to find a superior projection method (see the section entitled Other Variants of MIP).

Other effects are more subjective. For example, MIP images are often viewed by angiographers who compare them with conventional angiograms, which are similar to average projections through the entire volume, or at least through the vasculature (digital subtraction angiography [DSA]). However, conventional angiograms provide cues that are not available with MIP. The first cue results from the sensitivity of x-ray projections to vessel cross-section (54). Note that with an x-ray projection, the perceived vessel attenuation is a function of the length of the x-ray path through the vessel. As shown by Fig. 19-9, a vessel with a given normal lumen cross-section will exhibit higher attenuation than a vessel with the same normal cross-section but stenosed in the projection direction. This is not true with MIP, as only one voxel will be used per ray. Similarly, in conventional angiograms vessel loops or crossings attenuate the x-ray beam more than single vessels. MIPs do not provide this cue. However, since reprojections of volume data are performed retrospectively, MIP's lack of sensitivity to vessel cross-sections can be compensated for by generating views from multiple viewing directions. These views are often replayed on a video monitor in a movie loop to simulate a rotating viewing direction, providing cues as to eccentric stenoses and crossing or looping vessels.

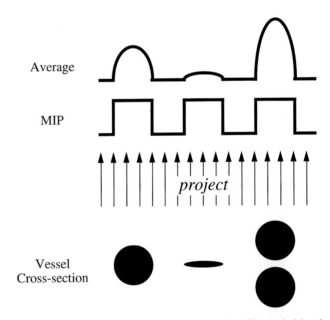

FIG. 19-9. Sensitivity to vessel cross-section. Example blood vessel cross-sections are shown at bottom, and results of MIP and average projections in the direction shown are above. Note that the average projection gives results similar to those afforded by conventional angiography with respect to vessel cross-section and overlap, yet MIP does not. For example, MIP gives the same result for elliptical and circular cross-sections; the average projection, on the other hand, projects less intensity in the direction shown for the elliptical vessel. Also, MIP is incapable of distinguishing two vessels positioned as shown at right; the average projection provides twice as much intensity in this case as it would for a single vessel.

Increase of Background Mean

Because MIP selects maxima from the distribution of intensities along each ray, the mean or average background value of the reprojected image increases as a function of projection thickness. (Fig. 19-10.) This phenomenon has been quantitatively analyzed (53,54), and several important clinical implications are exemplified in ref. 13 with regard to MRA. Because blood vessel conspicuity is directly related to the contrast-to-noise ratio, any effect that reduces this ratio will diminish the visibility of the vessel. That is, if the background mean rises, the contrast drops and, depending on the noise level, the vessel may become indistinguishable from the background. Thus the basic problem caused by an increase in background mean is the potential loss of blood vessel definition in regions where the blood "signal" is low.

In CTA, if the bolus of contrast material is administered correctly and the timing is successful, 200–400 HU (20% to 40%) of enhancement above the background may be expected. For large vessels (compared with the in-plane resolution) that run generally perpendicular to the acquired sections, the partial volume effect will decrease this contrast only at the edge of the vessel. However, in highly stenotic regions, partial volume can greatly diminish intensity within the vessel. Additional loss of contrast caused by MIP-induced background elevation may then cause the stenotic portion to disappear entirely. Flow distal to the disruption may be a clue that the "occlusion" is not real; restriction of the MIP to a small subvolume or inspection of the acquired sections may reveal a hidden "string sign." Note that the contrast of even normal vessels that course parallel to the transaxial plane and are small compared with the section

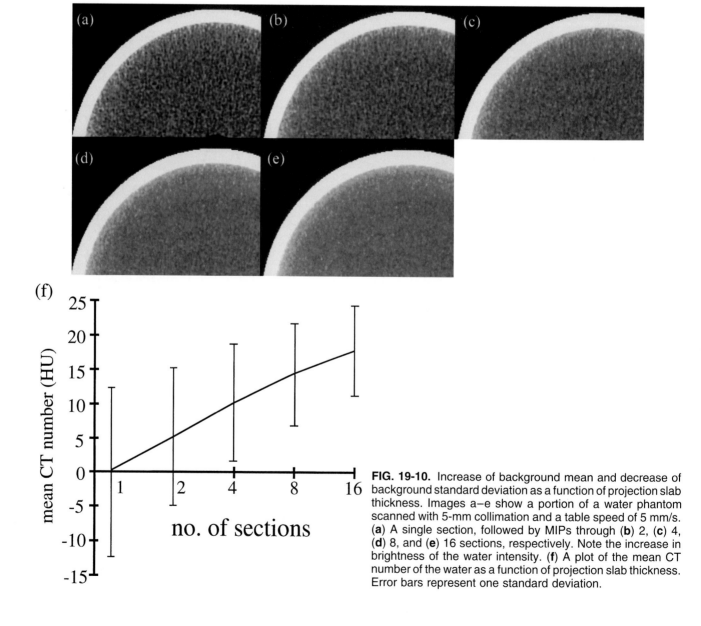

FIG. 19-10. Increase of background mean and decrease of background standard deviation as a function of projection slab thickness. Images a–e show a portion of a water phantom scanned with 5-mm collimation and a table speed of 5 mm/s. (**a**) A single section, followed by MIPs through (**b**) 2, (**c**) 4, (**d**) 8, and (**e**) 16 sections, respectively. Note the increase in brightness of the water intensity. (**f**) A plot of the mean CT number of the water as a function of projection slab thickness. Error bars represent one standard deviation.

thickness may also suffer from this effect and become invisible in MIPs through a large volume.

In CTA, background enhancement may also occur due to parenchymal perfusion and venous enhancement. Because the bolus is injected over an extended period of time, the slices that are acquired later in the sequence may have higher background values than earlier ones, and MIP will select them if they become higher than the vessel intensity. This effect is particularly common in the kidneys, where intrarenal arterial branches may become invisible. Also, CTAs of the circle of Willis in the brain almost always exhibit enhancement of the dural sinuses.

Resampling and MIP Artifacts

Cross-sectional imaging modalities fill a voxel grid with samples of an underlying distribution of intensities. Ideally, one would prefer to make the voxels as small as possible to be certain that the underlying structure is adequately represented. However, practical constraints, such as scanning time, adequate signal-to-noise ratio, and so on, serve to set a lower bound on voxel size. Today's CT scanners can reconstruct in-plane pixels as small as 0.5 mm, but the section thickness is never less than 1 mm and, using spiral CT, it is often three to five times larger than that.

To make matters worse, 3D reconstruction algorithms must resample the already sampled image data. This resampling operation can result in additional artifacts in the 3D images. The most common artifact, one of a class of artifacts known as "aliasing," can have a beaded or stair-step appearance of vessels that pass through the volume obliquely with respect to the voxel matrix (55). Resampling the voxel matrix using a finer grid than that given by the reconstructed voxels may reduce the aliasing, although this will greatly increase reconstruction time (13).

Maximum-intensity projection images often suffer from resampling artifacts. However, similar-appearing artifacts may also occur due to modulation of partial volume as a small vessel courses through the voxel grid. The cause of this so-called MIP artifact is illustrated by Fig 19-11. Acquiring and reconstructing the CT data on a finer grid will minimize resampling and MIP artifacts. However, once the data have been acquired and CT images reconstructed, not much can be done to eliminate the MIP artifact. Certainly, acquisitions in which there are gaps between acquired sections or in which the section profile is not "square" may exacerbate the effect. Reconstruction of overlapping sections, a particular strength of spiral CT for reduction of partial volume effects, may be the most effective means of minimizing this artifact. (See Chapter 1 for details.)

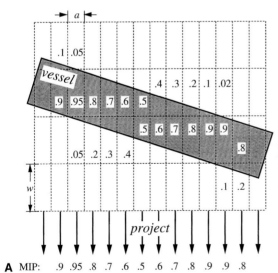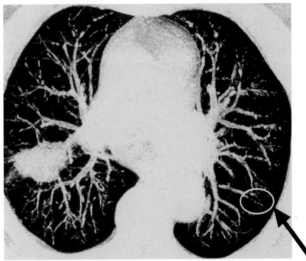

FIG. 19-11. (A) Two-dimensional illustration of the cause of MIP artifact. Suppose the gray rectangle represents a vessel passing through the stack of reconstructed images obliquely and that a MIP is computed down the columns of the pixel grid. *w* is the section width and *a* is the in-plane pixel size. Even if the vessel were uniform in intensity, the partial volume effect in the reconstructed images causes pixels to be computed with a fraction of the full intensity as shown. (Unlabeled pixels have zero intensity.) Thus the MIP has no choice but to pick out reduced maximum intensities that vary as a function of the percentage of the slice "filled" by the vessel at each position. Note that the example vessel has a width on the order of the section width size; larger vessels at this orientation to the grid may not show this effect. The width required to eliminate the artifact is dependent on the vessel orientation. **(B)** Example of a MIP through a 4-cm slab (collimator width: 1 mm; table speed: 1 mm/s) demonstrating the beaded appearance of MIP artifact. Note, for example, the vessel pictured within the white oval.

Sliding Thin-Slab (STS) MIP

Cross-sectional imaging, by its very nature, involves preselection of a volume of interest for scanning. If this is done properly, it may obviate the need for a great deal of preprocessing prior to MIP or other 3D rendering techniques. This is because selection of the volume to scan as a subset of the entire patient anatomy creates a window that, in some instances, may be free of overlying bone or other obscuring tissues. Consider, for example, the 1.6-cm slab of the circle of Willis portrayed using MIP in Fig. 19-12. Peering into the volume along the craniocaudal direction reveals much of the cerebral vasculature without the need for bone suppression. It is only the vessels near the skull that, because of the curvature of the skull, are obscured in the non-bone-suppressed MIP image. The individual acquired sections or, for that matter, any thin reformatted planes, also show blood vessels relatively unobscured. However, as stated previ-

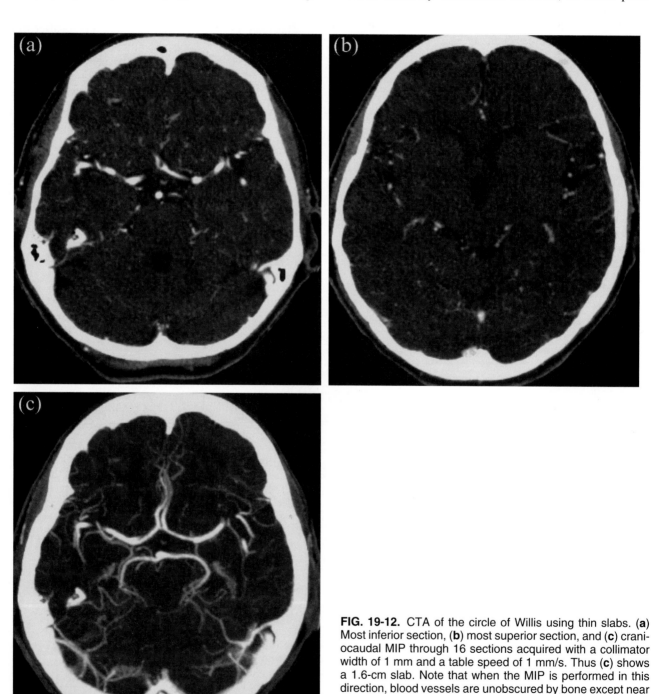

FIG. 19-12. CTA of the circle of Willis using thin slabs. **(a)** Most inferior section, **(b)** most superior section, and **(c)** craniocaudal MIP through 16 sections acquired with a collimator width of 1 mm and a table speed of 1 mm/s. Thus **(c)** shows a 1.6-cm slab. Note that when the MIP is performed in this direction, blood vessels are unobscured by bone except near the skull. Sliding thin-slab MIP exploits this possibility by reconstructing a sequence of overlapping thin-slab MIP images (typical slab width and overlap are 5 mm and 4 mm, respectively) for rapid movie-mode paging on a computer monitor.

ously, vascular anatomy is difficult to comprehend from cross-sectional images. This is primarily because blood vessels that are perpendicular or oblique to the section appear only as small circles or ellipses, and their connections to other structures and vessels are not generally visible in an individual section. A traditional method for overcoming this is to view the individual sections on a video monitor and rapidly page back and forth through the volume. By doing this, one attempts to mentally integrate the paths of vessels into a larger picture of vascular anatomy.

Sliding-thin-slab MIP (STS-MIP) (56), described in Fig. 19-13, is a technique that computes overlapping MIPs of limited depth to improve apparent vessel coherence when paged on a video monitor. As such, STS-MIP presents a compromise between spatial paging of this section and MIP of the entire acquired volume (including the necessity of preprocessing to suppress bone). A MIP over a few acquired sections has a contrast-to-noise ratio similar to that of each individual section (53), but vessels that transect the input sections at oblique angels are displayed over greater portions of their lengths. Though STS-MIP's major applications have been in the chest (57–59), the technique is also useful in other parts of the body (60,61). In its simplest form, thin slabs are comprised of a relatively small number of acquired transaxial sections. However, as shown by Fig. 19-13, slabs may also be oriented obliquely, with the possibility of interactive adjustment of slab orientation, position, and thickness.

Other Variants of MIP

The apparent simplicity of MIP and its attendant pitfalls have caused almost all users of the technique to search for a better algorithm. Two broad categories that may be used to organize the discussion are (a) preprocessing prior to MIP (similar to the techniques described in the next section) and (b) modifications or alternatives to MIP. The following paragraphs highlight some of these approaches and point the interested reader to relevant literature.

Approaches in the preprocessing category are based on image segmentation (i.e., the classification of voxels in the volume into categories of tissue). For CTA, we are interested in determining, prior to MIP, which voxels correspond to blood vessels and which do not. Vessel-tracking techniques (62,63) are similar to the connectivity-based approaches described under "Automatic Editing." However, rather than testing voxels adjacent to operator-selected "seed points" against a preset threshold, they adaptively adjust the threshold based on the statistics of the environment surrounding the voxel under test. The "connected voxel" algorithm (64) first divides the data set into cubical subsets and computes different thresholds for each. Voxels surviving the threshold are then grouped into a set of contiguous objects and objects smaller than a certain size are eliminated. Each object retains its unique identity and may be chosen (or not chosen) to be included in the MIP operation. Two other techniques, the "data adaptive reprojection technique (DART)" (65) and

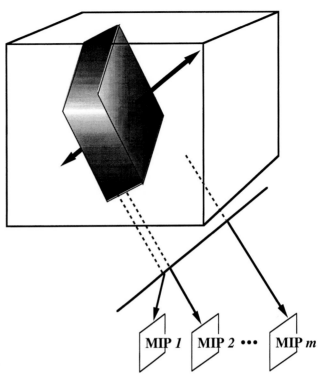

FIG. 19-13. Illustration of sliding thin-slab MIP (STS-MIP) in an oblique orientation. The operator first chooses an orientation and a thickness (mm) for the slab. Next, the computer produces a sequence of overlapping MIP images ("MIP 1," "MIP 2," etc.) by advancing the slab along the chosen axis. The MIP images have contrast-to-noise ratios similar to those for individual oblique sections, but vessels are visible over greater portions of their lengths. Playback of the resulting sequence in a movie-loop on a computer monitor can be an effective and simple alternative to extensive editing for appreciation of vascular anatomy and viewing of conventional rotating MIP sequences. In addition, interactive location, orientation, and thickness of the slab is an effective method for generating single images portraying desired vascular anatomy (61).

the "summed intensities or maximum projection (SIMP)" method (66), combine thresholded segmentation with both integral projection and MIP. "Traced ray by array processor (TRAP)" (67) uses a soft thresholding technique to weight voxels based on their probability of being contained within flow structures. Other preprocessing strategies are summarized in ref. 13.

Other algorithms are based on modifications to the MIP operation itself. For example, "intensity depth cueing" (52) weights voxel intensities in proportion to their distance from the observer. This weighting can be applied prior to or following MIP of each ray, with differing effects. The "consistent spatial perspective projection" algorithm (68) combines prior segmentation with MIP of only the vessels closest to the observer's viewpoint. Projection of various statistics (68,69) and the maximum spatial gradient (70) have also been explored. It is worth noting, however, that to date, none of these MIP variants has enjoyed the popularity of MIP for

MRA applications. Also, none of these approaches has yet been applied in the context of CTA. Because of the remaining problems with MIP, these and other approaches are likely to be developed further.

Preprocessing Techniques

For angiography, a primary advantage of volume data compared with projection data is the sheer amount of information available; however, this can also be a disadvantage if the additional information makes it hard to see the blood vessels of interest. Accordingly, much effort goes into what is loosely called "spatial editing" (i.e., the removal of tissues that obscure the structures of interest). In the next sections we illustrate these techniques for making usable CT angiograms out of properly timed, IV-enhanced CT volume data. Note that angiographic displays using MIP often require these preprocessing techniques to reduce the effects of obscuration by bone; however, generalized VRs and SSDs can benefit from their use as well.

Targeted Subvolume

The most obvious solution to the problem of over- or underlying bone is to eliminate it from the data set prior to the rendering operation. One can often simply "crop" the volume to isolate interior structures. User selection of the subvolume can be facilitated by providing an uncropped VR or MIP in an appropriate direction. A rectangle (or other simple shape) can then be drawn or traced on this reference image to represent the boundaries of a 3D solid object formed by "extruding" the tracing through the volume data in the direction perpendicular to the plane of the reference. Voxels of the volume that are outside the boundaries of the solid can then be ignored by the rendering algorithm. Figure 19-14 shows examples of using this method of subvolume selection to isolate different circulations in the circle of Willis prior to MIP. Targeting subregions in this way not only isolates the vessels of interest, but reduces the increase of the background intensity (see the preceding section entitled "Data Loss") and greatly speeds up the calculation. Note, however, that this technique may be inadequate for structures that curve in the direction of extrusion (e.g., the spine and the abdominal aorta).

Automatic Editing

Extrusion of simple shapes through a stack of reconstructed CT slices may not always result in complete elimination of unwanted structures. Another approach for removing calcified structures prior to reprojection is to exploit their high density and attempt to suppress them automatically. Simple thresholding (i.e., setting all pixels in the volume with density greater than some predetermined threshold to an arbitrarily low value, such as the "air" value of $-1,000$ HU, may be effective). However, it is not always possible to set the threshold low enough to suppress bones without suppressing vascular structures as well. If the threshold is too high, edges of bony structures with reduced intensity due to partial volume and other effects will not be detected. It is not uncommon for the CT intensities at these edges to be comparable to those found in contrast-enhanced blood vessels; therefore edges of bony structures might interfere with the display of the blood vessels in MIP images. Lowering the threshold by enough to eliminate the bone edges may cause vascular structures to be suppressed and appear falsely stenotic or disappear entirely.

Extensions of the thresholding approach have been used to suppress bone and other dense structures prior to 3D rendering for CTA (71). These methods are based on algorithms for spatial connectivity (72,73) and mathematical morphology (74). In brief, an operator selects a "seed point" in an axial slice that lies on a bony structure of interest, as shown in Fig. 19-15. Starting at the seed point, the algorithm searches the volume for other points that satisfy two conditions: (a) the candidate point must be above a predetermined threshold, and (b) the candidate point must be adjacent to (in any of the three coordinate directions) either the initial seed point itself or another point that has previously satisfied these two conditions. Thus the algorithm "grows" a region of connected voxels that contain the desired structure. These voxels can be "tagged" and set to low values prior to the rendering operation. As with straight thresholding, the choice of threshold for connectivity algorithms requires careful thought. Here too if the threshold is too high, the edges of the bony structure may not be tagged. However, because of the constraint of connectedness, lowering the threshold will not suppress *all* pixels in the volume above the new threshold—only the pixels connected to the structure. A lower threshold will, though, increase the possibility that the algorithm might "leak" from bone into an adjacent blood vessel and tag it and all other vessels connected (within the volume) to it.

Once a set of connected voxels has been determined, it can be manipulated in three dimensions to attempt to eliminate residual bone edges. One example is to use the morphological dilation operator (74) to "grow" the identified volume in space. Dilation convolves the binary image formed by the set of identified voxels with a blurring function and thereby includes additional voxels at the edges of the object. Since this operation is independent of threshold, leakage into adjacent structures cannot occur. However, overdilation can cause a part of a vessel that touches bone to be tagged, and there is a danger that in the final MIP reconstruction this will be falsely interpreted as a stenosis. Generally, using the lowest threshold possible that doesn't "leak," followed by dilation of the connected voxels by the order of the inplane pixel size, eliminates the residual edges, with minimal danger of removing parts of blood vessels (71). (Note that this technique was used to suppress the skull prior to computing the MIP images shown in Fig. 19-14.) Region-growing algorithms also may be used for suppressing structures other

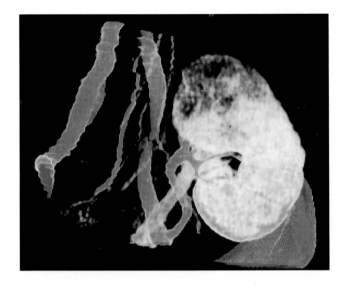

COLOR PLATE 13. Patent renal artery in a transplanted kidney. Spiral CT with 3D reconstruction demonstrates the patent renal artery anastomosis. Color enhancement can be helpful in select cases. Vessel patency could not be defined on the basis of axial images only.

CHAPTER 19

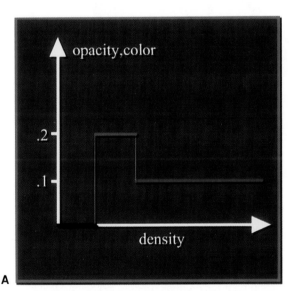

A

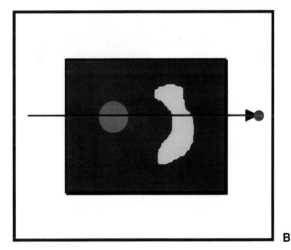

B

COLOR PLATES 14A and B. (**A**) Look-up table maps density to opacity and color; for example, in this case low-density voxels have zero opacity (i.e., are transparent), mid-density voxels have opacity of 0.2 per unit length and map to red, and higher-density voxels have opacity of 0.1 per unit length and map to blue. (**B**) Example of a ray passing through a single plane of voxels. Brighter shades of gray map to higher densities. According to look-up table (**A**), when the ray traverses the circle it accumulates twice the "amount" of red per voxel compared with the "amount" of blue it accumulates per voxel as it traverses the higher-density irregular shape. Other (low-density) tissue maps to zero opacity and therefore does not contribute to the exiting color and saturation. Assuming a ray does not saturate, the exit color is a mixture of red and blue. If the path length through the circle were large enough, ray could saturate before entering the irregular shape, resulting in an exit color of red. Note that look-up tables may be adjusted during rendering to adjust the relative visibilities of tissues with different densities.

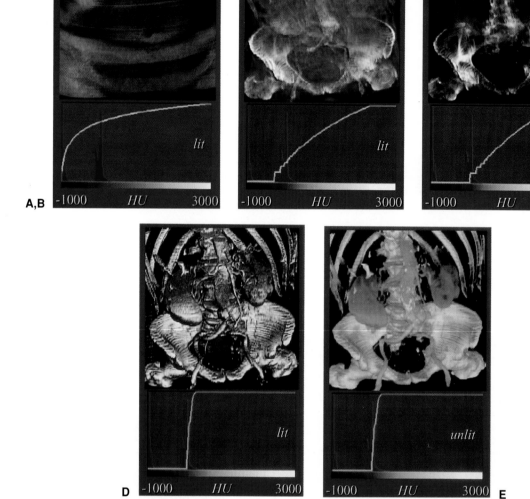

COLOR PLATES 15A, B, C, D, and E. Volume rendering with different opacity functions, color maps, and lighting. All images rendered at the same orientation in orthographic mode. Each sub-figure consists of a rendered image, voxel density histogram with superimposed opacity function, and color map, from top to bottom, respectively. First peak in histogram is air voxels, second is soft tissue, third is iodine/bone. (**A-D**) Lighting ON. (**E**) Lighting OFF. (**A**) Opacity map adjusted to saturate rays as soon as they enter soft tissue, thereby rendering skin surface. (**B**) Opacity map shifted to right makes soft tissue translucent and bone opaque. (**C**) Opacity map shifted further to right makes soft tissue transparent and bone/iodine translucent. (**D**) Steep opacity function near iodine peak renders iodine/bone/opaque. (**E**) Same as (d) but with lighting turned off.

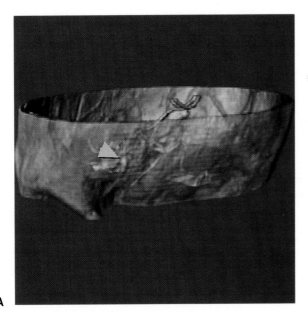

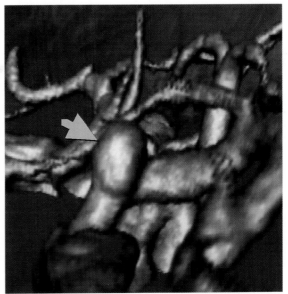

A

B

COLOR PLATES 16A and B. Example of perspective volume rendering in the circle of Willis. Image data is from a spiral CT scan of the brain following an IV injection of iodinated contrast material. Study parameters were: 1 mm collimation, 2 mm/s table speed for 25 s (covering 5 cm superiorly), image reconstruction interval 1 mm. (**A**) External perspective volume rendered view. Skull (rendered semi-transparently in shades of gray) obscures view of carotid artery aneurysm (arrow). (**B**) Internal perspective with observer positioned between the skull and the aneurysm (arrow). "Flying around" inside skull allows precise visualization of the neck of the aneurysm and determination of the best surgical approach. Both images were rendered with Voxel View 2.5.3 software (Vital Images, Inc., Fairfield, IA) with 40-degree field of view.

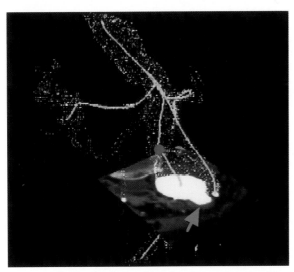

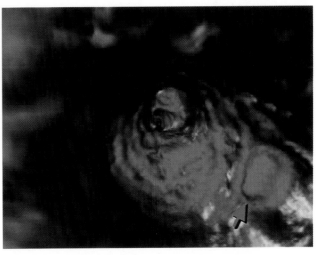

A

B

COLOR PLATES 17A and B. Example of use of perspective volume rendering for virtual angioscopy. (**A**) The technique proposed by Paik (85,86) starts by segmenting the blood vessel (cloud of white points) from its surroundings and iteratively thins the segmented vessel until only the central axis (*yellow lines*) remains. Next, a sequence of tomograms perpendicular to the path is generated; one such tomo-gram is shown through the ulcerated portion (*green arrow*) of an abdominal aortic aneurysm. In addition, the path is used to orient a sequence of internal perspective volume-rendered views. Virtual endoscopic view from the interior of the aneurysm at the blue dot in image A looking inferiorly along path. *Green arrow* shows ulceration matching green arrow on tomogram in image A. Image B is one frame of a movie sequence rendered along path with Voxel View 2.5.3 software (Vital Images, Inc., Fairfield, IA) with 70-degree field of view.

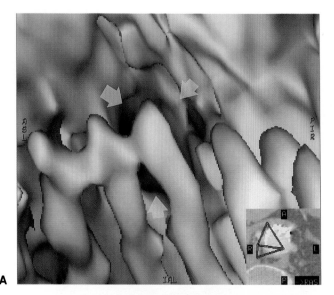

A

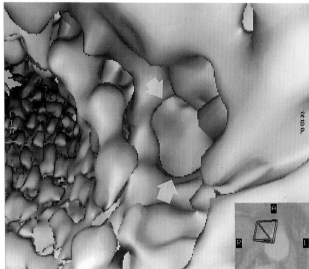

B

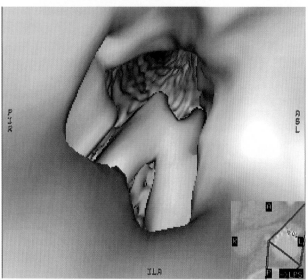

C

COLOR PLATES 18A, B, and C. Perspective SSD from a viewpoint 10 cm cephalad in the aorta, looking down on the renal artery origin, demonstrates how the steep angulation of the right renal artery origin preserves a conduit for right renal blood flow. The apparent degree of renal ostial occlusion is highly dependent on the view angle and overestimated by the CPRs. Perspective SSD from within the aorta looking right lateral demonstrates the metallic endoskeleton of the stent-graft (red) covering most the right renal artery osteum (*arrows*) View from within the right renal artery, looking out into the aorta, also demonstrates the pathway for flow around the stent-graft.

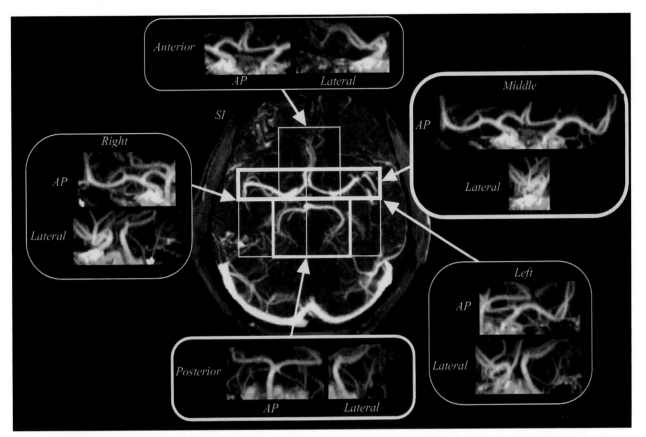

FIG. 19-14. Targeted reconstructions of the circle of Willis. The central image is a MIP performed through a 3-cm slab in the craniocaudal direction. Next, five rectangles representing the anterior, left, right, middle, and posterior circulations are superimposed on the superoinferior (SI) MIP and extruded through the volume. These rectangles are uniquely specified by 11 numbers representing the x and y coordinates of a subset of the corners of the set of rectangles. (For example, the y coordinate of the posterior aspect of the middle circulation is the same as the y coordinate of the anterior aspect of the posterior circulation.) Finally, a sequence of MIPs perpendicular to the SI axis over 180 degrees at 6-degree increments is calculated for each of the five circulations. These five sequences can be calculated in parallel in less than 5 min. The figure shows representative AP and lateral projections through the five targeted regions with the rounded-box outline thickness matching the appropriate rectangles drawn on the SI MIP. (Note that the connectivity/region growing algorithm, described under "Maximum Intensity Projection" was run to suppress the skull prior to MIP of the acquired volume data.)

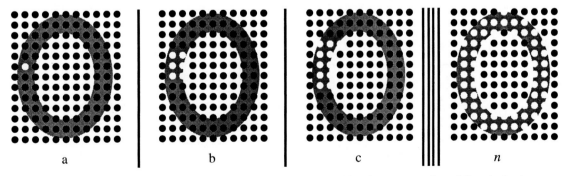

a   b   c   *n*

FIG. 19-15. Two-dimensional illustration of connectivity algorithm for suppression of the skull, shown in gray. (**a**) The operator selects a seed pixel, shown in white. (**b**) The algorithm identifies and tags any neighbors of the seed pixel that are above a preset threshold. These are shown in white. (**c**) The algorithm identifies all neighbors of all newly tagged pixels that are above the threshold, and tags these. (***n***) The algorithm continues until the entire "skull" is tagged. Extension of this 2D example to 3D is straightforward.

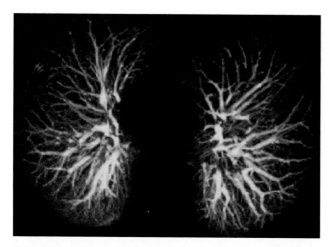

FIG. 19-16. Example of use of connectivity for suppression of chest and mediastinum prior to MIP in the superoinferior direction. The volume was acquired using two breath-held 30-s spiral acquisitions, each covering 9 cm along the superoinferior axis, for a total coverage of 18 cm.

than bone. For example, Fig. 19-16 illustrates tagging and suppressing the chest wall and mediastinum for a clearer view of the blood vessels of the lungs.

Different challenges exist for almost every clinical application of CTA display. As a result, many heuristic approaches have also been developed for specific tasks. For instance, Hentschel proposed a flood-fill and region growing technique to isolate the lungs and heart from a thoracic CT volume, and a rule-based and region growing technique to identify the spine and ribs for suppression in an abdominal CTA scan (75). Similar results have been reported by Fishman (76). Shiffman (77) proposed a semi-automated technique utilizing a neural network to classify voxels, followed by manual point-and-click editing of a small subset of the acquired sections for abdominal CTA (Fig. 19-17). Automated detection of the 3D contour of the liver has been demonstrated using elastic deformable models (78). Flexible registration and subtraction of a precontrast volume has also demonstrated potential utility for the segmentation of bolus-injected blood vessels (75,79).

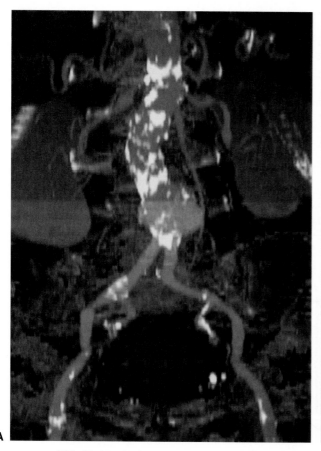
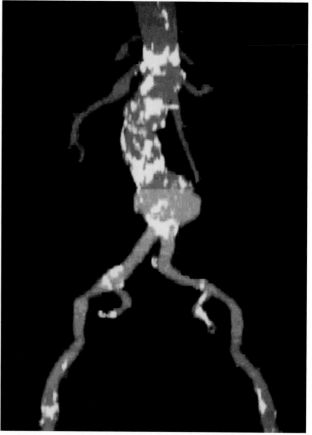

A   B

FIG. 19-17. Abdomen–pelvis CTA. Patient with abdominal aortic aneurysm. **(A)** Automated bone-editing using connectivity and dilation (71). Note that because of partial volume averaging, edges of spine and pelvic bone are not removed, nor are any soft-tissue components, which results in low image contrast. **(B)** Automated segmentation of aorta and branches using neural network and manual region selection on 5 of the 138 sections (77) results in complete removal of spine and soft tissue for higher vessel/background contrast.

Manual Editing

The preceding approaches are actually special cases of *volume editing:* the removal of structures from a volume. There may be instances where the suppression of undesired structures cannot be handled by targeting simple subvolumes or by the automatic techniques described earlier. As an example, consider Fig. 20-6, which shows several versions of CTA of the abdominal aorta. The MIP through the volume that has had only the spine suppressed shows a clear rendition of the lumen of this aortic aneurysm. But there is much more information in this study than that provided by a depiction of the opacified lumen. The cross-sectional image not only shows the lumen but also reveals intraluminal thrombus and aneurysm size, information which is clearly absent from the MIP. Figure 20-6E shows, on a representative slice, a region of interest (ROI) that was manually traced prior to computing the MIP shown in Fig. 20-6F. All pixels within the closed trace of (Fig. 20-6E) were retained, and the remaining pixels were set to a suitable low value. The CTA study consisted of 90 reconstructed CT sections; thus manual tracing was performed on 90 images prior to MIP—a nontrivial task requiring a steady hand, patience, and a knowledge of anatomy. Although this may not yet be practical to perform on a routine clinical basis, it does illustrate the wealth of information inherent in the CT slices that might be preserved should more efficient editing schemes become available. Virtually all the information that the vascular surgeon wants to know is present in the preedited MIP image: juxtarenal abdominal aortic aneurysm, 7-cm maximum extent, terminating superior to the iliac bifurcation.

Manual volume-editing programs are available on several scanners and workstation products that provide options for making the editing process more efficient than that described earlier. For example, one technique permits the assumption that there may be close similarities between traces on adjacent slices; it therefore lets the user copy a trace from one slice to the next, and modify it slightly if necessary, without having to redraw it in its entirety. Another technique allows the user to manipulate the stack of slices as a volume, adjust its orientation in three dimensions, and trace within planes of arbitrary orientation to surround or exclude voxels to be suppressed (80). Another very powerful technique, similar to the targeted subvolume approach described earlier, allows the user to compute and view an arbitrarily oriented MIP in real time while attempting to obtain a view angle in which the undesired structure can be removed by tracing a ROI on the MIP and extruding it through the reoriented volume.

Manual editing, can be *inclusive* or *exclusive. Inclusive* editing involves designation, by tracing or other means, of the volumes of interests to *include* in the MIP process. That is, all voxels outside these regions will be set to low values prior to rendering. On the other hand, *exclusive* editing involves the designation of volumes of interest to *exclude* from the rendering process. Thus all voxels within these regions will be suppressed prior to rendering. The choice of inclusive versus exclusive editing is usually based on expediency. For example, it is often simpler to use exclusive editing when one relatively small structure requires suppression for adequate visualization of another larger structure. Alternatively, inclusive editing would be chosen when the desired target structure is relatively small and simple to define. Both techniques require knowledge of anatomy and pathological possibilities, and each results in a different image. Thus it is important to consider the assumptions and implications of each technique, summarized in Table 19-2, before choosing an approach.

Use of Perspective

Shaded-surface display, generalized VR, and MIP techniques can be implemented in nonperspective and perspective modes. The nonperspective mode, which until recently was

TABLE 19-2. *Comparison and implications of inclusive and exclusive manual editing approaches*

Inclusive editing	Exclusive editing
Significance of Tracing Errors	
Since tracing occurs at the edges of target structures, great care must be exercised. Tracing errors of even a pixel may result in false stenotic appearance.	In general, tracing errors are less serious because they will not directly affect the target vessels. Exceptions occur when target vessels are adjacent to structures being removed; in this case, tracing errors can be as serious.
Reproducibility of Interpretation	
Since tracing occurs at the edges of target structures, inter- and intraoperator reproducibility may be lower than desired.	Because editing, in general, occurs at a distance from the target vessels, reproducibility may be less sensitive to tracing errors.
Image Contrast	
Displays tend to be of higher contrast, because by concentrating on only the target vessels, all other structures, including bone and soft tissue, are eliminated.	Because exclusive editing generally targets relatively small bright structures for removal, the remaining undesired soft tissue may result in displays with lower contrast.

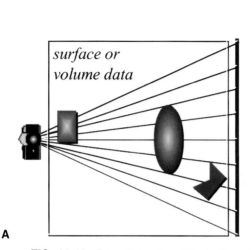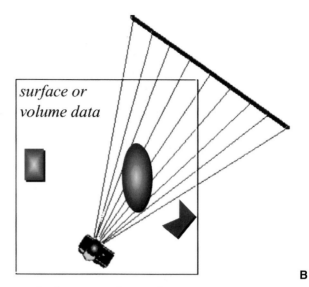

A
B

FIG. 19-18. Two-dimensional illustration of the geometry for perspective rendering, with observer at the camera and the rendering screen at the thick black line. The camera field of view is effectively the angle of the vertex at the observer. (**A**) Observer's view of the top portion of the ellipse is obscured by the rectangle. (**B**) Observer's viewpoint has moved to view ellipse from below; also, the rectangle no longer obscures the ellipse, which now fills more of the screen (and therefore appears larger) than it did from the prior viewpoint. The polygon is now outside of the field of view and is no longer a part of the image rendered on the screen. This type of "fly-around" may eliminate a major portion of the editing that is currently done for CTA; rather than attempting to identify and remove obscuring tissues, the user will simply move in to focus on the structure(s) of interest.

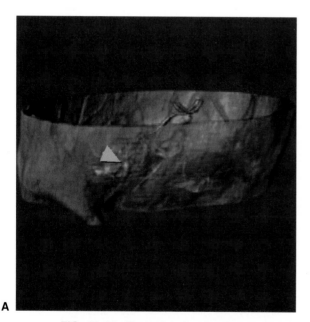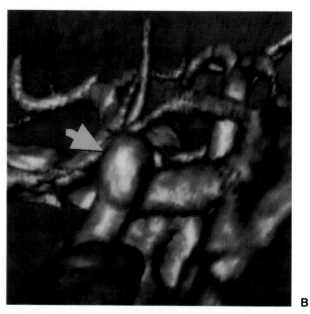

A
B

FIG. 19-19. Example of perspective volume rendering in the circle of Willis. Image data are from a spiral CT scan of the brain following an IV injection of iodinated contrast material. Study parameters were as follows: 1-mm collimation, 2-mm/s table speed for 25 s (covering 5 cm superiorly), image reconstruction interval 1 mm. (**A**) External perspective volume rendered view. Skull (rendered semitransparently in shades of gray) obscures view of carotid artery aneurysm (*arrow*). (**B**) Internal perspective with observer positioned between the skull and the aneurysm (*arrow*). "Flying around" inside skull allows precise visualization of the neck of the aneurysm and determination of the best surgical approach. Both images were rendered with Voxel View 2.5.3 software (Vital Images, Inc., Fairfield, IA) with 40-degree field of view.

vastly more popular in medical imaging applications, casts parallel rays along a chosen viewing direction to render a 2D image as it might be seen from that orientation. Parallel ray casting is mathematically equivalent to locating the observer at an infinite distance from the observed volume. It is simpler computationally than divergent ray casting, which is required if the observer is to be allowed to view the volume from finite distances, but does not simulate the human visual system. Figure 19-18 shows a 2D example of perspective rendering; it illustrates the ability of the observer to position him- or herself between an obscuring structure and an object of interest. The figure also illustrates the cues offered by the relative changes of the sizes of objects as the observer moves into the volume. Figure 19-19 shows an example of using perspective volume rendering in the circle of Willis to view a carotid artery aneurysm (see color plate 16 following p. 352).

Perspective rendering has created a whole new possibility for the exploration of 3D volume data that has been called virtual endoscopy (36,45,47,48,50). Figure 19-20 illustrates the use of this technique for angiographic applications (see color plate 17 following p. 351). Additional applications and examples can be found in Chapter 3.

Curved-Plane Reformatting

An alternative to reprojection for visualizing vascular anatomy is oblique-plane reformatting (OPR) (i.e., extracting an oblique plane from the volume data). The algorithm is simple: The output image is assumed to lie in a plane transecting the volume and, for each pixel on the plane, a value is interpolated from its nearest neighbors in the volume. An advantage of OPR is that it produces a cross-sectional image, much like a CT slice that might have been obtained if it were possible to orient the gantry to scan that plane directly. Thus voxels interior to a vessel are not hidden by the projection process, and as a result, OPR is particularly effective at revealing the vascular lumen within calcified vessel walls. However, because vessels seldom run in planes for significant portions of their lengths, an extension of OPR, called curved-plane reformatting (CPR), may be useful. This technique involves operator specification, usually by tracing a contour on an acquired slice or an SI MIP, of a curved surface, as shown in Fig. 20-15. Note, however, that the interpolation process used to extract pixels on the surface of the plane effectively averages neighboring voxels and therefore may result in reduced and spatially varying resolution. Also, because the surface is usually one pixel thick, the technique is particularly sensitive to tracing errors, whereby stenoses may be falsely implied because of the averaging of blood and surrounding tissue and the resulting apparent decrease in vessel intensity. Furthermore, CPR shows only a thin slice through a portion of the vessel. Thus a CPR image computed at one position or orientation along the axis of even a large vessel may not show important morphology that might be revealed by using a different position or orientation.

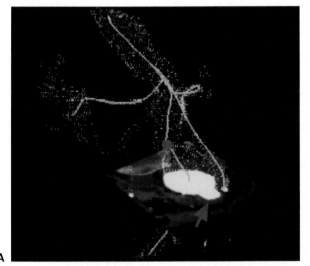

A

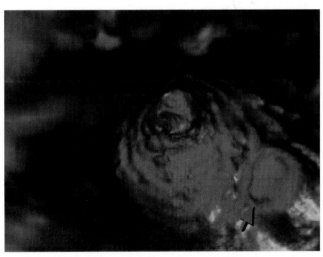

B

FIG. 19-20. Example of use of perspective volume rendering for virtual angioscopy. **(A)** The technique proposed by Paik (85,86) starts by segmenting the blood vessel (cloud of white points) from its surroundings and iteratively thins the segmented vessel until only the central axis (*yellow lines*) remains. Next, a sequence of tomograms perpendicular to the path is generated; one such tomogram is shown through the ulcerated portion (*green arrow*) of an abdominal aortic aneurysm. In addition, the path is used to orient a sequence of internal perspective volume-rendered views. **(B)** Virtual endoscopic view from the interior of the aneurysm at the blue dot in image A looking inferiorly along path. *Green arrow* shows ulceration matching green arrow on tomogram in **(A)**. Image **(B)** is one frame of a movie sequence rendered along path with Voxel View 2.5.3 software (Vital Images, Inc., Fairfield, IA) with 70-degree field of view.

SUMMARY

By increasing the number of sections that can be acquired per unit time, spiral CT has created the possibility for creating 3D angiograms from continuously acquired CT volume data (i.e., CT angiography). This chapter has described the technique, including bolus timing, protocol selection, and 3D reconstruction. Chapters 20 and 21 give examples of specific applications in the abdomen, neck, and brain. Investigations of other potential angiographic applications—including the lungs, thoracic aorta, pelvis, and the peripheral vasculature—are already in progress. Neither CTA nor any of several other vascular imaging techniques, such as Doppler ultrasound and magnetic resonance angiography, have yet unseated the "gold standard" of conventional intra-arterial angiography. But careful study over time may see one or several of these techniques replace conventional angiography in selected applications.

This chapter discussed many possibilities for 3D rendering of CT angiograms. After reading all of this, perhaps the most difficult question to answer is, "With the large number of images reconstructed for each patient, including both acquired sections and the many types of global and targeted 3D reconstructions, which images do I need to look at to make the proper interpretation?"

Our opening premise was that inspection of the acquired sections is not the most intuitive method for comprehending complex vascular structures. And 3D reconstructions, of which the most popular is MIP, are full of pitfalls, which can lead to false diagnosis. In the meantime, the job of the radiologist reading CTA exams is somewhat like that of the conventional angiographer, except that manipulations will be done retrospectively on computer data rather than prospectively on the patient. That is, it is necessary to explore the data from the suspect region in an attempt to confirm the presence of the pathological state, followed by use of one or more of the "tools" at hand to create views of the abnormality that demonstrate it best (50). These tools may include filmed images of MIPs and SSDs, rotating movie loops, STS-MIP movie loops, targeted subregion MIPs or SSDs, perspective "fly-around" or "fly-through" views, or even several of the acquired sections. Recall that all the information available is inherent and perhaps in its purest form in the acquired sections. These images can be used directly or for confirmation of a suspicion raised upon viewing the 3D renderings.

ACKNOWLEDGMENTS

I offer sincere thanks to my physician collaborators, including Michael D. Dake, Dieter R. Enzmann, Robert J. Herfkens, R. Brooke Jeffrey, Jr., David A. Katz, Michael P. Marks, Alexander M. Norbash, Geoffrey D. Rubin, and Gary K. Steinberg. In addition, I am grateful to David S. Paik, Ramin Shahidi, and Smadar Shiffman for technical contributions. I gratefully acknowledge support from Siemens Medical Systems, the Lucas Foundation, the Whitaker Foundation, and General Electric Medical Systems. Finally, thanks to my wife, Lyn Furness, my son Walt, and my daughter Madeline, who offer continued support and encouragement and put up with my frequent absences to get things like this done.

REFERENCES

1. Doby T. *Development of angiography and cardiovascular catheterization.* Littleton, MA: Publishing Sciences Group; 1976.
2. Dos Santos R, Lamas AC, Caldas JP. L'artériographie des membres de l'aorte et de ces branches abdominales. *Bull Soc Nat Chir* 1929;55: 587–601.
3. Seldinger SI. Catheter replacement of the needle in percutaneous arteriography: a new technique. *Acta Rad* 1953;87(suppl):1.
4. O'Donnell M. NMR blood flow imaging using multiecho, phase contrast sequences. *Med Phys* 1985;12:59–64.
5. Pelc NJ, Herfkens RJ, Shimakawa A, Enzmann DR. Phase contrast cine magnetic resonance imaging. *Magn Reson Quart* 1991;7:229–254.
6. Laub GA. MR angiography with gradient motion refocussing. *J Comput Assist Tomogr* 1988;12:377–382.
7. Runge VM, Gelblum DY. Future directions in magnetic resonance contrast media. *Top Magn Reson Imaging* 1991;3:85–97.
8. Holland GA, Dougherty L, Carpenter JP, et al. Breath-hold ultrafast three-dimensional gadolinium-enhanced MR angiography of the aorta and the renal and other visceral abdominal arteries. *AJR* 1996;166: 971–981.
9. Korosec FR, Frayne R, Grist TM, Mistretta CA. Time-resolved contrast-enhanced 3D MR angiography. Magn Reson Med 1996;36: 345–351.
10. Cloft HJ, Murphy KJ, Prince MR, Brunberg JA. 3D gadolinium-enhanced MR angiography of the carotid arteries. *Magn Reson Imaging* 1996;14:593–600.
11. Krinsky GA, Rofsky NM, DeCorato DR, et al. Thoracic aorta: comparison of gadolinium-enhanced three-dimensional MR angiography with conventional MR imaging. *Radiology* 1997;202:183–193.
12. Bass JC, Prince MR, Londy FJ, Chenevert TL. Effect of gadolinium on phase-contrast MR angiography of the renal arteries. *AJR* 1997;168: 261–266.
13. Siebert JE, Rosenbaum TL. Image presentation and post-processing. In: Potchen EJ, Haacke EM, Siebert JE, Gottschalk A, eds. *Magnetic resonance angiography: concepts and applications.* St. Louis: Mosby; 1993;220–245.
14. Mistretta CA. Relative characteristics of MR angiography and competing vascular imaging modalities. *J Magn Res Imag* 1993;3:685–698.
15. Abrams HL, ed. *Angiography,* Boston: Little, Brown; 1971.
16. Pelz DM, Fox AJ, Vineula F. Techniques and risks of cerebral angiography. In: Taveras JM, Ferrucci JT, eds. *Neuroradiology and radiology of the head and neck.* Philadelphia: JB Lippincott; 1986:1–14.
17. Chopra S, Ghiatas AA, Encarnacion CE, et al. Transjugular intrahepatic portosystemic shunts: assessment with helical CT angiography. *Radiology* 1997;202:277–280.
18. Alberico RA, Patel M, Casey S, Jacobs B, Maguire W, Decker R. Evaluation of the circle of Willis with three-dimensional CT angiography in patients with suspected intracranial aneurysms. *Am J Neuroradiol* 1995;16:1571–1578; discussion 1579–1580.
19. Wilms G, Guffens M, Gryspeerdt S, et al. Spiral CT of intracranial aneurysms: correlation with digital subtraction and magnetic resonance angiography. *Neuroradiology* 1996;38(suppl 1):S20–S25.
20. Katz DA, Marks MP, Napel SA, Bracci PM, Roberts SL. Circle of Willis: evaluation with spiral CT angiography, MR angiography, and conventional angiography. *Radiology* 1995;195:445–449.
21. van Erkel AR, van Rossum AB, Bloem JL, Kievit J, Pattynama PM. Spiral CT angiography for suspected pulmonary embolism: a cost-effectiveness analysis. *Radiology* 1996;201:29–36.
22. Remy-Jardin M, Remy J, Deschildre F, et al. Diagnosis of pulmonary embolism with spiral CT: comparison with pulmonary angiography and scintigraphy. *Radiology* 1996;200:699–706.
23. Schnyder P, Chapuis L, Mayor B, et al. Helical CT angiography for traumatic aortic rupture: correlation with aortography and surgery in five cases. *J Thorac Imaging* 1996;11:39–45.
24. Hunink MG, Boss JJ. Triage of patients to angiography for detection of aortic rupture after blunt chest trauma: cost-effectiveness analysis of using CT. *AJR* 1995;165:27–36.

25. Rieker O, Duber C, Schmiedt W, von Zitzewitz H, Schweden F, Thelen M. Prospective comparison of CT angiography of the legs with intraarterial digital subtraction angiography. *AJR* 1996;166:269–276.

26. Rubin GD, Dake MD, Napel S, et al. Spiral CT of renal artery stenosis: comparison of three-dimensional rendering techniques. *Radiology* 1994;190:181–189.

27. Galanski M, Prokop M, Chavan A, Schaefer CM, Jandeleit K, Nischelsky JE. Renal arterial stenoses: spiral CT angiography. *Radiology* 1993; 189:185–192.

28. Liang Y, Kruger RA. Dual-slice spiral versus single-slice spiral scanning: comparison of the neuroradiology and radiology of the head and neck: physical performance of two computed tomography scanners. *Med Phys* 1996;23:205–220.

29. van Hoe L, Marchal G, Baert AL, Gryspeerdt S, Mertens L. Determination of scan delay time in spiral CT-angiography: utility of a test bolus injection. *J Comput Assist Tomogr* 1995;19:216–220.

30. Wright AR, Collie DA, Williams JR, Hashemi-Malayeri B, Stevenson AJ, Turnbull CM. Pulmonary nodules: effect on detection of spiral CT pitch. *Radiology* 1996;199:837–841.

31. Rubin GD, Napel S. Increased scan pitch for vascular and thoracic spiral CT [Letter]. *Radiology* 1995;197:316.

32. Diederichs CG, Keating DP, Glatting G, Oestmann JW. Blurring of vessels in spiral CT angiography: effects of collimation width, pitch, viewing plane, and windowing in maximum intensity projection. *J Comput Assist Tomogr* 1996;20:965–974.

33. Mankovich NJ, Robertson DR, Cheeseman AM. Three-dimensional image display in medicine. J Digit Imaging 1990;3:69–80.

34. Strong AB, Lobregt S, Zonneveld FW. Applications of three-dimensional display techniques in medical imaging. *J Biomed Eng* 1990;12: 233–238.

35. Henri CJ, Pike GB, Collins DL, Peters TM. Three-dimensional display of cortical anatomy and vasculature: magnetic resonance angiography versus multimodality integration. *J Digit Imaging* 1991;4:21–27.

36. Davis RE, Levoy M, Rosenman JG, et al. Three-dimensional high-resolution volume rendering (HRVR) of computed tomography data: applications to otolaryngology—head and neck surgery. *Laryngoscope* 1991;573–582.

37. Levoy M. Methods for improving the efficiency and versatility of volume rendering. *Prog Clin Biol Res* 1991;363:473–488.

38. Kuszyk BS, Heath DG, Ney DR, et al. CT angiography with volume rendering: imaging findings. *AJR* 1995;165:445–448.

39. Johnson PT, Heath DG, Kuszyk BS, Fishman EK. CT angiography with volume rendering: advantages and applications in splanchnic vascular imaging. *Radiology* 1996;200:564–568.

40. Magnusson M, Lenz R, Danielsson PE. Evaluation of methods for shaded surface display of CT volumes. *Comput Med Imaging Graph* 1991;15:247–256.

41. Cline HE, Lorensen WE, Souza SP, et al. 3D surface rendered MR images of the brain and its vasculature. *J Comput Assist Tomogr* 1991; 15:344–351.

42. Link J, Mueller-Huelsbeck S, Brossmann J, Grabener M, Stock U, Heller M. Prospective assessment of carotid bifurcation disease with spiral CT angiography in surface shaded display (SSD)-technique. *Comput Med Imaging Graph* 1995;19:451–456.

43. Liang EY, Chan M, Hsiang JH, et al. Detection and assessment of intracranial aneurysms: value of CT angiography with shaded-surface display. *AJR* 1995;165:1497–1502.

44. Halpern EJ, Wechsler RJ, DiCampli D. Threshold selection for CT angiography shaded surface display of the renal arteries. *J Digit Imaging* 1995;8:142–147.

45. Rubin GD, Beaulieu CF, Argiro V, et al. Perspective volume rendering of CT and MR images: applications for endoscopic viewing. *Radiology* 1996;199:321–330.

46. Davis CP, Ladd ME, Romanowski BJ, Wildermuth S, Knoplioch JF, Debatin JF. Human aorta: preliminary results with virtual endoscopy based on three-dimensional MR imaging data sets. *Radiology* 1996; 199:37–40.

47. Napel S, Rubin GD, Beaulieu CF, Jeffrey Jr. RB, Argiro V. Perspective volume rendering of cross-sectional images for simulated endoscopy and intra-parenchymal viewing. *Medical Imaging '96*. Newport Beach, CA: SPIE; 2707:75–86.

48. Lorensen WE, Jolesz FA, Kikinis R. The exploration of cross-sectional data with a virtual endoscope. In: Satava RM, Morgan K, Sieburg HB,

Mattheus R, Christensen JP, eds. *Interactive technology and the new paradigm for health care: medicine meets virtual reality. III Proceedings.* Amsterdam: IOS Press; 1995:221–230.

49. Lacroute P, Levoy M. Fast volume rendering using a shear-warp factorization of the viewing transformation. In: *Computer graphics proceedings.* New York: SIGGRAPH Conference Proceedings; 1994:451–458.

50. Rubin GD, Napel S, Leung AN. Volumetric analysis of volumetric data: achieving a paradigm shift. *Radiology* 1996;200:312–317.

51. Keller PJ, Drayer BP, Fram EK, Williams KD, Dumoulin CL, Souza SP. MR angiography with two-dimensional acquisition and three-dimensional display. *Radiology* 1989;173:527–532.

52. Siebert JE, Rosenbaum TL. Projection algorithm imparting consistent spatial perspective. 9th Society of Magnetic Resonance in Medicine, 1:60, New York, 1990.

53. Brown DG, Riederer SJ. Contrast-to-noise ratios in maximum intensity projection images. *Magn Reson Med* 1992;23:130–137.

54. Cline HE, Dumoulin CL, Lorensen WE, Souza SP, Adams WJ. Volume rendering and connectivity algorithms for MR angiography. *Magn Reson Med* 1991;18:384–394.

55. Anderson CM, Saloner D, Tsuruda JS, Shapeero LG, Lee RE. Artifacts in maximum-intensity-projection display of MR angiograms. *AJR* 1990;154:623–629.

56. Napel S, Rubin GD, Jeffrey RB Jr. STS-MIP: a new reconstruction technique for CT of the chest. *J Comput Assist Tomogr* 1993;17: 832–838.

57. Bhalla M, Naidich DP, McGuinness G, Gruden JF, Leitman BS, McCauley DI. Diffuse lung disease: assessment with helical C: preliminary observations of the role of maximum and minimum intensity projection images [see comments]. *Radiology* 1996;200:341–347.

58. Remy-Jardin M, Remy J, Gosselin B, Copin MC, Wurtz A, Duhamel A. Sliding thin slab, minimum intensity projection technique in the diagnosis of emphysema: histopathologic-CT correlation. *Radiology* 1996;200:665–671.

59. Remy-Jardin M, Remy J, Artaud D, Deschildre F, Duhamel A. Diffuse infiltrative lung disease: clinical value of sliding-thin-slab maximum intensity projection CT scans in the detection of mild micronodular patterns [see comments]. *Radiology* 1996;200:333–339.

60. Yen SY, Rubin GD, Napel S. Fast sliding thin slab volume rendering. IEEE Symposium on Volume Visualization, 1:79–86, San Francisco, 1996.

61. Yen SY, Rubin GD, Napel S. Sliding thin slab visualization of CT and MR angiograms. RSNA-EJ; (http://ej.rsna.org)1:1997.

62. Hu X, Alperin N, Levin DN, Tan KK, Mengeot M. Visualization of MR angiographic data with segmentation and volume-rendering techniques. *J Magn Reson Imaging* 1991;1:539–546.

63. Lin W, Haacke EM, Smith AS, Clampitt ME. Gadolinium-enhanced high-resolution MR angiography with adaptive vessel tracking: preliminary results in the intracranial circulation. *J Magn Reson Imaging* 1992;2:277–284.

64. Saloner D, Hanson WA, Tsuruda JS, van Tyen R, Anderson CM, Lee RE. Application of a connected-voxel algorithm to MR angiographic data. *J Magn Reson Imaging* 1991;1:423–430.

65. Korosec FR, Weber DM, Mistretta CA, Turski PA, Bernstein MA. A data adaptive reprojection technique for MR angiography. *Magn Reson Med* 1992;24:262–274.

66. Keller PJ, Wilkenfeld M, Abrahams E. SIMP: an integrative combination with MIP. Tenth Society of Magnetic Resonance in Medicine, 1: 201, San Francisco, 1991.

67. Listerud J. First principles of magnetic resonance angiography. *Magn Reson Quart* 1991;7:136–170.

68. Siebert JE, Rosenbaum TL. Automated segmentation and presentation algorithms for 3D MR angiography. 10th Society of Magnetic Resonance in Medicine, 2:758, San Francisco, 1991.

69. Souza SP, Adams WJ, Dumoulin CL. Improved 3D MR angiography by statistical projection. 9th Society of Magnetic Resonance in Medicine, 2:487, New York, 1990.

70. Napel S, Rutt BK, Dunne S. Minimum voxel and maximum gradient Re-projection for MR angiography (abst). *Magn Reson Imaging* 1990; 8:108.

71. Napel S, Marks MP, Rubin GD, et al. CT angiography with spiral CT and maximum intensity projection. *Radiology* 1992;185:607–610.

72. Cline HE, Dumoulin CL, Hart HR Jr, Lorensen WE, Ludke S. 3D reconstruction of the brain from magnetic resonance images using a connectivity algorithm. *Magn Reson Imaging* 1987;5:345–352.

73. Cline HE, Lorensen WE, Kikinis R, Jolesz F. Three-dimensional segmentation of MR images of the head using probability and connectivity. *J Comput Assist Tomogr* 1990;14:1037–1045.

74. Serra J. *Image analysis and mathematical morphology*. New York: Academic Press; 1982.

75. Hentschel D, Ezrielev J, Fisler R, et al. Techniques for editing and visualizing CT angiographic data. *Proceedings of the Fifth Conference on Visualization in Biomedical Computing* 1:307–318, Rochester, 1994.

76. Fishman EK, Liang CC, Kuszyk BS, et al. Automated bone editing algorithm for CT angiography: preliminary results. *AJR* 1996;166:669–672.

77. Shiffman S, Rubin GD, Napel S. Semiautomated editing of computed tomography sections for visualization of vasculature. Conference Proceedings: Society for Optical Engineering Medical Imaging Conference, SPIE2707:140–151, Newport Beach, CA, 1996.

78. Gao L, Heath DG, Kuszyk BS, Fishman EK. Automatic liver segmentation technique for three-dimensional visualization of CT data. *Radiology* 1996;201:359–364.

79. Ter har Romeny BM, Bastin FH, Steenbeck J, Zuiderveld KJ, Viergever MA. Three-dimensional CT subtraction angiography. *Proceedings of the Fifth Conference on Visualization in Biomedical Computing* 1: 262–271, Rochester, 1994.

80. Ney DR, Fishman EK. Editing tools for 3D medical imaging. *IEEE Computer Graphics and Applications* 1991;11:63–71.

81. Hankey GJ, Warlow CP, Sellar RJ. Cerebral angiographic risk in mild cerebrovascular disease. *Stroke* 1990;21:209–222.

82. Earnest FI, Forbes G, Sandok BA, et al. Complications of cerebral angiography: prospective assessment of risk. *AJR* 1984;142:247–253.

83. Leow K, Murie JA. Cerebral angiography for cerebrovascular disease: the risks. *Br J Surg* 1988;75:428–430.

84. Foley JD, van Dam A, Feiner SK, Hughes JF. *Computer graphics*. Boston: Addison Wesley; 1990.

85. Napel S, Rubin GD, Beaulieu CF, Jeffrey RB SS Jr. Automated flight path planning for guided virtual endoscopy. 82nd RSNA, *Abstract in Radiology,* 201P:293, Chicago, 1996.

86. Paik DS, Jeffrey RB Jr, Beaulieu CF, Rubin GD, Napel S. Automated flight path planning for guided virtual endoscopy. *Med Phys* 1998 25(5).

CHAPTER 20

3D Spiral CT Angiography of the Aorta and Its Branches

Geoffrey D. Rubin

Perhaps nowhere has spiral CT revolutionized CT scanning more than in the vascular system. Just 5 years after its clinical introduction, CT angiography has become a minimally invasive imaging alternative for many applications traditionally performed with conventional angiography. CT angiography (CTA) is made possible by the rapid, volumetric acquisition of spiral CT obtained during an accurately timed high-flow peripheral intravenous injection of iodinated contrast material. The resultant images are processed with various computed rendering techniques to generate multiplanar and three-dimensional (3D) images of the vasculature. The rapid acquisition time of spiral CT enables an entire vascular territory to be imaged within a single 30–40-s breath-hold, thus freeing the resultant images from ventilatory misregistration (1). An additional advantage of the short acquisition time is that imaging can be timed to coincide with the arterial or venous phase of a peripheral intravenous contrast injection. As a result, 3D CTA can be performed quicker, less invasively, and at lower cost than conventional arteriography (2). Successful CTA requires a customized scan prescription that accounts for the orientation and size of the target vessels, the imaging volume of interest, the patient's breath-holding ability, and circulation time. A thorough understanding of the relative advantages and disadvantages of multiplanar and 3D rendering techniques is also important. This chapter augments the discussion of technical considerations for CTA presented in Chapter 19 by discussing clinical scenarios and specific protocol considerations; it subsequently reviews the range of disease states for which CTA can be valuable in the chest, abdomen, and pelvis.

PROTOCOL SELECTION CONSIDERATIONS

Successful CTA requires a customized scan prescription that optimizes the tradeoffs between spatial resolution, image noise, anatomic coverage, and contrast utilization.

Anatomic Coverage

Three fundamental variables determine the selection of spiral CT parameters: the anatomic coverage, the scan duration, and the gantry rotation period. Anatomic coverage is determined from preliminary unenhanced localizing sections that are acquired with a low-resolution spiral CT protocol using 10-mm collimation, pitch 2.0, and a 10-mm reconstruction interval. To minimize radiation exposure to the patient and overheating of the x-ray tube prior to acquiring the CTA, a low tube potential and current are selected (80 kV, 80 mA). These sections should liberally include vascular anatomy at the extremes of the anticipated scan volume. For example, when assessing the thoracic aorta, the entire thoracic aorta and its branches should be included in these preliminary sections, which are acquired from well above the thoracic inlet to the upper abdomen to ensure that unsuspected lesions of the brachiocephalic arteries or intra-abdominal extension are fully imaged on the CTA. For abdominal aortoiliac CTA, the preliminary sections should extend from the diaphragm to the lesser trochanters of the femora (femurs).

Scan Duration

Once the anatomic coverage has been determined as the table travel distance required to image the relevant anatomy, the scan duration must be ascertained. In the thorax and abdomen the scan duration is typically governed by the patient's breath-holding ability. Virtually all patients without severe respiratory dysfunction will maintain a 30-s breath-hold, provided that it is preceded by a period of hyperventilation. In fact, many patients will be capable of a 40-s breath-hold. Longer breath-holding is preferable because it will enable either greater scan coverage at the same longitudinal spatial resolution or greater longitudinal spatial resolution with the same scan coverage. When imaging is extended into the pelvis, the scan duration becomes independent of breath-holding capabilities, because there is minimal respiratory induced misregistration below the pelvic rim. As a result, the scan duration may approach 50–60 s for aortoiliac scans. The patient is instructed to hold their breath for the first 30–40 s, then to slowly exhale and breathe quietly during the duration of the scan through the iliac arteries. Two factors may alter this approach. First, on some CT scanners the use of a prolonged spiral acquisition results in substantially diminished tube output, which may result in unacceptable image noise levels in all but the thinnest patients. Second, longer scan durations require that greater volumes of intravenous contrast medium be administered to maintain arterial opacification. If a patient is azotemic and large volumes of contrast medium should not be administered, then the scan duration may be reduced to maintain opacification with less contrast medium at the expense of scan coverage or longitudinal spatial resolution.

We have found it valuable for technologists to practice the 30–40-s breath-hold, preceded by hyperventilation, with the patient prior to performing the spiral scan. Patient cooperation is critical for obtaining an optimized CTA. Various depths of inspiration can shift pertinent anatomy as much as 3–5 cm. It is imperative that the patient be coached to obtain the same degree of inspiration during localizing sections as during the spiral CT acquisition, lest the anatomy of interest be shifted out of the imaging volume.

Gantry Rotation Period

One final variable must be defined prior to selecting the scan parameters for the CTA: the gantry rotation period (GRP), or time required for the gantry to complete a 360-degree revolution. For the majority of scanners in clinical use in 1998, the GRP is 1 s per gantry rotation (GR); however, at the time of this writing, two manufacturers have subsecond GRP scanners available with 0.75-s/GR (Siemens Medical Systems, Iselin, NJ) and 0.85-s/GR (General Electric Medical Systems, Milwaukee, WN). It is likely that more scanners will become available with the capability for subsecond scanning and that the GRP will fall below 0.75 s/GR in the future. To understand the benefit of subsecond scanning, one need only calculate the difference in scan coverage resulting from a 1-s/GR versus a 0.75-s/GR scanner. If we allow the scan coverage to be the same, then a 40-s scan performed with a 1-s/GR scanner could be completed in 30 s with a 0.75-s/GR scanner. Alternatively, 33% greater scan coverage is possible in the same amount of time with a 0.75-s/GR scanner. Is there any penalty for subsecond scanning? The answer is no if the x-ray tube is capable of producing an increase in tube current so that the milliamperage is constant. Therefore, assuming the same kV, a 250-mA tube current would have to be increased to 333 mA to maintain the same exposure with a 0.75-s/GR scan, as compared with a 1-s/GR scan. A concomitant increase in tube current to maintain the signal-to-noise ratio when a shorter GRP is selected is most important when noise is a problem, as when imaging large patients and at the thoracic inlet or bony pelvis. In a comparison of routine thoracic spiral CT scans obtained with 0.75 s/GR versus 1.0 s/GR, three independent and blinded reviewers found that the quality of mediastinal images was superior with 0.75 s/GR, in spite of the same 290 mA used for both GRP settings (3).

Acquisition Parameters

With the scan duration, scan coverage, and GRP determined, the CTA acquisition parameters can be selected. The table speed is first determined as:

$$\text{Table speed (mm/GR)} = (\text{Scan coverage [mm]}$$
$$\div \text{Scan duration [s]}) \times \text{Gantry rotation period (GRP)}$$
$$(1)$$

Once the table speed has been determined, the collimation and scan pitch can be determined. These two parameters, together with the interpolation algorithm, determine the longitudinal resolution of the scan (4). The pitch is defined as the number of collimator widths that the table advances in the time required for the gantry to complete one revolution, or

$$\text{Pitch (collimator widths/GR)} = \text{Table speed (mm/GR)}$$
$$\div \text{Collimation (mm/collimator width)}$$
$$(2)$$

For CTA, using the most widely available interpolation algorithm (180-degree linear interpolation), selection of a high pitch value (up to 2.0) allows collimation to be minimized, resulting in scan parameters that optimize the longitudinal resolution. This is because, with 180-degree linear interpolation, the effective section thickness (EST), as defined by the full width at half maximum of the section profile, is equal to the collimator width for pitch 1.0 scans and 1.3 times the collimator width for pitch 2.0 scans (4,5). Therefore the collimation can be determined as

$$\text{Collimation (mm/collimator width)}$$
$$= \text{Table speed (mm/GR)}$$
$$\div \text{Pitch (collimator widths/GR)}, \quad (3)$$

where pitch is selected to be as close to 2.0 as possible, such that the calculated collimation is consistent with the scanner presets. This approach specifies the minimum collimation to image the required anatomic coverage within the selected scan duration without allowing the pitch to rise above 2.0.

The importance of narrow collimation for visualizing the renal arteries has been demonstrated by Zeman and colleagues (6). Visualization of the renal arteries was possible in six of nine patients imaged with 5-mm collimation and 14 of 14 patients with 3-mm collimation. Although an increase in scan pitch at the same collimator width would not affect the noise, the concomitant decrease in collimation increases the noise. Because vascular structures imaged with spiral CT have a high degree of contrast, a greater amount of noise is tolerable as compared with routine abdominal

CT, where the detection of low-contrast parenchymal lesions may be limited.

This information is best consolidated with some examples:

A. Anatomic coverage = 180 mm, scan duration = 30 s, GRP = 1 s. Using Eq. (1), table speed = (180 ÷ 30) × 1 = 6 mm/GR. Therefore using Eq. (3) with pitch = 2.0, collimation = 6 ÷ 2 = 3 mm, and the scan is performed with 3-mm collimation, pitch 2.0, EST ~ 3.9 mm.

B. Anatomic coverage = 200 mm, scan duration = 40 s, GRP = 1 s. Using Eq. (1), table speed = (200 ÷ 40) × 1 = 5 mm/GR. Therefore using Eq. (3) with pitch = 2.0, collimation = 5 ÷ 2 = 2.5 mm (not allowed), but using Eq. (2) with the next higher allowable collimation (3 mm) results in pitch = 5 ÷ 3 = 1.7, and the scan is performed with 3-mm collimation, pitch 1.7, EST ~ 3.6 mm.

C. Anatomic coverage = 200 mm, scan duration = 40 s, GRP = 0.75 s. Using Eq. (1), table speed = (200 ÷ 40) × 0.75 = 3.8 mm/GR. Therefore using Eq. (3) with pitch = 2.0, collimation = 3.8 ÷ 2 = 1.9 mm (not allowed), but using Eq. (2) with the next higher allowable collimation (2 mm) results in pitch = 3.8 ÷ 2 = 1.9, and the scan is performed with 2-mm collimation, pitch 1.9, EST ~ 2.6 mm.

D. Anatomic coverage = 100 mm, scan duration = 40 s, GRP = 1.0 s. Using Eq. (1), table speed = (100 ÷ 40) × 1.0 = 2.5 mm/GR. Therefore using Eq. (3) with pitch = 2.0, collimation = 2.5 ÷ 2 = 1.3 mm (not allowed), but using Eq. (2) with the next higher allowable collimation (2 mm) results in pitch = 2.5 ÷ 2 = 1.3, and the scan is performed with 2-mm collimation, pitch 1.3, EST ~ 2.2 mm.

E. Anatomic coverage = 100 mm, scan duration = 40 s, GRP = 0.75 s. Using Eq. (1), table speed = (100 ÷ 40) × 0.75 = 1.9 mm/GR. Therefore using Eq. (3) with pitch = 2.0, collimation = 1.9 ÷ 2 = 1 mm, and the scan is performed with 1-mm collimation, pitch 2.0, EST ~ 1.3 mm.

Comparing examples A with B and D with E illustrates the advantage of subsecond scanning as compared with a 1-s GRP. With a constant anatomic coverage and scan duration, the EST could be decreased by 38% and 70%, respectively.

Special Considerations for Imaging the Abdominal Aorta and Iliac Arteries

Special attention should be devoted to optimized technique for evaluating abdominal aortic aneurysms with CTA. The importance of accurately evaluating the position and patency of the celiac, superior mesenteric, and renal arteries requires narrow collimation (≤3 mm) (6,7); however, determination of the distal extension of the aneurysm and the presence of associated iliac occlusive disease is equally important for surgical planning (8). To maintain narrow collimation for imaging the proximal aortic branches yet cover an adequate scan length to image the distal aorta, Zeman and co-workers combined 3-mm collimation through the renal arteries followed by 7-mm collimation through the aortic bifurcation (6). The scan was divided into a 16–20-s spiral acquisition with 3-mm collimation, followed by a 7-s interruption for a breath, and then 12–16-s spiral acquisition with 7-mm collimation. Using this protocol, up to 16 cm of the aorta was imaged during two breath-holds. An alternative approach with similar results for visualizing proximal aortic branches, while enabling up to 18 cm of the aorta to be imaged within a single 30-s breath-hold, is to acquire 3-mm collimation with pitch 2.0 (9). Neither of these protocols can be expected to image distal to the proximal 1–3 cm of the common iliac arteries. Abdominal aortic aneurysm extension into the iliac arteries, coexistent iliac artery aneurysms, or significant iliac occlusive disease will not be imaged. Our current protocol for imaging abdominal aortic aneurysms with a 1-s GRP scanner takes advantage of both a variable collimation acquisition and increased pitch to image from the celiac origin to the inguinal ligament in a single acquisition (10). Three-millimeter collimation, pitch 2.0 (effective section thickness = 3.9 mm), is used to the level of the renal arteries (typically 10–15 s). This is followed by a required 5-s interruption to change collimation and the table to reposition. Patients maintain their breath-hold throughout the 5-s scan interruption. The scan is resumed with 5-mm collimation, pitch 2.0 (effective section thickness = 7.5 mm) for an additional 20–40 s until the inguinal ligament is reached. The patient is instructed to begin quiet ventilation after a total of 30 s breath-holding has been achieved. The scanner is invariably imaging within the pelvis at this time, where respiratory misregistration is not significant (Fig. 20-1). Alternatively, using a subsecond scanner, it is possible to image the entire aortoiliac system with 3-mm collimation, pitch 2.0, during a single 40–50-s exposure.

One final reported protocol relies upon two separate scans separated by a 15–20-s breath-holding period to image up to 60 cm in the abdomen and pelvis. The first scan is performed with 3-mm collimation and 1.3 pitch, whereas the second scan is 5-mm collimation with 1.5 pitch. A total of 200 mL of contrast is injected in two 100-mL boluses injected at 3 mL/s (11). Although this approach introduces the possibility for misregistration between the spiral scans due to differences in the level of inspiration or patient motion between acquisitions, it may be the only reasonable approach to imaging a large volume with a CT scanner that requires more than 5 s between spiral acquisitions.

Contrast Administration

CTA is performed with nonionic iodinated contrast (300–350 mg I/mL) injected into a peripheral vein. We use nonionic contrast to minimize idiosyncratic reactions that

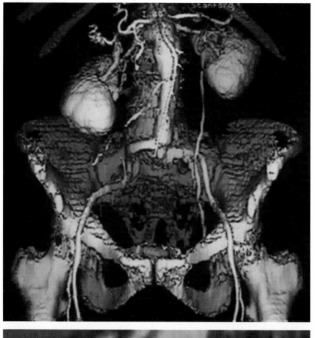

A

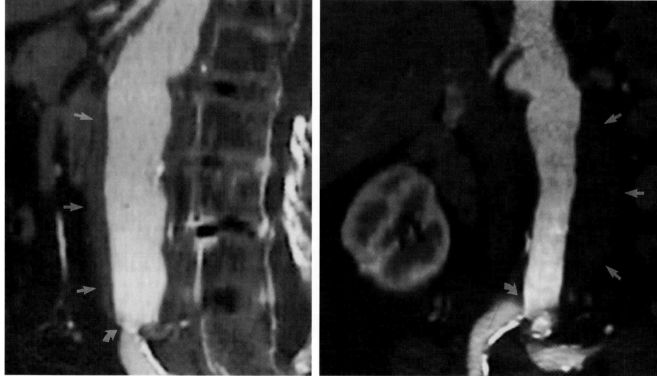

B   C

FIG. 20-1. The entire aortoiliac system can be imaged with 1.0 s GRP when a variable collimation and an increased pitch protocol is used. This examination was performed with 40 s of imaging within a 45-s period. The supraceliac aorta to below the renal arteries was scanned for 20 s (3-mm collimation, 2.0 pitch, 2-mm interval). The patient continued to maintain suspended ventilation for 5 s while the collimation changed. A second helical scan began from the end of the first scan through the lesser trochanters of the femurs (5-mm collimation, pitch 2.0, 3-mm interval). The patient was instructed to breathe quietly after a total breath-hold of 30 s (once the helical scan had reached the pelvic brim, where respiratory misregistration is minimal). 180 mL of contrast (300 mg I/mL) was injected at 4 mL/s. (**A**) Frontal shaded-surface display demonstrates a juxtarenal aortic aneurysm. *(continued)*

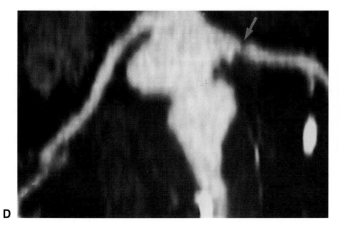

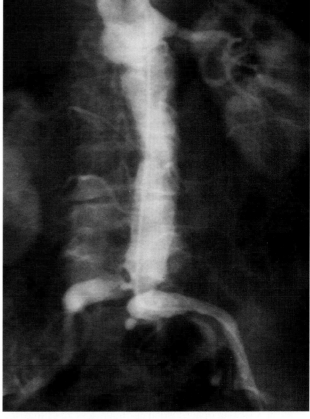

FIG. 20-1. *Continued.* The exact origin of the aneurysm neck can be difficult to appreciate from a shaded-surface display, because the thrombosed portions of the aneurysm are not visualized. Sagittal (**B**) and coronal (**C**) curved planar reformations through the right iliac artery allow visualization of the thrombosed (*straight arrows*) as well as the patent portions of the aneurysm. There is a moderate stenosis of the origin of the right common iliac artery (*curved arrow*). A curved planar reformation (**D**) through the renal arteries demonstrates a left renal artery stenosis. Correlative aortogram (**E**) demonstrates the right renal artery stenosis and iliac artery stenoses. (Reprinted from Rubin GD. Spiral (helical) CT of the renal vasculature. *Semin Ultrasound CT MR* 1996;17:374–397)

might jeopardize patient immobility during the CTA acquisition and to diminish morbidity if extravasation occurs. To maximize target vascular opacification and minimize venous and parenchymal opacification throughout the duration of the spiral scan, contrast delivery must be synchronized with the acquisition of the CTA. By imposing a bolus duration that is equivalent to the scan duration, the likelihood that contrast medium is wasted by opacifying the target vasculature before imaging has begun or after imaging is complete is minimized. There is no question that the hemodynamics of intravascular iodinated contrast media are complex and incompletely understood. However, our experience performing more than 1,000 aortic CTAs suggests that this approach is reliable.

To ensure that the contrast bolus duration is equivalent to the scan duration, one of two related equations is solved after the acquisition parameters have been selected:

$$\text{Contrast medium volume (mL)} = \text{Contrast medium flow rate (mL/s)} \times \text{Scan duration (s)} \quad (4)$$

or

$$\text{Contrast medium flow rate (mL/s)} = \text{Contrast medium volume (mL)} \div \text{Scan duration (s)} \quad (5)$$

In general and for a specific iodine concentration, the flow rate of the contrast medium dictates arterial opacification. Therefore for most aortic CTAs, we use Eq. (4) to calculate the volume of contrast medium required. For normal adults weighing between 60 and 120 kg, a flow rate of 4 mL/s should reliably opacify the thoracic aorta to a level that is greater than 200 HU (2). Patients with very abnormal hemodynamics associated with sepsis (high cardiac output, low systemic vascular resistance) may opacify the systemic arteries unpredictably; however, this is rarely a problem for CTA applications in the aorta. For adults weighing < 60 kg or > 120 kg, flow rates of 3.5 mL/s and 5 mL/s, respectively, are typically satisfactory. Flow rates of up to 4 mL/s can be comfortably administered through a 3-cm, 22-gauge antecubital intravenous catheter, and up to 7 mL/s can be comfortably administered through a 3-cm, 20-gauge IV catheter. In children or patients whose iodine dosage must be limited because of azotemia, Eq. (5) is used to calculate the flow rate required to deliver the dose of contrast medium in a bolus of equivalent length to the scan duration. For children we typically deliver 2–3 mL of 300 mg I mL^{-1} solution kg^{-1}. When performing CTA on children as small as 3 kg, we find that a power injector is always preferable to hand injection for controlling the bolus duration, particularly when flow rates as low as 0.2 mL/s are required.

For thoracic aortic CTA, injection into the right antecubital vein is preferable to the left, as a left antecubital injection results in opacification of the left brachiocephalic vein and the resultant perivenous artifact can substantially degrade visualization of the brachiocephalic artery origins. We perform most injections via the right antecubital vein, but when a catheter is present within the superior vena cava, injection into the superior vena cava results in a tighter bolus and greater arterial opacification because of less contrast medium pooling within the veins.

Although we have found that dilution of 300 mg I/mL solutions of contrast medium to near iso-osmolar levels (150 mg I/mL) results in significantly greater arterial enhancement and less perivenous artifacts than the same dosage of iodine delivered in 300 mg I/mL solution (12), we do not use dilute solutions for aortic CTA. Our study focused only upon performance of routine thoracic spiral CT, where the required vascular opacification is much less than that for CTA. Additional investigation is required to establish if the relationships between iodine concentration, perivenous artifact, and arterial enhancement determined for low iodine dosages (15–22.5 g) are similarly applicable at the higher doses required for CTA. Further, the typical capacity of power injectors is 200 mL, making delivery of typical CTA doses of 40–50 g I in a 150-mg I/mL solution impossible. For this reason we use 300 mg I/mL nonionic contrast medium for all aortic CTA.*

To ensure synchronization of the contrast medium bolus with the scan acquisition, a preliminary test of the time required to opacify the aorta at the anticipated initiation point of the CTA is measured (7,13). The optimal delay time between the initiation of the intravenous contrast bolus and commencement of spiral scanning cannot be predicted from the patient's blood pressure, heart rate, or other noninvasive physiological measures; rather, it must be individually determined for the selected target anatomy. Only 10 mL is required for bolus timing to the thoracic aorta in adults, and 15 mL is required for timing into the abdominal aorta. For children, we use approximately 1 mL for ever 5 kg of body weight up to 10 mL. The injection is administered at the same rate as the CTA, typically 4 mL/s. Five-millimeter collimated sections (80 kV, 80 mA) are acquired every 2 s at the anticipated initiation point of the CTA for a total of 20 images. In adults, imaging commences 8 s after the injection begins. Shorter delays are required in children and depend

upon the site of intravenous access. A time–density curve is generated from a region of interest drawn within the main artery imaged, usually aorta, to accurately determine the appropriate scan delay time for individual patients (Fig. 20-2). Although the circulation time to the aorta will be 20 ± 8 s in 80% of adult patients, it is typically impossible to predict which patients will have substantially delayed circulation, which can be caused by elevated cardiac filling pressures, poor cardiac output, tricuspid regurgitation, and venous stenoses. When present, these lesions can prolong the arrival of contrast to the aorta by up to 45 s. Once the images are acquired, visual inspection typically identifies the time of greatest opacification; however, for many patients the creation of a time–density curve is the most reliable means for

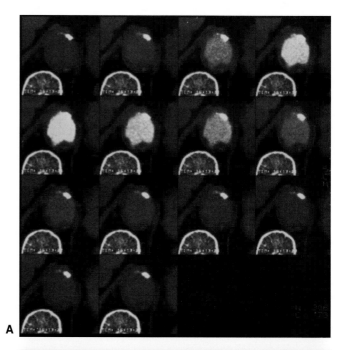

A

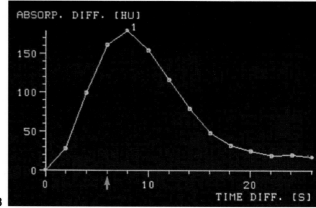

B

FIG. 20-2. (A) Axial CT sections obtained at the level of the supraceliac aorta every 2 s. The first image was obtained 8 s following initiation of a 20-mL contrast bolus injected at 5 mL/s. **(B)** Time–density curve generated by placing a region of interest within the aorta. Time zero on the curve represents the point where imaging began (8 s after initiation of the 20-mL bolus). The peak of the curve (16 s in this case) is selected as the postinjection CTA scan delay.

---

*A bolus of mL of saline delivered immediately after the iodine injection has been found prolong aortic enhancement (12a).

finding this peak. We select the time to greatest opacification as the delay for the CTA acquisition.

Recently, software has become available that automatically triggers the CT scan after a user-defined threshold of enhancement is detected within the aorta. Use of this technique eliminates the need for a preliminary test injection.*

Spiral Scan Reconstruction

Critical to maximal longitudinal spatial resolution and optimized multiplanar and 3D visualization of the CTA data is the generation of overlapping transverse reconstructions. In general, a reconstruction interval of one-half of the collimator width is a satisfactory compromise between an unwieldy number of reconstructed sections and the improved longitudinal resolution. Sections generated with a low-noise reconstruction kernel (''standard'' or ''soft'') will result in superior 3D renderings than reconstructions using higher spatial frequency kernels (''bone''), which tend to be unacceptably degraded by image noise. A targeted field of view of 18–25 cm results in improved in-plane resolution as compared with larger fields of view used for routine thoracic or abdominal applications. It is not advisable to reconstruct the data with fields of view that are smaller than the total table travel distance, as many workstations will not display 3D renderings or multiplanar reformations generated parallel to the longitudinal axis (coronal, sagittal, and intermediate obliquities) in their entirety.

Alternative Visualization

Detailed discussions of the various methods for alternative two- and three-dimensional visualization of CTA data is presented in Chapters 3 and 19, and salient advantages and

---

*Variations in the implementation of this technique by CT scanner manufacturers result in differing durations of the transition period between enhancement detection and scan initiation. Longer transition periods may result in an unacceptably long delay before imaging the contrast bolus. Transition periods of eight seconds or less are acceptable using a trigger threshold of 40 HU enhancement within the aorta.

disadvantages of the most commonly used visualization techniques are summarized in Table 20-1. Although volume rendering is not included in this table, it is a technique that is becoming increasingly available and has substantial advantages over MIP and SSD. It is discussed in detail in Chapter 3. Specific applications of these visualization techniques are included in the subsequent discussions of the various lesions assessed with CTA. It is important to stress, however, that the quality of multiplanar reformations and 3D renderings is primarily influenced by the quality of the CT data. A thorough understanding of spiral CT principles is required for optimal creation of multiplanar and 3D renderings, and no amount of sophisticated rendering and image segmentation can resurrect a poor acquisition.

Artifacts

Before reviewing the current clinical applications for aortic CTA, it is important to address the two artifacts that result in the majority of interpretative limitations of aortic CTA, both of which have primary relevance in the thorax: perivenous streaks and arterial pulsation. Both of these artifacts tend to have their greatest influence on the visualization of the ascending aorta and therefore are particularly important to bear in mind when assessing patients suspected of aortic dissection.

Perivenous streaks are likely caused by a combination of beam hardening and motion caused by transmitted pulsation to veins carrying undiluted contrast medium to the heart. Strategies designed to minimize this artifact include the use of dilute contrast medium solutions (12,14), caudal-to-cranial scan direction, and femoral venous injection (15). In practice, perivenous streaks are rarely confused with intimal dissection in the ascending aorta as their orientation typically varies from section to section and they typically extend beyond the confines of the aortic wall. The most problematic region for perivenous artifacts is the origin of the supra-aortic branches adjacent to an opacified left brachiocephalic vein. Perivenous streaks in this region can mask extension of intimal flaps into these branches as well as occlusive disease

---

TABLE 20-1. *Advantages and disadvantages of most commonly used visualization techniques*

	Muti/curved planar reformation	Maximum-intensity projection (MIP)	Shaded-surface display (SSD)
Advantages	"Slices" through the center of the vessel to show lumen; useful with arterial stents or eccentric calcifications	Differentiates calcification or stents from contrast column and mural calcium	Displays complex anatomic relationships in regions of vessel overlap or tortuosity
Disadvantages	Inaccurate curve drawing can falsely imply lesions not present	Confusing in regions of vessel overlap Cannot image interior of metallic stent	Cannot differentiate metallic stent or mural calcium from the intra-arterial contrast column. Incorrect threshold selection can falsely imply or exclude lesions
Prerendering editing	None	Minimum: removal of bones Preferred: removal of all structures other than the target vessels	Minimum: none Preferred: removal of all structures other than the target vessels
Time required	2 min	10–60 min	5–60 min

caused by atherosclerotic plaque at their origins. If detected at the time of initial section reconstruction (within 2 min of bolus initiation), then delayed sections can be rapidly prescribed to enable reimaging during a second pass of arterial contrast prior to the equilibrium phase. Other than this rapid intervention or reinjection of contrast, there are no techniques to adequately overcome obscured brachiocephalic arterial origins once the equilibrium phase has begun. The best prevention of this limitation is ensuring that peripheral venous access is from the right upper extremity.

Arterial pulsation has been recognized as a cause of false-positive aortic dissection on conventional and spiral CT scans. The increasing acquisition speed of spiral CT scanners may ultimately result in the elimination of this artifact; however, in the meantime there is an intervention that can be retrospectively applied to the raw scan data to minimize these artifacts. Segmented or weighted half-scan reconstruction is an alternative interpolation technique that minimizes the amount of projection data required to generate a cross section. As implemented by General Electric, this results in a reduction of projection data required to reconstruct a cross-section from the standard 360 degrees to 225 degrees. For a 1-s GRP, segmented reconstruction effectively improves the temporal resolution of the CT scan from 1 s to 0.6 s. This has been demonstrated to eliminate artifacts that might be misconstrued as intimal flaps on conventional CT scans (16). It is available for spiral scans as well. Its use is typically required if an equivocal finding is present on a single image and should not be considered necessary when linear filling defects are visualized entirely within the confines of the aortic wall on sequential reconstructions—an indication of a true intimal flap.

CLINICAL APPLICATIONS

Although conventional arteriography has long been considered the standard for arterial imaging, spiral CT may be superior for assessing the arteries of the thorax and abdomen, for several reasons. First, the volumetric acquisition of spiral CT enables clear delineation of the aorta, tortuous arterial branches, and adjacent aneurysms and pseudoaneurysms. Because conventional arteriography is a projectional technique, the typical overlap of these structures can confound their visualization and delineation of anatomic relationships, particularly at branch ostea. Second, blood pool imaging provided by the intravenous administration of iodinated contrast media allows simultaneous visualization of true and false luminal flow channels, intramural hematomas communicating with the aortic lumen, and slow perigraft flow around aortic stent-grafts. Finally, the aortic wall and non-communicating intramural collections are directly visualized. These advantages, together with the rapid, noninvasive means with which CTA is acquired, have resulted in CTA challenging conventional arteriography for the assessment of many arterial abnormalities.

Aortic Aneurysm

Aneurysm size dictates therapy; therefore the analysis of any CT scan demonstrating an aortic aneurysm must include accurate aneurysm sizing. Because of the tortuosity and curvature of the aorta in the setting of aneurysmal disease, aneurysm sizing is performed most accurately when double-oblique tomograms are generated perpendicular to the aortic flow lumen (Fig. 20-3). The challenge of such an approach is that data concerning the risk of aneurysm rupture and expansion rate are based upon measurements made from transverse sections, where true diameters can be overestimated. Further, the measurement technique must be reproducible to assess the rate of aneurysm expansion on sequential studies. Until analysis tools are available to automatically identify the center of the flow channel, create true perpendicular tomograms, and compute accurate cross-sectional areas and mean diameters (16a), the creation of true vessel cross-sections is probably not practical for routine applications unless sizing endoluminal prostheses as described subsequently.

The most sensitive measure of aneurysm size, however, is the determination not of true aortic diameters or even cross-sectional area, but of aneurysm volume. This approach has substantial drawbacks. Although the volumetric data of spiral CT should be excellent for determining aneurysm volume, both patent, thrombosed, and atheromatous elements of the aorta must be accurately segmented from the adjacent structures to make this determination. Currently, the only technique available to perform this is a painstaking manual segmentation performed by drawing regions of interest around the aorta on each cross-section. Furthermore, until now aneurysm expansion has been studied primarily in terms of radial expansion of the aorta. Although aneurysm volume determination is an attractive measure of aneurysm growth based upon theoretical considerations, data concerning the risk of aneurysm rupture and guidelines for intervention are based upon traditional transverse diameter measurements (17,18).

With respect to aneurysm visualization, SSDs typically provide the best overall appreciation of aortic tortuosity and the relationship of the aorta and its branch origins to the aneurysm (Fig. 20-4). Although of limited utility in the thorax (Fig. 20-5) (19), maximum-intensity projections (MIPs) can be very helpful in the abdomen to display occlusive lesions of the aortic branches, extent of mural calcification (particularly in the iliac arteries, where graft anastomoses to heavily calcified vessels can be challenging), and mural thrombus (Fig. 20-6). The extent of segmentation or editing performed on the axial images prior to 3D rendering determines the amount of information conveyed, particularly on MIPs. If no segmentation is performed, then the spine will obscure the aorta on a frontal projection (see Fig. 20-6A,B). If the bones are removed through 3D connectivity or 2D region-of-interest drawing, then the contrast-filled aortic lumen is visualized. However, the true diameter of the aorta is masked by overlapping soft tissues (Fig. 20-6C,D). If editing is performed to exclude all structures except the aorta and its branches, then a unique 3D appreciation of both mural

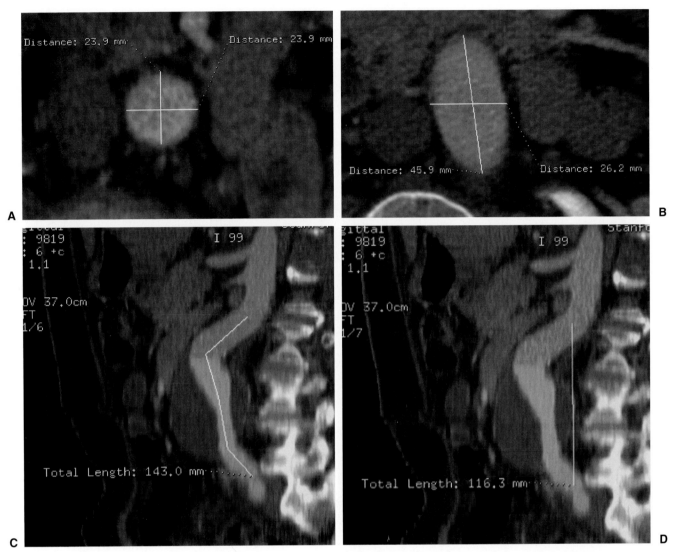

FIG. 20-3. (**A**) Double-oblique cross-section of an aortic aneurysm proximal neck, manually created perpendicular to the flow channel. The AP and lateral diameter measurements are identical (23.9 mm). (**B**) Transverse tomogram corresponding to the center of the aorta in image A. Both axes are overestimated (92% for the major axis and 10% for the minor axis). (**C**) Curved path manually drawn through the center of the aortic flow lumen from the top of the proximal aneurysm neck (inferior margin of the inferior renal artery) to a point 2 cm distal to the aneurysm. This distance should correspond to the appropriate length of an endoluminal prosthesis deployed through this aneurysm. (**D**) Standard craniocaudal determination of path length, typically determined from transverse sections, underestimates the appropriate length by 26.7 mm (23%).

thrombus and the contrast-filled residual lumen is appreciated. Thus delineation of extent of the aneurysm and position of the aneurysm neck with respect to aortic branches is better than that obtained with conventional arteriography (Fig. 20-6E,F). This latter approach is the most time-consuming and may be impractical for a busy CT department. In general, we do not edit our routine aortic aneurysms section by section, but favor a more rapid region-growing-based bone-removal process to create MIPs that we augment with curved planar reformations (CPR) through the aorta and all its branches. These CPRs clearly display mural thrombus relative to aortic branches and the enhancing flow lumen but do not necessitate preliminary segmentation. Because of the

limited view of eccentric lesions that single CPRs provide, we always create two orthogonal CPRs through each aortic branch (e.g., curved coronal and sagittal reformations of the aorta and iliac arteries, curved coronal and curved transverse reformations of the renal arteries, and curved sagittal and curved transverse views of the celiac axis and superior mesenteric artery).

Most aortic aneurysms are abdominal, but thoracic aortic aneurysms when present can be a substantially more difficult lesion to treat and are associated with greater morbidity and mortality. Because the issues concerning the imaging of thoracic and abdominal aneurysms tend to be different, they are discussed separately.

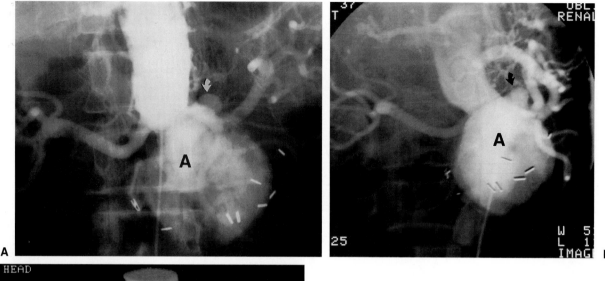

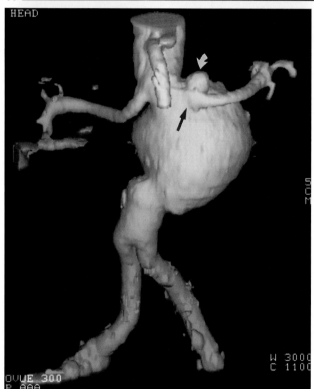

FIG. 20-4. Advantage of shaded-surface display CT angiography of a juxtarenal abdominal aortic aneurysm. Anteroposterior screen-film **(A)** and left anterior oblique digital subtraction **(B)** aortograms demonstrate the difficulty that can be encountered in delineating the renal artery origins when the aneurysm neck is juxtarenal. A saccular aortic aneurysm (A) has developed superior to an aortobiiliac bypass graft. Although the right renal artery origin is clearly delineated, the origin of the left renal artery and its possible involvement with a 1-cm saccular aneurysm (*curved arrow*) cannot be definitively determined. **(C)** Shaded-surface display CT angiogram clearly delineates the origin of the left renal artery (*straight arrow*) and the 1-cm saccular aneurysm just distal to its origin (*curved arrow*). Reprinted from Rubin GD. Three-dimensional spiral CT angiography. *Radiographics* 1994;14:905–912.

Thoracic Aortic Aneurysm

The application of CTA to lesions of the thoracic aorta is robust. In fact, most lesions can be accurately diagnosed from the primarily reconstructed transverse sections alone. Quint and colleagues reviewed spiral CT scans of 49 patients with a variety of thoracic aortic lesions (36 thoracic aortic aneurysms) who all underwent open operative repair (20). In comparing consensus interpretations of transverse sections versus multiplanar reformations, they found that multiplanar reformations did not alter the accuracy of diagnosis of aortic lesion type, which was determined to be 92% (45/49 lesions).

The four misdiagnosed lesions included two of five aortic dissections requiring surgery and two patients in whom intramural hematomas were identified, but an associated ulceration could not be identified. These lesions are specifically addressed in the upcoming sections corresponding to dissection and intramural hematoma.

CTA is useful for diagnosing thoracic aortic aneurysms, determining their extent, and predicting appropriate management (20). Although the diagnosis of aortic aneurysms is readily made from transverse sections, an assessment of the extent of the lesion, particularly when the brachiocephalic branches are involved, is facilitated by an assessment of

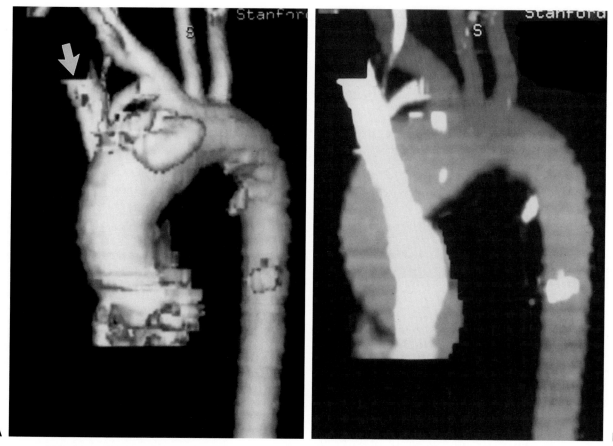

FIG. 20-5. (A) Shaded-surface display of a CTA demonstrates a pseudoaneurysm of the ascending aorta. The ascending aorta obscures most of the superior vena cava (*arrow*). If a view of the superior vena cava were desired, then an image from the right would show the superior vena cava obscuring the ascending aorta. **(B)** Maximum-intensity projection of the same data from the same angle fails to demonstrate the pseudoaneurysm, because it overlaps the ascending aorta. Furthermore, the higher-attenuation superior vena cava obscures the ascending aorta. A 180-degree rotated view would be right-left reversed; otherwise it would appear identical. The only way to prevent obscuration of the ascending aorta by the superior vena cava would be to edit it from the cross-sections prior to rendering. Because of the extensive overlap of vascular structures in the thorax, MIPs are less useful than SSDs for evaluating the thoracic aorta. (Reprinted from Rubin GD. Helical CT angiography of the thoracic aorta. *J Thorac Imaging* 1997;12 (*in press*).

curved-planar reformations (CPRs) and shaded-surface displays (SSDs) (Fig. 20-7).

In general, thoracic aortic aneurysms greater than 5 cm are at an increased risk for rupture. Although thoracic aortic aneurysms expand at a slower rate than abdominal aortic aneurysms, surgical repair is contemplated when thoracic aneurysms reach a diameter of 5–6 cm (17,18). In fact, Quint and colleagues found that an analysis of transverse sections and multiplanar reformations were 94% accurate with a positive predictive value of 95% and a negative predictive value of 93% for successfully predicting the need for intraoperative hypothermic circulatory arrest. With the exception of the elimination of one false-negative result, the addition of multiplanar reformations did not alter the predictions made from the transverse sections alone. Three-dimensional renderings were not evaluated in this study (20).

Abdominal Aortic Aneurysm

Aortography has traditionally been obtained prior to resection of abdominal aortic aneurysms (AAA) to define: (a) the relationship of the aneurysm to main and accessory renal, iliac, superior, and inferior mesenteric arteries; (b) extension of the aneurysm into the common, external, or internal iliac arteries to determine the type and length of prosthetic graft utilized; and (c) detect the presence of coexistent iliac or renal occlusive disease (21,22).

Computed tomography has been advocated in the preoperative evaluation of abdominal aortic aneurysm (21). It is less invasive than angiography, more accurate than conventional angiography for predicting abdominal aortic aneurysm size (23,24), and superior to angiography in its ability to demonstrate mural thrombus, inflammatory aneurysms, perianeurysmal blood due to contained rupture (21,23), and coexis-

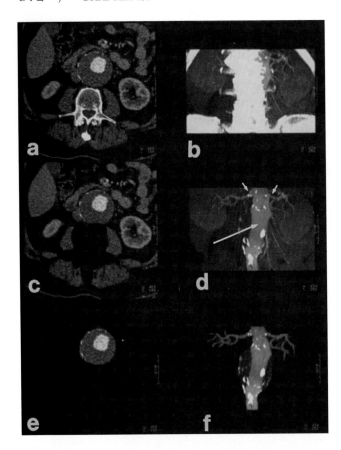

FIG. 20-6. (A) Axial CT section from spiral CT angiographic study at the level of an infrarenal abdominal aortic aneurysm. No editing has been performed. (B) Frontal maximum-intensity projection through the entire data set of 90 axial images demonstrates obscuration of the aneurysm by the spine. (C) Axial CT section shown in (A) following removal of the spine via manual segmentation. (D) Frontal MIP demonstrates the contrast-filled lumen (*long arrow*) and origins of the renal arteries (*short arrows*); however, the thrombosed portion of the aneurysm cannot be differentiated from the background. (E) Identical axial section as seen in (A) and (C); however, all structures other than the aorta and renal arteries have been excluded via manual segmentation. (F) Associated maximum-intensity projection now demonstrates both the patent and thrombosed portions of the aneurysm, allowing for a more accurate depiction of the aneurysm extent.

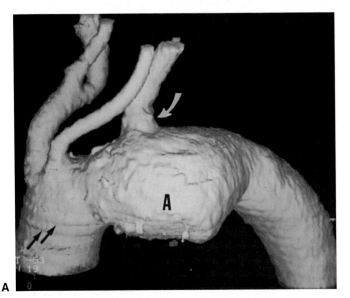

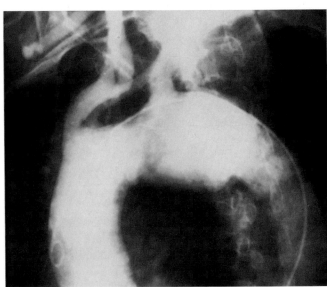

FIG. 20-7. (A) SSD-CTA demonstrates a large aneurysm of the aortic arch (A) originating 5 mm distal to the origin of the left common carotid artery. The left subclavian artery (*curved arrow*) originates from the wall of the aneurysm. Irregularities demonstrated in the wall of the ascending aorta (*straight arrows*) correspond to artifact resulting from transmitted cardiac pulsation. (B) Correlative conventional arteriogram.

tent nonvascular abdominal disease (21). The ability of conventional CT to accurately demonstrate juxtarenal or suprarenal extension of the aneurysm has been controversial. Some authors have reported predictive values as low as 13% for suprarenal extension (25); others have reported infrarenal localization of the aneurysm neck in as many as 94% (21). Data such as this must be interpreted carefully with consideration of the pretest probability that an abdominal aortic aneurysm will be infrarenal in approximately 95% of cases. Conventional CT has been considered inadequate for assessing the position and patency of aortic branch origins and stenoses and for detecting accessory renal arteries (21,24–26). Identification of these coexistent abnormalities is critical to optimizing surgical repair of abdominal aortic aneurysms.

Helical CT overcomes many of the limitations associated with conventional angiography. Specifically, the elimination of ventilatory misregistration enables an accurate depiction of the aneurysm neck relative to aortic branch vessels as well as an evaluation of the aortic branch vessels themselves (see Fig. 20-19). In a preliminary study of nine aortic aneurysms, CTA correctly determined the relationship of the proximal aspect of the aneurysm relative to renal artery branches in all cases (7). Zeman and colleagues studied the effects of overlapping versus nonoverlapping reconstruction and fixed versus variable collimation for determining the extent of abdominal aortic aneurysms on spiral CT sections. On axial sections alone, the determination of supra- versus infrarenal extension of the aneurysm was correctly diagnosed in 23 of 23 patients, whereas with nonoverlapping reconstruction, there was false-positive suprarenal extension in one patient. Van Hoe and colleagues studied 38 patients with AAA and a high prevalence of juxta- ($n = 8$) and suprarenal ($n = 7$) proximal necks. In comparison to measurements made during open repair, they found that digital subtraction angiography (DSA) correctly characterized only 12/15 (80%) aneurysms with juxta- or suprarenal necks, whereas spiral CTA performed with 2-mm collimation correctly characterized 14/15 (93%) (27). The greater accuracy of CTA can be attributed to its ability to detect the outer wall of the aorta and not just the flow lumen. Juxta- and suprarenal extension of AAA can be missed on DSA because of the presence of mural thrombus and atheroma at the proximal neck.

Regarding distal AAA involvement of the iliac arteries, Zeman et al. found that transverse CTA sections reconstructed with overlapping reconstructions resulted in four of 23 misdiagnoses (three false positive; one false negative), whereas nonoverlapping sections resulted in five of 23 incorrect diagnoses (four false-positive iliac involvement; one false negative) (6). It is likely that these diagnostic errors would have been reduced if multiplanar and 3D renderings were used in association with the axial sections for interpretation.

The ability of CTA to identify renal artery stenosis in the presence of abdominal aortic aneurysms has been assessed in two studies. Using spiral CT with 3D rendering, four of four greater than 50% diameter renal artery stenoses were detected in nine abdominal aortic aneurysms, with no false-positive diagnoses of renal artery stenosis (7). Of 83 arteries identified in Van Hoe and colleagues series, hemodynamically significant stenoses or occlusion were present in 17 on DSA and detected with 94% sensitivity and 96% specificity with CTA (27).

The influence of optimized CT angiographic technique (small effective section thickness and overlapping reconstructions) has been suggested by Zeman and co-workers, in a study of 23 patients with abdominal aortic aneurysms, seven of which were associated with greater than 50% renal artery stenosis. Renal artery stenosis was detected by spiral CT in one of two patients imaged with 5-mm collimation, and in four of five patients imaged with 3-mm collimation. Further, stenotic renal arteries were correctly identified in only two of seven patients with stenoses on nonoverlapping sections, whereas on overlapping sections stenoses were correctly identified in five of seven patients. Moreover, none of the four accessory renal arteries present in the aneurysm population was seen with nonoverlapping sections; however, two of four were seen with overlapping sections (6).

Helical CT provides the same information regarding aneurysm size and extent of mural thrombus available with conventional CT; however, the volumetric acquisition allows multiplanar and 3D renderings to be generated perpendicular to the long axis of the aneurysm, resulting in greater accuracy of the aneurysm size measurements.

Postoperative Assessment

Vascular clips, sternal wires, and graft materials typically result in relatively little artifact on spiral CT scans. As a result, spiral CTA is an excellent means for assessing the aorta for perianastomotic complications following aortic or coronary artery bypass graft placement and complications relating to placement of access canulas for cardiopulmonary bypass (Fig. 20-8).

Endoluminal Stent-Grafts

An application perfectly suited to CTA is the evaluation of endoluminal metallic stents and stent-grafts used for treatment of aortoiliac occlusive and aneurysmal disease. The metallic structure of the stents precludes their evaluation with magnetic resonance imaging (MRI) (7,9,28,29). In imaging more than 150 patients with aortoiliac or renal artery stents or stent-grafts, we have found that spiral CT provides an exquisite depiction of the lumen of both stents and stent-grafts as well as surrounding structures.

For the evaluation of aortoiliac and renal artery occlusive disease treated with arterial stents, the stent patency is easily determined with spiral CT, and neointimal hyperplasia

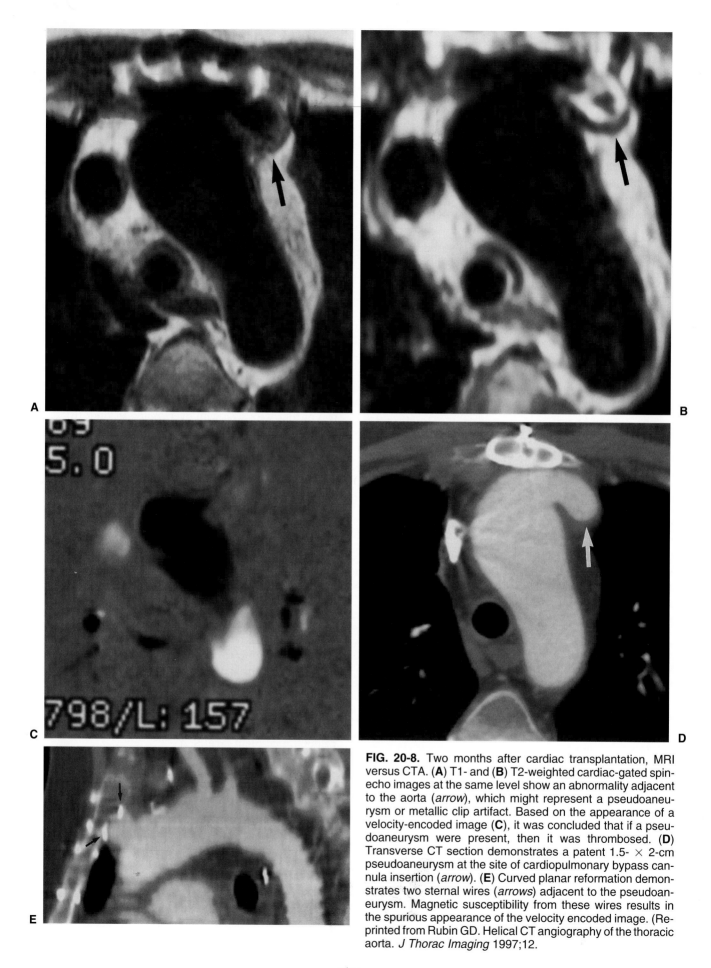

FIG. 20-8. Two months after cardiac transplantation, MRI versus CTA. (**A**) T1- and (**B**) T2-weighted cardiac-gated spin-echo images at the same level show an abnormality adjacent to the aorta (*arrow*), which might represent a pseudoaneurysm or metallic clip artifact. Based on the appearance of a velocity-encoded image (**C**), it was concluded that if a pseudoaneurysm were present, then it was thrombosed. (**D**) Transverse CT section demonstrates a patent 1.5- × 2-cm pseudoaneurysm at the site of cardiopulmonary bypass cannula insertion (*arrow*). (**E**) Curved planar reformation demonstrates two sternal wires (*arrows*) adjacent to the pseudoaneurysm. Magnetic susceptibility from these wires results in the spurious appearance of the velocity encoded image. (Reprinted from Rubin GD. Helical CT angiography of the thoracic aorta. *J Thorac Imaging* 1997;12.

within the stents can be visualized (28). Helical CT may represent a minimally invasive alternative to angiography for establishing stent patency in patients with recurrent symptoms following endoluminal metallic stent placement.

An exciting development in the therapy of aortic aneurysms is the development of endoluminal deployment of covered stents or stent-grafts typically deployed through a femoral arterial cut-down. The anticipated treatment of aortic aneurysms with stent-grafts places demands on imaging that are greater than those with conventional repair, because the opportunity for direct morphological characterization and quantification during open repair does not exist. As a result, accurate aortic quantification is critical preprocedurally to determine both the size of the prosthesis to be deployed and the most appropriate access route for endoluminal deployment. For the purpose of pre-stent-graft planning we divide the aorta into four primary zones: proximal neck, aneurysm body, distal neck, and access route. Pertinent data differ between these zones. Critical assessments of the proximal and distal aneurysm necks include true cross-sectional diameter measurements length along the median axis of the aorta, angulation relative to adjacent segments, mural atheroma/thrombus, and degree of tapering. The aneurysm body is assessed primarily for length and patent branches such as accessory renal arteries or unusually large lumbar or inferior mesenteric arteries originating from the aneurysmal segment. The access route (typically one of the iliac arteries) is assessed for minimal diameter, tortuosity, and extent of calcification. Although these three factors likely influence the ease with which the device can be advanced to its deployment position with minimal morbidity, the relative contribution of these three iliac properties and appropriate boundary conditions for their use have not been determined. Substantial investigation remains to determine the best means for quantifying the aorta and iliac arteries for optimally sizing and deploying stent-grafts.

One critical factor when quantifying the aorta that has been underappreciated to date is that measures of aortic diameter and length cannot be based solely upon an analysis of transverse cross-sections. Because the aorta rarely courses perpendicular to the transverse plane, oblique cross-sections perpendicular to the medial axis of the aorta and curved path lengths conforming to the course of the aorta in three dimensions must be used to avoid highly inaccurate estimations of these critical morphological features (30–32). The volumetric data of spiral CT should provide the most accurate for aortoiliac quantification (see Fig. 20-3), superior to the limited two-dimensional projections of conventional arteriography and the potentially arbitrary orientation of intravascular ultrasound. The proof of this statement is forthcoming.

CTA is also very useful for assessing the success of endoluminal stent-graft deployment (33). The success of aneurysm treatment by stent-graft deployment is dependent upon ensuring that the aneurysm has been completely excluded.

Perigraft flow can be very slow and thus during flush aortography may be undetected. Because spiral CTA relies upon generalized arterial opacification from an intravenous injection rather than on a local aortic injection, opacification of perigraft channels is frequently detected on postdeployment CTAs, when aortography suggested complete exclusion. Additionally, CTA with 3D rendering clearly depicts the position of the stent-graft relative to aortic branches and the aneurysm (9). Because the origins of the brachiocephalic branches are typically tortuous in the setting of thoracic aortic aneurysm, it can be challenging to demonstrate the relationship of the stent-graft and the brachiocephalic arterial origins arteriographically. When aortic branches are covered, thrombosis of the branches can be documented (Figs. 20-9, 20-10) (see color plate 18 following p. 352). Spiral CT is a useful means of serially evaluating patients with stent-grafts to confirm progressive thrombosis of the aneurysm. As new devices are developed for endoluminal treatment of aneurysmal disease of the abdominal aorta and its branches, spiral CT will play an important role in assessing the adequacy of these devices, both immediately after deployment and over the long term.

Aortic Dissection

The critical clinical issue required of any imaging test applied to a patient suspected of having an aortic dissection is the identification of an intimal flap and its localization to the ascending (type A) or descending (type B) aorta. This fundamental diagnostic feature that determines the need for emergent repair can be addressed by at least four imaging modalities: angiography, CT, MRI, and transesophageal echocardiography (TEE). The relative accuracy of these modalities has been debated in the medical literature and is confounded by the fact that technical improvements in CT, MRI, and TEE have outpaced our ability to compare them in appropriately designed prospective trials. Recent opinion has shifted toward MRI or TEE as the most sensitive tests for aortic dissection (34). Unfortunately, much of this opinion is based upon comparative studies where state-of-the-art MRI or TEE is compared with relatively primitive conventional CT technique (35,36). In 1989, Erbel and colleagues studied 164 consecutive patients with suspected aortic dissection. All patients were studied with transthoracic echocardiography and TEE, 85 patients were studied with CT, and 96 patients were studied with aortography. The technique for CT scanning involved the use of 10-mm-thick sections acquired at 20–40-mm intervals through the chest. Details of how iodinated contrast was administered are not given. Not surprisingly, CT was found to be less sensitive (77%) than echocardiography (98%) and aortography (89%) in those patients with surgical proof (35).

In 1993 Nienaber and co-workers compared 110 patients with suspected aortic dissection who underwent at least two of three imaging tests—TEE, CT, or MRI. CT was found to have lower sensitivity (93.8%) than TEE (97.7%) and MRI

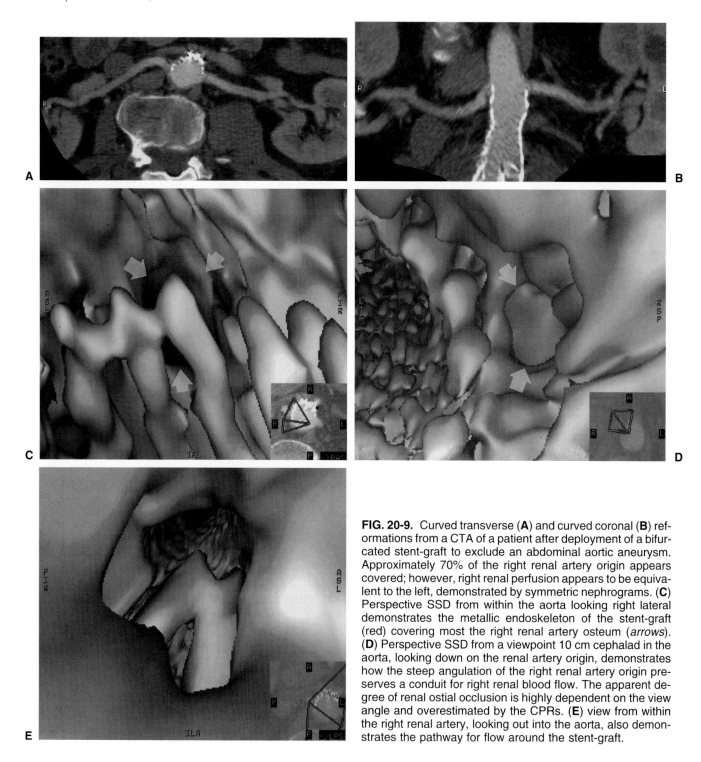

FIG. 20-9. Curved transverse (**A**) and curved coronal (**B**) reformations from a CTA of a patient after deployment of a bifurcated stent-graft to exclude an abdominal aortic aneurysm. Approximately 70% of the right renal artery origin appears covered; however, right renal perfusion appears to be equivalent to the left, demonstrated by symmetric nephrograms. (**C**) Perspective SSD from within the aorta looking right lateral demonstrates the metallic endoskeleton of the stent-graft (red) covering most the right renal artery osteum (*arrows*). (**D**) Perspective SSD from a viewpoint 10 cm cephalad in the aorta, looking down on the renal artery origin, demonstrates how the steep angulation of the right renal artery origin preserves a conduit for right renal blood flow. The apparent degree of renal ostial occlusion is highly dependent on the view angle and overestimated by the CPRs. (**E**) view from within the right renal artery, looking out into the aorta, also demonstrates the pathway for flow around the stent-graft.

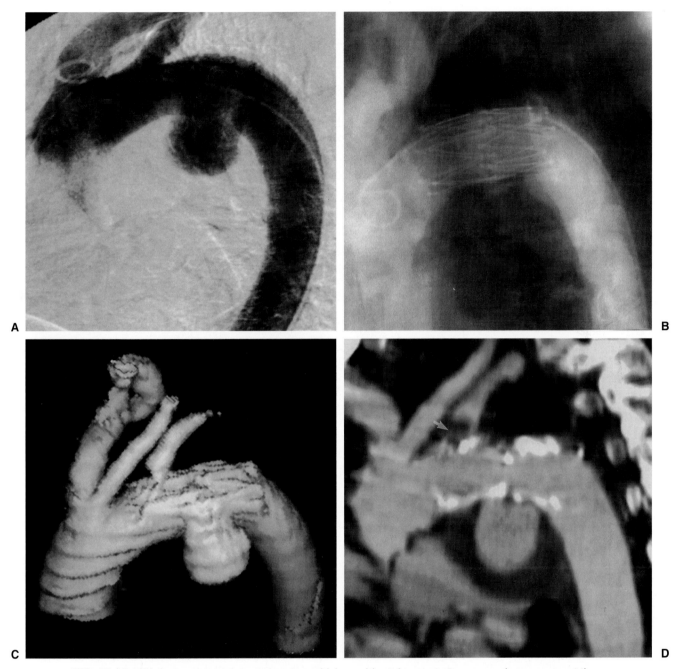

FIG. 20-10. **(A)** Aortogram status post motor vehicle accident demonstrates a pseudoaneurysm at the aortic isthmus. **(B)** The pseudoaneurysm appears to be completely thrombosed following deployment of a stent-graft (Dacron-covered modified Z stent). **(C)** SSD and **(D)** CPR CTA obtained 4 hours after stent-graft deployment demonstrates that the pseudoaneurysm is still patent. Additionally, the stent-graft covers the origin of the left subclavian artery, and a thrombus (*arrow*) has formed in the proximal left subclavian artery. The patient underwent transection of the left subclavian artery approximately 5 cm from its origin through a limited incision in the neck. The distal left subclavian artery was transplanted onto the left common carotid artery. *(continued)*

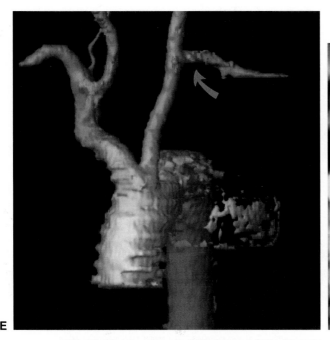

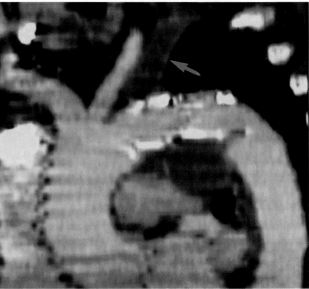

E   F

FIG. 20-10. *Continued.* SSD (**E**) and CPR (**F**) CTA performed 10 days later demonstrate spontaneous thrombosis of the pseudoaneurysm. The distal left subclavian artery originates from the left common carotid artery (*curved arrow*), and the proximal left subclavian artery has completely thrombosed (*straight arrow*). (Reprinted from Rubin GD. Helical CT angiography of the thoracic aorta. *J Thorac Imaging* 1997; 12 (*in press*).

(98.3%), and to have lower specificity (87.1%) than MRI (97.8%). For this study, 80–100 mL of contrast medium were administered during the course of 5–15-min CT scans that were performed with section intervals of 20 mm (36).

To date there have been no comparisons of spiral CT to either MRI or TEE. In comparison to conventional CT, Spiral CT substantially improves visualization of intimal dissections, associated pseudoaneurysms, branch involvement, and identification of sites of communication between the true and false lumina (Fig. 20-11). Although advances have occurred in CT imaging, TEE and MRI have undergone further improvements as well. The one modality that has not substantially improved has been conventional angiography. Currently, the primary indication for diagnostic arteriography of acute aortic dissection is in the setting of arrhythmia or ECG abnormalities suggestive of coronary artery involvement and myocardial ischemia. It is likely that in appropriately skilled hands, the accuracy of TEE, CT, and MRI will be nearly identical for the diagnosis of aortic dissection. Access to these three modalities is another issue, however.

Because patients suffering from acute aortic dissection are typically critically ill and potentially in need of an emergent operation, expediency of diagnosis is important. In a medical center where experienced cardiologists are available to perform state-of-the-art TEE in the emergency room to identify the presence of an intimal flap in the ascending aorta, TEE will probably be the preferred first-line imaging test. An additional advantage of TEE over CT acutely is its ability to identify aortic valvular insufficiency, which in the setting of acute aortic dissection will indicate the need for emergent valve replacement in addition to aortic repair. When high-quality TEE is unavailable, however, in most institutions CT will be the modality that is most accessible and staffed to handle potentially hemodynamically unstable patients.

When considering the clinical utility of a diagnostic test, it is useful to evaluate the likelihood that a test will suggest an alternative diagnosis when the primary diagnosis is not present. Figure 20-12 illustrates a case where acute chest pain and diminished right brachial and radial pulses were highly suggestive of aortic dissection. Following Spiral CT, dissection was not identified; however, a high-grade stenosis of the brachiocephalic artery origin and an occluded bypass graft originating on the anterior surface of the ascending aorta and inserting onto a proximally stenosed left anterior descending coronary artery was found on CTA. It is unlikely that either of these abnormalities would have been detected with TEE.

Abdominal aortic dissection is typically caused by direct inferior extension of thoracic aortic dissection. In the absence of trauma, particularly iatrogenic, isolated abdominal aortic or iliac artery dissection is quite rare. In the setting of abdominal aortic dissection, other imaging issues emerge that cannot be addressed by TEE. These include clinically relevant aortic branch involvement, which typically is in the intra-abdominal region, where acute mesenteric ischemia, acute renal ischemia (manifest by uncontrolled hypertension), and lower-extremity claudication indicate extension into or occlusion of mesenteric, renal, and iliac arteries, re-

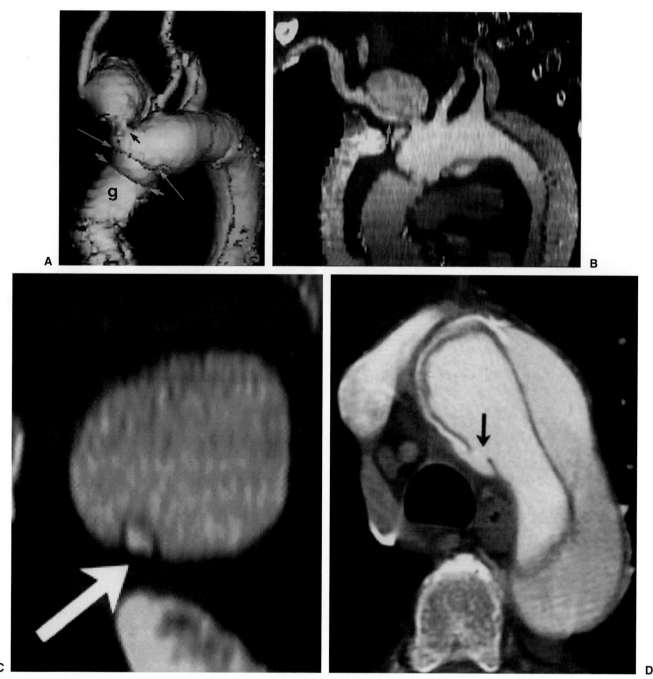

FIG. 20-11. Diminished arm pulses bilaterally after ascending aortic grafting for type A aortic dissection. **(A)** Shaded-surface display CTA demonstrates the anastomosis (*short arrows*) of the ascending aortic graft (g) to the aortic true lumen. A second line (*long arrows*) delineates the anterior extent of a circumferential false lumen that is directly supplying (*small black arrow*) a 3-cm false aneurysm of the brachiocephalic artery. An intimal flap is present within the left subclavian artery and extends inferiorly through the descending aorta. Curved planar **(B)** and oblique **(C)** reformations demonstrate the degree of brachiocephalic artery true luminal compression (*white arrow*) by the false luminal pseudoaneurysm. Unlike the shaded-surface display, the true and false lumina can be differentiated by their attenuation, which is lower in the false lumen at the cranial aspect of the scan and gradually becomes greater at the caudal aspect because of the slower flow into the false lumen. **(D)** Transverse section at the aortic arch demonstrates the site of communication (fenestration) between the true and false lumina (*arrow*). Note that the differential enhancement between true and false lumina equalizes closest to the fenestration and gradually increases posteriorly. *(continued)*

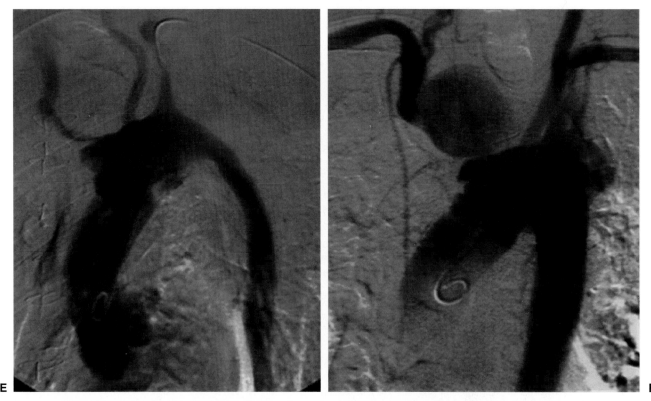

E   F

FIG. 20-11. *Continued.* **(E,F)** Two images from a correlative aortogram demonstrating the delayed filling of the pseudoaneurysm. The inability to simultaneously visualize and differentiate the true and false lumina on the aortogram makes the complex circumferential dissection around the aortic arch difficult to appreciate. (Reprinted from Rubin GD. Helical CT angiography of the thoracic aorta. *J Thorac Imaging* 1997;12 (*in press*).

spectively. Intervention, either surgically or using catheter-based techniques, may be required. Spiral CT provides excellent visualization of abdominal aortic branch involvement, displaying dissection flaps within the branches, restriction of flow into aortic branches from compression of the aortic true lumen by the false lumen, and intimal flap fenestrations, where true and false luminal blood communicate (Fig. 20-13). Visualization of these phenomena can be superior to that provided by the limited-view angle, single lumen opacification of conventional arteriography. When considering catheter-based interventions, preprocedural CT can be very useful. The simultaneous visualization of all aortic lumina can help to avoid confusion in the angiography suite that results from opacification of only one of three or more lumina in a complex dissection. The CT scan can also help identify the best route for achieving access to aortic branches and can be useful for assessing the success of endoluminal interventions aimed at reconstituting blood flow to ischemic organs (Fig. 20-14).

Although the superior spatial resolution and improved aortic enhancement provided by spiral CT result in substantially better images than conventional CT, some pitfalls persist. Pulsation in the ascending aorta can mimic an intimal flap. This artifact tends to be less of a problem with spiral CT because the generation of closely overlapping sections in the region of the suspected artifact or intimal flap, displayed

sequentially as a cine loop, usually establishes the artifact as rotating or moving relative to the aorta. Examination of wide windows may document extension of artifacts beyond the aortic wall. Also, as previously discussed, the use of retrospective segmented reconstruction of the spiral scan data may eliminate motion artifacts observed on standard reconstructions (16).

Differential flow in the true and false lumina can result in the spurious appearance of a thrombosed false lumen when scan delay is based upon a timing study directed to the true lumen of the aorta. In the setting of suspected aortic dissection, bolus timing should be performed just below the aortic arch, where transverse cross-sections of the distal ascending and proximal descending aorta can be evaluated. A region of interest is placed in both the true and false lumina and two curves are generated. A delay time that assures some false luminal opacification is selected, and the bolus duration is then extended by the number of seconds between the true luminal peak and the selected delay time. This assures true and false luminal opacification for the duration of the spiral acquisition. Other potential pitfalls of CTA are illustrated by two missed aortic dissections in Quint's series. One was in a patient with hematoma surrounding the ascending aorta but no identifiable aortic lesion on CT. At surgery, a short ascending aortic intimal tear was noted with a thrombosed false lumen that simulated mediastinal hematoma on CT.

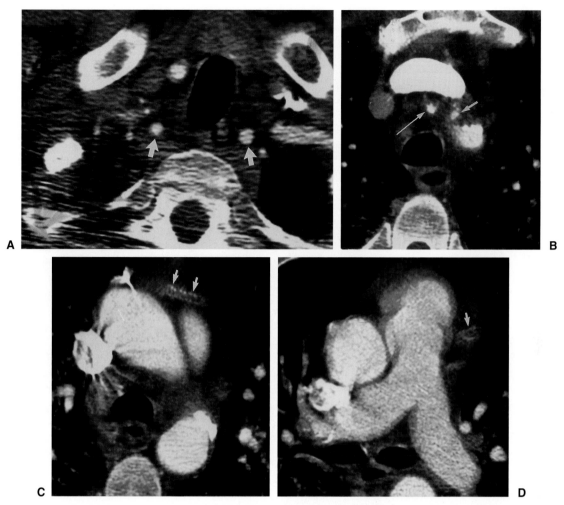

FIG. 20-12. (A–D) Transverse sections acquired with 3-mm collimation, 2.0 pitch in a patient with acute chest pain and diminished right brachial and radial pulses. One centimeter above the aortic arch (**B**), there is a high-grade stenosis of the brachiocephalic artery origin (*long white arrow*) and a narrow left common carotid artery origin (*short white arrow*). At the thoracic inlet (**A**) the left common carotid artery is completely occluded. Note that both vertebral arteries (*wide arrows*) are large in this patient with unsuspected, although substantial, flow limitation into the right and no flow into the left common carotid arteries. Below the aortic arch (**C,D**) a thrombosed coronary artery bypass graft (*arrows*) from the ascending aorta to the left anterior descending coronary artery is demonstrated. The findings were confirmed arteriographically and serial enzymes established the diagnosis of acute myocardial infarction. (Reprinted from Rubin GD. Helical CT angiography of the thoracic aorta. *J Thorac Imaging* 1997;12 (*in press*).

The other misdiagnosed case of aortic dissection was in a patient with an intimal tear on the underside of the aortic arch associated with partial thrombosis of the false lumen, which mimicked a small penetrating ulcer with associated intramural hematoma on CT (20).

When considering alternative visualization techniques in the setting of aortic dissection, it should not be surprising that MIPs are limited because they will not demonstrate the intimal flap unless it is oriented perpendicular to the MIP. Curved planar reconstructions can be very useful for displaying the flap within the center of the vessel and evaluating true versus false luminal blood supply (7,37) (Fig. 20-15), whereas shaded-surface displays depict the interface of the

intimal flap with the aortic wall. The use of raysum projections has also been advocated for intimal flap depiction (38).

Intramural Hematoma

Although initially identified pathologically in 1920, intramural hematoma has only recently been recognized as a distinct clinical entity from aortic dissection. Several mechanisms have been proposed, including spontaneous rupture of vasa vasorum, intimal fracture of an atherosclerotic plaque, and intramural propagation of hemorrhage adjacent

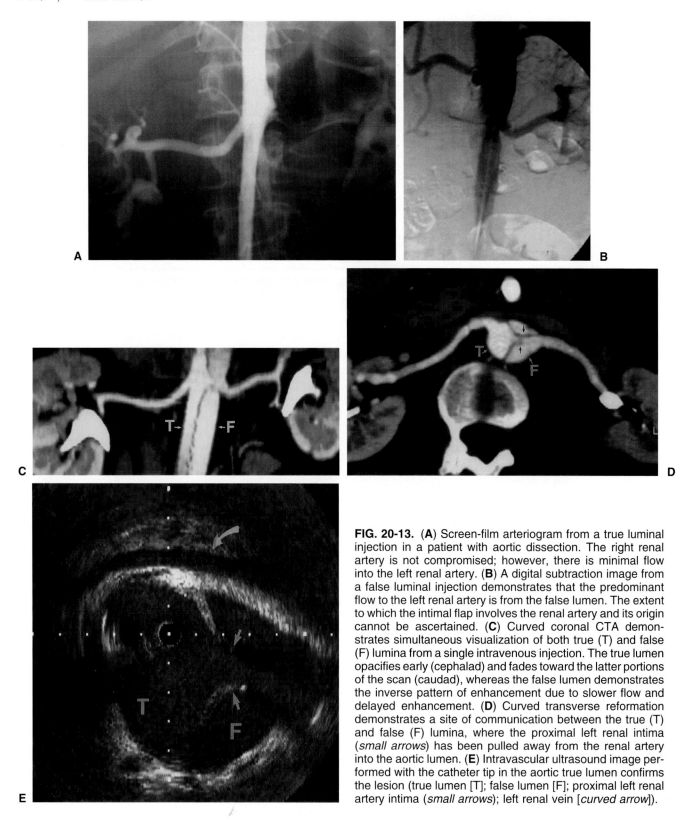

FIG. 20-13. (A) Screen-film arteriogram from a true luminal injection in a patient with aortic dissection. The right renal artery is not compromised; however, there is minimal flow into the left renal artery. **(B)** A digital subtraction image from a false luminal injection demonstrates that the predominant flow to the left renal artery is from the false lumen. The extent to which the intimal flap involves the renal artery and its origin cannot be ascertained. **(C)** Curved coronal CTA demonstrates simultaneous visualization of both true (T) and false (F) lumina from a single intravenous injection. The true lumen opacifies early (cephalad) and fades toward the latter portions of the scan (caudad), whereas the false lumen demonstrates the inverse pattern of enhancement due to slower flow and delayed enhancement. **(D)** Curved transverse reformation demonstrates a site of communication between the true (T) and false (F) lumina, where the proximal left renal intima (*small arrows*) has been pulled away from the renal artery into the aortic lumen. **(E)** Intravascular ultrasound image performed with the catheter tip in the aortic true lumen confirms the lesion (true lumen [T]; false lumen [F]; proximal left renal artery intima (*small arrows*); left renal vein [*curved arrow*]).

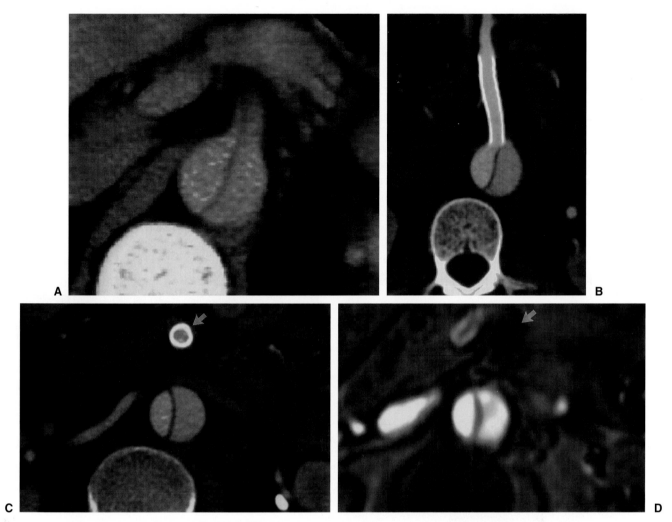

FIG. 20-14. (**A**) Transverse CT section from a patient with acute mesenteric ischemia demonstrates an intimal flap entering the superior mesenteric artery. (**B**) Curved transverse reformation of a CTA performed following deployment of a Wall stent into the true lumen of the SMA. The intimal flap has been displaced to the right and true luminal supply from the aorta restored. The lumen of the stent is not significantly obscured by the metallic stent. (**C**) Transverse CTA section and (**D**) gradient-echo MRI demonstrate the relative extent with which the metal of the stent interferes with luminal visualization (*arrows*). The SMA is completely obscured on the MR examination. The magnitude of this magnetic susceptibility artifact is influenced by the echo time (11 milliseconds in this case) and may diminish with shorter echo times.

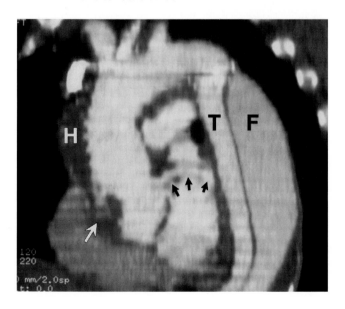

FIG. 20-15. Curved planar reformation from a patient with a descending aortic dissection (T = true lumen; F = false lumen) and an ascending aortic intramural hematoma (H) with extravasation of contrast through an ulceration just distal to the aortic root (*white arrow*). The left main and proximal circumflex coronary artery are illustrated (*black arrows*). (Reprinted from Rubin GD. Techniques of reconstruction in spiral CT of the chest. In: Remy-Jardin M. and Remy J., eds. Berlin: Springer-Verlag; 1996.)

to a penetrating atherosclerotic ulcer. Regardless of the cause, patients with intramural hematomas exhibit signs and symptoms as well as risk profiles that are virtually identical to classic aortic dissection (39).

The CT appearance of intramural hematomas caused by penetrating atherosclerotic ulcers was described in detail by Kazerooni and co-workers, based upon an analysis of conventional CTs in 16 patients. In addition to the visualization of at least one ulcer in 15 out of 16, the intramural hematoma was visualized in all 16, and its subintimal location was confirmed by the observation of displaced intimal calcifications in 13 (40). Although intramural hematomas associated with ulceration tend to predominate in the descending aorta (40), the distribution of all intramural hematomas was 48% ascending aortic, 8% aortic arch, and 44% descending aortic in one series (39).

The advantage of spiral CT for the assessment of intramural hematomas hasn't been specifically reported; however, the thinner collimation, volumetric acquisition, and superior aortic enhancement are likely to improve the identification and characterization of small atherosclerotic ulcerations over conventional CT and possibly aortography (Fig. 20-16). In Quint's series two patients in whom intramural hematomas were identified but an associated ulceration could not be identified were scored as false-negative examinations. Recognizing that intramural hematoma formation has two proposed mechanisms: (a) extension of a penetrating ulcer into the media with subsequent bleeding into the aortic wall, and (b) primary disruption of vasa vasorum without penetrating ulcer formation (40,41)—the diagnoses in these cases may have been correct, given a primary intramural bleed as the mechanism for intramural hematoma formation, which need not be associated with ulceration.

One useful observation that may help differentiate intramural hematomas from the thrombosed false lumen of a classical intimal dissection is that the latter tend to longitudinally spiral around the aorta, whereas the former tend to

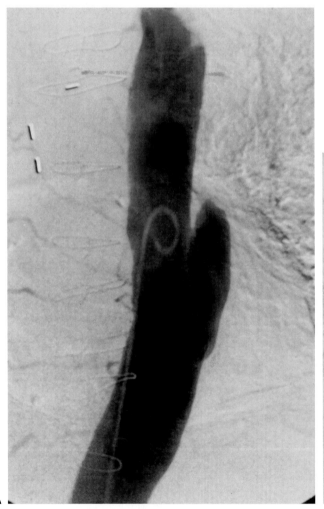

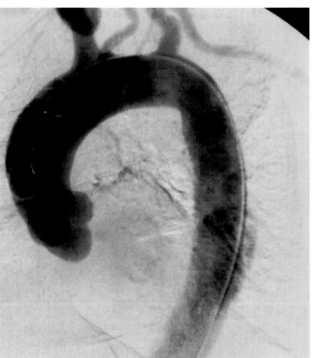

A

B

FIG. 20-16. **(A)** Descending thoracic aortogram performed in a 70-year-old man with acute chest pain demonstrates a penetrating ulcer on the posterior wall of the aorta with flattening of the posterior aortic lumen proximal to the ulceration consistent with intramural hematoma. **(B)** Arch aortogram is normal, suggesting that the lesion is limited to the descending aorta. *(continued)*

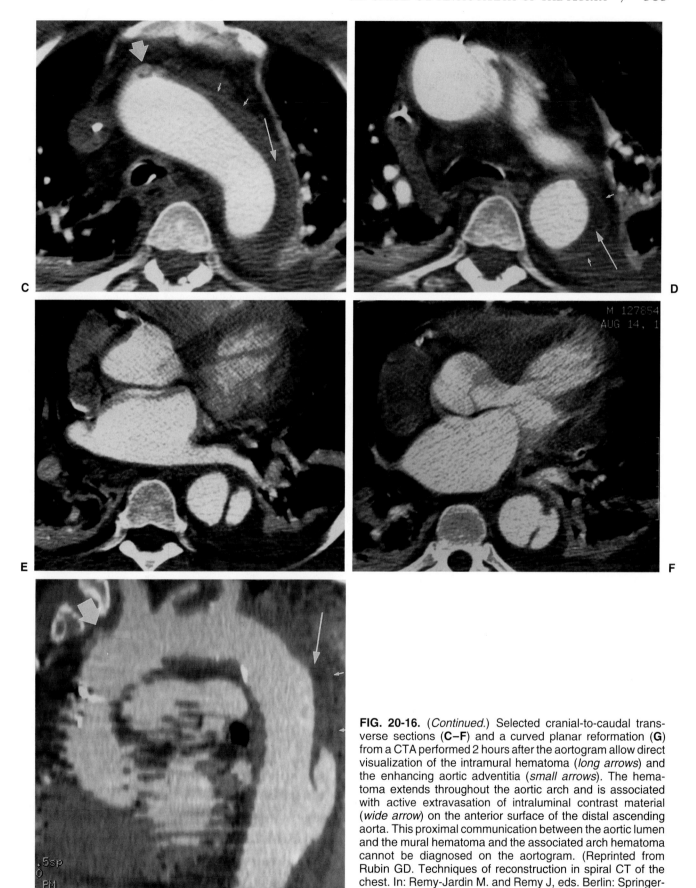

FIG. 20-16. (*Continued.*) Selected cranial-to-caudal transverse sections (**C–F**) and a curved planar reformation (**G**) from a CTA performed 2 hours after the aortogram allow direct visualization of the intramural hematoma (*long arrows*) and the enhancing aortic adventitia (*small arrows*). The hematoma extends throughout the aortic arch and is associated with active extravasation of intraluminal contrast material (*wide arrow*) on the anterior surface of the distal ascending aorta. This proximal communication between the aortic lumen and the mural hematoma and the associated arch hematoma cannot be diagnosed on the aortogram. (Reprinted from Rubin GD. Techniques of reconstruction in spiral CT of the chest. In: Remy-Jardin M. and Remy J, eds. Berlin: Springer-Verlag; 1996.)

maintain a constant circumferential relationship with aortic wall. Another finding that can be seen in the setting of intramural hematoma is intense enhancement and thickening of the aortic wall external to the hematoma, which may represent adventitial inflammation .

OCCLUSIVE DISEASE NOT CAUSED BY DISSECTION

Atherosclerosis, vasculitis, and fibromuscular dysplasia represent common causes of symptomatic aortic branch occlusive disease, with atherosclerosis being the most common cause in North America, Europe, and many parts of Asia. The most extensive investigations of the utility of CTA for assessing arterial occlusive disease have been directed toward the renal arteries.

Renal Arteries

An important indication for directed renal artery imaging is the assessment of patients with suspected renal vascular hypertension to exclude hemodynamically significant renal artery stenosis. Although major renal vascular disease accounts for less than 1% of all cases of hypertension (42), the identification of hemodynamically significant renal artery stenosis may represent the only curable cause of acute hypertension. Conventional angiography has been considered the reference standard for diagnosing renal artery stenosis; however, there has been a long-standing interest in developing less invasive techniques for reliably demonstrating renal artery stenosis. A 70% stenosis of the renal arteries is typically considered sufficient to alter renal arterial flow and is thus a criterion for intervention with either percutaneous transluminal angioplasty or surgery (43–45). Spiral CT allows simultaneous assessment of renal parenchymal abnormalities as well as arterial lesions.

Because the renal arteries course in-plane, they are more susceptible to partial volume artifact than through-plane vessels, such as the abdominal aorta. CT angiographic technique is similar to that of the abdominal aorta; however, collimation and pitch should be minimized to optimize resolution and diminish partial volume effects. Based on data generated with a renal artery model, it has been suggested that collimation greater than 2 mm results in inaccurate depiction of stenotic renal arteries (46). In another renal artery model, Davros and co-workers concluded that 1-mm collimation with pitch 2.0 substantially improved the depiction of modeled renal artery stenoses over 3-mm collimation (47). Use of 2-mm collimation with a pitch of 2.0 allows for borderline anatomic coverage 12 cm of table travel in 30 s and 16 cm of table travel in 40 s, assuming a 1-s GRP. Unfortunately, many spiral CT scanners do not offer 2-mm collimation. Use of 1-mm collimation and a pitch of 2.0 on a 1-s scanner allows for 6 cm of table travel in 30 s and 8 cm of table travel in 40 s. Many patients are too large to undergo renal artery CTA with 1-mm collimation without having the exam-

ination substantially degraded by image noise. With subsecond rotation speeds (750 ms GRP), however, the use of 2-mm collimation, when available, becomes practical as more than 21 cm can be covered in 40 s with a pitch of 2.0.

Because accessory renal arteries have been reported to arise as cranial as the inferior phrenic artery and as caudal as the median sacral artery (48,49), anatomic coverage should be substantially longer than the anticipated location of the main renal arteries. For practical purposes, 99% of renal arteries originate from the aorta, below the superior mesenteric artery origin, to the common iliac bifurcation (50). These are the landmarks we rely on for our renal CTA. This distance ranges between 20 and 25 cm in most people. Unless scanning with subsecond GRPs, 3-mm collimation must be used to cover this distance within a single breathhold. Fortunately, preliminary clinical data suggest that use of 3-mm collimation enables detection of accessory renal arteries and accurate grading of most renal artery stenoses (13,51). Although we comfortably rely on 3-mm collimated images to assess the renal arteries, we reduce the collimation to 1 or 2 mm whenever possible.

The accuracy of spiral CT for detection of hemodynamically significant stenoses has been assessed by several investigators. Galanski and colleagues studied 22 patients with suspected renal vascular hypertension with both CTA and intra-arterial DSA (13). Twenty-two of the 54 renal arteries assessed were noted to have renal artery stenosis with DSA. In 20 of these stenoses or occlusions, the site of disease was within the proximal one-third of the renal artery. Stenoses were identified in the middle or distal third of the renal artery in only two cases, one patient with fibromuscular dysplasia and a second with a transplanted kidney and renal artery. All renal artery stenoses and occlusions were detected with spiral CT, and grading was identical to DSA in all but four patients. In three of these four patients, the degree of renal artery stenosis was overestimated with spiral CT, suggesting 75% to 99% stenosis where DSA identified 50% to 75% stenosis. In the fourth case, a short renal artery occlusion was underestimated and diagnosed as a 75% to 99% stenosis with spiral CT.

We studied 73 renal arteries in 31 patients with both CTA and conventional arteriography, analyzing a subpopulation of 33 renal arteries in 14 patients with at least one hemodynamically significant renal artery stenosis (51). The analysis was performed as a blinded interpretation of CT angiograms and conventional arteriograms by three independent reviewers. Twenty-eight main and five accessory renal arteries were graded on a four-point stenosis scale. Using MIP-CTA, 80% of gradings were concordant with conventional angiography, with 3% undergraded and 17% overgraded. The tendency for overgrading of renal artery stenoses is likely attributable to partial volume effects with surrounding low-attenuation retroperitoneal fat, accentuated by the MIP. Grading accuracy would have likely been improved had multiplanar or transverse images been included with the MIP for assessment.

A recent study examined 131 renal arteries in 50 hypertensive patients. With a sensitivity of 88% and a specificity of 98% for the detection of more than 50% renal artery stenoses (52). Substantial differences in acquisition technique and data analysis were employed in this study, which makes comparison of these results with the two previous reports difficult (13,51–54).

The identification of ancillary findings such as nephrographic abnormalities or poststenotic dilation can improve the specificity of identifying hemodynamically significant renal artery stenoses. Nephrographic abnormalities can be global or regional. In our series, the identification of poststenotic dilatation or nephrogram asymmetries was highly specific (86% and 98%, respectively) for coexistent renal artery stenosis of more than 70% (51). In Galanski's series, abnormal renal cortical enhancement was noted in five cases, all associated with more than 50% renal artery stenosis (13). However, hemodynamically significant renal artery stenoses frequently occur without coexistent poststenotic dilatation or nephrographic abnormalities. We found the sensitivity for renal artery stenoses of more than 70% to be 50% for poststenotic dilatation and 53% for nephrographic abnormalities (51). Similarly, Galanski and co-workers found that five patients with renal artery stenoses of more than 50% had no renal parenchymal abnormalities (13). Nevertheless, when these signs are used in combination with direct visualization of the stenotic segment, overall grading accuracy should improve by reducing false-negative results.

These signs can be particularly helpful in the setting of calcified renal arteriosclerosis. The identification of mural calcium on CT angiographic images by itself is not a useful indicator of hemodynamically significant stenosis because 65% of renal arteries with mural calcification were not demonstrated to have greater than 70% stenoses. A study of incidental renal artery calcifications in patients undergoing abdominal CT and angiography for a variety of clinical indications found that the presence of calcium clumps of more than 3 mm in diameter on CT was associated with renal artery stenosis in 44% of arteries. Smaller calcium clumps were associated with renal artery stenosis in 30% of arteries, and renal arteries free of CT-detectable calcium were stenotic in 17% (55).

The assessment of transverse CT sections is frequently conclusive; however, renal artery CTAs are better assessed when transverse sections are reviewed in association with multiplanar reformations, MIPs, and SSDs. Galanski found this to be true in 15 of their 22 patients (13). Our initial experience with renal artery CTA has led us to never interpret these images without reformatted or three-dimensionally rendered images. The value of direct visualization of the third dimension (craniocaudal) cannot be understated when renal arteries are tortuous, have a steep craniocaudal course, or are associated with calcified plaque. It is important to understand the advantages and disadvantages of each rendering technique prior to relying on them for diagnosis (Fig. 20-17).

We found that SSDs were only 59% sensitive, whereas MIP-CTAs were 92% sensitive for the detection of greater than 70% stenosis. Both techniques were of equal specificity (82% to 83%) (51). The overall accuracy of stenosis grading was 80% with MIP and 55% with shaded-surface display. The poor performance of shaded-surface displays relative to MIPs can be explained by two features that limit surface displays: (a) calcification associated with stenoses will not be visualized with shaded-surface displays and cause underestimation of stenosis, and (b) partial volume averaging in regions of stenosis will be accentuated by the thresholding process and result in arterial discontinuities that overestimate stenosis. As a result of these data, we never assess aortic branch occlusive disease with SSDs.

Since publishing these data, we have come to rely on curved planar reformations as an additional means for visualizing renal artery stenoses. Although there are no published data, it appears as though curved planar reformations, when created in both the transverse and coronal planes, may be superior to MIPs, when lesions are associated with calcified plaque (Fig. 20-18), when high-grade stenoses manifest as arterial discontinuities, or when there is poor differential enhancement between the renal artery and an overlying renal vein (56). In Galanski's series, opacification of the left renal vein prevented adequate visualization of the left renal artery with MIP in six cases (13). Curved planar reformations are quicker to create than MIPs, because no editing is required; however, the reliability of the resultant images is highly dependent on the accuracy of the curve drawing (10). As our data indicate, shaded-surface displays tend to be the least informative for the routine assessment of renal artery stenosis. However, they can be useful in regions of complicated anatomy, including transplanted kidneys (57).

Mesenteric Arteries

Chronic mesenteric ischemia, though uncommon, should be suspected in elderly patients with chronic postprandial mid-abdominal pain (58). Atherosclerotic narrowing or occlusion of at least one and often several major mesenteric vessels is the typical cause of chronic mesenteric ischemia. The significance of a single vessel stenosis depends on the degree of collateral pathway formation (59). CTA is well suited for the evaluation of the celiac and superior mesenteric artery origins where atherosclerotic occlusive disease is likely to occur (Fig. 20-19). CTA is additionally capable of demonstrating major collateral pathways in patients with high-grade stenoses or occlusions.

The techniques of mesenteric CTA are similar to those of renal CTA, as the celiac branches and superior mesenteric artery origin course in plane also. If mesenteric ischemia is suspected, a high-resolution examination with 2-mm collimation (pitch 1.5) or 3-mm collimation (pitch 1.0) during a 30-s spiral exposure will result in a 9-cm scan, which ensures inclusion of the celiac and superior mesenteric artery origins as well as their proximal branches and regions where signifi-

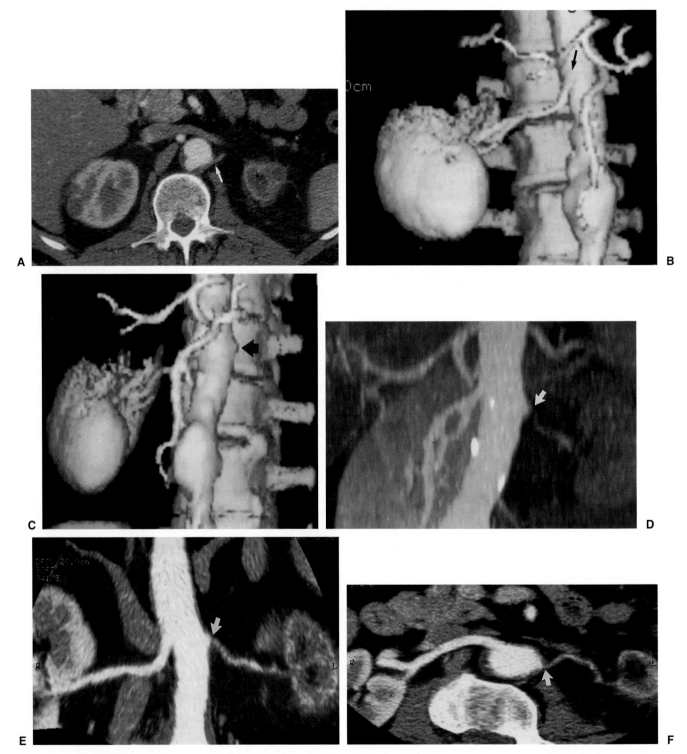

FIG. 20-17. Left renal artery stenosis. (**A**) Transverse CT section demonstrates the proximal portion of the left renal artery (*arrow*). There appears to be a high-grade stenosis at its origin; however, its appearance may be spurious due to the oblique course of the vessel if the origin of the renal artery is present on adjacent sections. Note that the size and attenuation of the left renal nephrogram is considerably less than that of the right. (**B**) Frontal (**C**) 30-degree left anterior oblique shaded-surface displays clearly show the right renal artery origin (*thin arrow*). The left renal artery and kidney have been lost due to thresholding and segmentation. A subtle contour irregularity (*wide arrow*) indicates the position of the left renal artery origin. (**D**) Maximum-intensity projection demonstrates a discontinuity in the proximal left renal artery (*arrow*). High-grade renal artery stenosis, rather than complete occlusion, is inferred by the observation that there is filling of the distal vessel without obvious collateral supply. The discontinuity is observed because overlying soft tissues have similar attenuation to the highly stenotic region of the left renal artery, resulting in this region being indistinguishable from the background. The nephrographic asymmetries, both size and attenuation, are clearly evident. (**E**) Curved coronal and (**F**) curved trans-

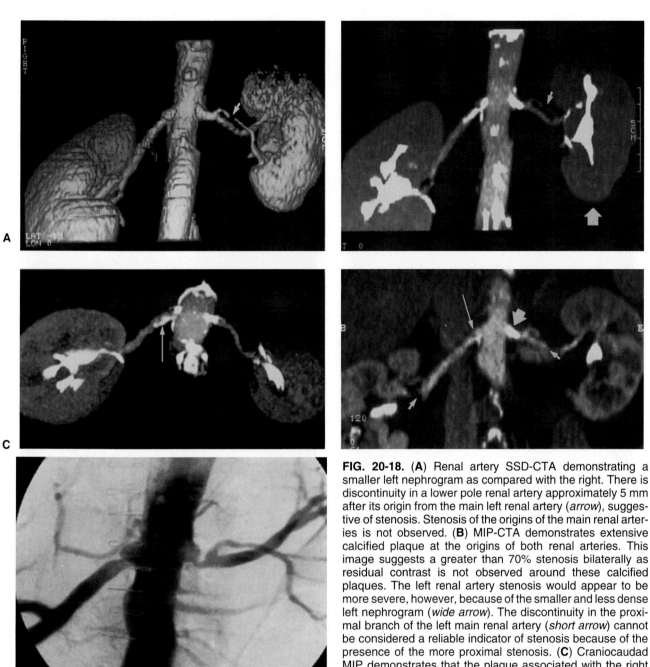

FIG. 20-18. (A) Renal artery SSD-CTA demonstrating a smaller left nephrogram as compared with the right. There is discontinuity in a lower pole renal artery approximately 5 mm after its origin from the main left renal artery (*arrow*), suggestive of stenosis. Stenosis of the origins of the main renal arteries is not observed. **(B)** MIP-CTA demonstrates extensive calcified plaque at the origins of both renal arteries. This image suggests a greater than 70% stenosis bilaterally as residual contrast is not observed around these calcified plaques. The left renal artery stenosis would appear to be more severe, however, because of the smaller and less dense left nephrogram (*wide arrow*). The discontinuity in the proximal branch of the left main renal artery (*short arrow*) cannot be considered a reliable indicator of stenosis because of the presence of the more proximal stenosis. **(C)** Craniocaudad MIP demonstrates that the plaque associated with the right renal artery is eccentrically located posteriorly (*arrow*) and contrast can be seen within the adjacent arterial lumen, indicating that this is a mild to moderate stenosis. A contrast column cannot be demonstrated adjacent to the left renal artery origin plaque, indicating severe stenosis. **(D)** Curved planar reformation, a one-voxel-thick section, which allows visualization of the calcified plaque along the inferior margin of the proximal right renal artery while contrast flows through the patent lumen superiorly (*long arrow*). No contrast is observed adjacent to the calcified origin of the left renal artery (*wide arrow*). Curved planar reformations are exceedingly operator dependent, and inaccurate curve drawing can result in spurious vascular discontinuities (*short arrows*). **(E)** Digital subtraction conventional arteriogram demonstrates an approximately 50% stenosis of the right renal artery and 80% stenosis of the left renal artery. The left lower polar renal artery branch is not stenotic.

verse planar reformations demonstrate the degree of renal artery stenosis best. Curved planar reformation should always be created in two perpendicular planes to avoid under- or overestimation of the stenosis in the presence of eccentric plaque. Note that no discontinuities are observed throughout the course of the left renal arteries although a high-grade left renal artery origin stenosis is present (*arrow*). (Reprinted from Rubin GD. Spiral [helical] CT of the renal vasculature. *Semin Ultrasound CT MR* 1996;17:374–397.)

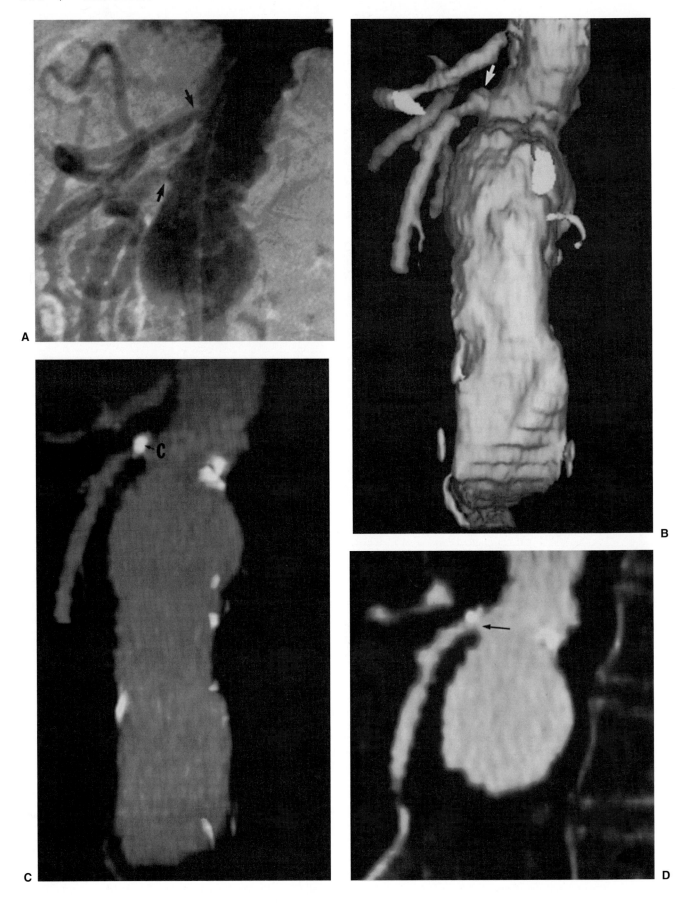

A

B

C

D

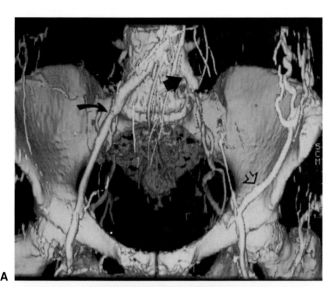

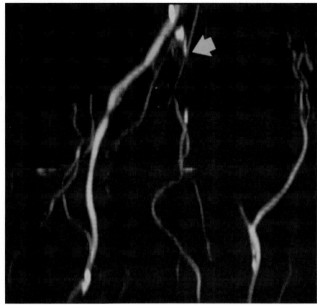

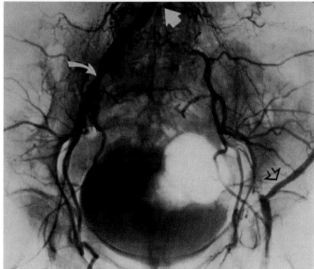

FIG. 20-20. (**A**) SSD-CTA demonstrates a long-segment occlusion of the left common and proximal external iliac arteries with reconstitution by an enlarged circumflex iliac artery (*open arrow*). The proximal portion of the common iliac artery (*straight arrow*) appears patent. An approximate 50% stenosis of the distal right common iliac artery is demonstrated (*curved arrow*). (**B**) MIP-CTA demonstrates that the entire left common iliac artery is occluded with the proximal segment, apparently patent on the SSD-CTA, being occluded by calcified atheroma (*arrow*). (**C**) Conventional arteriogram confirms the left common iliac occlusion (*wide arrow*), the right common iliac artery stenosis (*curved arrow*), and the large left circumflex iliac collateral supplying the distal left external iliac artery.

FIG. 20-19. (**A**) Digital subtraction conventional arteriogram demonstrating stenosis at the origin of the celiac axis and superior mesenteric artery (*arrows*). (**B**) SSD-CTA confirms the celiac stenosis; however, the superior mesenteric artery appears patent with an ectatic origin (*arrow*). (**C**) MIP-CTA demonstrates calcified plaque (c) overlying the superior mesenteric artery. The contrast-filled lumen is obscured by the calcium. (**D**) Oblique reformation (one pixel thick) demonstrates calcified plaque on the superior aspect of the SMA; however, intraluminal contrast is observed within the inferior portion of the vessel (*arrow*).

cant atherosclerosis is likely to occur. Data concerning the accuracy of CTA for detecting hemodynamically significant mesenteric arterial stenoses are scant and largely come from series of CTA directed toward primary aortic disease (7,11,27). The results suggest an accuracy for significant occlusive disease detection that is similar to that of renal arterial CTA.

Iliac Arteries

CTA of lower-extremity occlusive disease is limited by its inability to image the lower-extremity inflow and runoff vessels in a single setting with less than or equal to 3-mm collimation. Although preliminary reports of CTA of the lower extremities have been promising, more data are required. In an initial study, Lawrence and co-workers found that CTA, performed with 5-mm collimation, correctly detected greater than 50% stenoses or occlusions of the lower-extremity arteries with a sensitivity of 93% and specificity of 96% when compared to conventional arteriography (60). In the setting of lower-extremity claudication with noninvasive examinations suggestive of inflow disease, CTA readily displays the location and length of aortoiliac stenoses and important routes of collateral arterial supply (Fig. 20-20). In an early report of CTA for the detection of occlusive lower-extremity in-flow disease, we diagnosed five of five more than 50% atherosclerotic stenoses demonstrated by conventional angiography. These included two external iliac intimal dissections and one stenosis resulting from Takayasu arteritis with no false-positive diagnoses. Collateral pathways from the internal iliac, lumbar, intercostal, and contralateral iliac arteries were readily demonstrated (61). More data must be published in substantially larger groups of patients before we can ascertain the accuracy of CTA for detecting these lesions.

TRAUMA

Aortic injury occurs most commonly in the thoracic aorta at the aortic isthmus. Although most aortic transections never make it to medical centers for diagnosis and treatment prior to death, for the minority of patients who have a contained rupture and present to the emergency department alive, diagnosis must be accurate, and triage to the operating room must be rapid.

The use of CT scanning for the detection of aortic injury is controversial (62–64). The principal application of conventional CT is the detection of mediastinal hemorrhage. A recently published meta-analysis of 18 previously published series of post-traumatic thoracic CT revealed that mediastinal hemorrhage had a specificity of 87.1% and a sensitivity of 99.3% for predicting aortic injury (63). Furthermore, reliance on CT for triaging patients to angiography only when CT was suspicious resulted in an overall cost savings of more than $365,000 in Mirvis et al's own series of 677 trauma patients with chest radiographic abnormalities warranting aortic imaging (63). Although these results are impressive, some have argued that the confident identification of mediastinal hematoma, particularly on unenhanced CT, is extremely difficult (62).

The application of spiral CTA to suspected aortic trauma offers a new and important dimension to CT studies in these patients (Figs. 20-21, 20-22). Although initial reports have not relied on the use of high-resolution spiral acquisitions coupled with high-flow iodinated contrast injections, the results are encouraging. Gavant and colleagues published the first spiral CTA series of aortic injury. Using 7-mm collimation and a contrast medium flow rate of 1.5–2.0 mL/s, they found that the sensitivity of CT was greater than that of conventional arteriography (100% versus 94.4%), but the specificity and positive predictive values were less than those of conventional arteriography (81.7% and 47.4%, respectively, for CT, versus 96.3% and 81% for aortography) in a subset of 127 out of 1,518 patients with nontrivial blunt thoracic trauma who underwent both CT and aortography. Perhaps the most encouraging result of this study was that no false-negative results occurred in the 21 patients with aortic injury (65). This remains the only published comparative series of spiral CTA of blunt thoracic aortic trauma to date.

Gavant subsequently described the CT appearance of 38 thoracic aortic or great vessel injuries in 36 patients identified with spiral CT and confirmed with aortography or surgery. Six (17%) of these cases were found to have either no or difficult-to-detect para-aortic or mediastinal hematoma. Transverse sections showed either an intimal flap or a thrombus protruding into the aortic lumen in all cases. Of 28 injuries to the descending aorta, 23 (82%) were associated with a pseudoaneurysm. In subjectively comparing the value of the reconstructed transverse sections to multiplanar reformations and 3D renderings, the authors felt that the transverse sections were best for depicting the proximal and distal extent of the lesion, and aside from the fact that multiplanar reformations and 3D renderings portray the thoracic aortic lumen in a familiar light did not contribute substantially to the identification and characterization of aortic injury (66).

Some caution should be exercised when interpreting the very impressive reported sensitivity of spiral CT for aortic injury. In the previously mentioned study, iodinated contrast medium was only administered to patients with evidence of mediastinal hematoma. This of course assumes that the sensitivity of mediastinal hematoma on CT is 100% for detecting aortic injury. Although many authors believe this to be true, the negative predictive value of CT for aortic injury has not been proven (67). The definitive answer to this issue requires a prospective trial where both CT and angiography are performed in all patients who would undergo aortography on the basis of clinical and chest radiographic criteria. According to Trerotola, this would require approximately 1,500 patients, assuming 98% negative predictive value with 98% statistical power (67).

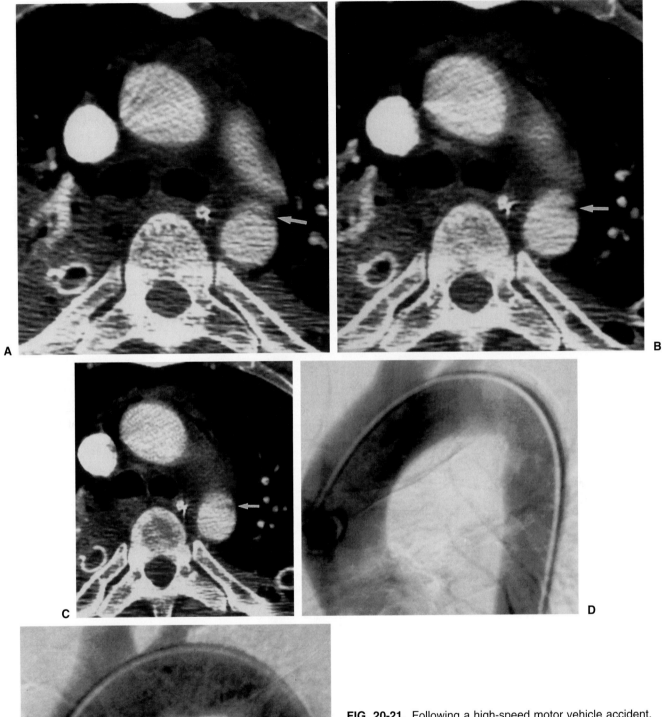

FIG. 20-21. Following a high-speed motor vehicle accident, subtle aortic injury was seen. (**A–C**) Consecutive transverse helical CTA reconstructions obtained with 3-mm collimation, 2.0 pitch, and 2-mm reconstruction intervals demonstrate a subtle intimal injury of the aortic isthmus (*arrow*). Because of other injuries and skeptical trauma surgeons, an aortogram was not obtained until 3 months later. No abnormality was detectable on the standard left anterior oblique view (**D**); however, based on the CT appearance, a true lateral view (**E**) was obtained that revealed the development of a small pseudoaneurysm (*arrow*). The injury was confirmed in the operating room. (Reprinted from Rubin GD. Helical CT angiography of the thoracic aorta. *J Thorac Imaging* 1997;12 [*in press*].)

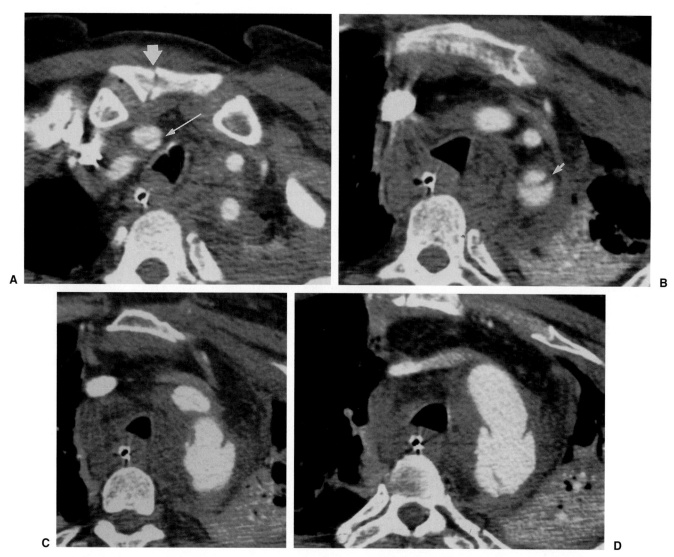

FIG. 20-22. Following a high-speed motor vehicle accident, gross aortic injury was seen. **(A–D)** Transverse helical CTA sections every 1 cm demonstrate aortic injury with pseudoaneurysm formation at the aortic isthmus. An intimal injury extends into the left subclavian artery (*short arrows*). An isolated intimal dissection in the right common carotid artery (*long arrow*) is additionally demonstrated deep to a vertical fracture of the manubrium (*wide arrow*). There is extensive mediastinal hematoma. The findings were confirmed in the operating room. (Reprinted from Rubin GD. Helical CT angiography of the thoracic aorta. *J Thorac Imaging* 1997;12.)

ORGAN TRANSPLANT EVALUATION

The detection of accessory renal arteries was reported to be 100% by the two preliminary investigations of renal artery stenosis (11 out of 11 accessory renal arteries in each reference) (13,51). The initial success of accessory renal artery detection led us to investigate the applicability of spiral CT as a single screening evaluation for living related renal donors. Twelve potential living related renal donors were imaged with spiral CT and conventional arteriography. In addition to determining the appropriate levels for CTA, initial noncontrast-enhanced localizing sections were used to screen for renal calculi. Subsequently, spiral CTA was performed from the superior mesenteric artery inferiorly to the aortic bifurcation. Five minutes following the iodinated contrast injection for CTA, a frontal projection was obtained for the purpose of visualizing renal collecting system anomalies. The interpretation of axial CT sections alone was compared with that of 3D rendered CTA with shaded-surface display and MIP. Both axial sections and 3D CTAs were 100% sensitive for identifying seven accessory renal arteries in these 12 patients (68) (Fig. 20-23). Platt and co-workers, in a subsequent study of 24 potential renal donors undergoing CTA and correlative DSA, found that three very small accessory renal arteries of the 19 identified in their population were only seen with transverse images (69). Since publishing our

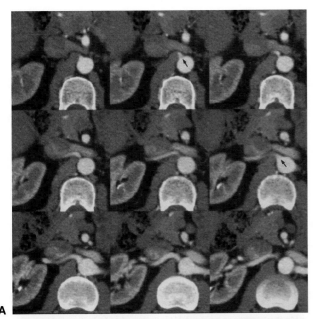

A

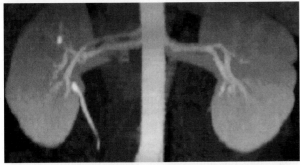

B

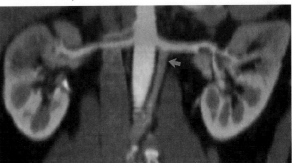

C

D

FIG. 20-23. Potential living renal donor. (**A**) Transverse CT angiogram sections (3-mm collimation; 2.0 pitch; 2.0-mm interval) demonstrate two renal arteries to the right kidney. The origins of the renal arteries are 6 mm apart (*arrows*). Careful scrutiny is required lest these two vessels be misdiagnosed as a single renal artery. (**B**) MIP allows identification of the two renal arteries easier than the transverse sections. Images such as this are very useful for illustrating arterial variants to clinicians accustomed to conventional arteriograms. (**C**) Curved planar reformation demonstrates the presence of two right renal arteries but also shows the posterior component of a circumaortic left renal vein (*white arrow*). The posterior portion originates from the main left renal vein just lateral to the aorta and extends posteriorly for 7 cm before passing posterior to the aorta and entering the inferior vena cava (*black arrow*) (**D**). (Reprinted from Rubin GD. Spiral (helical) CT of the renal vasculature. *Semin Ultrasound CT MR* 1996; 17:374–397.)

report, we have found that very small accessory renal arteries may not be depicted with surface displays or MIPs that are not subjected to extensive source image editing. Because extensive editing is impractical and the evaluation of transverse sections is most reliable for identifying accessory renal arteries, we rely exclusively on transverse sections for the identification of accessory branches except when there is a question of two separate renal arterial origins versus prehilar branching within several millimeters of a single renal arterial origin (70). Three-dimensional renderings and curved planar reformations, especially for small accessory renal arteries, are particularly useful for communicating these anatomic variants to our referring transplant surgeons.

Another important renal arterial variant is prehilar branching of the main renal arteries (less than 2 cm from the renal artery origin) (71–75). In our study, transverse CTA was only 14% sensitive for identifying five prehilar renal artery branches, whereas 3D CTA was 93% sensitive for identifying the five prehilar renal artery branches ($p < .001$). Of 11 patients with prehilar branching in the series of Platt and colleagues, three were detected with 3D renderings only (69). These results indicate the importance of generating 3D renderings for an accurate interpretation of complex arterial anatomy. Although all the information required to identify prehilar branching is available on transverse sections, considerable experience interpreting transverse sections for prehilar branching and correlation with 3D renderings is required prior to confidently relying on transverse sections for identifying prehilar branches in most cases.

An additional advantage of spiral CT evaluation is that the renal parenchyma and renal veins can be assessed for the presence of masses, calculi, or anomalies (68–70).

It has been estimated that the classic description of a single hepatic arterial supply via the proper hepatic artery from the common hepatic artery originating from the celiac trunk occurs in only 55% of humans, and there are 10 standard variations of this classical description. Spiral CT has demonstrated exceptional ability in delineating this variant anatomy (76). As a result, CT angiography has been proposed as a replacement for conventional arteriography in the evaluation of the arterial anatomy of patients being considered for hepatic transplantation. In a study of variant hepatic arterial supply in 33 patients with either conventional arteriographic or surgical correlation, 32 out of 33 had concordant results and CT was found to be as accurate as conventional angiography (77).

CONGENITAL ANOMALIES

Clinically relevant congenital anomalies of the aorta typically involve the thoracic aorta and its branches. These anomalies are readily visualized with spiral CT. Although the complex motion of the heart precludes the assessment of cardiac structures with current-generation spiral CT scanners, vascular rings, aberrant supra-aortic branching, coarctation (Fig. 20-24), and enlarged bronchial arteries or major

aortopulmonary collateral arteries (MAPCAs) are easily diagnosed and characterized (78,79). The use of conventional angiography for the diagnosis and characterization of lesions such as pulmonary sequestration should no longer be necessary if a thin-section volumetric acquisition is appropriately acquired with adequate contrast enhancement (19). The simultaneous visualization of the airways complements vascular visualization by allowing a direct determination of the specific structures responsible for tracheobronchial narrowing and the presence of aberrant airways. Although aortic stenosis secondary to coarctation is clearly demonstrated and enlarged intercostal arteries can be visualized as well, further study must be performed to determine the extent with which the thin webs that often are present in these lesions can be identified and the degree of aortic stenosis determined.

CT ANGIOGRAPHY VERSUS MR ANGIOGRAPHY

Recent advances in MRI technology have substantially improved the quality of thoracic and abdominal magnetic resonance angiography (MRA) (80,81). The introduction of higher-gradient-strength systems has allowed pulse sequence optimization, which has resulted in 3D acquisitions with repetition times below 10 ms and echo times approaching 1 ms. When combined with a dynamic injection of gadolinium, 60 1–1.5-mm sections can be acquired during a 30-s breath-hold (Fig. 20-25). The resulting data are volumetric, heavily T1-weighted blood pool images that do not suffer from the intravoxel dephasing or saturation effects seen with traditional time of flight due to the very short echo times and independence of vascular opacification on flow-related enhancement. When combined with phase contrast techniques, quantitative flow mapping can provide information that is unattainable from CTA. Initial reports using these ultrafast blood pool MR techniques have been encouraging. Although it has not been subjected to the same clinical scrutiny as CTA, MRA serves as an attractive alternative to CTA in patients who should not receive iodinated contrast medium. However, our experience suggests that a substantial number of patients with vascular pathology warranting evaluation are elderly and poorly tolerant of MR examinations because of subcutaneous cardiac pacemakers or defibrillators and back pain. Another difficulty facing the widespread adoption of MRA is the substantially greater variability in capabilities among imaging systems in clinical use. Although the fastest gradient systems are currently producing impressive results, they are not available on most sited MRI systems without expensive upgrades. The diversity of imaging capabilities results in a substantially greater variability in the quality of MRA that can be performed in community practices. Spiral CT technology, although subject to some variation, is not nearly as variable, and specific indices such as maximum scan time, x-ray tube output, and GRP serve to clearly delineate the capabilities of an imaging system.

Although MRA has the potential of assessing the postop-

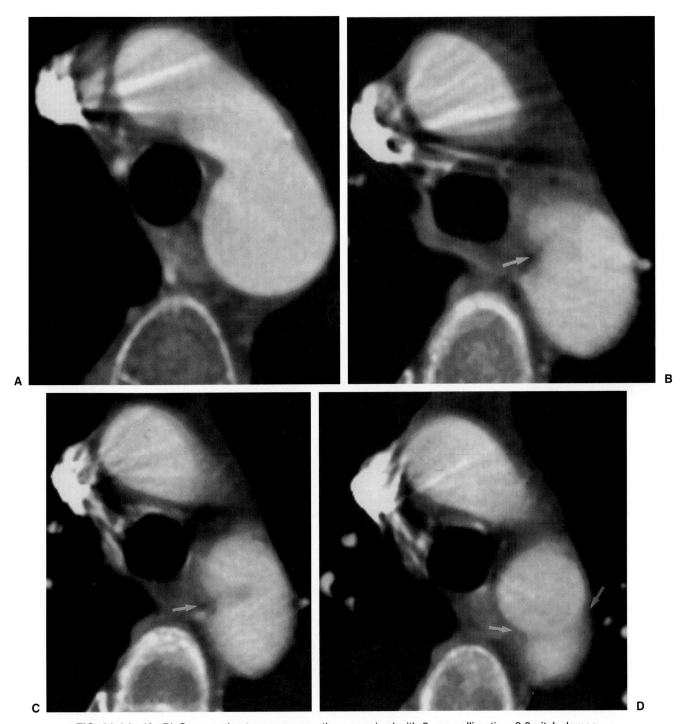

FIG. 20-24. **(A–D)** Consecutive transverse sections acquired with 3-mm collimation, 2.0 pitch demonstrates a linear filling defect in the proximal descending aorta (*arrows*). The lesion is difficult to characterize from the transverse sections alone. *(continued)*

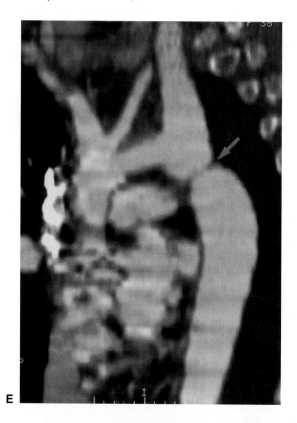

E

FIG. 20-24. *Continued.* (**E**) Curved planar reformation demonstrates a very short region of aortic coarctation (*arrow*) and a hypoplastic aortic arch with bovine branching pattern and enlarged left subclavian artery. (Reprinted from Rubin GD. Helical CT angiography of the thoracic aorta. *J Thorac Imaging* 1997;12.)

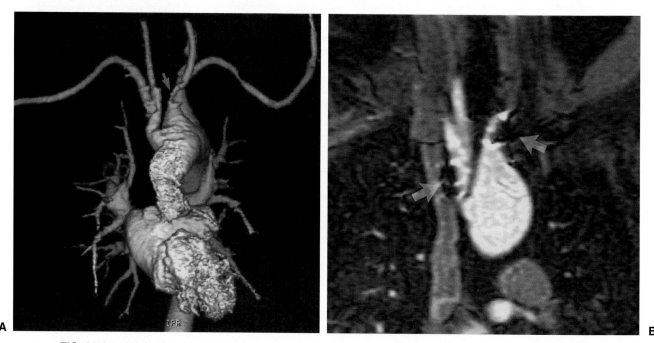

A   B

FIG. 20-25. (**A**) Surface display from a magnetic resonance angiogram obtained in 28 s (gradient echo acquisition of 60 2-mm-thick coronal images, TR = 5 ms, TE = 1 ms, 512 × 192 matrix) during the arterial phase of a 40-mL intravenous injection of gadolinium DTPA demonstrates the excellent image quality that is attainable with current state-of-the-art techniques. There appears to be a high-grade stenosis at the origin of the left common carotid artery (*arrow*). *(continued)*

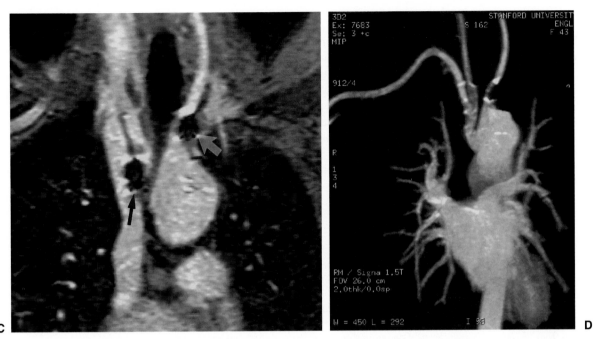

C

D

FIG. 20-25. (*Continued.*) Single coronal image from the arterial phase (**B**) and subsequent venous phase (30 s later) (**C**) demonstrates the presence of magnetic susceptibility artifacts arising from metallic clips lateral to the left common carotid artery and between the superior vena cava and the brachiocephalic artery (*arrows*). These result in a spurious appearance of stenosis on the SSD, where the segments are nonanalyzable because of the susceptibility artifact. Although the magnitude of these artifacts diminishes with shorter echo times, it remains a substantial limitation even with a 1-ms echo time. (**D**) MIP of these data do not demonstrate clues to the presence of this artifact, and unlike CTA, where metallic clips or calcium can be differentiated from the contrast-opacified lumen with a MIP, the presence of this artifact can only be deduced from a review of the original cross-sections.

erative vasculature, metallic clips or stents can produce considerable magnetic susceptibility artifact. CTA provides a clear depiction of the relationship of metallic stents and clips to the vessel lumen (28). CTA can be very helpful in evaluating patients who have undergone previous aortic reconstruction and branch reimplantation or revascularization. Most vascular clips cause minimal interference on CTAs, which can be a significant advantage for evaluating these patients when compared with MRI (7,37) (see Figs. 20-5, 20-15, 20-25).

Limitations of CT Angiography

When compared with both screen-film and DSA, CTA is a relatively low-resolution examination. This is primarily due to partial volume effects, as well as to the considerably lower intravascular iodine concentrations achieved with a peripheral intravenous injection. The resolution of CTA may be adequate for many diagnostic applications, if visualization of vessel luminal diameters of less than 2 mm is not required. The introduction of x-ray tubes with higher heat capacities, allowing a higher current during the 30–50-s acquisition, could result in improved CTA. The signal-to-noise ratio would increase, enabling collimator width reduction,

thus increasing spatial resolution. To maintain coverage, scanners capable of shorter GRPs or of acquiring data from multiple locations during a single GR will be necessary.

In patients with larger body habitus, spiral CT performed with narrow collimation can have an unacceptably low signal-to-noise ratio. This is predominantly due to a requirement for lower tube currents to perform spiral CT than are necessary with conventional CT. This requirement results from the absence of an interscan delay in spiral CT, which allows for some tube cooling to occur during a conventional CT examination. The maximum allowable milliamperage for spiral CT depends on the spiral scan duration. Improved tube outputs and greater detector efficiencies could help to overcome this limitation and enable the use of narrower collimation within the abdomen and pelvis.

Up to 170 mL of iodinated contrast material is required for diagnostic CTA in the abdomen and pelvis. This may be unacceptable in severely azotemic patients. Thoracic CTA may be performed with as little as 90 mL. Contrast dose may diminish, as tube output and detector efficiency increases, but the requirement for iodinated contrast medium is likely to remain an important limitation of CTA for the minority of patients with severe hypersensitivity or limited renal function.

CONCLUSIONS

Spiral CTA is a rapidly maturing technology for minimally invasive diagnosis of many thoracic, abdominal, and pelvic vascular abnormalities, previously attainable through conventional arteriography alone. Advantages of CTA over conventional arteriography include diminished patient morbidity, cost, and time as well as lessened physician time requirements. The single 3D acquisition of spiral CT enables visualization of lesions from an innumerable number of viewing angles, resulting in a superior assessment of some vascular lesions when compared with conventional arteriography.

ACKNOWLEDGMENTS

I am grateful for the support of R. Brooke Jeffrey, Sandy Napel, Michael D. Dake, Charles P. Semba, R. Scott Mitchell, D. Craig Miller, Christopher K. Zarins, and Laura Logan, who have contributed greatly toward CTA becoming an important clinical tool at Stanford University. I am also appreciative of the support from the RSNA Research and Education Fund, the General Electric/AUR Radiology Research Fellowship, Siemens Medical Systems, and General Electric Medical Systems. Finally, many thanks to my wife Rhesa and children—Rainier, Magellan, Giulianna, and Elka—for their patience with a crazy schedule and book chapter deadlines.

REFERENCES

1. Vock P, Soucek M, Daepp M, Kalender WA. Lung: spiral volumetric CT with single-breath-hold technique. *Radiology* 1990;176:864–867.
2. Rubin GD, Dake MD, Napel SA, McDonnell CH, Jeffrey RBJ. Abdominal spiral CT angiography: initial clinical experience. *Radiology* 1993;186:147–152.
3. Rubin GD, Leung AN, Robertson VJ, Stark P. Does subsecond spiral CT scanning affect the quality of thoracic CT images? *Radiology* 1996;201(P):401.
4. Polacin A, Kalender WA, Marchal G. Evaluation of section sensitivity profiles and image noise in spiral CT. *Radiology* 1992;185:29–35.
5. Rubin GD, Napel S. Increased scan pitch for vascular and thoracic spiral CT. *Radiology* 1995;197:316–317.
6. Zeman RK, Silverman PM, Berman PM, Weltman D, Davros WJ, Gomes MN. Abdominal aortic aneurysms: evaluation with variable-collimation helical CT and overlapping reconstruction. *Radiology* 1994;193:555–560.
7. Rubin GD, Walker PJ, Dake MD, et al. 3D spiral CT angiography: an alternative imaging modality for the abdominal aorta and its branches. *J Vasc Surg* 1993;18:656–666.
8. Schwarcz TH, Flanigan DP. Repair of abdominal aortic aneurysms in patients with renal, iliac, or distal arterial occlusive disease. *Surg Clin North Am* 1989;69:845–857.
9. Rubin GD, Dake MD, Napel S, Jeffrey RBJ. Three-dimensional CT angiography as an alternative to conventional arteriography in planning and in vivo evaluation of aortic stent grafts. *Radiology* 1993;189(P):112.
10. Rubin GD, Silverman SG. Helical CT of the retroperitoneum. *Radiol Clin North Am* 1995;33:903–932.
11. Raptopoulos V, Rosen MP, Kent KC, Kuestner LM, Sheiman RG, Pearlman JD. Sequential helical CT angiography of aortoiliac disease. *AJR* 1996;166:1347–1354.
12. Rubin GD, Lane MJ, Bloch DA, Leung AN, Stark P. Optimization of contrast enhanced thoracic spiral CT. *Radiology* 1996;201:785–791.
12a. Hopper KD, Kasales CJ, et al. Thoracic Spiral CT: delivery of contrast material pushed with injectable saline solution in a power injector. *Radiology* 1997;205:269–271.
13. Galanski M, Prokop M, Chavan A, Schaefer CM, Jandeleit K, Nischelsky JE. Renal arterial stenoses: spiral CT angiography. *Radiology* 1993;189:185–192.
14. Remy-Jardin M, Remy J, Wattinne L, Giraud F. Central pulmonary thromboembolism: diagnosis with spiral volumetric CT with the single-breath-hold technique. Comparison with pulmonary angiography. *Radiology* 1992;185:381–387.
15. Prokop M, Schaefer CM, Leppert AGA, Galanski M. Spiral CT angiography of thoracic aorta: femoral or antecubital injection site for intravenous administration of contrast material? *Radiology* 1993;189(P):111.
16. Posniak HV, Olson MC, Demos TC. Aortic motion artifact simulating dissection on CT scans: elimination with reconstructive segmented images. *AJR* 1993;161:557–558.
16a. Rubin GD, Paik DS, Johnston PC, Napel S. Measurement of the Aorta and its branches with helical CT. *Radiology* 1998;206:823–829.
17. Masuda Y, Takanashi K, Takasu J, Morooka Y, Inagaki Y. Expansion rate of thoracic aortic aneurysms and influencing factors. *Chest* 1992;102:461–466.
18. Dapunt L, Galla JD, Sadeghi AM, et al. The natural history of thoracic aortic aneurysms. *J Thorac Cardiovasc Surg* 1994;107:1323–1333.
19. Rubin GD. Helical CT angiography of the thoracic aorta. *J Thorac Imaging* 1997;12 (*in press*).
20. Quint LE, Francis IR, Williams DM, et al. Evaluation of thoracic aortic disease with the use of helical CT and multiplanar reconstructions: comparison with surgical findings. *Radiology* 1996;201:37–41.
21. Papanicolaou N, Wittenberg J, Ferrucci JT, et al. Preoperative evaluation of abdominal aortic aneurysms by computed tomography. *AJR* 1986;146:711–715.
22. LaRoy LL, Cormier PJ, Matalon TAS, Patel SK, Turner DA, Silver B. Imaging of abdominal aortic aneurysms. *AJR* 1989;152:785–792.
23. Bandyk DF. Preoperative imaging of aortic aneurysms. *Surg Clin North Am* 1989;69:721–735.
24. Pavone P, Di Cesare E, Di Renzi P, et al. Abdominal aortic aneurysm evaluation: comparison of US, CT, MRI, and angiography. *Magn Reson Imaging* 1990;8:199–204.
25. Vowden P, Wilkinson MB, Ausobskky JR, Kester RC. A comparison of three imaging techniques in the assessment of an abdominal aortic aneurysm. *J Cardiovasc Surg* 1989;30:891–896.
26. Crawford JL, Stowe CL, Safi HJ, Hallman CH, Crawford ES. Inflammatory aneurysms of the aorta. *J Vasc Surg* 1985;2:113–124.
27. Van Hoe L, Baert AL, Gryspeerdt S, et al. Supra- and juxtarenal aneurysms of the abdominal aorta: preoperative assessment with thin-section spiral CT. *Radiology* 1996;198:443–448.
28. Rubin GD, Dake MD, Napel S, Jeffrey RBJ. Renal stent position and patency: evaluation with spiral CT angiography. *Radiology* 1992;185(P):181.
29. Rubin GD, Dake MD, Semba CB. Current status of three-dimensional spiral CT scanning for imaging the vasculature. *Radiol Clin North Am* 1995;33:51–70.
30. Moritz JD, Rotermund S, Keating DP, Oestmann JW. Infrarenal abdominal aortic aneurysms: implications of CT evaluation of size and configuration for placement of endovascular aortic grafts. *Radiology* 1996;198:463–466.
31. Verbin C, Scoccianti M, Kopchok G, Donayre C, White RA. Comparison of the utility of CT scans and intravascular ultrasound in endovascular aortic grafting. *Ann Vasc Surg* 1995;9:434–440.
32. Baskin KM, Kusnick CA, Shamsolkottabi S, et al. Geometry analysis of tortuous and eccentric abdominal aortic aneurysms. *Radiology* 1996;201(P):317.
33. Rubin GD, Dake MD, Semba CP, Napel SA, Jeffrey RB. Helical CT angiography for evaluation of endovascular intervention. *Radiology* 1994;193(P):379.
34. Cigarroa JE, Isselbacher EM, DeSanctis RW, Eagle KA. Medical progress: diagnostic imaging in the evaluation of suspected aortic dissection— old standards and new directions. *AJR* 1993;161:485–493.
35. Erbel R, Daniel W, Visser C, Engberding R, Roelandt J, Rennollet H. Echocardiography in diagnosis of aortic dissection. *Lancet* 1989;March 4:457–461.
36. Nienaber CA, Kodolitsch Yu, Nicolas V, et al. The diagnosis of thoracic aortic dissection by noninvasive imaging procedures. *N Engl J Med* 1993;328:1–9.
37. Rubin GD. Three-dimensional helical CT angiography. *Radiographics* 1994;14:905–912.
38. Zeman RK, Berman PM, Silverman PM, et al. Diagnosis of aortic

dissection: value of helical CT with multiplanar reformation and three-dimensional rendering. *AJR* 1995;164:1375–1380.

39. Nienaber CA, Kodolitsch Yu, Petersen B, et al. Intramural hemorrhage of the thoracic aorta: diagnostic and therapeutic implications. *Circulation* 1995;92:1465–1472.

40. Kazerooni EA, Bree RL, Williams DM. Penetrating atherosclerotic ulcers of the descending thoracic aorta: evaluation with CT and distinction from aortic dissection. *Radiology* 1992;183:759–765.

41. Gore I. Pathogenesis of dissecting aneurysm of the aorta. *Arch Pathol Lab Med* 1952;53:142–153.

42. Hillman BJ. Imaging advances in the diagnosis of renovascular hypertension. *AJR* 1989;153:5–14.

43. May AG, Berg vd L, DeWeese JA, Ros CG. Critical arterial stenosis. *Surgery* 1963;54:250–259.

44. Bookstein JJ. Appraisal of arteriography in estimating the hemodynamic significance of renal artery stenoses. *Invest Radiol* 1966;1: 281–294.

45. Detection, evaluation, and treatment of renovascular hypertension: final report, Working Group on Renovascular Hypertension. *Arch Intern Med* 1987;147:820–829.

46. Brink JA, Lim JT, Wang G, Heiken JP, Deyoe LA, Vannier MW. Technical optimization of spiral CT for depiction of renal artery stenosis: in vitro analysis. *Radiology* 1995;194:157–163.

47. Davros WJ, Obuchowski NA, Berman PM, Zeman RK. A phantom study: evaluation of renal artery stenosis using helical CT and 3D reconstructions. *J Comput Assist Tomogr* 1997;21:156–161.

48. Edsman G. Angionephrography and suprarenal angiography. *Acta Radiol Suppl* 1957;155:5–139.

49. Merklin RJ, Michels NA. The variant renal and suprarenal blood supply with data on the inferior phrenic, ureteral, and gonadal arteries. *J Int Coll Surg* 1958;29:41–76.

50. Boijsen E. Angiographic studies of the anatomy of single and multiple renal arteries. *Acta Radiol Suppl* 1959;183:1–99.

51. Rubin GD, Dake MD, Napel S, et al. Spiral CT of renal artery stenosis: comparison of three-dimensional rendering techniques. *Radiology* 1994;190:181–189.

52. Beregi JP, Elkohen M, Deklunder G, Artaud D, Coullet JM, Wattinne L. Helical CT angiography compared with arteriography in the detection of renal artery stenosis. *AJR* 1996;167:495–501.

53. Rubin GD, Napel S. Helical CT of renal artery stenosis. *AJR* 1997; 168:1109–1110.

54. Beregi JP. Reply. *AJR* 1997;168:1110–1111.

55. Siegel CL, Ellis JH, Korobkin M, Dunnick NR. CT-detected renal arterial calcification: correlation with renal artery stenosis on angiography. *AJR* 1994;163:867–872.

56. Rubin GD, Costello P. Three-dimensional spiral CT angiography. In: Taveras JM, Ferrucci JT, eds. *Radiology: diagnosis, imaging, and intervention.* Philadelphia: JB Lippincott; 1994:1–16.

57. Mell MW, Alfrey EJ, Rubin GD, Scandling JD Jr, Jeffrey RBJ, Dafoe DC. Use of spiral computed tomography in the diagnosis of transplant renal artery stenosis. *Transplantation* 1994;57:746–748.

58. Morano JU, Harrison RB. Mesenteric ischemia: angiographic diagnosis and intervention. *Clin Imaging* 1991;15:91–98.

59. Odurny A, Sniderman KW, Colapinto RF. Intestinal angina: percutaneous transluminal angioplasty of the celiac and superior mesenteric arteries. *Radiology* 1988;167:59–62.

60. Lawrence JA, Kim D, Kent KC, Stehling MK, Rosen MP, Raptopoulos V. Lower extremity spiral CT angiography versus catheter angiography. *Radiology* 1995;194:903–908.

61. Rubin GD, Dake MD, Napel S, Jeffrey RBJ. 3D CT arteriography of the pelvis aortic to femoral bifurcations. *AJR* 1993;160(suppl):22.

62. Raptopoulos V. Chest CT for aortic injury: maybe not for everyone. *AJR* 1994;162:1053–1055.

63. Mirvis SE, Shanmuganathan K, Miller BH, White CS, Turney SZ. Traumatic aortic injury: diagnosis with contrast-enhanced thoracic CT— five year experience at a major trauma center. *Radiology* 1996; 200:413–422.

64. Brasel KJ, Weigelt JA. Blunt thoracic aortic trauma: a cost-utility approach for injury detection. *Arch Surg* 1996;131:619–626.

65. Gavant ML, Manke PG, Fabian T, Flick PA, Graney MJ, Gold RE. Blunt traumatic aortic rupture: detection with helical CT of the chest. *Radiology* 1995;197:125–133.

66. Gavant ML, Flick P, Manke P, Gold RE. CT aortography of thoracic aortic rupture. *AJR* 1996;166:955–961.

67. Trerotola SO. Can helical CT replace aortography in thoracic trauma? *Radiology* 1995;197:13–15.

68. Rubin GD, Alfrey EJ, Dake MD, et al. Spiral CT for the assessment of living renal donors. *Radiology* 1995;195:457–462.

69. Platt JF, Ellis JH, Korobkin M, Reige KA, Konnak JW, Leichtman AB. Potential renal donors: comparison of conventional imaging with helical CT. *Radiology* 1996;198:419–423.

70. Rubin GD. Spiral (helical) CT of the renal vasculature. *Semin Ultrasound CT MRI* 1996;17:374–397.

71. Derauf B, Goldberg ME. Angiographic assessment of potential renal transplant donors. *Radiol Clin North Am* 1987;25:261–265.

72. Riehle RA Jr, Steckler R, Naslund EB, Riggio R, Cheigh J, Stubenbord W. Selection criteria for the evaluation of living related renal donors. *J Urol* 1990;144:845–848.

73. Strauser GD, Stables DP, Weil R. Optimal technique of renal arteriography in living renal transplant donors. *AJR* 1978;131:813–816.

74. Sherwood T, Ruutu M, Chisholm GD. Renal angiography problems in live kidney donors. *Br J Radiol* 1978;51:99–105.

75. Kjellevand TO, Kolmannskog F, Pfeffer P, Scholz T, Fauchald P. Influence of renal angiography in living renal donors. *Acta Radiol* 1991; 32:368–370.

76. Winter TC, Nghiem HV, Freeny PC, Hommeyer SC, Mack LA. Hepatic arterial anatomy: demonstration of normal supply and vascular variants with three-dimensional CT angiography. *Radiographics* 1995;15: 771–780.

77. Winter TC, Freeny PC, Nghiem HV, et al. Hepatic arterial anatomy in transplantation candidates: evaluation with three-dimensional CT arteriography [see comments]. *Radiology* 1995;195:363–370.

78. Katz M, Konen E, Rozsenman J, Szeinberg A, Itzchak Y. Spiral CT and 3D image reconstruction of vascular ring and associated tracheobronchial anomalies. *J Comput Assist Tomogr* 1995;19:564–568.

79. Hopkins KL, Patrick LE, Simoneaux SF, Bank ER, Parks WJ, Smith SS. Pediatric great vessel anomalies: initial clinical experience with spiral CT angiography. *Radiology* 1996;200:811–815.

80. Prince MR, Narasimham DL, Jacoby WT, et al. Three-dimensional gadolinium-enhanced MR angiography of the thoracic aorta. *AJR* 1996; 166:1387–1397.

81. Krinsky GA, Rofsky NM, DeCorato DR, et al. Thoracic aorta: comparison of gadolinium-enhanced three-dimensional MR angiography with conventional MR imaging. *Radiology* 1997;202:183–193.

CHAPTER 21

Spiral CTA of the Cerebrovascular Circulation

Michael P. Marks

Advances in noninvasive or minimally invasive imaging studies such as duplex sonography, magnetic resonance angiography (MRA), and computed tomographic angiography (CTA) have led to their increasing use in the cerebrovascular circulation. Spiral CTA has some unique attributes that makes it well suited to the evaluation of the patient with cerebrovascular disease. A bolus enhanced scan is obtained that can then be reconstructed as a volume data set for three-dimensional (3D) images. Select regions of interest can be evaluated and the spiral CTA 3D images can be viewed at any angle. If the contrast bolus is properly timed, the inherent contrast between the intravascular space and surrounding soft tissue allows vessel lumina to be well visualized. Because visualization depends upon the contrast in the vessel at the time of imaging and not the physics of flow (as with current MRA), CTA provides good visualization even in areas of disturbed or irregular blood flow. This is true in regions of stenoses and aneurysm formation, where flow may be highly disordered, stagnant, and accelerated even in the same imaging data set.

Scan durations with CTA are typically on the order of 30 s, helping to minimize the risk of motion artifact and maximize the likelihood of obtaining useful imaging in the uncooperative patient. In addition, the larger available gantry and the use of CT technology allow for the imaging of patients who may have relative or absolute contraindications to evaluation with MRA, such as claustrophobia or metallic implants. Since the publication of the first edition of this text a host of papers have reported initial results and results of some blinded analyses of the efficacy of CTA in the evaluation of cerebrovascular disease. This has certainly extended our confidence in the use of the technique in the intra- and extracranial circulations.

TECHNIQUE

Scanning and Contrast Bolus

Extracranial Circulation

The carotid bifurcation lies between C2 and C3 in 91% of cases (1). We have found that initial identification of the

bifurcation site and prior timing of the contrast bolus to the carotid bifurcation optimizes the CTA examination. Contrast is timed as accurately as possible to maximize arterial enhancement and minimize parenchymal and venous opacification. To localize the bifurcation, noncontrast serial axial scans are obtained every 5 mm from C2 to C6. The scanner is then positioned to start the CTA evaluation of the common carotid artery 2—3 cm below the carotid bifurcation with axial scans. A preliminary bolus injection of 20 mL of nonionic contrast (Iohexol, 300 mg I/mL) is administered via a power injector over 5 s (4 mL/s) using a 20-gauge antecubital vein catheter. Following an 8-s scan delay, 12 5-mm-thick axial images are performed without table movement. These are done at a rate of two scans per second using 100 kVp and 140 mA (to minimize tube heating). A time–density curve is plotted from this data and used to determine the time delay for beginning scanning after a bolus is injected (Fig. 21-1). We have found that the optimal scan delay is approximately 1 s prior to peak enhancement on the time–density curve.

Although preliminary timing of the bolus clearly does optimize arterial opacification, many authors have recently adopted a set timing protocol for all patients using a predetermined delay to start scanning (2–4). Their results suggest that a predetermined delay may not adversely affect the degree of opacification to the point of significantly altering the results observed. However, there has not been a controlled series comparing the two techniques. In addition, contrast opacification is critical in obtaining good diagnostic studies. For example, one report found a much lower rate of correlation between CTA and angiography for the detection of carotid stenosis (5). Subsequent investigators have pointed out that one of the major differences in this study is that it utilized only 60 mL of contrast administered at 2 mL/s. The author of this report has separately reported that alteration of this protocol (which included increasing the contrast bolus to 90 mL at 3 mL/s) markedly improved the sensitivity of CTA (6).

All extracranial scanning is performed from inferior to superior to follow the direction of the bolus. If possible, a

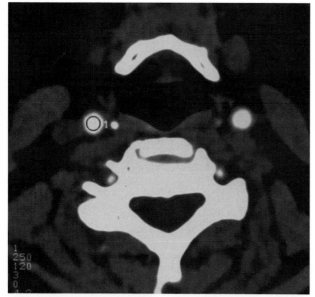

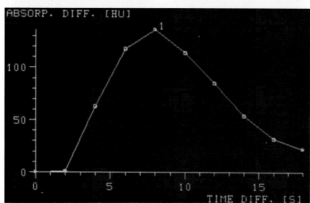

FIG. 21-1. Time–density curve for determining peak arterial enhancement and proper scan delay. **(A)** Axial CT scan of neck (5-mm collimation) at peak arterial enhancement following test bolus (20 mL). Imaging is at most inferior aspect of volume to be scanned (2–3 cm below the carotid bifurcation). Region of interest (*circle*) is in right common carotid lumen. **(B)** Change in density in Hounsfield units (*y* axis) versus time in seconds (*x* axis) during test bolus. The zero time is routinely started 8 s after the bolus began being injected. Scan delay used is the time 1 s prior to peak enhancement plus 8 s.

single breath-hold is used to minimize patient motion. Following the predetermined delay, scanning is started using 3-mm/s table speed and a 2-mm slice thickness (pitch 1.5). Scanning is carried out over 30 s, giving 9 cm total coverage. A total of 100 mL of contrast is given during 25 s (4 mL/s). Other scan parameters include 120 kVp, maximum milliamperage allowed (minimum 220), 22-cm field of view (FOV). Use of faster table speed or greater slice thickness does allow more anatomic coverage, but at the expense of spatial resolution. In addition, the scan time can be lengthened, but only with increased contrast administration, and scan times should be as short as possible to reduce the likelihood of a dense venous filling.

Intracranial Circulation

As with the carotid examination, timing of the bolus to the region of the circle of Willis optimizes the examination. To accomplish this, a preliminary test bolus of 20 mL non-ionic contrast (Iohexol, 300 mg I/mL) is administered via power injector at 3 mL/s through a 20-gauge catheter in the antecubital vein. Scanning is started after an 8-s delay, as with the carotid technique. The axial scan plane is placed at the upper portion of the sella. Ten 5-mm-thick images are obtained every 1 s with 1-s interscan delay. A region of interest (ROI) is selected from either of the carotid arteries or the basilar artery and a time–density curve is plotted, as is done with the carotid artery studies. The spiral CTA scanning is set to start 1 s prior to peak enhancement (after including the 8-s delay used for the test bolus scanning).

The angiogram is obtained by scanning inferior to superior. Ninety milliliters of contrast are administered for 30 s (3 mL/s). Scan parameters include 120 kVp, maximum milliamperage allowed (220–280 mA), and 22 cm FOV. A 1-mm slice thickness is used with 1.3 mm/s table speed (pitch 1.3) and scanning is continued for 40-s scan time, giving total coverage of 5.2 cm. This allows us to image from the mid-basilar artery and cavernous portions of the carotid arteries to approximately 2.5 cm above the genu of the anterior and middle cerebral arteries. The selection of 1-mm slice thickness for studies of the circle of Willis (as compared with 2 mm for the intracranial circulation) leads to improved spatial resolution needed for clearer visualization of extracranial aneurysms and stenoses.

Image Reconstruction

In the extracranial circulation axial images are reconstructed every 1–2 mm, yielding 45–90 images. In the intracranial circulation axial images are reconstructed every 0.5 mm to create 104 axial images. These transaxial images are interpreted as part of the patient's examination and may provide important additional information when coupled with the 3D reconstructions. The 3D reconstructions that are obtained from these data sets provide for multiple viewing directions and generally restrict imaging to the enhanced vascular structures that are selected.

The axial CT data are usually cropped to exclude bone and other unwanted structures prior to doing the 3D reconstruction. We have utilized manual editing and automatic editing using a connectivity algorithm. These techniques are more fully described in Chapter 19. For the circle of Willis we usually eliminate bone density structures in the skull base region using a semi-automated algorithm that requires the identification of seed points representing high-attenuation regions in the skull. The algorithm then sets all voxels that are spatially connected to these seed points at −1,000 Hounsfield units (HU).

Two 3D techniques have generally been used for CTA in the cerebrovascular circulation. These are maximum-intensity projection (MIP) and shaded-surface display (SSD). The MIP images allow for bone and calcium to be differentiated from the contrast-filled vessel lumina. The SSD technique uses the preset threshold to develop a surface display. With this technique, density differences between calcified structures and contrasts are lost. We are also utilizing curved planer reformatting (CPR) as an alternative to these projection techniques. This technique allows us to specify a contour that may follow the curved surface of a vascular structure. In addition to these 3D reconstruction techniques, we have more recently begun to use perspective display, particularly for evaluation of intracranial aneurysms. All these reconstruction display techniques are more fully explained, along with their inherent advantages and disadvantages, in Chapter 19.

EXTRACRANIAL VASCULAR DISEASE

The greatest demand for extracranial cerebrovascular imaging comes in the evaluation of the carotid bifurcation. This is the most common site for atherosclerotic disease in the cerebrovascular circulation (7). Most lesions are located at or within a few centimeters of the bifurcation (8). Reports from collaborative trials have described a benefit, with improved stroke and death outcome when surgery is performed on both symptomatic (9,10) and asymptomatic (11) carotid disease. All these studies have used well-defined screening measurements of carotid stenosis (usually determined by digital subtraction angiography [DSA]) to include patients for randomization between surgical therapy and medical therapy. The studies define a stenosis that would benefit from surgical therapy, which is >60% to 70%. In addition, one study (10) reported that patients with symptomatic carotid disease with <29% stenosis did not benefit from surgical therapy. Considered together, these trials set clearly defined goals for noninvasive imaging to accurately measure stenosis and thereby identify that subgroup of patients that will benefit from surgery.

Three-Dimensional Spiral CT Angiography

The spatial resolution and contrast-to-noise ratio available with spiral CT generally give an accurate picture of the carotid bifurcation and the degree of stenosis present in the carotid artery (Figs. 21-2, 21-3). Calcifications present in the region of carotid bifurcation are common with atherosclerotic lesions. There is enough variation in the attenuation to clearly differentiate between calcification in the wall of the atherosclerotic vessel and intraluminal contrast using MIP reconstructions (see Fig. 21-3). However, when these calcifications are present in a concentric or nearly concentric fashion, the degree of stenosis is often difficult to determine from the available 3D MIPs. In these cases, we have found that the source images (the initial contrast-enhanced two-dimensional studies) provide accurate information regarding the degree of stenosis (Fig. 21-4). A connectivity algorithm

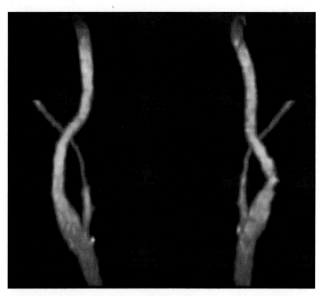

FIG. 21-2. Normal spiral CT angiogram of carotid bifurcation (collimation 2 mm, table speed 3 cm, pitch 1.5). Region of interest was selected to include both right and left carotids in this MIP reconstruction.

also can be used to remove calcifications in the vessel wall (12,13).

Several studies have presented blinded evaluations of CTA when compared with DSA for the assessment of carotid stenosis requiring endarterectomy. These are shown in Table 21-1.

The studies outlined in this table generally used criteria for stenosis described by the North American Symptomatic Carotid Endarterectomy Trial (9). Stenosis was classified as mild (<30%), moderate (30% to 69%), or severe (70% to 99%), with occlusion considered as a separate group. There was an 82% to 95% agreement for all categories of disease. For surgical disease (70% to 99% stenosis) these studies showed a high sensitivity (82% to 100%) and specificity (94% to 100%). Three of the studies outlined in Table 21-1 utilized SSD and three used MIP coupled with axial images. One study (2) did evaluate SSD, MIP, and axial images from CTA separately as compared with DSA. Axial images alone correctly scored 37 of 39 (95%) carotid arteries. Neither MIP nor SSD was able to evaluate 10 arteries because of circumferential calcification. Of the remaining 29 arteries MIP correctly evaluated 28 (96%) and SSD correctly evaluated 23 (79%). SSD was found to generally underestimate stenosis. As explained in Chapter 19, SSD is strongly affected by the choice of threshold, and it will underestimate stenosis if a lower threshold is selected.

The identification of ulceration may also prove important in the evaluation of patients with ischemic symptoms. Plaque ulcerations can act as a site for the formation of platelet–fibrin clots, which can embolize distally into the intracranial circulation. Deep or severe ulceration has been found to increase the incidence of ischemic symptoms and stroke (17).

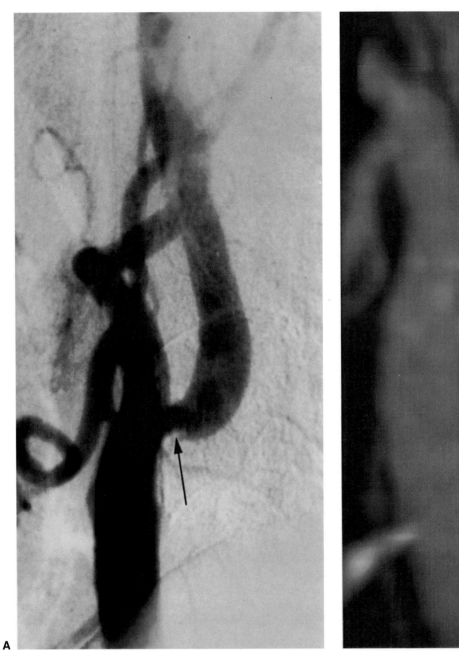

FIG. 21-3. Moderate carotid stenosis in 56-year-old man with symptoms of transient ischemic attacks. **(A)** Conventional carotid angiogram (lateral projection) showing moderate internal carotid bulb stenosis (*arrow*). **(B)** Lateral projection spiral CT angiogram (collimation 2 mm, pitch 1.5) of carotid bifurcation showing moderate stenosis. Higher-intensity calcification within the plaque was not seen on conventional angiogram (*white arrows*). Jugular venous return is seen between external and internal carotid (v.) and was easily differentiated from carotid arteries using multiple viewing angles.

TABLE 21-1. *CT angiography of carotid stenosis**

Study	Arteries in study	Overall agreement (%)	Arteries 70–99% stenosis	Sensitivity (%)	Specificity (%)
Schwartz et al. (13)	40	92	20	100	100
Dillon et al. (14)	50	82	17	82	94
Marks et al. (15)†	28	89	6	100	96
Cumming et al. (2)	70	83	17	94	100
Leclerc et al. (3)†	39	95	13	100	100
Link et al. (44)†	92	85	30	91	100

* From reference 16.
† Using MIP reconstructions and axial reconstructions.

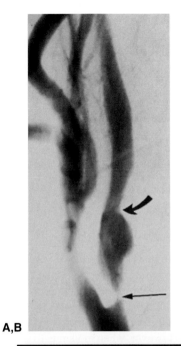 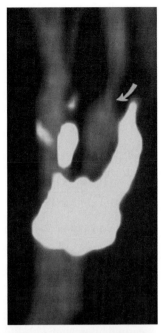

A,B

FIG. 21-4. Calcified high-grade stenosis of proximal right internal carotid artery in an 83-year-old man with a right hemisphere infarct. (**A**) Lateral common carotid conventional angiogram showing a proximal high-grade stenosis (*arrow*). There is also irregularity and stenosis (*curved arrow*) distal to the short-segment high-grade stenosis. (**B**) Right carotid lateral CT angiogram (collimation 2 mm, pitch 1.5) shows extensive calcification obscuring proximal stenosis. More distal irregularity and stenosis are well seen above the calcified portion of the plaque (*curved white arrow*). (**C**) Axial source image for B at level of high-grade stenosis showing arterial wall calcification extending around approximately half the circumference of the carotid artery (*short arrows*), contrast in residual severely narrowed lumen (*long arrow*). (**D**) Two-dimensional time-of-flight MRA shows no signal in the region of the high-grade stenosis with MRA (*segment between arrows*). MRA is able to diagnose severe stenosis because signal is seen in the more distal cervical portion of the internal carotid artery (beyond the signal void); however, the exact degree and true length of the stenosis are obscured.

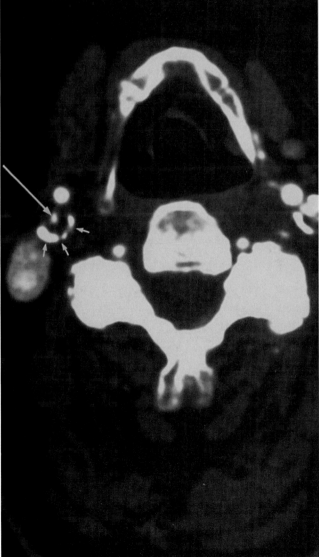

C

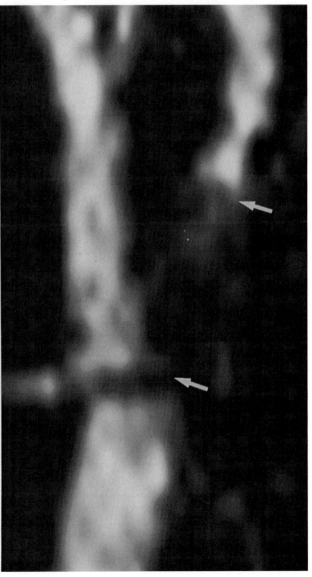

D

The most accurate evaluation of the true luminal margins and depiction of plaque morphology may be helpful in the evaluation of the patient with carotid bifurcation atherosclerotic disease. Prior studies using surgically proven ulceration as a gold standard have shown that a significant number of ulcers can be missed even with conventional angiography. Eikelboom et al. correlated angiographically determined ulceration with surgically proven ulceration and found that angiography had a sensitivity of 73% and a specificity of 62% (18). Similarly. Edwards et al. found that angiography diagnosed 60% of the ulcers found at surgery (19). CTA with more limited spatial resolution (when compared with DSA) cannot accurately depict ulceration (4,13,14).

CTA has also proven capable of identifying those vessels that are completely occluded with a high degree of accuracy. This is a critical test of a presurgical screening tool to exclude patients with already occluded arteries and at the same time include those with a trickle of flow that would most benefit from endarterectomy. A number of studies have shown occlusion that is evaluated with 100% sensitivity and specificity (2–4,13,15). One study did report only seven of eight carotid occlusions were correctly evaluated, with one false-negative evaluation (14). The DSA study in this false-negative case was performed 28 days after the detection of severe stenosis by CTA, allowing ample time for the carotid in question to go on to occlusion and calling into question these data.

An additional cause for ischemic symptoms originating in the carotid artery is spontaneous or traumatic carotid dissection (20,21). These patients will often develop ischemic symptoms early in the course of dissection and require long-term therapy with anticoagulants. Follow-up imaging is obtaining over a period of months to assess healing or the development of further stenosis or aneurysmal enlargement of the vessel lumen (20). Conventional CT and MRI have been utilized to detect the initial subintimal hematoma that is seen with dissection. CTA can provide a noninvasive modality for evaluating the extent of luminal narrowing and for following the patient requiring repeated examinations for dissection (Fig. 21-5).

CTA and Other Noninvasive Modalities

Two other noninvasive techniques are currently available for evaluating the carotid bifurcation, MRA and duplex sonography, both of which have have inherent advantages and limitations. MRA has been shown to have a high degree of sensitivity for the detection of significant stenoses in the carotid bifurcation (22–26). However, when moderate to severe stenosis is present, the degree of stenosis is often overestimated with MRA, because of complex flow and intravoxel dephasing (22–26). These factors also lead to overestimation of the length of involved vessels when a severe stenosis is present, as the signal void extends beyond the exact length of stenosis on the MRA images (22,25). This inability of MRA to accurately depict the lumen in

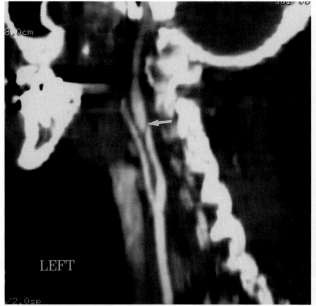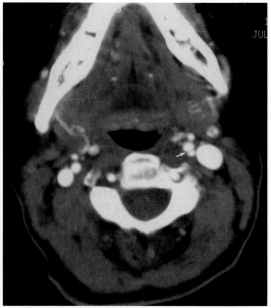

FIG. 21-5. Forty-four-year-old woman with a known left internal carotid artery dissection. (**A**) Sagittal view from a curved planar reformatted image through the internal carotid artery (ICA). Spiral CTA was performed several months after the initial angiogram to assess for continued dissection. The proximal portion of the intimal flap is well shown (*arrow*). In addition, there is an aneurysmal dilatation in the carotid distal to the beginning of the dissection. (**B**) Axial image from the spiral CTA examination showing the ICA dissection. The *arrow* in (**B**) indicates the intimal flap. Compare this with the normal internal carotid artery seen on the opposite side.

areas where there is perturbed flow makes evaluation of the morphology of the atherosclerotic plaque difficult when moderate to severe stenoses are present (see Fig. 21-4). In addition, regions of dense calcification may create magnetic field inhomogeneities leading to overestimation of stenosis. CTA, which relies on contrast opacification, is not susceptible to these flow perturbations. Recently, contrast enhanced MRA has been suggested as an alternative that will eliminate many of the pitfalls seen with conventional time-of-flight or phase-contrast studies. However, at the time of this writing, blinded evaluations comparing contrast-enhanced MRA with other imaging modalities have not been performed.

Duplex ultrasound has also been shown to have a high degree of accuracy for the detection of stenosis of greater than 50% in the carotid artery with sensitivities in the range of 80% to 90% (27–29). There are some imaging pitfalls for this technique, however. Differentiation between a preocclusive, severely stenosed carotid artery and a truly occluded vessel is often difficult because velocities are greatly reduced as the stenosis becomes very severe (30,31). As explained previously, this distinction between low flow and complete occlusion is important in the presurgical evaluation of the carotid stenosis patient. In addition, the examination can be nondiagnostic because of dense calcification in the carotid bifurcation region in up to 10% of cases (32). Recently, a combined noninvasive examination to include ultrasound and MRA has been suggested to replace DSA in the evaluation of carotid stenosis. CTA has many inherent advantages and could easily be considered an alternative noninvasive modality. In such a scheme combining MRA and ultrasound, CTA would be able to augment or even replace a modality such as MRA.

INTRACRANIAL VASCULAR DISEASE

Spiral CTA through the circle of Willis in the region of the base of the brain will yield images that clearly depict the arterial anatomy well beyond the A1, M1, and P1 segments of the intracranial cerebral arteries (Fig. 21-6). The 3D MIP reconstruction can be used to select regions of interest that preferentially evaluate the anterior (carotid), posterior circulation (vertebrobasilar), or right and left hemisphere circulations. CTA must utilize a small enough region of interest to exclude bone from the skull base region or have a proper bone suppression technique that results in clear depiction of the vessels without the bony edges of the skull base. The semi-automated seed point algorithm that we employ results in contour artifacts, but these are usually readily differentiated from vascular anatomy (see Fig. 21-6). Contour artifacts are also clearly separated from normal vascular anatomy when a rotating or rocking cine sequence is employed.

Occlusive Vascular Disease

Clear depiction of the intracranial carotid arteries and the arteries in the region of the circle of Willis is often helpful

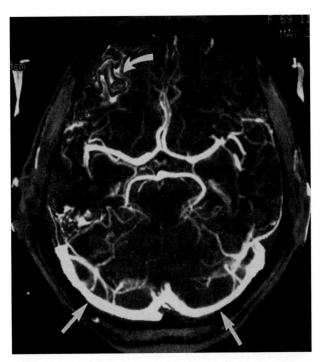

FIG. 21-6. Normal circle of Willis spiral CT angiogram (collimation 1 mm, pitch 1.3) in a 69-year-old woman with a right cerebellar infarct. Arterial anatomy within the circle, including anterior and posterior communicating arteries, is clearly demonstrated. Branching arteries well beyond the immediate circle of Willis are also well seen. Enhancement of transverse and sigmoid dural venous sinuses (*arrows*) is also noted. Also note contour artifacts seen after bone removal artifact (*curved arrow*), easily differentiated from vascular anatomy.

in the evaluation of the patient ischemic symptoms. The presence of a tandem stenosis in the intracranial circulation may preclude performing an endarterectomy of the extracranial circulation at the carotid bifurcation. Fixed atherosclerotic stenotic lesions in the extracranial circulation are certainly far less common than at the carotid bifurcation. Primary atherosclerosis of the middle cerebral artery (MCA) has been found to be the cause of an MCA territory infarct in less than 10% of cases (33,34). However, tandem stenoses can occur. For example, Marzewski et al. found that 54% of patients with intracranial carotid stenoses of greater than 50% had extracranial stenoses (35). In addition, emboli can be present in the circle of Willis, having originated from atherosclerotic lesions more proximal or in association with pathological cardiac conditions such as arrhythmias and endocarditis. Newer treatment modalities for acute stroke such as thrombolysis may be benefited by a rapidly performed examination that leads to the early diagnosis of thromboembolic occlusion or stenosis. Initial experience with spiral CTA suggests that this technique may be helpful in the evaluation of circle of Willis anatomy and the diagnosis of fixed stenotic lesions in the intracranial circulation.

We have compared CTA with phase-contrast MRA in the evaluation of circle of Willis arteries and found similar sensitivities for the detection of these vessels making up the circle (36). CTA had an 88.5% sensitivity and that of MRA was 85.5%, with most of the arteries missed by either modality being <1 mm. These smaller arteries were usually the anterior or posterior communicating arteries. One preliminary evaluation of MCA stenosis and occlusion has found a high correlation with transcranial ultrasound (37), but further analysis of CTA sensitivity and specificity will be needed to validate such findings. An example of the use of CTA for intracranial stenosis is shown in Fig. 21-7.

Preliminary evaluation of progressive occlusive conditions such as moya-moya disease can also be performed with spiral CTA. Moya-moya disease results in an intimal thickening that leads to progressive occlusion of intracerebral arteries. It can have a variable age of onset but is more frequently seen in children. It usually affects the distal carotid artery as well as the anterior and middle cerebral arteries first, but it may affect the posterior circulation in later stages (38). Angiography has been described as indispensable for the diagnosis; however, we have found that spiral CTA provides good initial information regarding the status of the vessels of the circle of Willis (Fig. 21-8). One report has also successfully used CTA to evaluate the surgical anastamoses done to treat Moya-Moya disease (39).

Intracranial Aneurysms

Background

Large autopsy series show that in the general population intracranial aneurysms are quite prevalent, with an incidence of 3% to 8% (40). Aneurysms often originate in areas of vessel branching and are therefore most common in the circle of Willis or at the MCA trifurcation. This reduces the geographic area that needs to be searched to make it likely that an aneurysm will be detected. However, approximately 15% to 20% of patients harboring intracranial aneurysms will have them at multiple sites (41), requiring visualization of the major branching points of all skull base vessels. Patients usually present with subarachnoid hemorrhage, although they may develop signs and symptoms of mass effect, including cranial neuropathies, seizures, or headaches. In addition, the aneurysm may act as a source of emboli, causing ischemic symptoms. Therapeutic management options include surgical clipping or endovascular treatment, generally with coil occlusion. Clear depiction of the aneurysm, location, shape, and neck are all critical for the management decisions related to the treatment of a patient with an aneurysm. For this reason conventional angiography, with its inherent improved spatial resolution, has been the study of choice when evaluating a patient with a suspected aneurysm.

Subarachnoid Hemorrhage

The development of subarachnoid hemorrhage represents the most common presentation of intracranial aneurysms, with the majority of nontraumatic subarachnoid hemorrhage being due to an underlying sacular aneurysm. In North America each year there are approximately 28,000 cases of subarachnoid hemorrhage caused by aneurysmal bleeding (42). Approximately 50% of patients succumb following subarachnoid hemorrhage, and those who survive often have poor outcomes (43). About one-third of these patients who have subarachnoid bleeds die before hospitalization. The international cooperative study on the timing of aneurysm surgery reported an additional 26% rate of death in those patients surviving to be admitted to a major neurosurgical unit, with only 58% making a complete recovery (43). Patients may succumb following hospitalization to ischemia secondary to vasospasm, rebleeding from the aneurysm, or medical and surgical complications of their disease. This necessitates rapid and accurate diagnosis of the etiology of the subarachnoid hemorrhage so that if an aneurysm is present, prompt treatment can occur. Of nontraumatic subarachnoid hemorrhage, 80% to 90% is due to aneurysm rupture (44). However, other etiologies—including arteriovenous malformations, arterial dissecting, bleeding disorders, substance abuse, or a cervical source of the hemorrhage—may give a pattern of diffuse subarachnoid bleeding (45). In addition, a more limited pattern of perimesencephalic bleeding can be seen following symptomatic presentation that may relate to bleeding from perforating arteries or venous/capillary bleeding (46,47).

Noncontrast CT remains the mainstay for diagnosis of acute subarachnoid hemorrhage. It follows that a contrast-enhanced study to supplement the noncontrast CT capable of evaluating for possible aneurysms would significantly add to the clinical work-up of such patients. High-resolution nonspiral contrast-enhanced CT has been used in the setting of both unruptured and ruptured aneurysms (48–50). Two of these studies were retrospective, direct comparisons between contrast CT and angiography with limited patients (48,50). One study was performed as blinded prospective comparison in 102 patients with a sensitivity of 90.8% for contrast CT detection of an aneurysm (49). None of these authors suggested, based upon their experience, that contrast CT should replace conventional angiography. However, the technique might be used as the sole preoperative diagnostic tool in a life-threatening clinical setting such as that of a patient with a rapidly expanding intracranial hemorrhage demonstrating a well-localized aneurysm adjacent to the hemorrhage. In such a situation the contrast CT would allow the patient to be sent directly to surgery without delay for angiography.

Three-Dimensional CT Angiography

Recently, a host of papers have begun to evaluate both spiral and nonspiral 3D reconstructions of enhanced axial CT images with SSD and MIP reconstructions (51–58). Some of the earlier or initial experiences have been limited retrospective reports with direct comparison to digital angiography (51–53). However, in the past few years blinded compari-

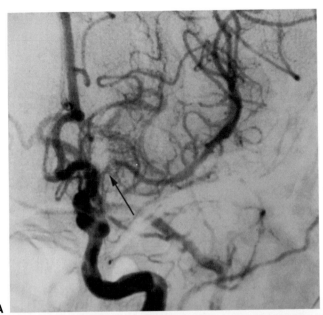

FIG. 21-7. High-grade left middle cerebral artery (MCA) stenosis in a 30-year-old woman with left MCA territory ischemic disease. (**A**) Posteroanterior view of left internal carotid arteriogram shows a high-grade stenosis of proximal MCA M1 segment (*arrow*). (**B**) Frontal view of spiral CT angiogram with ROI selected to include both carotid circulations. Right and left internal carotid arteries (*arrows*) (collimation 1 mm, pitch 1.3). Tight stenosis of left MCA shown (*curved arrow*) adjacent to the left internal carotid bifurcation. (**C**) Frontal-view 3D phase-contrast MRA with ROI selected to include both carotid circulations (TR 23/TE 7.8, 40 cm/s velocity encoding). Right and left carotid arteries (*arrows*). Signal voids in proximal left anterior cerebral artery (*short open arrow*) and left MCA (*curved arrow*). Note longer segment of flow void in MCA segment compared with angiogram or CTA.

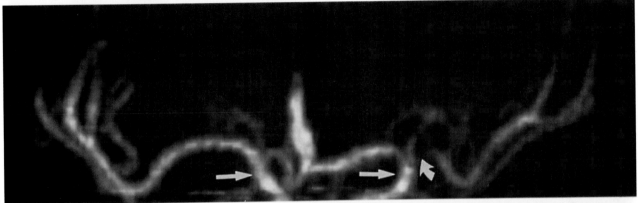

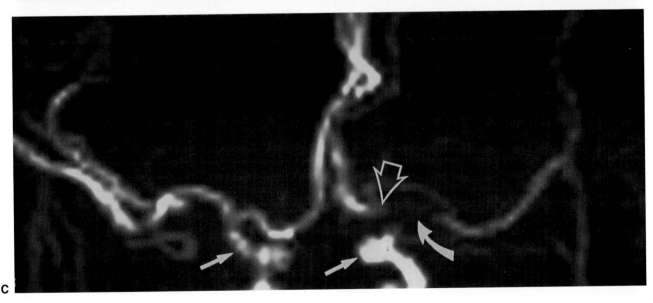

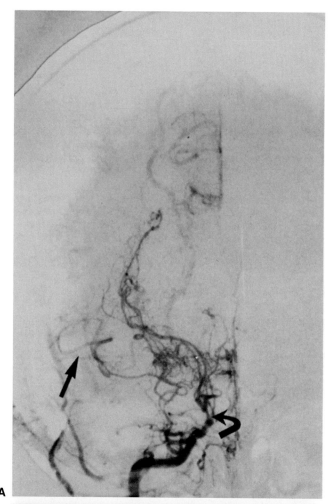

A

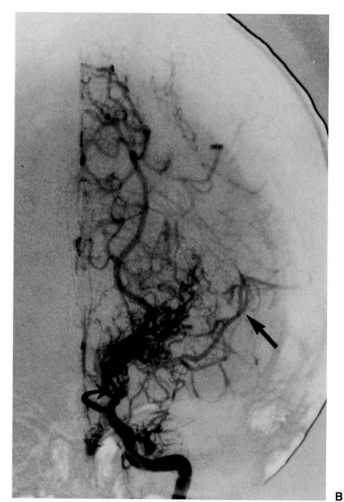

B

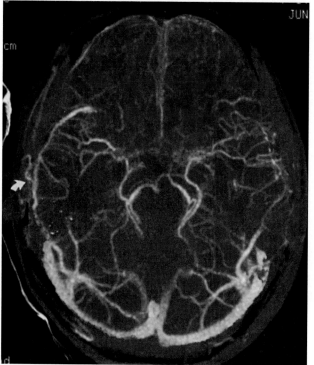

C

FIG. 21-8. Moya-moya disease in a 14-year-old girl who has had bilateral superficial temporal artery to middle cerebral artery bypass grafts. (**A,B**) Anterior views of right (A) and left (B) carotid artery conventional angiograms. Occlusions of right and left middle and anterior cerebral arteries are noted. Bilateral opercular MCA branches are also noted to fill slowly via collaterals (*arrows*). Stenoses are also noted at both the internal carotid bifurcations (*curved arrows*). (**C**) Craniocaudal view of spiral CT angiogram (collimation 1 mm, pitch 1.3) showing lack of filling bilateral proximal middle and anterior cerebral arteries. Distal MCA opercular branches do have filling, and partial filling is from bypass grafts. Transcranial portion of bypass is seen on right (*curved arrow*).

sons between 3D CTA and conventional DSA have been performed (54,56–58). These studies have suggested a high degree of sensitivity for the detection of aneurysms (67% to 96%) that rivals those sensitivities reported for MRA. When aneurysm data are stratified by size using either a spiral or nonspiral technique, most of the aneurysms that go undetected are 4 mm or less. For example, the recently published paper by Ogawa et al. (57) evaluated 73 aneurysms with two blinded observers. Eighteen of the total 73 aneurysms were overlooked by both observers and 15 of these 18 aneurysms were 4 mm or less in diameter. Similar results are seen for the other major noninvasive technique used to evaluate for aneurysms, MRA, where recent reports have suggested that the sensitivity for aneurysm detection falls off sharply for the aneurysm that is less than 5 mm (59,60).

Although nonspiral CTA has been used in this setting of aneurysm detection, spiral CTA has certain inherent advantages. Because the spiral exam is a volumetric acquisition, overlapping reconstructions can be performed. This can be done without additional radiation dose and scanning time, unlike nonspiral acquisitions, which would require overlapping acquisitions to create overlapping reconstructions. In addition, spiral CTA can be performed much more rapidly along the longitudinal plane. This allows the contrast bolus volume and rate to be maximized so that peak arterial enhancement can be maximized during the short scan time. Nonspiral protocols have typically called for slower scanning times of 1 mL/s for 100–120 s (51,57), whereas spiral protocols have allowed 3 mL/s to be bolused in 27–45 s (54,56). In addition, more rapid coverage along the longitudinal plane affords more opportunity to expand the imaging volume. A problem with false-negative determinations has been found with nonspiral CTA missing aneurysms that were outside the imaging volume (57,58). Indeed, spiral CTA has been suggested as a solution to missing aneurysms outside the imaging volume by some of the authors working with the nonspiral technique (57,58).

Some workers have recently used minimally invasive studies such as MRA to screen for aneurysms in patients who may be at increased risk because of underlying diseases such as polycystic kidney disease (61). These noninvasive techniques may have a role in the evaluation of patients with conditions known to be associated with intracranial aneurysms such as polycystic kidney disease, Ehlers-Danlos, Marfan's syndrome, and of patients with a family history of aneurysms. However, the difficulty with lower detection rates in smaller aneurysms (<4–5 mm) and the need to clearly show the aneurysm neck and relation to surrounding vasculature currently limit the role on these noninvasive techniques to a screening tool in certain settings.

In the setting of subarachnoid hemorrhage or to more definitively work up a known aneurysm prior to therapy, conventional DSA is generally the study of choice. As has been pointed out, MRA and CTA have similar sensitivities for the detection of aneurysms when compared with conventional DSA (59,60,62). There are certain limitations to MRA

that may not be as profound as those with CTA. With the time-of-flight MRA, larger aneurysms with slower flow may contain saturated protons resulting in loss of signal and inaccurate depiction of the aneurysm morphology. In addition, thrombus may be hyperintense on T1-weighted images and may inaccurately be interpreted as an area of flowing blood (62,63). The detection of giant aneurysms (where slow flow and hyperintense clot within the aneurysm are often present) can usually be made with MR or CT imaging alone. Spiral CTA may, however, more clearly depict the morphology of the aneurysm lumen in such cases, as it is not limited by slower flow. Our experience with spiral CTA suggests that with moderately sized aneurysms following 3D reconstructions we are able to clearly depict the aneurysm and accurately describe the morphology for treatment planning (Figs. 21-9, 21-10).

Vascular Malformations

Vascular malformations are congenital lesions and are generally categorized into four subtypes based upon histological and morphological criteria (64). These four types have significantly different radiological and clinical courses. They are arteriovenous malformations (AVMs), venous malformations, cavernous malformations, and capillary telangiectasias.

Intracranial AVMs are high-flow lesions containing abnormal shunts between the arterial and venous components of the cerebral circulation. These are usually identified easily on MRI or CT imaging alone (65). However, complete evaluation of an AVM depends upon the accurate depiction of vascular characteristics within the AVM that include feeding vessel aneurysms, intranidus aneurysms, feeding arteries, draining veins, and stenoses within the feeding or draining vessels. AVMs are treated with embolization, radiosurgery, and conventional microsurgery (or combinations of these therapies). Prior to making management decisions, however, a detailed vascular map of the AVM (including the previously mentioned vascular characteristics) is necessary. Many of these vascular characteristics have also proven to be of prognostic value in determining risk of hemorrhage or neurological deficit (66,67).

Conventional angiography can image with a rapid film sequence and therefore can be temporally resolved during viewing of the length of the film sequence. This generally allows for separate evaluation of the arterial phase, the structure of the AVM nidus, and the venous drainage if filming is rapid enough. MRA and CTA do not allow for such temporal resolution. In addition, conventional angiography has a greater inherent spatial resolution than MRA or CTA and therefore is the study of choice for the evaluation of these lesions. However, some authors have shown that noninvasive imaging with MRA does add to the early understanding of these lesions, giving added information over conventional MRI such as vascular supply to the AVM (68,69). Spiral CTA is also capable of depicting the feeding arteries, AVM

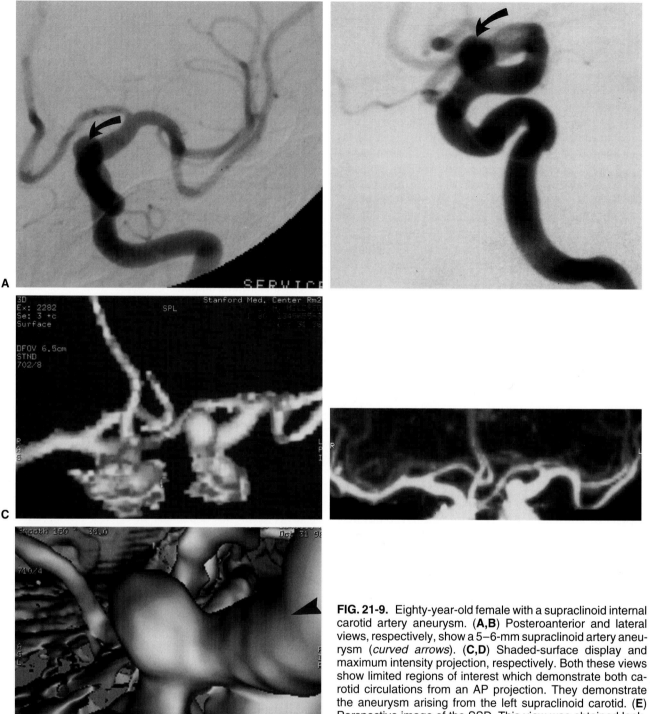

FIG. 21-9. Eighty-year-old female with a supraclinoid internal carotid artery aneurysm. (**A,B**) Posteroanterior and lateral views, respectively, show a 5–6-mm supraclinoid artery aneurysm (*curved arrows*). (**C,D**) Shaded-surface display and maximum intensity projection, respectively. Both these views show limited regions of interest which demonstrate both carotid circulations from an AP projection. They demonstrate the aneurysm arising from the left supraclinoid carotid. (**E**) Perspective image of the SSD. This view was obtained looking down the supraclinoid carotid artery from the point of its bifurcation into the anterior and middle cerebral arteries. The *arrowhead* shows this direction of view down the supraclinoid carotid as we are looking at the aneurysm. Compare this with the angiogram as shown in (**A**) to understand this perspective from the top of the supraclinoid carotid.

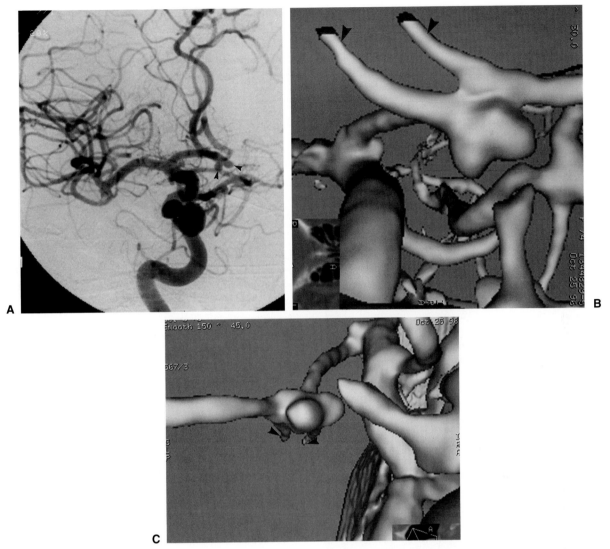

FIG. 21-10. Seventy-five-year-old female with a bilobed anterior communicating artery aneurysm. (**A**) Posteroanterior projection from a right internal carotid artery angiogram demonstrates an anterior communicating artery aneurysm with two lobes pointing inferiorly (*small arrowheads*). (**B,C**) Two views from a perspective image obtained with shaded-surface display technique. Image **B** shows the aneurysm with both lobes projecting inferiorly. We are looking from a frontal projection in **B**. In **C** we are looking from the inferior upward to the aneurysm. This shows the aneurysm from below and slightly to the right with the two lobes seen projecting inferiorly. The A2 segments are marked in both images (*small arrowheads*). They are well seen in the frontal projection (**B**) but are foreshortened as we look from below (**C**).

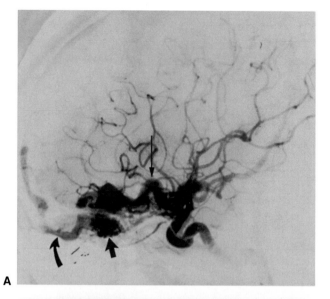

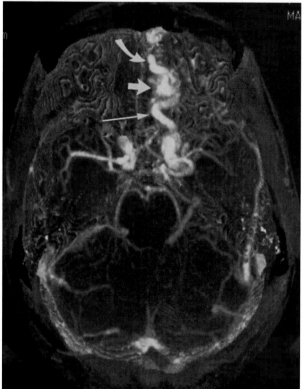

FIG. 21-11. Left inferior frontal lobe gyrus rectus arteriovenous malformation in a 32-year-old woman. (**A**) Lateral view of left internal carotid arteriogram showing AVM nidus (*arrow*) with large feeding fronto-orbital artery (*long arrow*) and enlarged draining vein (*curved arrow*). (**B**) Craniocaudal view of spiral CT angiogram (collimation 1 mm, pitch 1.3) also showing frontal AVM nidus (*arrow*) with large fronto-orbital feeding artery (*long arrow*) and enlarged draining vein (*curved arrow*).

nidus, and draining veins with similar spatial resolution to MRA (Fig. 21-11). Other vascular malformations such as cavernous malformation, developmental venous anomalies, and capillary telengeictases do not have rapid blood flow and will therefore probably continue to be more easily diagnosed and assessed with MRI or conventional CT imaging.

REFERENCES

1. Lasjaunias P, Berenstein A. Arterial anatomy: introduction. In: *Surgical neuroangiography.* Berlin: Springer-Verlag; 1980(1):1–32.
2. Cumming MJ, Morrow IM. Carotid artery stenosis: a prospective comparison of CT angiography and conventional angiography. *AJR* 1994; 163:517–523.
3. Leclerc X, Godefroy O, Salhi A, Lucas C, Leys D, Pruvo JP. Helical CT for the diagnosis of extracranial internal carotid artery dissection. *Stroke* 1996;27(3):461–466.
4. Link J, Brossmann J, Grabener M, et al. Spiral CT angiography and selective digital subtraction angiography of internal carotid artery stenosis. *AJNR* 1996;17:89–94.
5. Castillo M. Diagnosis of disease of the common carotid artery bifurcation: CT angiography vs catheter angiography. *AJR* 1993;161:395–398.
6. Castillo M, Wilson JD. CT angiography of the common carotid artery bifurcation: comparison between two techniques and conventional angiography. *Neuroradiology* 1994;36:602–604.
7. Mohr JP, Gautier JC, Pessin MS. Internal carotid artery disease. In: Barnett HJM, Mohr JP, Stein BM, Yatsu FM, eds. *Stroke: pathophysiology, diagnosis, and management,* 2nd ed. New York: Churchill Livingstone; 1992:285–336.
8. Fisher CM, Gore I, Okabe N, et al. Atherosclerosis of the carotid and vertebral arteries: extracranial and intracranial. *J Neuropathol Exp Neurol* 1965;24:455.
9. Barnett HJM, Taylor DW. Beneficial effect of carotid endarterectomy in symptomatic patients with high-grade carotid stenosis. *N Engl J Med* 1991;325:445–453.
10. European Carotid Surgery Trialists' Collaborative Group: MRS European carotid surgery trial: interim results for symptomatic persons with severe (70–99%) or with mild (0–29%) carotid stenosis. *Lancet* 1991; 337:1235-1243.
11. Executive Committee for the Asymptomatic Carotid Atherosclerosis Study: endarterectomy for asymptomatic carotid artery stenosis. *JAMA* 1995;273:1421-1428.
12. Napel S, Marks MP, Rubin GD, et al. CT angiography with spiral CT and maximum intensity projection. *Radiology* 1992;185:607–610.
13. Schwartz RB, Jones KM, Chernoff DM, et al. Common carotid artery bifurcations: evaluation with spiral CT. *Radiology* 1992;185:513–519.
14. Dillon EH, van Leeuwen MS, Fernandez MA, et al. CT angiography: application to the evaluation of carotid artery stenosis. *Radiology* 1993; 189:211-219.
15. Marks MP, Napel S, Jordan JE, Enzmann DR. Diagnosis of carotid artery disease: preliminary experience with maximum-intensity-projection spiral CT angiography. *AJR* 1993;160:1267–1271.
16. Marks MP. Computed tomography angiography. *Neuroimaging Clin North Am* 1996;6(4):899–909.
17. Moore WS, Boren C, Malone JM, et al. Natural history of non-stenotic asymptomatic ulcerative lesions of the carotid artery. *Arch Surg* 1978; 113:1352.
18. Eikelboom BC, Riles TR, Mintzer R, et al. Inaccuracy of angiography in the diagnosis of carotid ulceration. *Stroke* 1983;14(6):882–885.
19. Edwards JH, Kricheff II, Riles T, Imparato A. Angiographically undetected ulceration of the carotid bifurcation as a cause of embolic stroke. *Radiology* 1979;132:369–373.
20. Anson J, Crowell RM. Cervicocranial arterial discussion. *Neurosurgery* 1991;29:89-96.
21. Mokri B, Sundt TM Jr, Houser OW, et al. Spontaneous dissection of the cervical internal carotid artery. *Ann Neurol* 1986 19:126-138.
22. Litt AW, Eidelman EM, Pinto RS, et al. Diagnosis of carotid artery stenosis: comparison of 2DFT time-of-flight MR angiography with contrast angiography in 50 patients. *AJNR* 1991;12:149–154.
23. Massaryk AM, Ross JS, DiCello MC, et al. 3DFT MR angiography of the carotid bifurcation: potential and limitations as a screening examination. *Radiology* 1991;179:797–804.

24. Heiserman JE, Drayer BP, Fram EK, et al. Carotid artery stenosis: clinical efficacy of two-dimensional time-of-flight MR angiography. *Radiology* 1992;182:761–768.

25. Polak JF, Bajakian RL, O'Leary DH, et al. Detection of internal carotid artery stenosis: comparison of MR angiography, color Doppler sonography, and arteriography. *Radiology* 1992;182:35–40.

26. Huston J III, Lewis BD, Wiebers DO, et al. Carotid artery: prospective blinded comparison of two-dimensional time-of-flight MR angiography with conventional angiography and duplex ultrasound. *Radiology* 1993;186:339–344.

27. Jackson VP, Kuehn DS, Bendick PJ, et al. Duplex carotid sonography: correlation with digital subtraction angiography and conventional angiography. *J Ultrasound Med* 1985;4:239–249.

28. Jacobs NM, Grant EG, Shellinger D, et al. Duplex carotid sonography: criteria for stenosis, accuracy, and pitfalls. *Radiology* 1985;154:385–391.

29. Robinson ML, Sacks D, Perlmutter GS, et al. Diagnostic criteria for carotid duplex sonography. *AJR* 1988;151:1045–1049.

30. Bornstein NM, Alatko GB, Norris JW. The limitations of diagnosis of carotid occlusion by Doppler ultrasound. *Ann Surg* 1988;207:315–317.

31. Bridgers SL. Clinical correlates of Doppler/ultrasound errors in the detection of internal carotid artery occlusion. *Stroke* 1989;20:612–615.

32. Polak JF, Dobkin GR, O'Leary DH, Wang AM, Cutler SS. Internal carotid artery stenosis: accuracy and reproducibility of color-Doppler-assisted duplex imaging. *Radiology* 1989;173:793–798.

33. Fisher CM. Cerebral ischemia-less familiar types. *Clin Neurosurg* 1971;12:267.

34. Lhermitte F, Gautier JC, Derouesne C. Nature of occlusions of the middle cerebral artery. *Neurology* 1970;20:82.

35. Marzewski DJ, Furlan AJ, St. Louis P, et al. Intracranial internal carotid artery stenosis: long-term prognosis. *Stroke* 1982;13:821.

36. Katz DA, Marks MP, Napel SA, Bracci PM, Roberts SL. Circle of Willis: evaluation with spiral CT angiography, MR angiography and conventional angiography. *Radiology* 1995;195:445–449.

37. Wong KS, Liang EY, Lam WWM, Huang RK. Spiral computed tomography angiography in the assessment of middle cerebral artery occlusive disease. *J Neurol Neurosurg Psychiatry* 1995;59:537–539.

38. Suzuki J, Kodama N. Moyamoya disease: a review. *Stroke* 1983;14(1):104–109.

39. Kukuchi M, Asato M, Sugahara S, et al. Evaluation of surgically formed collateral circulation in Moyamoya disease with 3-D CT angiography: comparison with MR angiography and X-ray angiography. *Neuropediatrics* 1996;27:45–49.

40. Fox JL. The incidence of intracranial aneurysms. In: Fox JL, ed., *Intracranial aneurysms.* New York: Springer-Verlag; 1983(1):15–18.

41. Vajda J. Multiple intracranial aneurysms: a high risk condition. *Acta Neurochir (Wien)* 1992;118:59–75.

42. Kassell NF, Drake CG. Timing of aneurysm surgery. *Neurosurgery* 1982;10:514–519.

43. Kassell NF, Torner JC, Haley EC, et al. The International Cooperative Study on the Timing of Aneurysm Surgery, part 1: overall management results. *J Neursurg* 1990;73:18–36.

44. Suzuki S, Kayama T, Sakurai Y, et al. Subarachnoid hemorrhage of unknown origin. *Neurosurgery* 1987;21:310–313.

45. Rinkel GJE, van Gijn J, Wijdicks EFM. Subarachnoid hemorrhage without detectable aneurysm. *Stroke* 1993;24(9):1403–1409.

46. Rinkel GJE, Wijdicks EFM, Vermeulen M, et al. Nonaneurysmal perimesencephalic subarachnoid hemorrhage: CT and MR patterns that differ from aneurysmal rupture. *AJNR* 1991;12:829–834.

47. Duong H, Melancon D, Tampieri D, Ethier R. The negative angiogram in subarachnoid haemorrhage. *Neuroradiology* 1996;38:15–19.

48. Asari S, Satoh T, Sakurai M, Yamamoto Y, Sadamoto K. Delineation of unruptured cerebral aneurysms by computerized angiotomography. *J Neurosurg* 1982;57:527–534.

49. Schmid UD, Steiger HJ, Huber P. Accuracy of high resolution computed tomography in direct diagnosis of cerebral aneurysms. *Neuroradiology* 1987;29:152–159.

50. Newell DW, LeRoux PD, Dacey RG, Stimac GK, Winn HR. CT infusion scanning for the detection of cerebral aneurysms. *J Neurosurg* 1989;71:175–179.

51. Aoki S, Sasaki Y, Machida T, Ohkubo T, Minami M, Sasaki Y. Cerebral aneurysms: detection and delineation using 3-D-CT angiography. *AJNR* 1992;13:1115–1120.

52. Dorsch NWC, Young N, Kingston RJ, Compton JS. Early experience with spiral CT in the diagnosis of intracranial aneurysms. *Neurosurgery* 1995;36 (1):230–238.

53. Schwartz, RB, Tice HM, Hooten SM, Hsu L, Stieg PE. Evaluation of cerebral aneurysms with helical CT: correlation with conventional angiography and MR angiography. *Neuroradiology* 1994;192(3):717–722.

54. Alberico RA, Patel M, Casey S, Jacobs B, Maguire W, Decker R. Evaluation of the circle of Willis with three-dimensional CT angiography in patients with suspected intracranial aneurysms. *AJNR* 1995;16:1571–1578.

55. Grossi G, Romanze R, Macchia G, Ruffinengo UR, Calla S. Angio CT: a proposal for emergency diagnosis in subarachnoid hemorrhage as a preliminary to therapeutic choices. *Intervent Neuroradiol* 1995;1:43–57.

56. Liang EY, Chan M, Hsiang JHK, et al. Detection and assessment of intracranial aneurysms: value of CT angiography with shaded-surface display. *AJR* 1995;165:1497–1502.

57. Ogawa T, Okudera T, Noguchi K, et al. Cerebral aneurysms: evaluation with three-dimensional CT angiography. *AJNR* 1996;17:447–454.

58. Hope JKA, Wilson JL, Thomson FJ. Three-dimensional CT angiography in the detection and characterization of intracranial berry aneurysms. *AJNR* 1996;17:439–445.

59. Huston J III, Nichols DA, Luetmer PH, et al. Blinded prospective evaluation of sensitivity of MR angiography to known intracranial aneurysms: importance of aneurysm size. *AJNR* 1994;15:1607–1616.

60. Korogi Y, Takahashi M, Mabuchi N, et al. Intracranial aneurysms: diagnostic accuracy of three-dimensional, Fourier transform, time-of-flight MR angiography. *Radiology* 1994;193(1):181–186.

61. Huston J, Torres UE, Sullivan PP, Offord KP, Weibers DO. Value of magnetic resonance angiography for the detection of intracranial aneurysms in autosomal dominant polycystic kidney disease. *J Am Soc Nephrol* 1993;1871–1877.

62. Ross JS, Masaryk TJ, Modic MT, et al. Intracranial aneurysms: Evaluation by MR angiography. *AJNR* 1990;11:449–456.

63. Sevick RJ, Tsuruda JS, Schmalbrock P. Three-dimensional time-of-flight MR angiography in the evaluation of cerebral aneurysms. *J Comput Asst Tomogr* 1990;14(6):874–881.

64. McCormick WF. Pathology of vascular malformations of the brain. In: Wilson CB, Stein BM, eds. *Intracranial arteriovenous malformations.* Baltimore: Williams and Wilkins; 1984:44–63.

65. Kucharczyk W, Lemme-Pleghos L, Uske A, et al. Intracranial vascular malformations: MR and CT imaging. *Radiology* 1985;156:383–389.

66. Marks MP, Lane B, Steinberg GK, Chang PJ. Hemorrhage in intracerebral arteriovenous malformations: angiographic determinants. *Radiology* 1990;176:807–813.

67. Marks MP, Lane B, Steinberg GK, Snipes GJ. Intranidal aneurysms in cerebral arteriovenous malformation: evaluation and endovascular treatment. *Radiology* 1992;183:355–360.

68. Nussel F, Wegmüller H, Huber P. Comparison of magnetic resonance angiography, magnetic resonance imaging and conventional angiography in cerebral arteriovenous malformation. *Neuroradiology* 1991;33:56–61.

69. Edelman RR, Wentz KU, Mattle HP, et al. Intracerebral arteriovenous malformations: evaluation with selective MR angiography and venography. *Radiology* 1989;173:831–837.

Subject Index

419